THE INTERNET COMPENDIUM

SUBJECT GUIDES TO HEALTH AND SCIENCE RESOURCES

LOUIS ROSENFELD, JOSEPH JANES and
MARTHA VANDER KOLK

NEAL-SCHUMAN PUBLISHERS, INC.

New York   London

Published by Neal-Schuman Publishers, Inc.
100 Varick Street
New York, NY 10013

Copyright © 1995 by Louis Rosenfeld, Joseph Janes, Martha Vander Kolk

All rights reserved. Reproduction of this book, in whole or in
part, without written permission of the publisher is prohibited.

Printed and bound in the United States of America

Library of Congress Cataloging-in-Publication Data

Rosenfeld, Louis B.
    Internet compendium subject guides to health and sciences resources
/ edited by Louis Rosenfeld, Joseph Janes, Martha Vander Kolk.
       p.   cm.
    Includes index.
    ISBN 1-55570-219-8
    1. Medicine--Computer network resources.   2. Business--Computer
network resources.   3. Internet (Computer network).   4. Database
searching.   I. Janes, Joseph   II. Vander Kolk, Martha.
R859.7.D36R67   1995
025.06'574--dc20   95-2171
                                                                                CIP

To the Pioneers

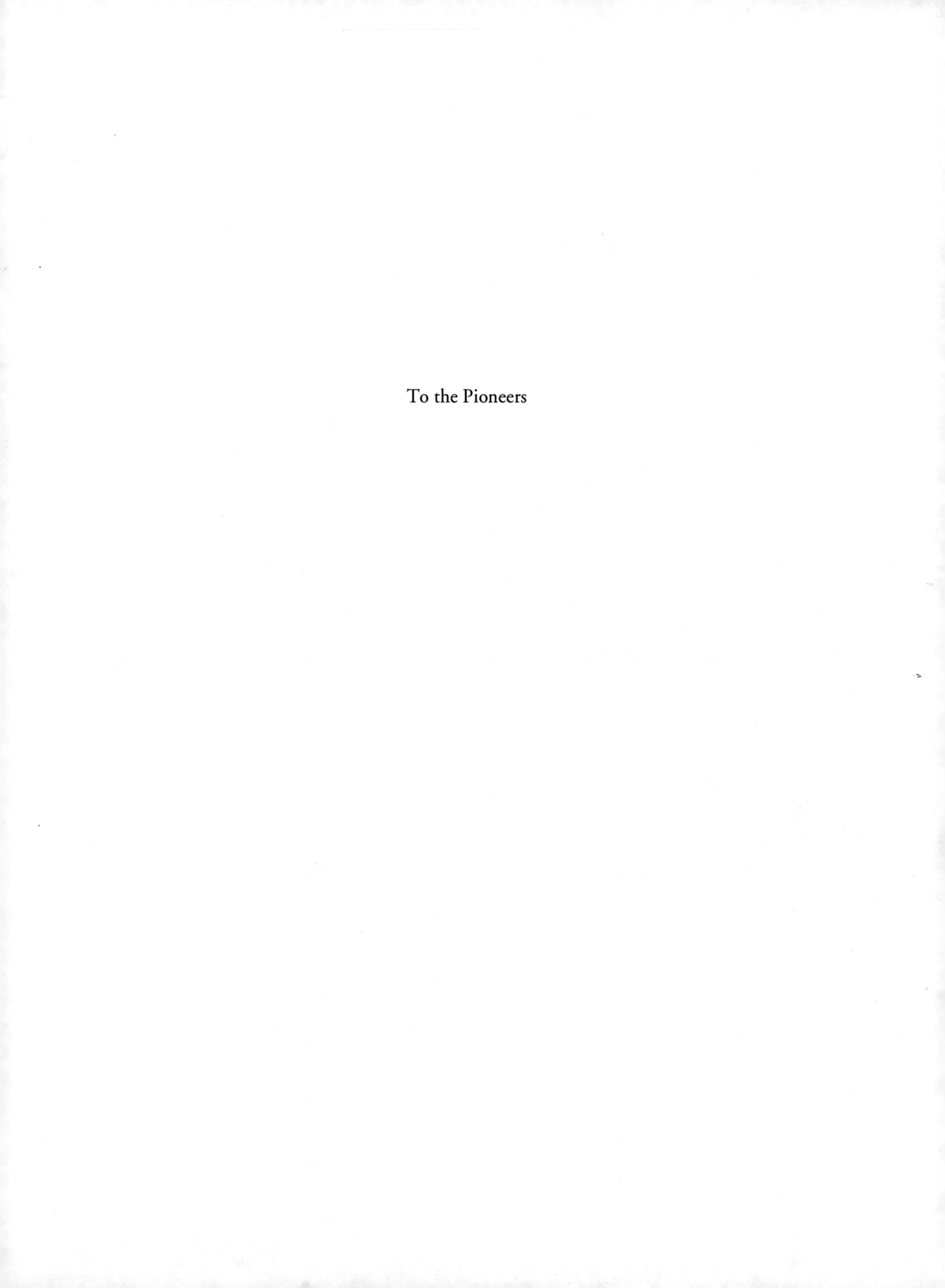

Table of Contents

About the Authors		vi
Acknowledgments		vii
Foreword		viii
Preface		vix

Part I How To Use This Book

	Chapter 1	Internet Addresses	3
	Chapter 2	Clients and Servers	7
	Chapter 3	Navigating: Tools and Resources	11
	Chapter 4	Communicating with Individuals and Groups	21

Part II Beyond This Book: Next Steps

	Chapter 5	Searching for Files to FTP: Archie	31
	Chapter 6	Searching for Gopher Resources: Veronica	35
	Chapter 7	WAIS: Wide Area Information Servers	39
	Chapter 8	Putting it all Together: Building your own Subject-Oriented Guide	43
	Chapter 9	The Clearinghouse for Subject-Oriented Internet Resource Guides	49

Part III Subject-Oriented Guides

	Chapter 10	Aerospace Engineering: A Guide To Internet Resources	53
	Chapter 11	The Electronic Zoo	71
	Chapter 12	Aquatic Biology Information Resources on the Internet	195
	Chapter 13	Some Chemistry Resources on the Internet	205
	Chapter 14	On-line Resources for Earth Scientists (ORES)	219
	Chapter 15	A Guide to Environmental Resources on the Internet	257
	Chapter 16	Health Sciences Resources	287
	Chapter 17	Guide to Molecular Biology Database	449
	Chapter 18	Neurosciences Internet Resource Guide	469
	Index	Recommended Resources	413
	Index	Subject	415

About the Authors

Lou Rosenfeld is, with Joe Janes, a partner in Argus Associates, Inc., an Internet publishing and marketing, training, research, and publishing company. Rosenfeld is also an instructor and doctoral student at the University of Michigan's School of Information and Library Studies, where he received his MILS in 1990. Prior to returning, he was a researcher at UM's College of Engineering and a librarian at the University Library. Rosenfeld founded and now administers the Clearinghouse for Subject-Oriented Internet Resource Guides. His hobbies are tinkering in his yard and dreaming of owning a computer.

Joseph Janes came to Ann Arbor from Oneida Castle, New York, with a ten-year stop in Syracuse where he picked up, among other things, three degrees. He is an Assistant Professor in the School of Information and Library Studies at the University of Michigan. Janes teaches courses in information technologies and their impacts, searching for information and statistics as well as a course (with Lou Rosenfeld) on the process of discovery, description, organization and design of networked information resources. His research interests include user's evaluation of information and the networked environment. Janes is the co-author of two other books: *Now What? Readings on Surviving (And Even Enjoying) Your First Experience at College Teaching,* with Diane Hauer (published by Copley Press); and *Online Retrieval: A Dialogue of Theory and Practice,* with Geraldene Walker (published by Libraries Unlimited). He enjoys bad science fiction movies, racquet sports, and receiving royalty checks.

Martha Vander Kolk, raised in a small town along the eastern shore of Lake Michigan, holds a Bachelor of Arts Degree in German from Hope College and a Master's Degree from the University of Michigan's School of Information and Library Studies. Vander Kolk is the co-author, with Deborah Torres, of the "Guide to Theater Resources on the Internet." Prior to her association with Argus Associates, she worked in the publishing industry in New York. Vander Kolk currently resides in Alexandria, VA where she remains connected to the rest of the world via a 2400-baud modem.

Acknowledgments

The Internet is as much about collaboration and cooperation as anything else, and this book symbolizes that kind of group effort. The Internet is also about serendipity: chance meetings—virtually, through Internet mailing lists and searches, and in person at conferences and happy hours—all helped build the diverse community of people who contributed to this book.

The editors played only a small role in its production; the greatest recognition is due to the authors of these guides. Often working alone and without much (if any) guidance, these authors took on the difficult task of making sense of the Internet's chaos, and were kind enough to share their labors with the rest of the Net community. At the University of Michigan, the University Library and the School of Information and Library Studies are to be credited for sponsoring the Clearinghouse for Subject-Oriented Internet Resource Guides, where these guides initially came together as a collection. And our publisher, Neal-Schuman, had the foresight to see the value in creating a reference series based on this collection.

At Argus Associates, the production crew of Martha Vander Kolk, Kristen Garlock, Lisa Wood, Peter Morville, and Phil Ray boldly took the initiative to ensure that the information in this book was current and that the book itself stood as a coherent whole. Without them, there would be no book. We'd also like to thank Patricia Schuman and Bettina Versaci at Neal-Schuman for their patience throughout an often ornery production process.

Others deserve much credit as well: Maurita Holland, Amy Warner, Dan Atkins, C. Olivia Frost, Mary Beth Cobbs, Nat Good, Jan Hartley, parents, pets, and host of others who through their friendship enabled us to achieve our goals.

Foreword

Ah! The Internet!

Thousands of powerful host computers, interconnected by cables, phone lines, satellites, and wireless communications. On them—for the asking, a plethora of full text electronic books, documents on every subject, graphics, movies, audio files, even software. Then there are the thousands of discussion lists, concerned with topics large and small, topics both weighty and frivolous. Some of them are populated with renowned subject specialists, who enlighten us with their insights, while rubbing their electronic elbows with those of mere mortals.

And what metaphors do we use for the Internet? We drive the electronic superhighway, we cruise the Internet sea lanes, we surf off into the fractal sunset and never look back.

But, Oh—the Internet!

Those computer connections? Sometimes they don't work. Hosts become unreachable. Favorite sites disappear, and new ones are built overnight. And how easy is it to use? Your mileage may vary. Depending on your type of connection, and conditions at your site, the Net can be clumsy, confounding, and user-antagonistic. Or, it can be easy, seamless, and almost effortless to use. Those alluring files? Anyone can put up a document and claim it's authoritative. Same thing with the folks on the discussion groups—there are real experts, self-acclaimed experts, and wannabe-experts. There are things on the Internet that will offend, disgust, mis-inform, and provoke you. Why do we put up with it? Because there are also things on the Internet that will astound, educate, amuse, and empower you.

Terabytes of information, all of it looking for readers. But how to find what is important to *you* on the Internet?

Hardy Franklin, Past-President of the American Library Association, says that when he comes into a library, he's looking for information, not a research project.

Toto, I don't think we're in a public library anymore.

The Net needs the services of reflective librarians and other "information people," sifting available electronic resources to find the authoritative voices, the quality materials, the most reliable hosts. This effort, until now, has been uneven.

Beyond that though, the Net needs the efforts of proactive folks, who don't just react to what has been, but create Internet tools and techniques and resources of their own.

This book is one of the latter. It is not Just Another Internet Book. It's the book that has done all that searching and sifting, and built something that real-end users (that's you) need. It will guide you and help you find out why the Internet may be important to *you*, your colleagues, your family, and your career.

And that makes all the difference.

Jean Armour Polly, MLS
Director of Public Services & Internet Ambassador, NYSERNet, Inc.

Author of *Surfing the Internet*
Jamesville, New York

Preface

Once upon a time, in the not-too-distant past, entering the publishing industry meant taking on large staffs, investing heavily in equipment outlays, and knowing at least a thing or two about the production of *quality* information. Suddenly, thanks to many powerful and amazingly cheap technologies, tens of thousands of institutions, organizations, and individuals have become publishers of information.

Nowhere is this more apparent than the Internet. College freshmen operate highly popular information systems from their dorm rooms. Fifth graders publish electronic documents describing their favorite colors. Immigration lawyers hawk green-card information. Everyone and his brother is getting into the act, and the result is a flood of predominantly low-quality information resources.

Of course, quality becomes an issue only if you first can determine whether any relevant information exists at all. Because it is highly decentralized, the Internet is as unfriendly to searching as an information environment can get. Completing an exhaustive search of the Internet is no piece of cake either; the Internet's searching tools are simply too primitive.

Despite the Internet's explosion of low quality information and the radical changes it witnesses almost every month, the situation is not hopeless. Many experienced citizens of the Internet have endeavored to identify and describe resources that are relevant to specific subjects, and, in many cases, they have evaluated the quality of those resources. This process of Internet resource discovery and evaluation is, for the reasons noted above, extremely difficult. The subject-oriented resource guides presented in this book make it possible for you to survive this difficult process alone. Instead, these guides serve as reference sources to enable you to maximize your use of the Internet and its information.

It may help to think of this as a travel book. What we've collected here are a group of road maps, each of which describes one small portion of the large territory known as cyberspace, or, more appropriately, the Internet. Like the real world, it's much easier to find your way around in cyberspace when you have some idea where you're going and how to get there. Sure, it's fun to just float around and see what's out there, but after a while, it's nice to have some sense of direction, especially if you're looking for something in particular. In fact, we hope that after reading and using these guides, you'll be encouraged to do some surfing, explore further and find new things. You might even get inspired to develop a new guide of your own on some topic. If you do, let us know...there's always a need for more good guides to the Net.

Part I

Introduction

WHAT THIS BOOK IS (AND ISN'T)

Most of the books about the Internet are useful for helping you learn how to do and understand specific things: installing and using Internet software, becoming familiar with the culture and customs of Internet communities, and so on. This series is different. Its goal is to help you access the *content* of what's out there on the Internet.

Instead of providing long and general lists of all known Gophers, Usenet newsgroups, or World Wide Web servers, like many other books do, this series describes and evaluates the Internet's resources *by subject*. So the reader with a specific, focused interest, such as aerospace engineering or theater materials, will find relevant Internet resources assembled in a single, easy-to-use chapter.

The chapters in this series were compiled by "power users" of the Internet. The authors are subject specialists and practitioners; most are librarians, faculty, and graduate students who have expertise in the subject at hand and are committed to making the subject's relevant Internet resources more accessible through their work to all.

Although our original intent was to publish a single book of these topical guides to the Internet, there was much more high quality material than we originally anticipated. Instead, there are now three volumes in this series. This volume covers Internet resources to health and science; in it you'll find a wide variety of topics, including chemistry, molecular biology, and aerospace engineering. You'll also note the interesting and somewhat patchwork coverage of health and the sciences; unfortunately, there simply aren't guides available on every imaginable topic at this time. The other two volumes in this series cover the social sciences and the humanities.

Each chapter in the series, and many more, is electronically available via the Internet from the Clearinghouse for Subject-Oriented Internet Resource Guides (described in Chapter 9). Created and maintained by one of the editors, the Clearinghouse is internationally recognized as one of the Internet's best and highest-quality resources for topical information, and serves hundreds of thousands of users every year. We have included a subset of the guides that we feel is the cream of the crop for the Clearinghouse. Some guides couldn't be published because they were difficult to use, out of date, or the authors didn't want to have their guides published at this time.

Why then are we making these guides available in print? There is still nothing like having this kind of useful information packaged in a handy, portable, and easy-to-use book. Plus we have provided some useful sections on how to use the Internet's still-primitive information searching and browsing software tools, and a chapter which will help you become a "power user" by actually applying these tools to identify and evaluate the Internet's information resources. We envision the volumes in this series located nearby computers used to access the Internet, providing ready reference for users and librarians alike.

We hope you will find this series indispensable, and look forward to your comments. Send them to `lou@argus-inc.com`!

How To Use This Book

We think there are three chief uses for this book and the guides it contains:

First, its primary intended use is functional, as a reference device to help people interested in specific subjects find resources in those areas that are available over the Internet. To be sure, not every subject of interest will be covered by guides you'll find here, but that's probably because no one has yet taken the time and trouble to create one. More about this in a moment.

Second, it could be used as a general orientation to the kinds of resources available in cyberspace. If you're not particularly interested in a specific topic but rather want to know what's out there in general, these guides will point you to some fascinating and diverse things.

Third, we hope that at least for some people it serves as a jumping-off point for further Internet exploration, discovery, and organization. You may find yourself working to extend the efforts of the authors represented here, going in to more detail on a narrower topic, or striking out on your own into new regions of the Net. We feel strongly that this will be a most effective way of improving access to and use of networked information resources.

No matter how you intend to use it, there are some basic things you should know before you proceed. If you are an experienced Internaut, then some of the next sections will be old hat to you. Feel free to skip them and get right to the good stuff. But if terms like "gopher" and "FTP" and "URL" are still a bit new to you, we've provided some instructions and context here to help you on the way. We can't provide a complete guide to all of the Internet tools and resources here, but we can give you a start. Once you get on and get going, a lot more will become clear as you gain experience. Enjoy!

When Things Don't Work

Those of you who are familiar with the Internet know that there are a lot of times things will go wrong, and with many possible explanations. For you novices, the explanations could include problems with one or more of the following:

- your computer
- the remote computer you're trying to connect to
- your local network
- the remote computer's network
- your connection to the Internet
- the remote network's connection to the Internet
- the connections between your network and the remote network

In the case of popular resources like Veronica, there often are too many people trying to access the same resource at the same time. Or in some cases, people responsible for maintaining a resource have been lazy, laid off, or laid to rest.

The authors of the guides in this book have tried to save you from dealing with these hassles, but there will be instances in which the addresses provided are inaccurate. This may be an error on the author's part, or simply due to the fact that the Internet is changing so quickly that it's difficult to keep up with. We can at least assure you that we've done our best to check and verify all the addresses provided in this book. In other cases, certain resources are described as non-functional. We've left references to those resources in this book because knowing what *doesn't* work can also keep you from going down some blind alleys.

Internet Addresses

The Internet is a vast series of interconnected computer networks. You can use the Internet to share information with millions of people all over the world via electronic mail, live discussions, and to access information resources organized in a number of ways. Nobody runs the thing; it just sort of happens based on the collective effort of a lot of people. The major reason it's able to work is because everyone agrees on a set of protocols (called Transmission Control Protocol (TCP) and Internet Protocol (IP)), by which data is sent and received. These protocols are fairly low-level; once you get connected, if you're a casual user, they will not be a part of your daily life. Suffice to say that these provide the environment in which things like electronic mail, Gophers, telnet and the World Wide Web can be developed and operate.

One of the best ways you have of orienting yourself in cyberspace is by use of addresses. These addresses are really just ways of referring to *computers* which are connected to the Internet, *people* who use these computers and *resources* which are located on them. An understanding of the structure and form of the addresses can be very helpful in making your way around.

ADDRESSES OF COMPUTERS: DOMAINS

Here are examples of a few *domain names*, or addresses of computers and networks:

```
madlab.sprl.umich.edu
info.cern.ch
zeus.esusda.gov
nyplgate.nypl.org
www.fsz.bme.hu
quake.think.com
```

These addresses are read and structured from left to right[1], but it might be best to start at the end to understand the structure. Take the first address as an example.

```
umich.edu
```

This tells us that the computer in question is part of a network at the University of Michigan (umich), which is an educational institution (edu). This last part, often called the *top-level* domain, gives the broadest information about the host. There were originally six of these:

- .com   commercial (business)
- .edu   educational
- .gov   US Government
- .mil   military
- .net   network
- .org   non-profit organizations

---

[1] The last two parts of the address are and actually pronounced, too—many people, when speaking, will say as many parts as possible of these addresses as words, like "yoo-mish" for umich, "ed-yoo" for edu and so on. The periods are usually said as "dot". So umich.edu becomes "yoo-mich dot ed-yoo".

Now, many more have been added for hosts outside the United States. These top-level domains consist of two letters. For example,

`.ca`	Canada
`.uk`	United Kingdom
`.il`	Israel
`.hu`	Hungary
`.hk`	Hong Kong
`.se`	Sweden

The part directly to the left of the high-level domain tells us what organization or company is responsible for a given computer.

`umich.edu`	University of Michigan
`cern.ch`	CERN, Switzerland
`nypl.org`	New York Public Library
`think.com`	Thinking Machines, Inc.
`esusda.gov`	Extension Service, US Department of Agriculture

As you move further to the left, you get more specific information yet—the names of networks or machines within these organizations. So `quake.think.com` is the name of a specific machine at Thinking Machines, and `madlab.sprl.umich.edu` is a machine called `madlab` on a network known as `sprl` at the University of Michigan (`sprl` stands for Space Physics Research Laboratory).

After a while, you get good at reading these. Often, the last two parts are pretty obvious (`oklahoma.edu`, `compuserve.com`, `whitehouse.gov`), but sometimes a bit of guesswork or foreknowledge helps (for example, `tamu.edu` is Texas A&M University, and `mtu.edu` is Michigan Technological University).

In point of fact, this isn't really how it works. The networks don't use domain names like `quake.think.com` when sending data back and forth. They use corresponding addresses composed of numbers, like `141.211.203.30`, which are called *IP addresses*. But the alphabetical addresses are much easier for us to understand. There are computers called Domain Name Servers out there which translate back and forth, so when we type `madlab.sprl.umich.edu`, it is converted automatically to `141.212.196.79`.

ADDRESSES OF HUMANS: ELECTRONIC MAIL

These domain names specify particular computers or networks. However, to find actual people on the Net, you need personal addresses for them on their local networks. The following email addresses will look pretty familiar to you now:

```
janes@sils.umich.edu
lou@umich.edu
president@whitehouse.gov
smith@cern.ch
```

The right-hand side of this is a domain name, as we've already seen. The left-hand side is new, and is called the *userid* (pronounced "user eye dee"), which identifies a particular person on a system. Joe's userid on the email system belonging to the School of Information and Library Studies at the University of Michigan is `janes`, so his email address is `janes@sils.umich.edu`.

ADDRESSES OF RESOURCES: URLs

For a large number of the resources described in this book, you'll see something that looks like this:

URL: `http://info.cern.ch/hypertext/DataSources/ByAccess.html`

A piece of this will look familiar to you; the `info.cern.ch` part. This is a domain name, as we've discussed previously. What about the rest of it, though?

The whole thing is called a *Uniform Resource Locator*, or just *URL*. URLs are unique addresses and identifiers for almost all resources available via the Internet. At the moment, you most often see URLs associated with the World Wide Web (about which more soon), but that is not exclusively the case. We have decided to provide URLs for as many resources in this book as possible, since they are a convenient and consistent way to describe and point to resources.

We will discuss the format of different kinds of URLs in more detail shortly. For now, you should know that a URL tells you the following information:

- what kind of resource you're dealing with (telnet, FTP, Gopher, World Wide Web)
- where it is located (for example, the domain name of the host)
- where it is located on that machine

Before we go into detail, it's necessary to introduce a couple of other concepts central to a good understanding of the Net: clients and servers.

Clients and Servers

2

At some point you will hear the phrase *client/server architecture* bandied about during discussions of the Internet and its software tools. Clients and servers refer to specialized portions of a software program that may be installed on different computers on a network.

Let's back up: you know that when you install your copy of WordPerfect, the whole program fits on your computer's hard drive. This makes sense; after all, you are the only person who will be using the software, and you're probably the only person who uses your computer. You probably don't share electronic versions of your WordPerfect documents with other folks much, and if you do, it's likely you just hand them a copy on a floppy disk.

So why would you want to take a perfectly good program and chop it up into parts? And then install some parts on some computers, and others elsewhere?

The Internet is really about *sharing*; it was originally set up to allow researchers to exchange data and share mainframe computers. And, of course, it grew and grew because so many other people wanted to share information. Over time, however, a few things changed. Besides having better and better access to the Internet, users had increasingly more powerful computers sitting on their own desks, with sophisticated and user-friendly graphical interfaces.

To take advantage of all this power, programmers found that they could break apart or *modularize* their software into different specialized parts. One part of the software, called a server, could live on a networked computer that stored useful data; the server would manage that data. Another part of the software, called a client, could sit on a user's powerful desktop computer, and could take advantage of its great capabilities. And thanks to such networks as the Internet, these separate software modules could communicate and work with each other, despite their physical distance.

For example, let's take Gopher.

```
gopher.lib.umich.edu
```

This is a Gopher server's address, in this case at the University of Michigan Library. All the files loaded there are managed by the UM Library's Gopher server software.

The Gopher client, on the other hand, might reside on any other computer directly connected to the Internet. In fact, there are tens of thousands of Gopher clients that have been installed all over the Internet. And there are different kinds of Gopher clients. For those with Macintosh host computers, TurboGopher is the choice. There are also Gopher clients designed to run on PC-compatibles running Microsoft Windows, and on UNIX computers too. Each takes advantage of the operating system it's been designed to run on. So TurboGopher has folders and icons, and allows users to save and print displayed files, just like any other Macintosh software.

So when you select a menu in Gopher, your Gopher client sends a message over the Internet to a Gopher server, which then processes the request and returns the data to the Gopher client, which then displays the data. The same set of data will be accessed and displayed by your Gopher client, regardless of what kind of clinet software you use. But if you've used Gopher before, you know that the data comes from many different places. This is because Gopher servers, like clients, can run on many different computer platforms; hence, there are thousands of Gopher servers connected to the Internet, all making different types of data available. So when you look over that Gopher menu, one item may point to data being served by a Gopher running on a UNIX computer in British Columbia, while the next item points to data coming from a Gopher on a DOS computer in Athens.

All of this works great—if your computer is *directly* connected to the Internet. That is, if your computer is a true host, with its own address. But if you're like many users of the Internet, you dial in from a home computer via a modem. If this is the case, you probably can't run a client on your computer at home; your computer simply doesn't have a valid Internet address or a fast enough connection.

For this reason, many organizations and institutions on the Internet provide *public clients*. Like FTP archives and public telnet sites, public clients make information stored in servers available to just about anyone. In the case of Gopher, you could telnet to a public Gopher client and use Gopher just as someone with their own client would, with a few exceptions. You wouldn't be able to save and print files easily, if at all. This will depend upon the capabilities of your telecommunications software to either download data or capture what scrolls across your screen.

Additionally, most public clients operate in what's called VT100 terminal emulation mode. VT100 is a simple way for a remote computer (such as the host you've accessed) to "draw" or control what's happening on your computer's screen. VT100 is sort of a "lowest common denominator" method of presenting information, so simple that just about any computer can understand it. Because it's so simple, it won't allow you to display any information other than plain (ASCII) text. Here is an example of what a screen looks like from a VT100 Gopher client, the kind that might be used as a public client:

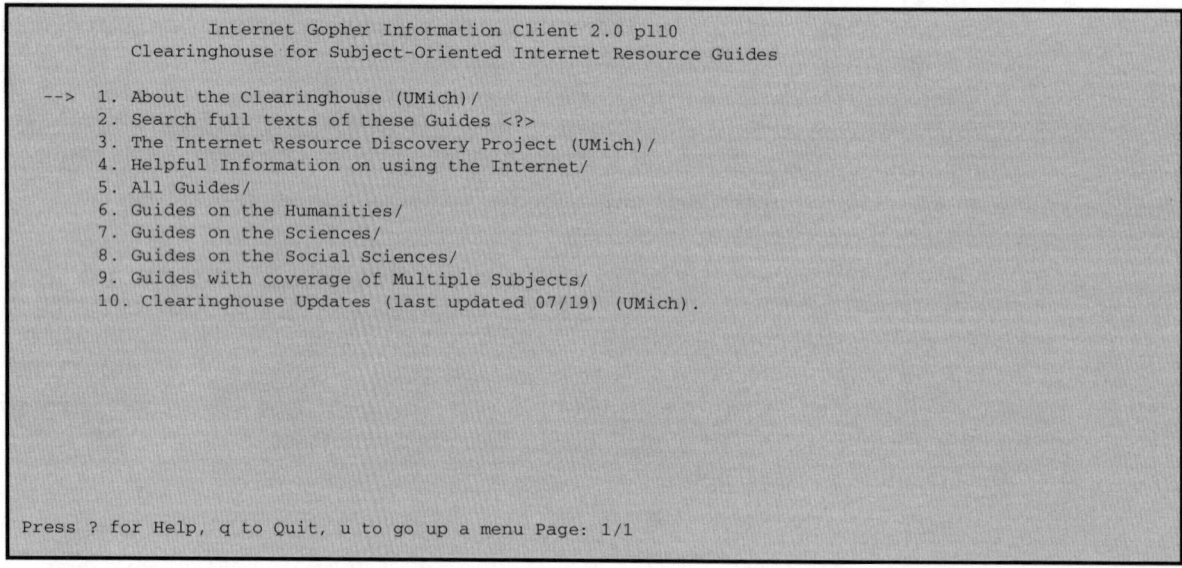

And here is how that same server would look from a non-VT100 Gopher client (this is TurboGopher, a popular client used on Macintosh computers):

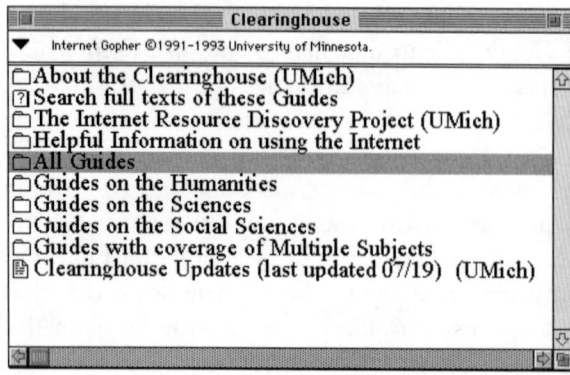

Following is a list of public Gopher and World Wide Web clients which you can telnet that don't require a password; all are at English-speaking institutions.

Gopher

Login as `gopher` unless otherwise specified.

`consultant.micro.umn.edu`
`seymour.md.gov`
`gopher.msu.edu`
`cat.ohiolink.edu`
`sunsite.unc.edu`
`panda.uiowa.edu`
`inform.umd.edu`
`info.anu.edu.au` (login as: `info`)
`gopher.brad.ac.uk` (login as: `info`)

World Wide Web

Login as `www` unless otherwise specified.

`www.njit.edu`
`ukanaix.cc.ukans.edu`
`gopher.msu.edu` (login as: `web`)
`sunsite.unc.edu` (login as: `lynx`)
`millbrook.lib.rmit.edu.au` (login as: `lynx`)

Navigating: Tools and Resources 3

As more and more people have joined the Internet community, systems have been developed which make the Net easier to use and make information easier to find. In this section, we will discuss four primary ways of moving around and getting data and how to get to a particular resource based on its URL. As we proceed, you'll notice that the tools will get more sophisticated and easier to use. By the time we get to the World Wide Web, all you'll have to do is type in the URL and you're there.

CONNECTING TO ANOTHER MACHINE: TELNET

Telnet (not to be confused with the commercial wide-area network called "Telenet") is an Internet facility that enables users to connect to another machine and use information resources located there. At various times over the last year or so, all three of us have connected to our email system in Ann Arbor from places all over the world: San Francisco, London, Prague, Washington. We did this by telnetting to our host machine from other computers connected to the Internet, and logging in as we normally do. This is possible because, using telnet, you can get just about anywhere from everywhere.

Even if you don't have an account on another system, you can telnet there if the system's administrators have provided for public telnetting. This is the case when they have an information resource that they want to make widely available. Most library catalogs on the Internet operate this way. Our example will be the Weather Underground system, maintained by the Department of Atmospheric, Oceanic and Space Sciences at the University of Michigan.

The URL for this telnet site is the following:

```
telnet://madlab.sprl.umich.edu:3000/
```

There are three parts to this URL as follows:

`telnet`	tells us that this URL refers to a telnet site
`madlab.sprl.umich.edu`	is the actual telnet address (domain name)
`3000`	is the site's port number to use in accessing the resource

Some of the structure of URLs is due to their use within the World Wide Web. If you're attempting to access this resource (or indeed, any resource) from the Web, just enter the URL at the appropriate place (Open URL menu choice in Mosaic, or type G in Lynx).

If, however, you're trying to access this resource directly from your Internet account's system prompt, type telnet followed by the address. If a port number is given (they aren't always), type a space, and then the port number. Then hit Enter or Return.

Here's an example: (characters in **bold face** are entered from the keyboard; the % is the system prompt)

```
%telnet madlab.sprl.umich.edu 3000
Trying 141.212.196.79...
Connected to madlab.sprl.umich.edu.
Escape character is '^]'.
---------------------------------------------------------------------------
*                          University of Michigan                         *
*                          WEATHER UNDERGROUND                            *
---------------------------------------------------------------------------
*                                                                         *
*            College of Engineering, University of Michigan               *
*            Department of Atmospheric, Oceanic, and Space Sciences       *
*            Ann Arbor, Michigan  48109-2143                              *
*            comments: sdm@madlab.sprl.umich.edu                          *
*                                                                         *
* With Help from:  The National Science Foundation supported Unidata Project *
*                  University Corporation for Atmospheric Research        *
*                  Boulder, Colorado  80307-3000                          *
*                                                                         *
*        This service is for educational and research purposes only.      *
*        Commercial users should contact our data provider, Alden         *
*        Electronics, 508-366-8851 to acquire their own data feed.        *
*                                                                         *
---------------------------------------------------------------------------
*   NOTE:---------> New users, please select option "H" on the main menu: *
*                   H) Help and information for new users                 *
---------------------------------------------------------------------------

Press Return for menu, or enter 3 letter forecast city code:syr

Weather Conditions at 7 AM EDT on 18 JUL 94 for Syracuse, NY.
Temp(F)    Humidity(%)    Wind(mph)     Pressure(in)     Weather
================================================================
  67           86%         EAST at 3       30.00       Partly Cloudy

LFPSYR

SYRACUSE AND VICINITY FORECAST...CORRECTED
NATIONAL WEATHER SERVICE SYRACUSE NY
1100 AM EDT MON JUL 18 1994

  THIS AFTERNOON...A MIX OF SUN AND CLOUDS WITH SCATTERED SHOWERS OR
THUNDERSTORMS.  HIGH ABOUT 80.  SOUTHWEST WIND 5 TO 15 MPH.
  TONIGHT...A 30 PERCENT CHANCE OF AN EVENING SHOWER OR THUNDERSTORM
THEN PARTLY CLOUDY WITH PATCHY FOG.  LOW NEAR 60.  LIGHT WIND.
  TUESDAY...PARLTY SUNNY.  HIGH 80 TO 85.

  ..BOATING AND RECREATIONAL FORECAST FOR ONEIDA AND ONONDAGA LAKES...
  THIS AFTERNOON...SOUTHWEST WIND 6 TO 12 KNOTS.  SCATTERED SHOWERS OR
THUNDERSTORMS.
  TONIGHT...VARIABLE WIND UNDER 8 KNOTS.  CHANCE OF AN EVENING SHOWER
OR THUNDERSTORM...THEN AREAS OF OVERNIGHT FOG.
  TUESDAY...NORTHWEST WIND 5 TO 12 KNOTS.  FAIR.

SWF
  EXTENDED FORECAST...
  WEDNESDAY...FAIR.  LOWS IN THE 60S.  HIGHS IN THE 80S.
  THURSDAY...VERY WARM AND HUMID WITH A CHANCE OF THUNDERSTORMS.
LOWS 65 TO AROUND 70.  HIGHS 85 TO AROUND 90.
  FRIDAY...  VERY WARM AND HUMID WITH A CHANCE OF THUNDERSTORMS.
LOWS 65 TO AROUND 70.  HIGHS 85 TO AROUND 90.

    Press Return to continue, M to return to menu, X to exit:x
```

Getting Files: File Transfer Protocol (FTP)

One of the earliest and most frequent uses for the Internet was to share files—data, software, images, and so on. The most efficient way to do this is via the File Transfer Protocol, known as FTP. To retrieve a file from an FTP archive,[1] you must know the address of the FTP server, the name of the file, and its location on that machine. A URL will give you all that information. The following is a sample:

`file://quartz.rutgers.edu/pub/humor/Python`

This happens to be a repository of Monty Python film scripts on a machine at Rutgers University. This URL also has three major parts, as follows:

`file:`	means that the URL refers to a file in an FTP archive
`quartz.rutgers.edu`	is the address of the FTP server
`pub/humor/Python`	is the directory path on that FTP server where the files are

Connecting to an FTP site and using anonymous FTP

Most of the time, you'll probably want to FTP documents from host computers on which you don't have an account. That's not a problem (usually), because many machines provide for public access to some resources. Other files on these machines will not be available to you, but they're also typically not going to be in guides or generally known, so it's a case of not knowing what you're missing. This public FTP capability is called *anonymous FTP*, and it is very widely used.

To connect to a machine with an FTP archive, you must first log in to your account. This is because the document has to have somewhere to go. You can't FTP without an account of your own on a machine with access to the Internet. From your system's prompt, type the following, where <hostname> is the address of the machine you wise to connect to.

`ftp <hostname>`

You'll get a message that you're connected, and then it will ask you for your name. Here you type anonymous. When you are asked for a password, you really needn't give it one, because this is public access. It is conventional (and considered good netiquette) to give it your email address. This allows the people who maintain the FTP site to know where the accesses are coming from. You could type guest or anonymous or anything else, but we encourage you to abide by the convention. As a security measure, this password will not appear on the screen.

Commands to view and move through directories

You are now at an FTP prompt. This tells you that you are connected to the remote machine via the file transfer protocol and are ready to begin downloading. Files in these archives are organized in much the same way that they are in DOS or Windows-based systems (in fact these are Unix-based systems), with directories and subdirectories in hierarchies. If you know the exact pathname, you can go directly to the file you want that way. Alternatively, if you've found a potentially interesting FTP site and you just want to explore it, you can examine the directories that way.

To move through directories, use the `cd` command (cd for change directory). To move to a directory called `library`, for example, type the following:

`ftp>`**`cd library`**

To move back up to the previous directory, (i.e., the one higher in the hierarchy), use

`ftp>`**`cd ..`**

To see the contents of a directory, use the `dir` command.

`ftp>`**`dir`**

---

[1] FTP can also be used to send files, but we won't go into that here.

Here's an example of several uses of these commands:

```
%ftp quartz.rutgers.edu
Connected to quartz.rutgers.edu.
220-QUARTZ.RUTGERS.EDU FTP ARCHIVE
220-enter 'anonymous' for username
220-enter email address as password
220-
220-
220 quartz.rutgers.edu FTP server (Version 2.1aWU(1) Sat Jul 3 15:53:35 EDT 1993
) ready.
Name (quartz.rutgers.edu:janes): anonymous
331 Guest login ok, send your complete e-mail address as password.
Password:
230-----------------------------------------------------------------------------
230-WELCOME TO THE QUARTZ.RUTGERS.EDU FTP ARCHIVE
230-
230-If your ftp program does not like quartz's ftp, reconnect and type
230-a dash as the first letter of your password, e.g. "-foo@bar.com"
230-All transfers are logged! If you don't like this, QUIT now!
230-
230-YOUR COMMENTS ARE APPRECIATED! Mail to: bbs@quartz.rutgers.edu
230-You may drop files off for the archive in the /incoming directory.
230-
230-See the file "COMPRESS" for information on how to uncompress our
230-GZIP format .z and .gz files! We have gzip software in directory
230-/gzip OR you can use the FTP server itself uncompress the files by
230-omitting the .z/.gz suffix when getting files.
230-----------------------------------------------------------------------------
230-Ftp server active at Mon Jul 18 13:57:50 1994 from sils.umich.edu.
230-
230 Guest login ok, access restrictions apply.
ftp> dir
200 PORT command successful.
150 Opening ASCII mode data connection for /bin/ls.
total 10
lrwxrwxrwx   1 root      21003          12 Jun 27  1993 COMPRESS -> pub/COMPRESS
-rw-r--r--   1 31630     21003         782 Jul  3  1993 README
drwxr-xr-x   2 root      21003         512 Nov 25  1993 bin
drwxr-xr-x   2 root      21003         512 Jun 24  1992 dev
drwxr-xr-x   2 root      21003         512 Sep 14  1993 etc
drwxr-sr-x   2 31630     21003         512 Jan 29 04:41 gzip
d-wxrwsrwx   2 ftp       21003         512 Jul 18 07:26 incoming
lrwxrwxrwx   1 root      21003           9 Nov 25  1993 ls-alR -> pub/FILES
drwxr-xr-x  35 31630     21003        1024 Jul 15 02:13 pub
drwxr-xr-x   3 root      21003         512 Jun 24  1992 usr
226 Transfer complete.
646 bytes received in 0.46 seconds (1.4 Kbytes/s)
ftp> cd pub/humor
250-Directory: /pub/humor
250-Humor files, silly!
250-Some are sorted, check the subdirectories.
250-
250 CWD command successful.
ftp> dir
200 PORT command successful.
150 Opening ASCII mode data connection for /bin/ls.
total 214
-rw-r--r--   1 31630     21003          85 Aug 17  1993 00.README
drwxr-xr-x   2 31630     21003        1024 Jul 15 02:12 Computer
drwxr-xr-x   2 31630     21003         512 Jul 15 02:12 Political
drwxr-xr-x   2 31630     21003         512 Jul 15 02:12 Python
drwxr-xr-x   2 31630     21003         512 Jul 15 02:12 Religion
drwxr-xr-x   2 31630     21003         512 Jul 15 02:12 School
drwxr-xr-x   2 31630     21003         512 Jul 15 02:12 Science
drwxr-xr-x   2 31630     21003        1024 Jul 15 02:12 Sex
drwxr-xr-x   2 31630     21003        1024 Jul 15 02:12 Tests
-rw-r--r--   1 31630     21003        2782 Feb 26  1993 antizodiac.gz
-rw-r--r--   1 31630     21003       10827 Nov 20  1992 ascii-art.gz
-rw-r--r--   1 31630     21003         654 Jul 14  1993 barney-episodes.gz
-rw-r--r--   1 31630     21003       19982 Nov 20  1992 blonde-jokes.gz
-rw-r--r--   1 31630     21003        1457 Nov  6  1992 braindamage.scale.gz
-rw-r--r--   1 31630     21003        4214 Dec 11  1992 cane-toads.gz
-rw-r--r--   1 31630     21003        1347 Dec 12  1992 carlin-tvwords.gz
-rw-r--r--   1 31630     21003        1926 Apr 21  1991 chicken.cross.gz
-rw-r--r--   1 31630     21003        1205 Jun 26  1993 childrens-books.gz
-rw-r--r--   1 31630     21003       44890 Jan 31  1992 compleat.cows.gz
-rw-r--r--   1 31630     21003       12909 Apr 11  1991 drunk.trek.gz
-rw-r--r--   1 31630     21003        2993 Nov 20  1992 dump-blind-date.gz
-rw-r--r--   1 31630     21003        1276 Oct 13  1991 fart.chart.gz
-rw-r--r--   1 31630     21003        2201 Feb 29  1992 first.aid.gz
```

```
-rw-r--r--   1 31630      21003         576 Sep 22  1991 gashlycrumb.gz
-rw-r--r--   1 31630      21003       11116 Feb 19  1993 lawyer.jokes.gz
-rw-r--r--   1 31630      21003        6710 Nov 20  1992 lightbulb-jokes.gz
-rw-r--r--   1 31630      21003        3391 Apr 11  1991 limericks.gz
-rw-r--r--   1 31630      21003        1214 Feb  2  1993 management-performance.gz
-rw-r--r--   1 31630      21003         895 Oct 13  1991 mens.room.gz
-rw-r--r--   1 31630      21003         810 Apr 11  1991 murphy.combat.gz
-rw-r--r--   1 31630      21003       11248 Jan 31  1992 murphy.gz
-rw-r--r--   1 31630      21003        2525 Feb  2  1993 new-cabling.gz
-rw-r--r--   1 31630      21003         980 Apr  4  1992 poopie.list.gz
-rw-r--r--   1 31630      21003        5311 Dec 12  1992 radar.game.gz
-rw-r--r--   1 31630      21003         894 May 16  1991 ru.fight.song.gz
-rw-r--r--   1 31630      21003        1762 Mar  3 03:19 slaw-lane.gz
-rw-r--r--   1 31630      21003        7340 Apr 11  1991 some.jokes.gz
-rw-r--r--   1 31630      21003       14649 Feb 26  1993 steven-wright-quotes.gz
-rw-r--r--   1 31630      21003        2307 Mar 25  1993 telemarketers.gz
-rw-r--r--   1 31630      21003        4109 Sep 20  1991 tourists.gz
-rw-r--r--   1 31630      21003        7021 Jan 21  1993 unnatural-inq.gz
-rw-r-----   1 31630      21003        2559 Nov  6  1992 wisconsin-app.gz
226 Transfer complete.
2923 bytes received in 1.1 seconds (2.5 Kbytes/s)
ftp> cd Python
250 CWD command successful.
ftp> dir
200 PORT command successful.
150 Opening ASCII mode data connection for /bin/ls.
total 102
-rw-r--r--   1 31630      21003       53127 Aug 15  1992 Holy_Grail.gz
-rw-r--r--   1 31630      21003        2950 Nov 20  1992 cheese-shop.gz
-rw-r--r--   1 31630      21003       11647 Nov 20  1992 life-of-brian.gz
-rw-r--r--   1 31630      21003       35386 Nov 20  1992 meaning-of-life.gz
226 Transfer complete.
296 bytes received in 0.033 seconds (8.7 Kbytes/s)
```

How to get files

When you've found the directory that contains the file you want, use the `get` command to download it.

```
ftp> get <filename>
```

You can end the FTP session with the `quit` command.

```
ftp> quit
```

```
ftp> get Holy_Grail.gz
200 PORT command successful.
150 Opening ASCII mode data connection for Holy_Grail.gz (53127 bytes).
226 Transfer complete.
local: Holy_Grail.gz remote: Holy_Grail.gz
53326 bytes received in 3.4 seconds (15 Kbytes/s)
ftp> quit
221 Goodbye.
```

When you have successfully downloaded the file, it will reside in the account from where you began the FTP session. If this is some account you regularly use, it is in that space and you can do anything you want to it: load it into a word processing or text editing package such as pico or Microsoft Word and edit it, print it out, send it somewhere else via email, whatever. If you logged into some other kind of account or if you have no home account, you may have to display the file again and transfer it using your telecommunications package. If this is the case, you'll probably want to ask for help.

A few words of advice

If you're just exploring an interesting site, you may find it useful to look at files called README or INDEX, or something like that. These are often files which describe the contents of the other files in the archives or give other information such as formats or compression mechanisms being used, etc.

Menus of Resources: Gopher

Gopher was the first attempt to provide some semblance of order to the chaos that is the Net. It gets its name from the Golden Gophers, the mascot of the University of Minnesota, where the protocol was developed. Before Gophers, it was necessary to know the precise Internet address of an information source to be able to telnet or FTP to it. If you didn't know the address, or had it wrong in any respect, you got nowhere. Further, there was a large number of resources that nobody knew about because there was no central catalog or index.

There still isn't, but Gophers have made finding and maneuvering between resources much easier. Gophers organize networked resources in hierarchical structures, and permit browsing and searching via menus. It's a great idea, and was a vast improvement over the previous situation. One of the best features of Gopher, apart from its simplicity of use and understanding, is that most Gophers are connected. So, if you start with almost any Gopher, you can pretty much get to any other one through a menu choice like "All the Gopher Servers in the World" or "Other Gophers". Pretty neat. You can see, from following paths like this, how surfing the Internet got its name.

Using Gopher, you do not need to know addresses,[2] and the interface is blindingly simple to learn and use. But it still has its limitations. There are two that are of primary importance to anyone trying to use Gophers to find specific information. First of all, while there are technical protocols for building Gophers, there are no standards for how the menus are organized or titled. Thus, a resource you really want might be underneath a menu choice with a title like "Really Cool Stuff" or "New Things" or "Everything Else" or who knows what else. Moreover, these menus change as new resources are added and old ones go away. That sort of thing is fine if you're just playing around, but if you're looking for a recent Supreme Court decision or a recipe for black bean chili you may well be out of luck. You are really at the mercy of the designer of the Gopher, and these people, largely, have no training in information work as we know it.

If you do know the address of a particular resource in Gopher, though, it can be even easier to access. Here's a sample Gopher URL, which is the address for information from the US Department of Agriculture meant to assist survivors of natural disasters:

```
gopher://zeus.esusda.gov/11/disasters/finances
```

Again, three parts:

`gopher`	means this refers to a Gopher
`zeus.esusda.gov`	is the address of the Gopher
`disasters/finances`	is the chain of menus you must follow to get to the resource

In this case, the path is a bit more complicated. With an FTP address, the path given is exactly the names of the directories and subdirectories on the host computer. Here, though, these are abbreviated versions of the menu choice you must make. Here's a series of screen images showing how you would move down to the menu you want:

---

[2] You don't need to know addresses, but you *can* find out where a particular resource is coming from. When you put a Gopher together, you only have to point to resources that are located on other machines; you don't have to have a copy on your local machine. This is done by creating a link file, which specifies where to go when a particular menu item is chosen. You can see this link file while you are using the Gopher. To do this, make sure the arrow is pointing at the item you're interested in, and hit the = key. This will display the link file. This will work in VT100 Gopher clients; if you're using some client software like TurboGopher for the Mac, you need to consult documentation to see how to display link files.

```
%gopher zeus.esusda.gov

              Internet Gopher Information Client 2.0 p110

                     Root gopher server: zeus.esusda.gov

         1.  About this Gopher -- Extension Service, USDA.
         2.  What's New in this Gopher -- Extension Service (ES), USDA.
         3.  FYI -- Extension Service (ES), USDA/
         4.  National Initiatives -- Extension Service (ES), USDA /
         5.  Educational Base Programs -- Extension Service (ES), USDA /
         6.  Policy and Strategic Directions--ECOP..-USDA(was: Ed. & Info. Tech) /
         7.  Information Servers -- Cooperative Extension System (CES)/
         8.  Internet Services and Information/
         9.  USDA and Other Federal Agency Information/
         10. Other Gopher Information Servers/
    -->  11. Disaster Relief Information (includes Flood, Hurricane info...)/
         12. White House and Congress (incl. Health Care, NAFTA, NII, NPR)/
```

Here we see the main menu for the USDA Extension Service Gopher. The URL indicated that the resource we're looking for was located on the path disasters/finances; it would appear that menu choice 11, Disaster Relief Information is the right one, so we use the down arrow to move to that line and hit return, taking us to the following screen:

```
              Internet Gopher Information Client 2.0 p110

         Disaster Relief Information (includes Flood, Hurricane info...)

         1.  About this Section.
         2.  ASCS Emergency Programs -- July 1993.
         3.  Center for Disease Control, Disaster and Emergency Activities/
         4.  Cleanup and Salvage -- Factsheets/
         5.  Disaster Info(U.S. and Int'l) Gopher--Volunteers in Tech Assistanc../
         6.  Disaster Preparedness -- Factsheets/
         7.  Disaster Reports and CES Responses/
         8.  Earthquake Relief Information/
         9.  Emotional Stress after Disasters/
    -->  10. Finances and Insurance Issues/
         11. Flood-Related Relief Information/
         12. Food and Water Safety -- Factsheets/
         13. Gardens, Crops, Pests -- Factsheets/
         14. Home Repairs and Renovation -- Factsheets/
         15. USDA 1993 Flood and Disaster Info/
```

Menu choice 10, here, would appear to be correct, so we follow the same procedure, taking us to this menu of financial and insurance issues for disaster survivors:

```
              Internet Gopher Information Client 2.0 p110

                          Finances and Insurance Issues

    -->  1.  Contracts.
         2.  Filing insurance claims.
         3.  Flood insurance and credit for disaster victims.
         4.  Good news about your homeowner's insurance policy.
         5.  Handling Insurance.
         6.  Protecting Valuable Records.
         7.  about.
         8.  he11400.wp.
         9.  he11500.wp.
```

MOVING THROUGH HYPERTEXT: THE WORLD WIDE WEB

The World Wide Web (or W3, or just "the Web") has been around for quite some time, but in the last year or so, since the introduction of a new client called Mosaic, it has become tremendously popular. It's a simple enough idea: use a hypertextual[3] system to provide links to resources that are similar or that someone feels should be related somehow, and let other people follow those links. Better still, let resources normally used with many different kind of tools be joined seamlessly and with a single interface: Gophers, FTP sites, telnet links as well as "native" Web documents. Advanced clients like Mosaic can in turn present all of this information via a graphical interface which can access images, audio, and video files, as well as plain text.

This wonderful idea has caused a great deal of excitement, both in the Net community and among professionals in libraries and information centers. Web documents (called "HTML documents" for the HyperText Markup Language used to create them) are quite easy to develop and allow people to become creative publishers of networked information resources with little difficulty.

Following is an HTML document as displayed by Lynx, a VT100 World Wide Web client. Notice the underlined links; you could use your arrow keys to move from one to another. Pressing the return or enter key would lead you to another Web document or Internet resource.

```
                                              Missing Children (p1 of 3)
   [IMAGE]
                         MISSING CHILDREN DATABASE
   _____

   This is a mirror site for the Missing Children's Forum on CompuServe.
   It contains known information about, and pictures of, children who
   are missing. The database is maintained by the National Center for
   Missing and Exploited Children (NCMEC). This mirror of the files
    contained in the CompuServe Forum is maintained as a public service
   by Maxwell Labs in order to provide access to this information for
   Internet users.

   Of course, if you have any information about any of these little
   tykes, please call the number below.

   Please DO NOT redistribute these pictures. Consider the feelings
   -- press space for next page --
   Arrow keys: Up or Down to move. Right to follow a link; Left to go back.
   H)elp O)ptions P)rint G)o M)ain screen Q)uit /=search [del]=history list
```

On the following page is the same document displayed by NCSA Mosaic (Macintosh version): note the addition of images and different sized typefaces, as well as buttons that can speed navigation. (The color that would normally also occur can't be duplicated here.)

Again, note that these are the same document; the only difference is they have been displayed by different World Wide Web clients. Here is its URL:

    `http://www.scubed.com:8001/public_service/missing.html`

Mosaic normally displays the URL for the current document at the top of the window. When running Mosaic, choose the menu choice Open URL, and type the URL in the box which pops up. This will take you directly to the resource you named. (In Lynx, type G for Go; you will then be prompted for the URL to Go to.) You will notice that when you are scanning a Web page from Mosaic, if you place the mouse over a link (links are usually in blue, or red if they've already been clicked on) that the URL for the document it represents will appear near the top of the screen. People now trade URLs—it's easy and fun!

---

3   Hypertexts are documents or sets of documents than are organized in a non-linear way. Hypertexts include words or phrases which serve as "live" links to other parts of the document, or to other documents. For example, an encyclopedia entry for 'Paris' might include terms such as 'cuisine' and 'France'. If 'cuisine' is a link, selecting it might cause an entry on Parisian cuisine to be displayed. Hypermedia refers to non-linearly arranged information which, besides text, could include images, audio, video, or combinations of those formats. So choosing the link 'France' might display a map of France. Selecting the southern portion of the map of France might display a detailed map of the Riviera, and so on.

NAVIGATING: TOOLS AND RESOURCES 19

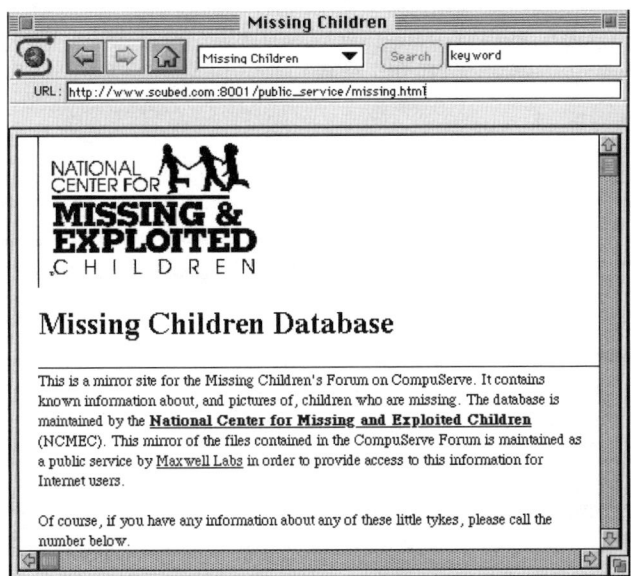

One of the great limitations of the Web, until quite recently, is that there was no good searching tool to find particular resources of interest. The best ways to find out what was good out there was (1) to ask other people, (2) to use the *Starting Points for Internet Exploration* or the *Resources by Subject* links on the *Mosaic Home Page*, each of which have a large number of links to stuff on the Web, and (3) to scan regularly the *What's New* page from the main Mosaic site at the University of Illinois. This page gives updates several times a week about new and interesting resources available on the Web. There's a new What's New page every month; old ones are still available; these provide a fascinating glimpse of the variety and diversity of activity on the Web. The URLs for these documents are the following:

NCSA Mosaic Home Page:
`http://www.ncsa.uiuc.edu/SDG/Software/Mosaic/NCSAMosaicHome.html`

NCSA What's New Page:
`http://www.ncsa.uiuc.edu/SDG/Software/Mosaic/Docs/whats-new.html`

If you aren't sure if the resources you need exist or what their URLs are, you might check any of the attempts at organizing the Web. Known as "virtual libraries," these documents organize the Web's resources by subject or by other schemes. Though they are useful, be careful: *they are rarely up-to-date, and are likely not comprehensive*. With this in mind, consider consulting any of the following virtual libraries:

- The World-Wide Web Virtual Library: Subject Catalogue (URL: `http://info.cern.ch/hypertext/DataSources/bySubject/Overview.html`)
- The Whole Internet Catalog (URL: `http://nearnet.gnn.com/wic/newrescat.toc.html`)
- EINet Galaxy (URL: `http://www.einet.net/galaxy.html`)
- Nova-Links (URL: `http://alpha.acast.nova.edu/start.html`)
- Joel's Hierarchical Subject Index (URL: `http://www.cen.uiuc.edu/~jj9544/index.html`)

You might also consider looking at a geographically organized list of known World Wide Web servers. The document *World-Wide Web Servers: Summary* is located at

URL: `http://info.cern.ch/hypertext/DataSources/WWW/Servers.html`

The searching tools that have emerged recently aren't bad, but aren't perfect either. The easiest one to use is JumpStation, developed in the UK. JumpStation allows you to search nearly all the known Web documents at one time. JumpStation provides searching of either *header* or *title* portions of World Wide Web documents. Documents have one title, and can have many headers, which often serve as section titles. Thus you will find that a title search will generally retrieve fewer documents than a header search.

After you enter your search, JumpStation will simply retrieve and provide you a list of documents that contain your keyword. Boolean or truncated searching are not available from JumpStation at this time.

URL: `http://www.stir.ac.uk/jsbin/js`

More searching tools for the World Wide Web are on the way, including World Wide Web Worm, Web Crawler, EINet Galaxy, LYCOS, and a host of others. Some are designed to search full texts of HTML documents on the Web, and others are designed for special purposes. Just remember that none are as truly stable and comprehensive as a commercial product might be. A good place to check out other Web searching tools is

URL: `http://cui_www.unige.ch/meta-index.html`

Communicating with Individuals and Groups 4

The Importance of People

The resources mentioned so far are all well and good, and can be of enormous usefulness, especially if you know where you're going. We'll discuss searching for resources shortly, but our experience has shown that one of the most important classes of resources available via the Internet is other people. Very often, the easiest way to find an answer to a question or a lead to a useful information resource is to ask someone. The problem can be finding the person to ask. Posting questions to discussion groups such as LISTSERVs and Usenet newsgroups can be an effective way around this, but there are still times when you want to be able to send email or a file to that very special someone.

There is not, as of yet, a single comprehensive directory of all Internet users. It's unlikely that there ever will be an Internet white pages, either. There are, however, a couple of tools which you can use to assist you in the quest for a individual email address.

Finding People

So you want to send email to someone—you need to know their Internet address. In many cases, the easiest way to find that out is to ask them, or to have them send you email so you can reply to it. There are also a couple of approaches to finding names which may be useful.

```
% finger polly@nysernet.org
[nysernet.org]
Login name: pstapley              In real life: Polly Stapley
Directory: /nyser3/k12/pstapley   Shell: /bin/csh
Last login Tue May  4, 1993 on ttyp6 from 192.77.9.2
Mail last read Thu Jul  7 12:31:56 1994
No Plan.

Login name: lpolly                In real life: Larry Polly
Directory: /nyser3/guest/lpolly   Shell: /bin/csh
Last login Thu Jun  2 19:23 on ttyp3 from micro.ec.hscsyr.
Mail last read Thu Jul  7 12:31:17 1994
No Plan.
Login name: lpolly                In real life: Larry Polly
Directory: /nyser3/guest/lpolly   Shell: /bin/csh
Last login Thu Jun  2 19:23 on ttyp3 from micro.ec.hscsyr.
Mail last read Thu Jul  7 12:31:17 1994
No Plan.

Login name: jpolly                In real life: Jean Armour Polly
Directory: /nyser2/staff/jpolly   Shell: /bin/csh
Last login Wed Jul  6 16:36 on ttyp9 from tv.lpl.org
New mail received Thu Jul  7 18:14:07 1994;
  unread since Thu Jul  7 18:03:38 1994
Project: Being an outrider on the Internet frontier.
```

```
Plan:
Director of User Services
315/ 453-2912 ext 224    FAX 315/ 453-3052

"Do Right; Fear Not."
- sign outside church, The Rocky Horror Picture Show

"Demand epiphany!" -- Pat Hunt, Mendocino Co. Library, California

"An idea can turn to dust or magic,
 depending on the talent that rubs against it." -- William Bernbach

"We are surrounded by insurmountable opportunity."-- Pogo

"If you practice an art, be proud of it and make it proud of you...
it may break your heart, but it will fill your heart before it breaks it;
it will make you a person in your own right." -- Maxwell Anderson

"Mom, aren't you off the computer YET??!!" -- Stephen Jade Polly, age 8
```

finger

If you are working on a Unix system or can connect to one, you may be able to use the `finger` command to find people. This command requires you to know at least the domain of the person you're fingering. To try and find out the email address of somebody, use finger, their name and the domain:

We find three listings containing the name "Polly" at `nysernet.org`, the third being Jean Armour Polly, our target. The text at the end of her listing is her plan—a file she maintains on her computer to tell people a bit more about herself, in this case including quotes she finds interesting. We know from this result that her email address is `jpolly@nysernet.org`.

Netfind

Another method which seems to best balance ease-of-use with comprehensiveness is called Netfind, a program created by Mike Schwartz and Panos Tsirigotis at the University of Colorado, Boulder. Netfind is particularly useful if you don't know the person's domain: if you can supply a person's last name and a rough description of where the person works, Netfind can often (not always) find an Internet e-mail address for that person. The simplest way to access NetFind is to telnet to the host `ds.internic.net` and login as `netfind`.

```
%telnet ds.internic.net
Trying 198.49.45.10...
Connected to ds.internic.net.
Escape character is '^]'.
            InterNIC Directory and Database Services

Welcome to InterNIC Directory and Database Services provided by AT&T.
These services are partially supported through a cooperative agreement
with the National Science Foundation.

First time users may login as guest with no password to receive help.

Your comments and suggestions for improvement are welcome, and can be
mailed to admin@ds.internic.net.

AT&T MAKES NO WARRANTY OR GUARANTEE, OR PROMISE, EXPRESS OR IMPLIED,
CONCERNING THE  CONTENT OR  ACCURACY OF THE  DIRECTORY  ENTRIES AND
DATABASE  FILES  STORED  AND  MAINTAINED  BY  AT&T.  AT&T EXPRESSLY
DISCLAIMS AND EXCLUDES ALL EXPRESS WARRANTIES AND IMPLIED WARRANTIES
OF MERCHANTABILITY AND FITNESS FOR A PARTICULAR PURPOSE.


************************************************************
DS0 will be rebooted every Monday morning between 8:00AM and 8:30AM est.

DS0 will be unavailable Wednesday August 3, 1994 from 8:00 to 8:30 am.

Please use DS1 or DS2 during this period.
```

```
SunOS UNIX (ds)

login: netfind
Last login: Tue Aug  2 09:36:01 from sils.umich.edu
SunOS Release 4.1.3 (DS) #3: Tue Feb 8 10:52:45 EST 1994

*****************************************************************************

              Welcome to the InterNIC Directory and Database Server.

*****************************************************************************


I think that your terminal can display 24 lines.  If this is wrong,
please enter the "Options" menu and set the correct number of lines.

Top level choices:
        1. Help
        2. Search
        3. Seed database lookup
        4. Options
        5. Quit (exit server)
--> 2
```

At the search prompt, we will search for the e-mail address of Ed Vielmetti at Msen, Inc., an Internet service provider in Ann Arbor, Michigan. Keep in mind that search terms are implicitly ANDed together; in other words, the more terms you search, the smaller the retrieval will be, and vice versa.

```
Enter person and keys (blank to exit) --> vielmetti msen ann arbor
Please select at most 3 of the following domains to search:
        0. msen.com (msen, inc, ann arbor, michigan)
        1. aa-unet.msen.com (msen, inc, ann arbor, michigan)
        2. aa.msen.com (msen, inc, ann arbor, michigan)
        3. clarkson.msen.com (msen, inc, ann arbor, michigan)
        4. demo.msen.com (msen, inc, ann arbor, michigan)
        5. dexter.msen.com (msen, inc, ann arbor, michigan)
        6. pnet.msen.com (msen, inc, ann arbor, michigan)
        7. research.msen.com (msen, inc, ann arbor, michigan)
        8. troy-unet.msen.com (msen, inc, ann arbor, michigan)
        9. troy.msen.com (msen, inc, ann arbor, michigan)
       10. whitl.msen.com (msen, inc, ann arbor, michigan)
Enter selection (e.g., 2 0 1) --> 0
( 1) SMTP_Finger_Search: checking domain msen.com
SYSTEM: msen.com
        Login: emv                              Name: Edward Vielmetti
        Directory: /usr/msen/emv                Shell: /bin/bash
        Office: Msen, 313-998-4562              Home Phone: 313-761-4248
        On since Tue Aug  2 09:14 (EDT) on ttyqa (messages off) from irx1
        Plan:
            Edward Vielmetti, vice president for research, Msen Inc. emv@Msen.com
            Msen Inc., 320 Miller, Ann Arbor MI  48103 +1 313 998 4562 (fax: 998 456
3)

Continue the search ([n]/y) ? -->
```

Our search was a bit too broad, as there are several Internet domains which include the terms 'msen', 'ann', and 'arbor'. We needed to narrow the list by choosing which domain to search. Enter the selections' number or numbers at the prompt. As we weren't sure which domain hosted Ed's account, we chose the broadest, most broad, generic address (0 -- msen.com), although we could have entered more than one address.

NetFind then proceeded to search the remote computers at the domain msen.com. After some garbage characters scrolled by, NetFind found Ed's e-mail address: emv@msen.com; we determine this by combining his login name (emv) and the domain name we started with (msen.com). Also found are his phone number and address, added bonuses. Now that we've found the information we were looking for, we can log out.

A few words of warning and advice: Netfind doesn't always work; in fact, it's pretty hit and miss. Here are some hints:

- You're often better searching as narrowly as you can to begin with (i.e., give as much information as you have about the domain; don't give first names), and then see what hosts you get as a result. Then pick the broadest domain you can, . . . unless you know better.
- If one of the hosts which are presented to you looks right (i.e., if your subject works for the Institute for Sensory Research at Syracuse University, and `isr.syr.edu` comes up, try that along with `syr.edu`
- If you know the domain name, give it rather than trying to search within the descriptive information given for each host. There are a lot of hosts with "university" and "california." If you do know the domain, enter it following the person's name, but don't use any periods—separate the parts with spaces instead.

Gopher

For people who are affiliated with organizations, especially colleges or universities, you may be able to access the organization's phone book or directory over the net, especially through a Gopher. There are two approaches here; either find that particular institution's Gopher, and see if it contains a directory, or go to a collection of such directories at a Gopher maintained at the University of Notre Dame.

You can get to this Gopher via the normal paths ("All the Gophers in the World") in almost any other Gopher. You can also do directly to it. The URL is as follows:

```
gopher://gopher.nd.edu:70/11/Non-Notre Dame Information Sources/Phone Books--Other
Institutions/North America
```

ELECTRONIC MAILING LISTS: LISTSERVS

Mailing lists enable email users to broadcast e-mail to groups of other e-mail users who share a common interest. These lists serve as forums for questions and answers, announcements, discussions, and often, spirited arguments (known as *flames*). For example, if you wanted to find out what Paul McCartney is doing these days, you might post a question to the address of one of the Beatles mailing lists, and thousands of devoted fans of Paul will read your query. Many of them will generate answers, post them to the list, and you (and everyone else on the list) will be able to read them.

This probably sounds like fun, but we should warn you: mailing lists can be extremely addictive. They are an easy way to *not* get work done. Also, as mailing lists are based on email, you may find yourself overwhelmed by the number of messages waiting for you in your mailbox, and subsequently be frustrated by how quickly your time fritters away. It is not rare to subscribe to a mailing list which generates over one hundred postings in a day.

There are thousands of electronic mailing lists. Often you'll hear them referred to as "LISTSERVs". LISTSERV is one specific software package designed to help mailing list administrators manage mailing lists; there are many others available. This is similar to how people use the brandname "Kleenex" to describe facial tissues in general.

To find a relevant mailing list, ask your friends and colleagues. It's likely that someone you know uses the Internet and shares some similar areas of interest, so you should ask them what mailing lists they recommend. Another way to find a mailing list is to search through guides such as those included in this book, or those stored in the Clearinghouse for Subject-Oriented Internet Resource Guides, described in another section. Lastly, you can also find LISTSERVs by sending to any LISTSERV address (e.g., `listserv@cunyvm.bitnet`) the following message via electronic mail (don't use a subject line or any other text in this message) where keyword is the term you're searching for.

```
list global/<keyword>
```

Keep in mind that the names of mailing lists are often abbreviated to save space, so if you're looking for "library" consider using the keyword "lib". The results of your search are an e-mailed list of LISTSERVs and their addresses. Here is the just the first few results from a search for "lib":

```
Date: Mon, 1 Aug 1994 18:48:46 -0400
From: BITNET list server at CUNYVM <LISTSERV@CUNYVM.CUNY.EDU>
To: lou@UMICH.EDU
Subject: File: "LISTSERV LISTS"

Excerpt from the LISTSERV lists known to LISTSERV@CUNYVM on 1 Aug 1994 18:48
Search string: LIB

Network-wide ID  Full address    List title
---------------  ------------    ----------
AACRL            AACRL@UABDPO    Alabama Association of College and Research
+
ACRL             ACRL@UICVM      Association of College and Research
Librarie+
ADAPT-L          ADAPT-L@AUVM    Library Adaptive Technology
ADVANC-L         ADVANC-L@IDBSU  ADVANC-L - Users of the Geac ADVANCE
Library+
AFAS-L           AFAS-L@KENTVM   African American Studies and Librarianship
AGRIS-L          AGRIS-L@IRMFAO01 The Food and Agriculture Organization
Libra+
AIBIBL           AIBIBL@PLEARN   ACADEMIC INITIATIVE IBM , PROJECT "LIBRARY
S+
AJCUILL          AJCUILL@GUVM    AJCU Law Librarians/Interlibrary Loan
Contac+
AJCULIB          AJCULIB@GUVM    AJCU Librarians
ALF-L            ALF-L@YORKVM1   Academic Librarian's Forum
ALHELA           ALHELA@UABDPO   Alabama Health Libraries Association
ALXFOCUS         ALXFOCUS@RUTVM1 Alexander Library Electronic Focus Group
ARCLIB-L         ARCLIB-L@IRLEARN Mailing List for Irish and UK Architectural
+
ARIZSLS          ARIZSLS@ARIZVM1 Library Science Conference
ARLIS-L          ARLIS-L@UKCC    ART LIBRARIES SOCIETY DISCUSSION LIST
ATLANTIS         ATLANTIS@HARVARDA ATLANTIS - American Theological Library
Disc+
ATLAS-L          ATLAS-L@TCUBVM  ATLAS-L  DRA Library systems interest list
AUTOCAT          AUTOCAT@UBVM    AUTOCAT: Library cataloging and authorities
```

To participate in a mailing list, you will need to subscribe to it, and remember: even though they call it "subscribing," there is no charge for joining a mailing list. The directions below describe the LISTSERV subscription process.

> Address a message to the LISTSERV software at that LISTSERV's address (as opposed to sending it to the name of the LISTSERV itself). So, if you wish to subscribe to `pacs-l@uhupvm1.uh.edu` (the Public-Access Computing Systems List), you would send a message to:
>
> `listserv@uhupvm1.uh.edu`
>
> NOT `pacs-l@uhupvm1.uh.edu`
>
> The text of the message should consist of the following text:
>
> `subscribe pacs-l Jane Smith` (or whatever your name is)

You should soon receive e-mail from the LISTSERV software confirming your subscription. Save this message, as it will provide you with important information, such as instructions on how to *unsubscribe* from the mailing list, as well as how to activate special features of some mailing lists, such as the digest feature and the vacation feature, which temporarily terminates the mail you receive from the LISTSERV. For more information on what a specific LISTSERV can do, send a message to it with the following text:

`help`

If you lose the instructions for unsubscribing from a mailing list, the following will usually do the trick:

Send a message to:

`listserv@uhupvm1.uh.edu`

With the text:

`unsubscribe pacs-l`

Again, you should receive a confirmation from the LISTSERV within minutes.

To send a posting to a LISTSERV, you should address it to the name of the LISTSERV, not its address. In other words, if you want to post to, for example, `pacs-l@uhupvm1.uh.edu`, send the message to:

`pacs-l@uhupvm1.uh.edu`

Or you can reply directly to a posting you received from that mailing list. Remember, your response goes directly to the whole list, not just the individual poster, so be careful of what you say.

USENET Newsgroups

Usenet *newsgroups* are similar to LISTSERVs and other mailing lists in terms of the content and tone of their postings. In fact, there are many more newsgroups (between five and ten thousand) than there are mailing lists. Their main difference is that Usenet doesn't deliver its postings as electronic mail messages. Instead, you log into Usenet using *newsreader* software and peruse the unread postings to the newsgroups you subscribe to. (Examples of newsreader packages are rn, trn, and Nuntius.) Just as with mailing lists, subscribing doesn't mean you pay for the information; it just means that the newsreader software you use knows which of those thousands of newsgroups you are interested in keeping up with.

Each Usenet newsgroup serves as a forum for discussion on a topic or sub-topic of collective interest. Like mailing lists, newsgroups may vary greatly in traffic; some are defunct, while others may disseminate hundreds of postings daily. Newsgroups are organized in a hierarchy; the top level of this hierarchy is shown below, and gives you a general sense of what broad categories Usenet newsgroups fit.

- `alt`   alternative
- `bit`   gatewayed BITNET mailing lists
- `biz`   business
- `comp`   computers
- `rec`   recreation
- `sci`   science
- `soc`   society
- `talk`   discussion

There are also other, less common top-level hierarchy names as well, including those related to specific nations (`can`, `aus`), institutions or organizations (`umich`, `ieee`), and technologies (`gnu`).

Parts of the hierarchy are used to name the groups; moving from left to right, the parts of the name indicate broader to narrower categories. Therefore, the newsgroup which discusses the Gopher information system software is called:

`comp.infosystems.gopher`

Some topics are so popular that they have spawned multiple newsgroups which discuss subtopics. Take, for example, the recreational activity of aviation:

```
rec.aviation
rec.aviation.announce
rec.aviation.answers
```

```
rec.aviation.homebuilt
rec.aviation.ifr
rec.aviation.military
rec.aviation.misc
rec.aviation.owning
rec.aviation.piloting
rec.aviation.products
rec.aviation.simulators
rec.aviation.soaring
rec.aviation.stories
rec.aviation.student
```

One of the best ways to use Usenet is as a source for the answers to especially tough questions. The following text is a real example of a question and its answer from `bit.listserv.buslib-l`, a newsgroup geared toward business librarians. Note the helpful and timely nature of the response.

Question:

```
bit.listserv.buslib-l #4686 (18 more)                                    [1]
Comments: Gated by NETNEWS@AUVM.AMERICAN.EDU                            -[1]
Approved-By: KANDERSO@UCS.INDIANA.EDU
Date: Thu Jul 28 15:25:13 EDT 1994
From: KANDERSO@ucs.indiana.edu
[1] electronics resources
Lines: 8

Can anyone recommend specific resources on electronics companies and the
overall industry?  I am looking for specialized items not the usual
industrial directories or D&B stuff.  I am trying to enhance our
international business collection into certain industry sectors, one of
which will be electronics.  Of special interest would be any publications
by international trade groups, etc.  I would the help on this.
K. Anderson
Indiana Center for Global Business
Indiana U. - Bloomington
End of article 4686 (of 4717) -- what next? [npq]
```

Response:

```
bit.listserv.buslib-l #4700 (17 more)                                    (1)
Comments: Gated by NETNEWS@AUVM.AMERICAN.EDU                            -[1]
Original_To: BITNET%"BUSLIB-L@IDBSU.BITNET"
Date: Fri Jul 29 12:15:00 EDT 1994
From: Dereck Brassington <BRASSING@VUVAXCOM.BITNET>
[1] Re: electronics resources
Lines: 9

One source I would recommend for industry information is the annual
_Electronic Market Data Book_ published by the Electronic Industries
Association (202-457-4900).  Most of the information covers the U.S.,
but there is a section on "International Electronics."  This section
provides brief profiles of U.S. electronics trade with a variety of
other countries.

Dereck Brassington
Villanova University
brassing@ucis.vill.edu
End of article 4700 (of 4717) -- what next? [npq]
```

Part II

Beyond This Book: Next Steps

The previous sections have discussed how to find and make use of the resources you'll find discussed in the guides in this book. As we said, though, we hope you will be interested in pursuing further development of new guides. Towards that end, we now will give you the fundamentals of searching for information using Internet tools (though don't forget the importance of people in groups such as mailing lists and Usenet newsgroups), followed by some tips on construction of guides and how to share them with the wider Internet community.

SEARCHING FOR INFORMATION

If you're accustomed to information searching tools of the kinds you find in libraries, you're in for a bit of a shock. Because the Internet is so decentralized and resources independently maintained, there are only very simple searching tools, as of now. They do work, and other than getting guidance from people in the know or stumbling on things by luck, they are the only ways of finding things. In each section here, we discuss the tools themselves and give some tips on searching them. Good luck!

Searching for Files to FTP: Archie

5

There are a number of Archie servers around the Net, and they index the filenames of files in many (but, significantly, not all) FTP archives. When you do an Archie search, you will get in response a list of archive addresses, pathnames and filenames which match the criteria you gave. You then must leave Archie, and FTP these files to your local system.

Archie servers and how to get into them

Here are the addresses of several Archie searchers:

archie.au	Australia
archie.funet.fi	Finland
archie.sogang.ac.kr	Korea
archie.nz	New Zealand
archie.luth.se	Sweden
archie.hensa.ac.uk	UK
archie.sura.net	US
archie.unl.edu	US
archie.ans.net	US
archie.rutgers.edu	US
ds.internic.net	US

It really doesn't matter which one you use, but if you try to use one and it doesn't work or seems to be going slowly, try another.

You begin the process by telnetting to an Archie site (login as `archie`):

```
% telnet archie.ans.net
Trying 147.225.1.10 ...
Connected to forum.ans.net.
Escape character is '^]'.

AIX telnet (forum.ans.net)

IBM AIX Version 3 for RISC System/6000
(C) Copyrights by IBM and by others 1982, 1991.
login: archie

# Bunyip Information Systems, 1993

# Terminal type set to 'vt100 24 80'.
# 'erase' character is '^?'.
# 'search' (type string) has the value 'exact'.
archie>
```

Searching

At the `archie>` prompt, you may begin the search or change the search parameters. The search command here is `prog`, and you follow it with what you want to find. Let's try a simple search first:

```
archie> prog clinton
# Search type: exact.
# Your queue position: 5
# Estimated time for completion: 01:01
working... \

Host etext.archive.umich.edu     (192.131.22.7)
Last updated 09:27 24 Feb 1994

     Location: /pub/CPSR
        DIRECTORY    drwxr-xr-x     1536 bytes  08:10  1 Nov 1993  clinton

     Location: /pub/CPSR/clinton/econplan
        DIRECTORY    drwxr-xr-x     1024 bytes  13:57 25 Oct 1993  clinton

     Location: /pub/CPSR/government_info
        DIRECTORY    drwxr-xr-x     1536 bytes  09:27 15 Nov 1993  clinton

     Location: /pub/CPSR/government_info/clinton/econplan
        DIRECTORY    drwxr-xr-x      512 bytes  09:45 15 Nov 1993  clinton

Host net.bio.net     (134.172.2.69)
Last updated 10:07 23 Feb 1994

     Location: /alt/politics
        DIRECTORY    drwxrwxr-x     6144 bytes  07:51 22 Feb 1994  clinton

     Location: /alt/president
        DIRECTORY    drwxrwxr-x     5120 bytes  07:06 22 Feb 1994  clinton

Host ftp.sunet.se     (130.238.127.3)
Last updated 13:10  3 Nov 1993

     Location: /pub/Internet-documents/sunet/sunetten/sunetten/sunetten92_6
        FILE     -r--r--r--      622 bytes  23:00 11 Jan 1993  clinton

     Location: /pub/Internet-documents/sunet/sunetten/sunetten/sunetten92_6/.cap
        FILE     -r--r--r--       42 bytes  23:00 11 Jan 1993  clinton
```

Let's see what each of the pieces of those results means:

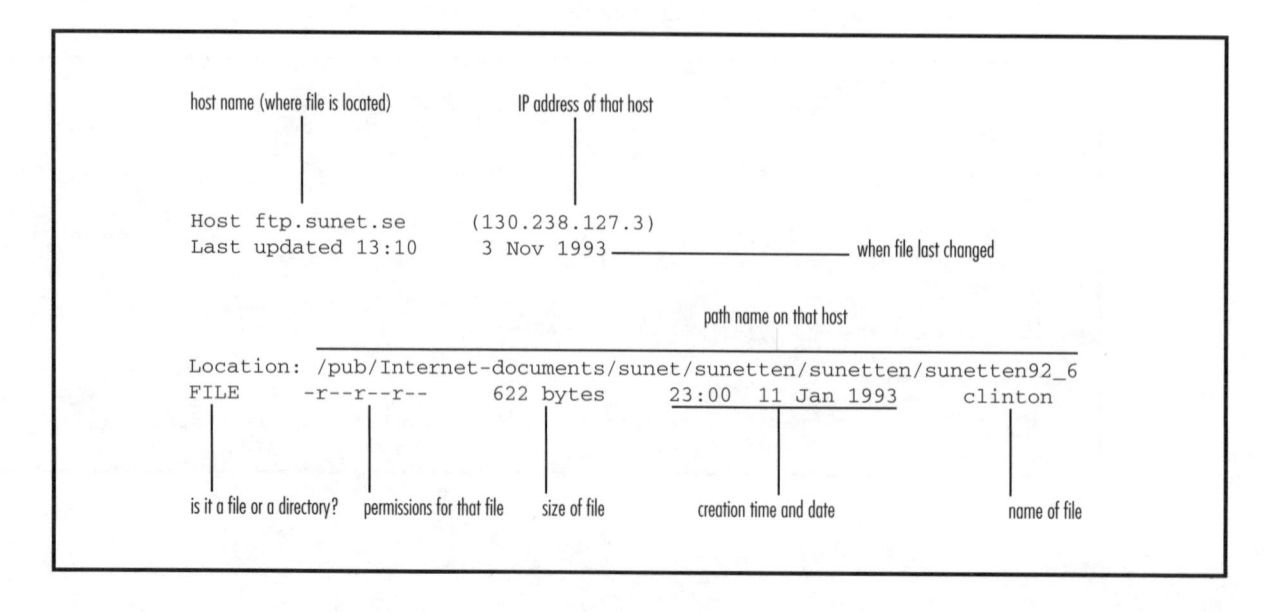

```
                host name (where file is located)        IP address of that host
                         |                                       |
                         |                                       |
                Host ftp.sunet.se          (130.238.127.3)
                Last updated 13:10          3 Nov 1993 ─────────── when file last changed

                                                  path name on that host
                                        ───────────────────────────────────────────────
                Location: /pub/Internet-documents/sunet/sunetten/sunetten/sunetten92_6
                FILE      -r--r--r--      622 bytes      23:00  11 Jan 1993      clinton
                  |            |              |                  |                  |
                  |            |              |                  |                  |
          is it a file or a directory?  permissions for that file   size of file   creation time and date   name of file
```

You see we found seven hits searching for the word "clinton". Well, that's all very fine and wonderful, but doesn't it seem that there should be more things than that out there? In fact, there are, and the results we got are a direct consequence of the way in which we searched and the nature of what we're able to search, both of which we'll discuss now.

What you get to search in Archie and why it's pretty poor

Not much. As we said, Archie "indexes" (and we use this term *very* loosely) the filenames of files in FTP archives. Well, if you've had any experience working with DOS or UNIX-based systems, you get an idea of what you're up against here. First of all, there is a very limited space available for these filenames—in most cases, only a very few characters are available, and most people don't use all of them. Second of all, people don't always give names to their files which are good indicators of content. Look at what we just got... what is a file named `clinton` likely to contain? It could be anything. Sometimes, the pathname (what follows `Location:` in the above examples) can give you a clue, but that's uncertain at best, and here they don't seem to be much help. Things are slowly getting better as people work out that cryptic filenames mean few if any accesses, but don't hold your breath.

Ways to search Archie: exact, substring, case sensitivity

You do have a bit of control over how the search is done. If you notice in the example above, it says that the search type was "exact;" that's the default method of searching in Archie, and it means that what you type must match *exactly* the filename or it won't be presented to you. You do have other options, though. You can ask for implicit truncation, that is, that you want to find any filename which contains the character string you ask for. In this case, a search for "clinton" would retrieve any file or directory which contains those seven characters in that order, but not those alone. You make this change by typing `set search sub` at the `archie>` prompt. This will make subsequent searches *substring* searches instead of exact searches.

Here's an example:

```
archie> set search sub
archie> prog clinton
# Search type: sub.
# Your queue position: 63
# Estimated time for completion: 75:31
working... /
```

I stopped this by hitting control-Z; you see the estimated time to complete the search was over 75 minutes! To change back to an exact search, type `set search exact` at the `archie>` prompt.

You can also ask for the search to be *case-sensitive*, which means that not only must characters match, but they must agree in terms of upper and lower case. In this situation, a search for `clinton` would match a file called `clinton` but not one called `Clinton` or `CLINTON`. It may seem that this makes an already restrictive search even worse, but there are situations in which this could come in quite handy, especially if you're searching for a known title and case is a part of it. The default, however, is a case-insensitive search, and that's usually the best way.

Getting the results mailed to you

If you get anything more than two or three retrievals from an Archie search, they have an annoying tendency to go flying off the top of the screen, which is fine if you can scroll back and see it, but that's not always the case. There is an alternative. The mail command will send a copy of the latest search to your email address. There are two ways you can do this:

1. If you only want to do this once or twice, just give the command at the prompt and the most recent search results will be sent to that email account.

```
archie>mail <email address>
```

2. If you will be doing a series of searches, you can give the following command which will set this as the address for all mailings.

```
archie>set mailto <email address>
```

After this, you can simply say the following and the results of the last search will be sent to the address you previously specified.

```
archie>mail
```

How to stop a search

If for any reason you want to stop an Archie search, type control-Z (hold the CONTROL or CTRL key down, and while holding it, hit Z).

Advice

How should you search Archie? With care and trepidation. With trepidation because this is such a poor way to search, but with care because it's the only game in town for searching FTP archives.

Come up with an initial strategy which you think will be productive but not overwhelming. If you get too many hits, try something more specific: a longer string, exact searching or even case sensitivity. If you get too few, broaden: try a smaller string or go to substring searching. Also keep in mind the environment in which you're working. There is always the possibility that what you're looking for isn't there, or that it has been given some completely unrecognizable name (`funstuff.exe` or some such thing) and you'll never find it.

Searching for Gopher Resources: Veronica

6

Veronica is very nice, and certainly helps enormously in finding things in gopherspace, but it's still a relatively unsophisticated searching mechanism. It has features Archie doesn't have (truncation and boolean searching) and is designed to search actual words and phrases rather than cryptic file names (which granted isn't Archie's fault but still is a pain in the neck), but it cannot do, for example, proximity or adjacency searching or anything more sophisticated than boolean. There is a simplistic form of field specification. And, like Archie, there's only just so much you can search. Veronica cannot search the texts or contents of resources available through Gopher; you are able only to search on menu titles.

Typically, you access Veronica through an "Other Gophers" menu choice. There are a number of Veronica sites throughout the world, so if one is busy, try another.

```
                Internet Gopher Information Client 2.0 p110

                       Search Gopherspace using Veronica

    -->  1.  How to compose veronica queries (from Nevada).
         2.  veronica server at NYSERNet <?>
         3.  veronica server at SUNET <?>
         4.  veronica server at U. of Manitoba <?>
         5.  veronica server at UNINETT/U. of Bergen <?>
         6.  Search Gopher Directory Titles at NYSERNet <?>
         7.  Search Gopher Directory Titles at SUNET <?>
         8.  Search Gopher Directory Titles at U. of Manitoba <?>
         9.  Search Gopher Directory Titles at UNINETT/U. of Bergen <?>
        10.  veronica FAQ (from Nevada).
```

When you choose one of these options, a box will open up asking for your query. Enter the words you want to search for here. You can use AND and OR, but don't get any more complicated than that; don't use parentheses or anything too complex. Veronica can be *very* slow at times, and a simple query will often be quicker. On the other hand, a single-word query may well get you hundreds of results after a several-minute search. So, once again, our advice is to search on the most specific word or words you think you can get away with, but no more. Searching here is not case-sensitive, so it doesn't matter whether you search with upper or lower case letters.

```
                Internet Gopher Information Client 2.0 p110

                       Search Gopherspace using Veronica

         1.  How to compose veronica queries (from Nevada).
    -->  2.  veronica server at NYSERNet <?>
         3.  veronica server at SUNET <?>
         4.  veronica server at U. of Manitoba <?>
         5.  veronica server at UNINETT/U. of Bergen <?>
         6.  Search Gopher Directory Titles at NYSERNet <?>
         7.  Search Gopher Directory Titles at SUNET <?>
         8.  Search Gopher Directory Titles at U. of Manitoba <?>
         9.  Search Gopher Directory Titles at UNINETT/U. of Bergen <?>
        10.  veronica FAQ (from Nevada).
```

```
+------------------------veronica server at NYSERNet------------------------+
|                                                                           |
| Words to search for                                                       |
|                                                                           |
|                                                                           |
|                                                                           |
|                 [Cancel: ^G] [Erase: ^U] [Accept: Enter]                  |
+---------------------------------------------------------------------------+
```

Here's an example of a search for materials on "entrepreneurship":

```
               Internet Gopher Information Client 2.0 pl10

             veronica server at UNINETT/U. of Bergen: entrepreneurship

 --> 1.  JBR Special Issue on Entrepreneurship.
     2.  Educating for entrepreneurship in outdoor recreation. .
     3.  Educating for entrepreneurship in outdoor recreation. .
     4.  Entrepreneurship, Creativity and Organization(BUS)(1518).
     5.  Entrepreneurship in Imperial Russia and the Soviet Union. G. Gurof...
     6.   Israel M. Kirzner, COMPETITION AND ENTREPRENEURSHIP.
     7.  COMM 468     ENTREPRENEURSHIP          M W    1400 1515.
     8.  Creation of a Technological Entrepreneurship Data Base.
     9.  Entrepreneurship (ENT).
     10. Entrepreneurship (ENT).
     11. AGEC 3454 SMALL BUSINESS MANAGEMENT AND ENTREPRENEURSHIP.
     12. MGT 3454 SMALL BUSINESS MANAGEMENT AND ENTREPRENEURSHIP.
     13. AGEC 3454 : SMALL BUSINESS MANAGEMENT AND ENTREPRENEURSHIP.
     14. MGT 3454 : SMALL BUSINESS MANAGEMENT AND ENTREPRENEURSHIP.
     15. badm346 entrepreneurship: small business formation..
     16. badm346 entrepreneurship: small business formation..
     17. badm346 entrepreneurship: small business formation..
     18. Center for Entrepreneurship and New Venture Management.
     19. ENTREPRENEURSHIP.
     20. 92590 Entrepreneurship and Business development.
     21. 92590 Entrepreneurship and Business development.
     22. (1153) 2420:227-001   ENTREPRENEURSHIP PROJ.
     23. Group= sbmanent  ( Management and Entrepreneurship ).
     24. Entrepreneurship Programs/
     25. Management and Entrepreneurship Department/
     26. SBC Network & Entrepreneurship in Kenya.
     27. Small Business Entrepreneurship (QUT)/
     28. ADM5010 L'entrepreneurship dans les industries technologiques.
     29. EDU8005 Education ' l'entrepreneurship.
     30. CORNELL TO CELEBRATE ENTREPRENEURSHIP APRIL...   (03/26/93).
```

You can add *truncation* to your searches in Veronica; the truncation operator is the asterisk *.

```
               Internet Gopher Information Client 2.0 pl10

                     Search Gopherspace using Veronica

     1.  How to compose veronica queries (from Nevada).
     2.  veronica server at NYSERNet <?>
     3.  veronica server at SUNET <?>
     4.  veronica server at U. of Manitoba <?>
 --> 5.  veronica server at UNINETT/U. of Bergen <?>
     6.  Search Gopher Directory Titles at NYSERNet <?>
     7.  Search Gopher Directory Titles at SUNET <?>
     8.  Search Gopher Directory Titles at U. of Manitoba <?>
     9.  Search Gopher Directory Titles at UNINETT/U. of Bergen <?>
     10. veronica FAQ (from Nevada).



+-------------------veronica server at UNINETT/U. of Bergen-----------------+
|                                                                           |
| Words to search for                                                       |
|                                                                           |
|  entrepreneur* not entrepreneurship                                       |
|                                                                           |
|                 [Cancel: ^G] [Erase: ^U] [Accept: Enter]                  |
+---------------------------------------------------------------------------+
```

```
           Internet Gopher Information Client 2.0 pl10

 veronica server at UNINETT/U. of Bergen: entrepreneur* not entrepreneurship

 -->  1.  Entrepreneurial Studies - Evening.
      2.  TEIC - TECHNION ENTREPRENEURIAL INCUBATOR CO. LTD.
      3.  Search Centre for the Development of Entrepreneurs <?>
      4.  Resource managers as policy entrepreneurs: Governance challenges .
      5.  ENTREPRENEURIAL STUDIES.
      6.  136.* Business Strategy and  Entrepreneurial Studies. .
      7.  Entrepreneur Program.
      8.  [Entrepreneurs: An American Adventure] Expanding America.
      9.  Entrepreneur hopes to save Garden State racetrack.
     10.  U.S. pledges $50 million for Romanian entrepreneurs.
     11.  Centre for the Development of Entrepreneurs (organizationalUnit)/
     12.  Page 3, Local firm sets up entrepreneur school.
     13.  Entrepreneur Information.
     14.  Centre for the Development of Entrepreneurs (organizationalUnit)/
     15.  Centre for the Development of Entrepreneurs (organizationalUnit)/
     16.  Entrepreneur's Exit Decisions: The Role of Threshold.
     17.  Entrepreneurs Contest Planned.
     18.  <INVENT> Inventors and entrepreneurs can get help in marketi.
     19.  Entrepreneurs in hardwoods: A study of small business strategies..
     20.       Softpub - Software Entrepreneur's Mailing List.
     21.  Female entrepreneurs focus on service businesses.
     22.  Entrepreneurial Studies/
     23.  Read Centre for the Development of Entrepreneurs entry.
     24.  Centre for the Development of Entrepreneurs (organizationalUnit)/
     25.  BECOMING AN INDEPENDENT ENTREPRENEUR IN THE INFORMAL SECTOR OF NOR...
     26.  Centre for the Development of Entrepreneurs (organizationalUnit)/
     27.  Search Centre for the Development of Entrepreneurs <?>
     28.  badm347 legal strategies for the entrepreneurial firm..
     29.  Corporate grocery impressario goes entrepreneurial.
     30.  Read Centre for the Development of Entrepreneurs entry.

 Press ? for Help, q to Quit, u to go up a menu              Page: 1/7
```

Another nice thing about Veronica is that, since the search is being executed from within Gopher, the results come to you as a menu of choices, as you see in a "regular" Gopher session, and you can pick and choose from them directly, and, most importantly, see them right then and there. You don't have to leave Veronica, and then enter Gopher. Again, this is different from the Archie/FTP situation, because these (Veronica and Gopher) are newer technologies, designed ever so slightly with the user in mind. Progress of a sort, you must admit.

For further information, see the Veronica FAQ compiled at the University of Nevada. It's available at the Veronica screen in most Gophers. We strongly suggest you get a copy of this because it's the best available documentation for Veronica.

WAIS

WAIS stands for Wide Area Information Servers. It is intended to be an easy-to-use, general-purpose retrieval mechanism for networked information resources. The basic structure of WAIS takes advantage of the client-server architecture underlying the Internet: people and organizations make resources available on various servers around the world. They are able to be searched remotely, via clients which have been freely and widely distributed. (For a resource to be searched this way, it must be appropriately prepared; this process is often called "WAISifying".) There are many hundreds of WAIS *sources*, and they cover a great number of subject areas; however, due to its distributed nature, there is no real consistency between resources nor a sense of completeness of coverage. In addition, as with the rest of the Net, the individual resources are only as good as the people who maintain them.

WAIS can be used for searching in one of two ways: a machine with a direct connection to the Internet can have WAIS client software loaded on it (WAISStation, for example), and search directly. Other machines without such a configuration can telnet to a public WAIS client; the best known of these is located at Thinking Machines, Inc., the company which housed early WAIS development efforts. The telnet address is `quake.think.com`; login as `wais`, and follow the directions provided to begin a search.

How to search using WAIS

Because there are many hundreds of WAIS sources, it is likely that a user will not know particular resources to search. (Those who do, of course, could proceed directly to such a search). Most WAIS clients provide an alphabetical list of available resources; these brief titles may be enough of an indication of content to provide a starting point.

```
SWAIS                           Source Selection                  Sources: 663
   #           Server                     Source                      Cost
 397:  [      munin.ub2.lu.se]  lolita-dator                          Free
 398:  [      munin.ub2.lu.se]  lolita-miljo                          Free
 399:  [        gopher.uwo.ca]  london-free-press-regional-inde       Free
 400:  [        zenon.inria.fr] lp-bibtex-zenon-inria-fr              Free
 401:  [       wais.fct.unl.pt] lp-proceedings                        Free
 402:  [       wais.ub2.lu.se]  Lund_University_thesis                Free
 403:  [             cs.uwp.edu] lyrics                               Free
 404:  [    next2.oit.unc.edu]  mac.FAQ                               Free
 405:  [  cmns-moon.think.com]  macintosh-news                        Free
 406:  [  cmns-moon.think.com]  macintosh-tidbits                     Free
 407:  [     gopher.stolaf.edu] MacPsych                              Free
 408:  [          wais.cic.net] mailing-lists                         Free
 409:  [           ftp.tic.com] matrix_news                           Free
 410:  [          nic.sura.net] matsci                                Free
 411:  [       wais.ub2.lu.se]  Medicine_Books_Lund_Pre1800           Free
 412:  [         nic.merit.edu] merit-archive-mac                     Free
 413:  [         nic.merit.edu] merit-nsfnet-linkletter               Free
 414:  [        zenon.inria.fr] meval-bibtex-zenon-inria-fr           Free

Keywords:

<space> selects, w for keywords, arrows move, <return> searches, q quits, or ?
```

In many instances, though, this may not be enough. There is a resource called the *Directory of Servers* which serves as a catalog of sorts of the available resources. It is not like a library catalog; rather, it is a list of descriptions of the sources, often provided by the maintainers. These descriptions will vary in length, quality, depth, vocabulary, and so on. They will generally be at a broader conceptual level, but some may be quite specific. Our advice is to search the *Directory of Servers* using the broadest concepts and terms which still are meaningful to you. For example, if you were searching for resources dealing with the *Iliad* and the *Odyssey*, you might search for "epic poetry" or "classical literature" or even "literature" in the *Directory of Servers*. After identifying potentially good resources, then you might search for the more specific terms in the sources themselves.

Here's an example:

```
SWAIS                          Source Selection              Sources: 663
   #            Server                   Source                     Cost
217:    [     munin.ub2.lu.se] cwis_list                            Free
218:    [      ds.internic.net] ddbs-info                           Free
219:    [          inet.ed.gov] Department-of-Education-Program     Free
220:    [      wais.digital.com] Digital-All                        Free
221:    [      wais.digital.com] Digital-Customer-Update            Free
222:    [      wais.digital.com] Digital-DTJ                        Free
223:    [      wais.digital.com] Digital-SOC                        Free
224:    [      wais.digital.com] Digital-SPD                        Free
225:    [cicg-communication.g] directory-grenet-fr                  Free
226:    [          irit.irit.fr] directory-irit-fr                  Free
227:  * [      quake.think.com] directory-of-servers                Free
228:    [        zenon.inria.fr] directory-zenon-inria-fr           Free
229:    [        zenon.inria.fr] disco-mm-zenon-inria-fr            Free
230:    [          wais.cic.net] disi-catalog                       Free
231:    [      munin.ub2.lu.se] dit-library                         Free
232:    [          doccenter.com] document_center_catalog           Free
233:    [          doccenter.com] document_center_inventory         Free
234:    [      dewey.tis.inel.gov] DOE-Interpretations-Guide        Free

Keywords: epic poetry poem poems

Searching: directory-of-servers
```

These are the sources WAIS retrieves in response to that initial query.

```
  #    Score      Source                 Title                    Lines
001:  [1000] (directory-of-se)  POETRY-index                        28
002:  [ 765] (directory-of-se)  poetry                              18
003:  [ 353] (directory-of-se)  ANU-Cheng-Tao-Ko-Verses             99
004:  [ 353] (directory-of-se)  ANU-Philippine-Studies              92
005:  [ 176] (directory-of-se)  ANU-Buddha-L                        80
006:  [ 176] (directory-of-se)  ANU-Dhammapada-Verses               91
```

The first two look quite promising (POETRY-index and poetry), so we search those using a much more specific set of keywords:

```
SWAIS                          Source Selection              Sources: 663
   #            Server                   Source                     Cost
469:    [   dewey.tis.inel.gov] OSHA-Standards                      Free
470:    [   dewey.tis.inel.gov] OSHA-Tech-Manual                    Free
471:    [pet1.austin.unimelb.]  oz-postcodes                        Free
472:    [ cmns-moon.think.com]  patent-sampler                      Free
473:    [        town.hall.org] patent                              Free
474:    [             calypso]  pc-sounds                           Free
475:    [stardust.jpl.nasa.go] PDS-Data-Prep-Workbook               Free
476:    [stardust.jpl.nasa.go] PDS_catalog                          Free
477:    [stardust.jpl.nasa.go] PDS_labels                           Free
478:    [stardust.jpl.nasa.go] PDS_standards                        Free
479:    [stardust.jpl.nasa.go] PDS_templates                        Free
480:    [     wais.ece.uiuc.edu] pegasus-mail-disc                  Free
481:  * [      sunsite.unc.edu] POETRY-index                        Free
482:  * [microworld.media.mit]  poetry                              Free
483:    [     wais.concert.net] posix.1003.2                        Free
484:    [  enslapp.ens-lyon.fr] Preprints-alg-geom                  Free
485:    [  enslapp.ens-lyon.fr] Preprints-cond-mat                  Free
486:    [  enslapp.ens-lyon.fr] Preprints-gr-qc                     Free

Keywords: iliad odyssey

Searching: poetry
```

```
SWAIS                           Search Results                  Items:    6
   #     Score      Source                 Title                          Lines
 001:    [1000] (          POETRY) The Odyssey          Andrew Lang     A    21
 002:    [1000] (    POETRY-index) William Logan - Volume 151   October 19   19
 003:    [1000] (    POETRY-index) Christpher Logue - Volume 160    April-S   4
 004:    [ 375] (          POETRY) Development          Robert Browning     128
 005:    [ 312] (          POETRY) Rain          Nicolas Guillen (translated 20
 006:    [ 312] (          POETRY) Battle-Scene            Sylvia Plath     48
```

Our results are less than stellar: the first document is a poem called "The Odyssey;" the second and third are articles about the Odyssey; the others are poems which mention Homer's *Odyssey* (we discover from this that the POETRY source here is full texts of poems).

```
SWAIS                         Document Display              Page:   1
Christpher Logue - Volume 160    April-September 1992 Page 157
       Kings:  An Account of Books 1 and 2 of Homer's Iliad
       (Review by William Logan)
```

WAIS can accept natural language searches (that is, you can type just about anything you want at it, and you'll get something back). However, the mechanism it uses to score and rank what it finds (see the "Score" column in the previous search) is not entirely clear, so you should use some caution in selecting words to search—not too many, not too specific, not too broad. The scores can be helpful in some situations, but you should not under any circumstances take this as anything other than gross indicators of how related something is to what you searched for.

WAIS is certainly a useful tool in some circumstances, but it is not yet (if it ever will be) a general-purpose information seeking tool. There are a lot of things available, but many more things aren't. It doesn't cover Gopher resources, FTPable resources, things available via the Web, etc. For these tools, you should use Veronica, Archie, and Web searching tools.

WAIS does have some advantages: it is the only Net searching mechanism (as of this writing) which permits searching of the full text of resources, as opposed to FTP file names, Gopher menu titles, and HTML headers. It will accept keyword searches (but there's no way to do boolean AND/OR/NOT searching), and the ranking can often be useful. Our best advice: it's probably worth a try, but don't be disappointed if you come up dry.

Putting it all Together: Building your own Subject-Oriented Guide 8

As you use the guides in this book, you might find that the guide to your subject area of interest just isn't as comprehensive as you'd like. Or maybe it reflects the author's bias too strongly. Perhaps there simply is no guide for your subject.

Whatever the case may be, you might decide to create your own subject-oriented Internet resource guide. Creating a meaningful information "product" is challenging, and your successful pioneering effort will benefit the greater community in many ways:

- your guide's users will be spared the frustration of going down the same blind alleys that you encountered in your search,
- writing a guide is a useful way to hone your Internet information searching skills,
- guides serve as useful "blueprints" for those building topical Gopher servers and World Wide Web documents,
- guides are useful as sources of content and examples for Internet workshops geared toward specific audiences (e.g., paralegals, a chemistry faculty, etc.), and
- most importantly, consider the fame and fortune writing a guide will bring you.

The following "12 step program" is the core of what we teach our students at the School of Information and Library Studies at the University of Michigan. These guidelines are quite general. Your experience may be different due to such variables as subject, audience, and the quantity, quality, and format of your subject's information resources.

1. determine your subject and audience

This step may seem obvious and is easy to take for granted, but the small amount of time you invest at this point will pay great dividends over the course of the guide building process. Information searching is by nature an iterative process, and the subject itself may be a moving target. It is preferable to avoid changing course in midstream; otherwise, you may need to repeat time-consuming steps in the search process.

You can alleviate the possibility of changing your focus by planning for it ahead of time. You can do this by determining and searching for interesting narrower and broader subjects related to your own. For example, if your intended subject is the U.S. space program, you might keep an eye open for items specific to the shuttle program or to the proposed space station. You might also be prepared to broaden your search to include the space exploration programs of other countries. In all cases, maintain a list of relevant keywords that can be used for searching.

It is also a good idea to determine who your audience is and what their specific requirements and restrictions are. For example, are they novices, or are they subject experts themselves? What levels of Internet access and skills do they possess? For example, if they cannot use NCSA Mosaic, you may not want to devote much time identifying and describing image, audio, and video files that cannot be displayed with less powerful tools.

2. determine what you already know

Record your current knowledge of the Internet's resources relevant to your subject in a single document. This document can serve as the starting point for your search. Ask yourself what you already know about each resource. How did you learn about it? Who maintains it? Is it valuable or not, and why? The answers will help you determine where else to look, whom to ask for assistance, and what characteristics to look for when evaluating a resource.

3. do a brief search

When you eventually ask other Internet citizens for assistance, you'll want to show that you are familiar with the best-known Internet resources in order to demonstrate that you're serious and at least somewhat facile with using the Internet. A brief search can also give you an initial sense of how much is out there on your subject; you may find this moment a good time to adjust the broadness or narrowness of your search.

At this point, you don't need to be an expert Internet searcher; using such basic Internet searching tools as Veronica and JumpStation is sufficient. A "quick and dirty" search will result in some of the more popular (and obvious) resources of interest. Also, check the Clearinghouse for Subject-Oriented Internet Resource Guides (described below) and other sources to see if anyone has already created a guide to your subject. If one already exists, don't give up; multiple "views" on the subject are useful, and yours may even complement the existing guide.

4. identify knowledgeable people, and ask them for help

Not everyone can be an expert, so consider finding some true subject specialists and enlisting their help. You might ask members of a professional association's local chapter, or faculty or librarians from a nearby college if they'd agree to help you evaluate the relevance and quality of the information you find on the Internet. They don't need to know much if anything about the Internet, as you'll be the expert in that area.

As stated previously, the most useful sources of information on the Internet itself are people. No information retrieval tool can approximate the knowledge stored in a community of interested users. Use the means of identifying relevant LISTSERVs and Usenet newsgroups described earlier to find electronic communities who might be willing to help you.

Before asking for assistance, "keep your ear to the ground." Don't intrude on the discourse of the community until you get a sense of what they are about. You may find, after a few days, that the discussion of a newsgroup which sounded especially promising turns out to be sophomoric flaming, or just plain defunct.

Once you feel comfortable with a few relevant communities, send them a message which briefly describes: 1) who you are; 2) what kind of information you are looking for; 3) where you have already looked; and 4) what you already know (this can be a short listing of resources identified in steps 2 and 3 above). If there is already a guide to your subject, state diplomatically why you feel another one would be useful. And perhaps most importantly, be sure to state that you will make the results of your search available to the Internet.

You may find that most of the responses are simply notes of encouragement, rather than descriptions of resources. However, in the face of this daunting task, you may need all the encouragement you can get. Remember that you may not receive responses immediately. As your message is forwarded around the Internet over the next few days or weeks, an awareness of your project will grow, and responses will trickle in from what may be some unexpected places.

5. use the tools you know best, then use the rest

As you learn about relevant resources from folks around the Internet, you should also make an effort to become very familiar with the Internet's information tools. This is the best time to learn the intricacies of Archie searching, or which Veronica servers are the least crowded. You quickly will find that certain tools are more useful than others for one or many reasons: better interfaces, faster response time, and higher quality retrievals. Concentrate your searching on those tools that work best for you, and spend less time on the others. Don't get bogged down in a wrestling match in an attempt to get one specific tool to work; you can always come back to it.

6. keep a journal of your travels

As you begin to identify Internet resources, you will want to take notes on how you reached them (e.g., the resource's URL, a Gopher server address and path) as well as any related conditions, such as time of day it was most accessible, etc. Your notes will prove invaluable when you come back to the resource in a week or a month to do a more detailed evaluation.

7. choose an appropriate categorization scheme

Whether you identify five or five hundred resources, your guide should have a logical organization that makes it easy for users to find the information they need. Traditionally, resources were categorized by tool; for example, a guide would have a section on LISTSERVs, another on FTP archives, and so on. This may have been appropriate in the days when there simply weren't many resources relevant to a specific subject. However, today there are so many resources relevant to most topics that the tool-based organization approach leaves a lot to be desired. Users of a guide to biology are likely more interested in a sub-topic, such a molecular biology, rather than a list of biology-related Gopher servers.

For this reason, we suggest you organize your guide by some scheme other than tool-based categories. Consider your subject, the volume of resources identified, and how your audience is most likely to use the information. Then choose from one of the following approaches: subject-based, geographical, or chronological. Or you might organize your guide into sections which range from most to least relevant. The most relevant resources would have more detailed descriptions, and vice versa.

You might want to record each resource you identify on a separate piece of paper, or better yet, a 3" x 5" card. When you come to the point of categorizing and organizing your resources, you might find it especially effective to spread your 3" x 5" cards on a table and group and order them in different ways until you find a logical scheme.

8. know what you're looking for with each resource

After you've identified a set of resources and chosen an organizational scheme, you'll want to go back to the resources you've chosen and begin to evaluate them. The evaluation process is important because it's no longer sufficient to simply identify what's out there of relevance to a subject. Users want to know what's actually valuable among those resources. For example, users don't want to go through the trouble of subscribing to a LISTSERV to find out that its traffic is overwhelming, or its discussion is irritating. Providing this kind of information ahead of time is what will make your guide especially useful.

When you are evaluating an Internet resource, assemble two types of information: descriptive and qualitative. Descriptive information includes: name of resource, address/location, maintainer's or contact's name and address, tool (e.g., HTML document, WAIS source), format (text, Postscript file), start date, update frequency, intended audience, and, in the case of mailing lists and Usenet newsgroups, average traffic volume. It obviously won't be possible to obtain this information for each resource, and, depending on the type of resource, you'll want to find different types of descriptive information.

The qualitative information you gather will require you to actually use or participate in the resources you've identified. Consider such issues as whether the resource functions regularly and dependably, is its source authoritative, is the information itself comprehensive and current. In the case of mailing lists and newsgroups, evaluate the resource's level of discussion: is it scholarly, friendly; do questions get answered; do discussions or announcements predominate? Although this may appear to be a lot of information to search for, remember that you likely won't be able to find it all. Including the descriptive and qualitative components, your resource descriptions may be only a paragraph or two long. And certainly, look in the Clearing house for Subject-Oriented Internet Resource Guides for examples of how other authors have evaluated their resources.

9. keep your community informed

During the guide-building process, you should maintain a presence in the communities of advisors and potential users you established contact with in step No. 4. Posting a periodic update which includes names of the resources you have found to date shows those communities that you're serious about your work and reminds them to let you know when they stumble across a relevant resource.

10. making your guide more usable: adding meta-information

At some point which is entirely up to you, you'll decide to stop the process of identifying, organizing, and evaluating resources. This may be due to a deadline you've imposed, or perhaps you are simply satisfied with the comprehensiveness of your work.

Unfortunately, you're not out of the woods. The best Internet guides include *meta-information* that describes the content of your guide and process of what you did. Meta-information should include:

- *information about you:* your name, your organizational affiliation, addresses, and other contact information
- *the purpose of your guide:* why you created it, the intended audience, and planned update frequency
- *what was involved in creating your guide:* which Internet tools were most useful, what keywords were used, the time period during which the information gathered, and a list of cited and related works
- *aids for using your guide:* a key to the resource descriptions, a table of contents, indices organized by tool and by other categorization schemes that might be useful
- *miscellaneous information:* disclaimers, acknowledgements, pointers to useful Internet books, and copyright statements

11. announce publication to your user communities

When version 1.0 of your guide is ready, you owe it to the people on the Internet who have helped you to let them know your guide is ready for release. You might send them the file directly as an electronic mail message. You also might make it available from an Internet site such as the Clearinghouse for Subject-Oriented Internet Resource guides (as described below), and simply send out an announcement to relevant mailing lists and newsgroups which includes access instructions for your guide.

12. update, update, update

You will soon find yourself recognized as *the* expert on your subject's Internet information resources. Questions will roll in, ranging from such requests as "How do I use FTP?" to "Would you be willing to present/teach a workshop/publish an article . . . ?".

Most of all, you'll receive many suggestions for modifications, corrections, and the inclusion of additional resources in your guide. This may seem frustrating, given the amount of work you've done just to complete the first version of your guide, but the Internet changes too quickly for any guide to be comprehensive. Guides are simply "snapshots" of what's out there at a particular moment; continuing the process of resource discovery, organization, and evaluation is the only way your guide will remain current.

The Clearinghouse for Subject-Oriented Internet Resource Guides   9

At the University of Michigan, the University Library and the School of Information and Library Studies have jointly created the Clearinghouse for Subject-Oriented Internet Resource Guides. The goals of the Clearinghouse are to:

- serve as a central location for subject-oriented Internet guides
- publicize the availability of these guides
- encourage the creation of additional guides

In order to reach the widest public, the most popular Internet tools are used to provide access, including anonymous FTP, Gopher, and WWW/Mosaic. The guides are also WAIS-indexed for full text searching. No profit is involved, and all work is voluntary.

The Clearinghouse may be especially useful to you as a general user of Internet information, as it provides the most up-to-date versions of the guides in this book, as well as many others. If you decide to author a guide, you can submit it for inclusion in the Clearinghouse. It will then have a stable home which you can publicize to your user communities. The Clearinghouse also provides guide authors with plenty of examples and models for guide building.

From the time of the Clearinghouse's inception in September, 1993, its collection of guides has grown from about 20 to about 140 in July, 1994. Over that period, the number of guide accesses has climbed from 7000 to almost 70,000. Some simple math indicates that, because each guide is used about 500 times per month, there must be some need for these efforts. For this reason, we highly encourage you to consider creating and submitting a guide for whatever subject interests you.

How To Access Guides From The Clearinghouse

Access to these guides is available via Anonymous FTP, Gopher, and World Wide Web browser such as Mosaic. Instructions are provided below. A searchable WAIS index of the full text of these guides is available via Gopher and World Wide Web.

using anonymous FTP:

host: `una.hh.lib.umich.edu`
path: `/inetdirsstacks`
(a key to the file names is available from the FTPable file `.README-FOR-FTP`)

using Gopher:

From the University of Minnesota's list of All Gophers, follow this menu progression:

```
=>>North America
 =>>USA
  =>>Michigan
   =>>Clearinghouse for Subject-Oriented Internet...
```

Or you can Gopher directly to:

```
gopher.lib.umich.edu
  =>>What's New and Featured Resources
   =>>Clearinghouse for Subject-Oriented Internet...
```

using World Wide Web:

Use one of these Uniform Resource Locators (URL):

```
http://http2.sils.umich.edu/~lou/chhome.html
http://www.lib.umich.edu/chhome.html
gopher://una.hh.lib.umich.edu/11/inetdirs
```

How To Submit Your Guide For Inclusion In The Clearinghouse

You can send your subject-oriented Internet resource guide directly to the following, or make it available via anonymous FTP and then notify that same address, so the Clearinghouse' administrators can download it.:

```
i-guides@umich.edu
```

Please handle updates in the same way.

There are no set requirements for what is included in the Clearinghouse, but the administrators do reserve the right to reject certain guides. Following are some recommendations that will improve your guide and its chances of inclusion in the Clearinghouse.

Highly recommended:

- Your guide should be subject-oriented. It should not be a list of all the library Gophers or WAIS sources that exist, but should instead try to at least sample various kinds of resources pertinent to a specific subject, e.g., interface design or classical studies.

- Please make it available (via e-mail or FTP) in the lowest common denominator format, i.e., plain ASCII text, no more than 60 characters wide. This will allow your guide to be made available to the broadest audience. In addition, HTML versions of your guide can now be pointed to from the Clearinghouse; just send the URL to the Clearinghouse address.

Also recommended:

- Please let the Clearinghouse know when you update your guide, or better yet, send the updates directly. The importance of currency can not be overemphasized.

- Using the template below, please attach the following descriptive information to your guide, preferably in the form of a header in the body of your text:

```
title:
version/edition:
update frequency:
date:
author/contact name:
author/contact e-mail address:
institution:
descriptive keywords:
intended audience:
```

- Consider contacting the listowners of relevant mailing lists and moderated newsgroups before including references to their lists in your guide. Many are concerned with the disruptions their communities may experience when exposed to increased publicity and new members.

Part III

Subject-Oriented Guides

Aerospace Engineering: A Guide To Internet Resources

10

David Dalquist and Christopher Poterala
School of Information and Library Studies
The University of Michigan, Fall, 1993

Permission to use, copy, and distribute this document in whole or in part for non-commercial purposes and without fee is hereby granted provided that this permission notice and appropriate credit to this document's authors be included in all copies. Commercial use of this document requires prior written consent from its authors. The authors assume no responsibilty for errors or omissions, or for the results of using the information contained herein.

TABLE OF CONTENTS

Index
Introduction
How to Use This Guide

FTP

Elroy	Jet Propulsion Lab anonymous FTP archives
Explorer	Ames Research Center anonymous FTP archives
Goddard-1	Goddard Space Flight Center FTP Archive
Goddard-2	Goddard Space Flight Center FTP Archive
Langley-FTP	NASA Langley Technical Reports
NSSDCA	National Space Science Data Center MultiNet Server

GOPHER

ARC	Ames Research Center gopher
GSFC-1	Climate and Radiation Server
GSFC-2	Goddard Space Flight Center (GSFC) gopher
GSFC-3	Allows you to search the GSFC gopher
GSFC-4	High Energy Astrophysics Science Archival Research Center (HEASARC)
GSFC-5	High Energy Astrophysics Science Archival Research Center (HEASARC)
GSFC-6	MU-SPIN (Minority Universities) Program
GSFC-7	NASA Shuttle Small Payloads Project
HQ	Office of Life and Microgravity Sciences and Applications
JSC	NASA/JSC Engineering Computational Facility
LARC	Langley Research Center (LaRC)
LERC	Lewis Research Center Gopher (LeRC)
NAIC	NASA Networked Applications and Information Center
STI	NASA Scientific and Technical Information (STI) gopher
Toronto	The University of Toronto Gopher USENET FAQs
Tech-Com	Mid-Continent Technology Transfer Center
SEDS	Students for the Exploration & Development of Space (SEDS) gopher
Brown	Brown Univ. gopher

Harvard	Harvard-Smithsonian Center for Astrophysics
NCSU	North Carolina State University Library gopher
Rice	The Rice University gopher
STSCI	Space Telescope Electronic Information System (STEIS)
Chicago	University of Chicago gopher
Omaha	The University of Nebraska at Omaha gopher
COSMIC	COmputer Software Management and Information Center (COSMIC)
HPCC	HPCC Case Studies
LOC	Library of Congress gopher
PATH-NET	Path-Net gopher

LISTSERV

AEFlow	Defunct
Aeronautics	Moderated version of the sci.aeronautics newsgroup
AIAA	American Institute of Aeronautics and Astronautics
Aircraft	Defunct
AV-Theory	Defunct
Aviation	Defunct
Space-Investors	List for the business side of aerospace

OPACs

Brief explanation, but no sites listed.

TELNET

NODIS	NODIS database
NAIC-TEL	NASA Network Applications and Information Center(NAIC)
COSLINE	COSMIC Online Information Services
Kansas	WWW site accessed via TELNET
NASANews	NASA Headquarters Daily News Brief
ESA	Data Dissemination Network of the European Space Agency

USENET Newsgroups

rec.aviation.answers	Newsgroup for questions and answers about the rec.aviation hierarchy
rec.aviation.military	Discussions about military aircraft
rec.aviation.misc	General aviation topics
rec.aviation.student	Learning to fly? Here's the place
sci.aeronautics	Mirrors the Aeronautics mailing list

WWW (World Wide Web)

Dryden	NASA Dryden Flight Research Facility
Goddard-WWW	NASA/Goddard Space Flight Center
Johnson	NASA Johnson Space Center
Kennedy	NASA Kennedy Space Center WWW Server
LaRC-WWW	Langley Research Center
NASA-HQ	NASA Information from Washington, DC
NASA-Info	NASA Information by Subject
WWW	NASA World Wide Web Home Page

GENERAL INFORMATION

Introduction

This is a guide to Internet resources that contains information pertaining to aerospace engineering. Our original intent was to cover the area of aerospace engineering as applied to lower atmospheric flight. Because of the nature of the subject area and the available resources, we found it difficult to narrow the sites down to specific subject areas. As the guide evolved, we necessarily found ourselves including sites with a broader scope of information going beyond aerospace engineering, e.g., there are easily as many sites that deal with astronomy. The guide is by no means comprehensive and exhaustive (except to us); there are sites that we have not included or are not aware of, and we welcome suggestions as to changes that should be made.

We provide additional information about who, what, where, when, why, and how at the end of this document.

Chris & Dave

How To Use This Guide

Organization

The organization of the guide revolves around the main types of access and navigation tools currently available on the Internet, i.e., FTP, GOPHER, LISTSERV, USENET, WAIS, and WWW. Within these groups, the sources are ordered alphabetically by the name of the organization. A short field-oriented identifier begins the description of each source. This identifier provides enough information for the user to quickly judge what the source is and how to access it. The identifier contains the information as shown below:

NAM: NAMe
ORG: ORGanization responsible for resource
URL: `resource://internet.address/directory/subdir/file.name`

"NA" means "Not Applicable." The indentifier may be followed by textual information that provides additional information about the resource, such as additional resource descriptions and quotes from a resource's introductory screens.

Quotations

Where possible, we have quoted information directly from the sources to avoid possibly distorting information through translation. Quotation marks identify this information.

Keyboard Commands

Specific keys to be pressed are enclosed in brackets—for example, <Esc>. Information to be typed is enclosed in brackets and quotation marks—for example, <"opac">.

FTP

Elroy

NAM: Jet Propulsion Lab anonymous FTP archives
ORG: NASA/JPL
URL: `ftp://elroy.jpl.nasa.gov`

Small site; SUN workstation help; contains the following directories:

```
SDC
eric
jpl
jpl.vicar
newsclient
plato
sendmail
sun.tuning
```

Explorer

NAM: explorer.arc.nasa.gov
ORG: NASA
URL: `ftp://explorer.arc.nasa.gov`

This archive is the home for the archives that were formerly at "ames.arc.nasa.gov."

The two main directories to look at are "cdrom" and "pub"; there's something for everyone here; check the "index" and "readme" files.

The "/cdrom/Magellan" directory contains information about data from the Magellan mission to Venus.

The "/cdrom/Viking" directory contains information about images from the Viking mission to Mars.

The "/cdrom" directory contains information about images from the Voyager missions to Jupiter, Neptune, Saturn, and Uranus.

The "/pub/hsewg" directory is intended to support the discussions and operation of the High Performance Computing and Communications Program (HPCC) Software Exchange Working Group (HSEWG).

Here's the list of subdirectories in "/pub/SPACE":

ANIMATION	HEADLINE.NEWS	PIONEER
ASTRO	HST	PRESS.RELEASE
BBXRT	JPEG	PROGRAMS
CASSINI	JPL	RADIO
COBE	LEI	SSFP
CONTRACT	LOGOS	StEphSACetc
CRAF	MAGELLAN	TOPEX
DXS	MARINERMARS.OBSERVER	UARS
EDUCATION	MARS.ROVER	UIT
FRR	NASA.SELECT	USMP
GALILEO	NTE	VICAR
GIF	PAYLOAD.STATUS	VOYAGER
GRO	PEGASUS	

Goddard-1

NAM: Goddard Space Flight Center FTP Archive
ORG: NASA/Goddard Space Flight Center
URL: `ftp://ftp.gsfc.nasa.gov/nic`

See the "AAAREADME.TXT" file in each directory for a description of that directory's contents. A general site with the following directories:

GENERAL.INFO	NREN	RFC
GSFC	ONLINE.SERVICES	SECURITY
IMAGES	OTHER_NETS	SOFTWARE
MAPS	PROTOCOLS	SOLICIT

Goddard-2

NAM: Goddard Space Flight Center FTP Archive
ORG: NASA/Goddard Space Flight Center
URL: `ftp://ftp.gsfc.nasa.gov/GSFC` or `ftp://ftp.gsfc.nasa.gov/pub`

Mac, VMS, UNIX directories; SUN, X11, and networking stuff; GIF images from the Hubble Space Telescope.

This archive also contains a program called ALEX: "The Automatic Login Executor (ALEX), a "portable" software utility which was conceived and designed at the Advanced Data Flow Technology Office of the NASA Goddard Space Flight Center. ALEX allows users to pick a remote host from among those in either the Internet Research Guide (copyright 1989 BBN Systems and Technologies Corporation) or the Network Information Center On-Line Aid System (NICOLAS) developed at NASA. ALEX then connects the user into the selected resource. When the user finishes his remote session, he returns to ALEX."

Langley-FTP

NAM: NASA Langley Technical Reports
ORG: NASA/Langley
URL: `ftp://techreports.larc.nasa.gov`

Move to the "/pub/techreports/" directory; also available through:

`http://techreports.larc.nasa.gov/ltrs/ltrs.html`

Reports available for the years 1989-1994

"The electronic reports are missing some, none, or all of their illustrations because the electronic files for these illustrations are not available. However, figure legends are present even when the illustrations are not."

NSSDCA

NAM: National Space Science Data Center MultiNet FTP Server
ORG: NASA
URL: `ftp nssdca.gsfc.nasa.gov`

The file "AAREADME.DOC" in the root directory contains a complete description of resources available; similarily, each subdirectory contains a "AAREADME.DOC" file:

"NSSDC maintains some of its most often requested data and information in directories publicly accessible over DECnet and Internet through the Anonymous user account on NSSDCA. Several flight projects at GSFC maintain directories on Anonymous for distribution of project-related data and information. In contrast to the NODIS system (NSSDC account), which provides specific user interfaces for each application, Anonymous users utilize network transfer protocols to read and retrieve files in the Anonymous directories."

This is the list of directories:

```
ACTIVE              ASM              CDM             CDROM
COBE                COHO             DATA_DIST       FITS
GRAPHICS_SOFTWARE   GSFCPID          HQ-NRAS
MD_DOCS             MODELS           MULTIDIS        NCDS
OPERATIONS          SFDU             SPACE_PHYSICS   SPDS
SYSTEM              TOOLS
```

GOPHER

ARC

NAM: Ames Research Center gopher
ORG: NASA/ARC
URL: `gopher://pathfinder.arc.nasa.gov`

The Pathfinder Sampler directory "contains samples of the data sets which one day will be available for the entire Pathfinder project. The data sets contained here are for a single day, March 20, 1988, the Vernal Equinox. The purpose of this sampler is to demonstrate the range of products available from the various Pathfinder instruments." Other directories provide access to a variety of environmental information sources.

GSFC-1

NAM: Climate and Radiation Server
ORG: NASA/GSFC
URL: `gopher://climate.gsfc.nasa.gov`

Discrete Ordinate Radiative Transfer Program
"The DISORT package consists of several files for performing 1-D radiative transfer in very general circumstances."

Guides To Writing Programs
"This subdirectory contains a variety of materials related to the process of writing scientific programs, with an emphasis on numerical modeling of physical phenomena."

Mie Scattering Program (e.m. scattering by a sphere) a link to the NCAR/UCAR Gopher which is "maintained by the Distributed Services Group in the Scientific Computing Division, National Center for Atmospheric Research, Boulder, CO."

GSFC-2

NAM: Goddard Space Flight Center (GSFC) Gopher
ORG: NASA/GSFC
URL: `gopher://gopher.gsfc.nasa.gov`

A general-purpose gopher with all kinds of information about NASA and GSFC; it also provides links to most other NASA sites.

Look at the directory "`About this Gopher/Navigating this gopher; What's here`" for a map of what this gopher offers.

Goddard Contact information: Centerwide Network Environment (CNE) Points of Contact
Other directories:

```
Networking
Science Information
US Government
FTP Archives
Virtual Reference Shelf
```

GSFC-3

NAM: GSFC 'What's new since...'
ORG: NASA/GSFC
URL: `gopher://gopher.gsfc.nasa.gov:5070/1`

Allows you to search the GSFC gopher

GSFC-4

NAM: High Energy Astrophysics Science Archival Research Center—HEASARC
ORG: NASA/GSFC
URL: `gopher://heasarc.gsfc.nasa.gov/1`

Points to <legacy.gsfc.nasa.gov> (see the next listing below).
This site now maintains a WWW server at:

`<http://heasarc.gsfc.nasa.gov:80>`

GSFC-5

NAM: High Energy Astrophysics Science Archival Research Center—HEASARC
ORG: NASA/GSFC
URL: `gopher://legacy.gsfc.nasa.gov`

Essentially an FTP server via gopher; check the README file for directory descriptions.

It should be noted that all Anonymous FTP accounts intended for public access on other Office of Guest Investigators (the OGIP: this is the umbrella organization that includes the HEASARC, the Compton Gamma-Ray Observatory Science Support Center, and the Guest Observer Facilities for the ROSAT, XTE, and ASCA (Astro-D) missions) machines such as ROSSERV will be shortly or already have been phased out, and their functionalities and data sets are all now available on LEGACY.

GSFC-6

NAM: MU-SPIN (Minority Universities) Program
ORG: NASA/GSFC
URL: `gopher://muspin.gsfc.nasa.gov`

For background information, see the "What is the MU-SPIN-Program? /Background" directory.

Short term: Transfer of advanced computer networking technologies to Historically Black Colleges and Universities/Other Minority Universities(HBCUs/MUs) and its use for supporting multi-disciplinary research.

Long term: Institutionalize network technology and scientific applications into the core of the universities such that faculty/students will have reliable access to computer systems as a basic tool of communicating with the NASA community. Create a mentor training environment within the MU-SPIN community in order to propagate network, scientific, and technical training.

GSFC-7

NAM: NASA Shuttle Small Payloads Project
ORG: NASA/GSFC
URL: `gopher://sspp.gsfc.nasa.gov`

NASA Space Shuttle small payloads programs.

HQ

NAM: Office of Life and Microgravity Sciences and Applications
ORG: NASA/HQ
URL: `gopher://gopher.olmsa.hq.nasa.gov`

> "It is the intent of the OLMSA Gopher to serve as an outreach server, providing our primary customers, the International scientific community, with electronic access to the most recent information available on Life Sciences, Microgravity Sciences, Gravitational Biology, Biotechnology, and Space Biomedical research efforts."

Time will tell; many of the links came back with "nothing available."

JSC

NAM: NASA/JSC Engineering Computational Facility
ORG: NASA/JSC
URL: `gopher://killerbee.jsc.nasa.gov`

An apparently young gopher; the README file emphasizes that it is a "prototype."

LARC

NAM: Langley Research Center (LaRC)
ORG: NASA/LaRC
URL: `gopher://gopher.larc.nasa.gov:7001/11/`

ISD (Information Systems Division) Customer List

Lots of computer stuff: schedules, bulletins, Cray, Fortran, documentation, graphics, parallel computers, and supercomputers.

Other directories:

```
Convex and Flight Simulation
Math Libraries
NAS Information, NASA Center Gophers
```

LERC

NAM: Lewis Research Center Gopher (LeRC)
ORG: NASA/LeRC
URL: `gopher://gopher.lerc.nasa.gov`

> "Information maintained in this gopher is intended to be generally useful for persons interacting specifically with the NASA Lewis Research Center and with NASA in general."

Other directories:

```
NASA Gopher and Other Information Services
Newsletters & Journals (DEC, Silicon Graphics, and SUN)
```

```
Telecommunications and Networking
Unix(tm) Workstation Support
Scientific and Engineering Workstation Catalogs
SEWP Information
```

NAIC

NAM: NASA Networked Applications and Information Center
ORG: NASA
URL: `gopher://naic.nasa.gov/11`

Pretty much everything that NASA has to offer description from gopher:

> "Located at NASA's Ames Research Center at Moffett Field, CA, the NAIC currently has three main areas of focus. *First*, the NAIC serves as a facilitator for a distributed network information center architecture that will colocate information services with NASA Centers' end users. Once such a system is in place, the NAIC will provide support to these Center NICs (CNICs).
>
> "*Second*, until a distributed system is in place, the NAIC will be responsible for providing the services formerly provided by the NASA Science Internet Network Information Center (NSI NIC), which was at Goddard Space Flight Center.
>
> "*Third*, the NAIC also supports several advanced applications developed by the Advanced Network Applications (ANA) group. Among these are support for X.500 implementations and mail applications, as well as hardcopy document distribution of manuals and guides to these applications."

STI

NAM: NASA Scientific and Technical Information (STI) gopher
ORG: NASA/STI
URL: `gopher://gopher.sti.nasa.gov`

There's a WWW version at

`http://www.sti.nasa.gov/STI-homepage.html`

NASA Selected Current Aerospace Notices (SCAN):

> "Selected Current Aerospace Notices (SCAN) is a current awareness publication, published on the first and the fifteenth of each month that brings to your attention recently issued report and journal literature pertaining to aeronautics and aerospace research. SCAN covers the full spectrum of aeronautics and aerospace information, but segments it into subject groupings or topics, which are narrower in scope than those provided by Scientific and Technical Aerospace Reports (STAR) and International Aerospace Abstracts (IAA)."

Toronto

NAM: The University of Toronto Gopher USENET FAQs
ORG: The University of Toronto
URL: `gopher://gopher.physics.utoronto.ca:70/11/FAQ/Faq_by_name`

The USENET archives has a section on "space"; move into the directory `<6. USENET News Frequently Asked Questions (FAQ)>` and go to number 1350 (or thereabouts) and you will find some FAQs on space.

Tech-Com

NAM: Mid-Continent Technology Transfer Center
ORG: A NASA Regional Technology Transfer Center
URL: `gopher://technology.com`

> "The mission of the Mid-Continent Technology Transfer Center is to serve the national interest by providing business, engineering, scientific, information and educational services

for the mid-continent region enabling public and private enterprises to acquire, develop and apply technologies from or with NASA, federal laboratories and other sources to expand the use of technology, promote commercialization and improve competitiveness."

Other directories:

```
Conference Calendar
Emerging Technology Reports
Federal Information
Technology Transfer Information
```

SEDS

NAM: Students for the Exploration & Development of Space (SEDS) gopher
ORG: Univ. of Arizona
URL: **gopher://seds.lpl.arizona.edu**

"Students for the Exploration and Development of Space was founded in 1980 at MIT and Princeton and consists of an international group of high school, undergraduate, and graduate students from a diverse range of educational backgrounds who are working to promote space as a whole."

Brown

NAM: Brown Univ. gopher
ORG: Brown Univ.
URL: **gopher://gopher.brown.edu:70/11/usr/subject/aero**

Provides access to several E-journals along with other links

Harvard

NAM: Harvard-Smithsonian Center for Astrophysics
ORG: Harvard Univ./Smithsonian
URL: **gopher://cfata4.harvard.edu**

Harvard-Smithsonian Center for Astrophysics Theory Group Gopher

```
Numerical Recipes Information
SLATEC (Public Domain) Common Mathematical Library
Preprint-Bulletin-Boards
```

NCSU

NAM: North Carolina State University Library gopher
ORG: North Carolina State University
URL: **gopher://dewey.lib.ncsu.edu:70/11/library/disciplines/astronomy**

Links to many NASA gophers

```
Astrophysics preprints (University of Chicago)
Includes a number of Telnet links:
ESA (European Space Agency) <TEL>
Lunar & Planetary Institute (Johnson Spaceflight Center) <TEL>
NASA Spacelink <TEL>
NASA online database <TEL>
NODIS—National Space Science Data Center <TEL>
Space Physics Analysis Network Information Center SPAN_NIC <TEL>
SpaceMet—Science/Space BBS <TEL>
US Naval Observatory Automated Data Service <TEL>
```

Rice

NAM: The Rice University gopher
ORG: Rice University
URL: `gopher://riceinfo.rice.edu/11/Subject/Aerospace`

This gopher contains links to many of the sites listed in this document. Many other gophers point to this list at Rice University.

STSCI

NAM: Space Telescope Electronic Information System (STEIS)
ORG: NA
URL: `gopher://stsci.edu`

Everything you ever wanted to know about the Space Telescope

Chicago

NAM: University. of Chicago gopher
ORG: University. of Chicago
URL: `gopher://granta.uchicago.edu:70/11/Preprints/astro-ph`

Astrophysics preprints

Omaha

NAM: The University of Nebraska at Omaha gopher
ORG: The University of Nebraska at Omaha
URL: `gopher://gopher.unomaha.edu:70/11/UNO Student Organizations/UNO Aviation`

General aviation gopher

COSMIC

NAM: COmputer Software Management and Information Center (COSMIC)
ORG: NASA/Univ. of Georgia
URL: `gopher://cossack.cosmic.uga.edu`

> "NASA's COmputer Software Management and Information Center (COSMIC) has been located at the University of Georgia since its beginning in 1966. We presently have over 800 computer programs that were originally developed by NASA and its contractors for the U.S. space program. Software is available for a number of areas of interest including: artificial intelligence, computational fluid dynamics, finite element structural analysis, scientific visualization, thermal and fluid flow analysis, and many more. Programs are priced on a cost-recovery basis and usually include source code. U.S. educational institutions are eligible for a substantial discount."

HPCC

NAM: HPCC Case Studies
ORG: National Coordination Office for High Performance Computing and Communications (HPCC)
URL: `gopher://gopher.hpcc.gov/11/blue94/case.studies`

Currently contains case studies such as:
> "Air flow past delta wing with thrust reverser jets in ground . . ."
> "Galaxy Formation"
> "Design and Simulation of Aerospace Vehicles."

LOC

NAM: Library of Congress gopher
ORG: Library of Congress
URL: `gopher://marvel.loc.gov/11/global/sci/astro`

Directories:

```
 1. Astronomy, Astrophysics, and Physics Journals/
 2. Guides to Astronomy, Astrophysics, & Physics on the Internet/
 3. Aerospace Directory from Rice U./
 4. American Astronomical Society/
 5. American Institute of Physics (AIP)/
 6. Astronomical Internet Resources Directory from STScI/
 7. Case Western Reserve Univ, Physics Gopher/
 8. Center for Extreme Ultraviolet (EUV) Astrophysics/
 9. Cold Fusion Bibliography <?>
10. Electromagnetic Wave Research Inst. of NRC (Florence, Italy)/
11. HST—Hubble Space Telescope Archive <TEL>
12. LANL Physics Info/
13. Lunar/Planetary Institute - Geology, Geophysics, Astro <TEL>
14. Mathematical Physics Preprint Archive (mp_arc)/
15. NASA—Goddard Space Flight Center/
16. NASA Extragalactic Database (Username: ned) <TEL>
17. NASA Network Applications and Information Center (NAIC)/
18. NASA, Earth Observing System (EOS)/
19. National Institute of Standards and Technology, U.S. (NIST)/
20. Physics Resource Directory from U.C. Irvine/
21. Space Telescope Electronic Information System
```

PATH-NET

NAM: NA
ORG: Pandora Systems (?)
URL: `gopher://path.net:8001/11/.subject/Aerospace`

Similar to the Rice University. gopher, it offers a comprehensive listing of Internet sites.

LISTSERV

AEFlow

When we attempted to subscribe to this list, we received the following reply:

```
>>From LISTSERV@TECHNION.AC.IL Ukn Nov 2 14:13:34 1993
>No LISTSERV distribution list by the name of "AEFLOW" is
>known to exist.
```

Aeronautics

NAM: Aeronautics: The Aeronautics Mailing List
ORG: University of Texas at Austin
URL: Send email to **majordomo@rascal.ics.utexas.edu** with the message SUBSCRIBE
AERONAUTICS "firstname" "lastname"

General discussion of aerospace engineering:
Maintainer: Robert Dorsett, rdd@rascal.ics.utexas.edu

Mary Shafer is the thematic moderator: she scans incoming traffic and decides what to post. The basic requirements are conciseness, accuracy, and relevance to the group charter. No class projects and no flames.

The group charter: "A moderated discussion-group dealing with atmospheric flight, specifically: aerodynamics, flying qualities, simulation, structures, systems, propulsion, and design human factors."

"The list is a news-to-mail feed from the sci.aeronautics newsgroup on USENET. Sci.aeronautics was created in 1989; from 1989 through Feb. 1993 the group was "unmoderated." A Digest version of the group was available as a mailing list, however. This message-based list replaces the Digest. This list, which has 200 subscribers, also serves the USENET group "sci.aeronautics" which has 15,000 subscribers. Posts are sent to both the newsgroup and the mailing list. Rascal is also home to the defunct Digest archives."

AIAA

NAM: AIAA (American Institute of Aeronautics and Astronautics)
ORG: University of Arizona
URL: Send email to **listserv@arizvm1.ccit.arizona.edu** with the message <SUBSCRIBE AIAA "firstname" "lastname">

General discussion of aerospace engineering.
Manager: pete@music.ame.arizona.edu (William Hojnowski, Sai Thallam)
   This list receives a substantial amount of business from its local members with the number of messages ranging from 2-10 per day. The discussions are active and varied.

Aircraft

We received the following reply when we tried to subscribe to this list:

>>From: LISTSERV%GREARN.BITNET@FRMOP11.CNUSC.FR Oct 12

>Sorry, list AIRCRAFT is closed.

AV-Theory

We received the following reply when we tried to subscribe to this list:

>>From: cmaeda@cs.washington.edu Ukn Nov 2 14:37:19

>av-theory is defunct

Aviation

NAM: Aviation
ORG: NA
URL: Send email to **listserv%brufpb.bitnet@uicvm.uic.edu** with the message SUBSCRIBE AVIATION "firstname" "lastname"

General aviation: There are approximately 180 list members.

Space-Investors

NAM: space-investors@cs.cmu.edu
ORG: NA
URL: Send email to **space-investors-request@cs.cmu.edu** with the message SUBSCRIBE AIAA "firstname" "lastname"

General aviation
Manager: Vince Cate: vac@cs.cmu.edu
   This list is for information relevant to investing in space related companies.

OPAC

Due to time and space limitations, we did not cover individual On-line Public Access Catalogs (OPACs) in this guide. OPACs receive relatively little attention in the Internet world, but they can be very helpful in the world of research, especially when one needs hard-to-find materials, materials your local library does not have, or citation information. Check with your local library about using Inter-Library Loan to obtain books that you find through OPACs.

Most of the university OPACs with ties to aerospace were located through a Veronica search ("aerospace and librar*") or are listed in the The College Blue Book: Degrees Offered by College and Subject, 23rd edition (New York: Macmillan Publishing Company, 1991) under the section "Aerospace Engineering."

Nearly all OPACs are available only through a Telnet connection, and, as with most Telnet systems, we STRONGLY recommend that users make use of the "Help" screens; they can make the difference between a good experience or a bad one. If you have access to a gopher, use it to find a listing of OPACSs. One very good site is the following:

`gopher://yaleinfo.yale.edu:7000/11/Libraries/by.place`

BTW, the Library of Congress gopher can be reached at the following:

`gopher://marvel.loc.gov`

TELNET

NODIS

NAM: NODIS
ORG: NASA/Space Physics Data Facility
URL: `telnet://nssdca.gsfc.nasa.gov;` login: nssdc

Provides access to databases in several subject categories with each category containing several subcategories to choose from:

```
0 - NODIS Overview
1 - Multi-Disciplinary Services
2 - Astrophysics Services
3 - Space Physics Services
4 - Planetary Science Services
5 - Earth Science Services
6 - Life Sci/Micrograv Services
```

NAIC-TEL

NAM: NASA Network Applications and Information Center (NAIC)
ORG: NASA/NAIC
URL: `telnet://naic.nasa.gov` login: naic password: naic

Provides a telnet connection to the NASA Network Applications and the following:

Information Center (NAIC) gopher server
Pretty much everything that NASA has to offer
Description from gopher as follows:

> "Located at NASA's Ames Research Center at Moffett Field, CA, the NAIC currently has three main areas of focus. *First*, the NAIC serves as a facilitator for a distributed network information center architecture that will colocate information services with NASA Centers' end users. When such a system is in place, the NAIC will provide support to these Center NICs (CNICs).
>
> "*Second*, until a distributed system is in place, the NAIC will be responsible for providing the services formerly provided by the NASA Science Internet Network Information Center (NSI NIC), which was at Goddard Space Flight Center.
>
> "*Third*, the NAIC also supports several advanced applications developed by the Advanced Network Applications (ANA) group. Among these are support for X.500 implementations and mail applications, as well as hardcopy document distribution of manuals and guides to these applications."

COSLINE

NAM: COSMIC Online Information Services
ORG: NASA/Univ. of Georgia
URL: `telnet://cosline.cosmic.uga.edu`

An information center and software database (approx. 1200 programs).

"This is an information service offered for the benefit of active and prospective customers of NASA's Computer Software Management and Information Center which is operated by the University of Georgia."

This site also contains information about conferences and technology transfer including names and addresses of contacts.

Kansas

NAM: The University of Kansas
ORG: The University of Kansas
URL: `telnet://www.cc.ukans.edu` login: `www`

A WWW server using LYNX which provides text only access to WWW sites and can be used over a modem using VT100 emulation.

For those that do not have access to Mosaic, this excellent site offers text-only access to World Wide Web sites. There are three logins provided at the introductory screen, but to immediately access WWW, users should type `www` at the login prompt. Most of the NASA servers may be found through the `by subjects` and `Aeronautics` links.

NASANews

NAM: NASANews
ORG: NASA Headquarters Washington, D.C.
URL: `finger nasanews@space.mit.edu`

Daily news brief from NASA

This utilizes the "finger" command to bring up a daily news brief of events concerning NASA.

ESA

NAM: Data Dissemination Network of the European Space Agency
ORG: European Space Agency
URL: `telnet://esrin.esa.it`

Provides access to the following databases:

```
ESAIRS    Information Retrieval Service
EMITS     Electronic Mail Invitation to Tender System (VT100/TTY)
EMITSWIN  Electronic Mail Invitation to Tender System Windows)
GDS       ESA Earth Observation Guide and Directory Service
DODIS     Official Document Distribution Service (VT100/TTY)
DODISWIN  Official Document Distribution Service (Windows)
CUIS      Columbus Utilisation Information System (VT100)
CUISWIN   Columbus Utilisation Information System (Windows, Mac)
EECF      Ers-1 European Central Facility
ERSUS     Ers-1 User Services
VAS       OSI Value Added Services
```

USENET

rec.aviation.answers

Aviation Usenet Newsgroup, The place for questions and answers about the REC.AVIATION hierarchy. Beginners to this area should start here. These newsgroups are not very tolerant of obvious questions. What is obvious?

rec.aviation.military

Military newsgroup. Historical questions can be answered here. Pretty lively discussion. This group provides a nice forum for novice Internet users to participate. Folks with historical interest in aviation participate alongside people with technical backgrounds.

`rec.aviation.misc`

All sorts of topics related to aviation discussed. Much more open discussion then many of the other groups. This is probably the best group for a beginner to participate. You're not sure about something in these newsgroups? Ask it here.

`rec.aviation.students`

Newsgroup for student pilots. This may be a better place then sci.aeronautics for aerospace students to ask questions. Focused around flying lessons, where, how, cost, etc. Again, this discussion is a great place for students/beginners to participate.

`sci.aeronautics`

The USENET version of the Aeronautics mailing list. Aerospace engineering, pretty technical, no flames, no class projects (why not?). This is not a group for the faint of heart. Dave and I were questioned as to what the heck we were doing when we first put this guide together. Where else would we go? The experts are here!

WWW

Dryden

NAM: NASA Dryden Flight Research Facility
ORG: NASA
URL: `http://mosaic.dfrf.nasa.gov/dryden.html`

This is the WWW page for the Dryden Flight Research Facility. NASA Dryden Flight Research Facility Center, named in honor of the first NACA director Dr. Hugh L. Dryden, is responsible for high-speed flight research, flight testing, and many other aspects of flight research.

Goddard-WWW

NAM: NASA/Goddard Space Flight Center
ORG: NASA
URL: `http://hypatia.gsfc.nasa.gov/GSFC_homepage.html`

Jumping off points for many GSFC resources gophers, wais servers, ftp sites and other NASA resources.

Johnson

NAM: NASA: Johnson Space Center
ORG: NASA
URL: `http://www.jsc.nasa.gov/JSC_homepage.html`

This is a re-vamped homepage that was supposed to be done by July 6, 1994. My visit earlier was successful. This server provides an excellent interface to the many directorates at Johnson. Very well organized.

Kennedy

NAM: NASA Kennedy Space Center WWW Server
ORG: NASA
URL: `http://www.ksc.nasa.gov/ksc.html`

Under construction, access to many KSC resources including gophers, ftp archives and space shuttle related items. Connectivity can be slow. Patience.

LaRC-WWW

NAM: Langley Research Center
ORG: NASA
URL: `http://mosaic.larc.nasa.gov/larc.html`

Information for the Langley Research Center. This site also contains the technical reports found at the following:

```
ftp://techreports.larc.nasa.gov.
```
To dial into them directly, use:
```
http://mosaic.larc.nasa.gov/ltrs/ltrs.html
```

NASA-HQ

NAM: NASA Headquarters
ORG: NASA
URL: `http://www.mtpe.hq.nasa.gov/HQ_homepage.html`

From the folks in Washington DC.

> This Web is run by staff at NASA Headquarters in Washington, DC. It points to other information servers and resources at HQ, Internet resources of interest to HQ personnel, other NASA affiliates, as well as the NASA homepage and the NCSA Mosaic homepage.

NASA-Info

NAM: NASA Information by Subject
ORG: NASA
URL: `http://hypatia.gsfc.nasa.gov/nasa_subjects/nasa_subjectpage.html`

> This site contains a prototype by NASA to provide ". . . access point[s]for NASA WWW information organized by subject. The subject catagories follow those used by NASA's Science & Technical Information Program. As a prototype, it is not likely to be complete, and it is subject to frequent changes and updates."

WWW

NAM: NASA World Wide Web Home Page
ORG: NASA
URL: `http://hypatia.gsfc.nasa.gov/NASA_homepage.html`

A jumping off point to the other NASA WWW homepages. Think of this the place to start and the Information by Subject site as the index system to these sites.

General Information

About this Guide

This guide was created by David Dalquist and Chris Poterala as a project for ILS 606, "Internet: Resource Discovery & Organization," a class offered by the School of Information and Library Studies at the University of Michigan. We created it to aid students, faculty, and others who have a general interest in aerospace engineering. We hope to help Internet users shortcut the normal searching process that they must often go through to find subject resources.

This guide concentrates on resources that may be obtained freely; fee-based information resources are growing steadily, but are not within the scope of this guide (or our wallets). Also, several new and sophisticated Internet searching and navigation tools have arrived and will continue to evolve. Unfortunately, many Internet users do not have the computer or financial resources required to support some of the new systems. With that in mind, we have elected to categorize this guide in terms of Internet access tools. This way, users who have limited access or computer resources can still locate sources easily. The one drawback to this is that some sources may be duplicated in different areas of the guide.

Internet Access Tools Used

For those people who are curious, our most productive finding aids were Gophers, WWW/Mosaic, currently available resource guides, and other people. Some of the ways we used them may not be so obvious—for example, if you press the equal (=) key while in a gopher directory, it responds with information about the site of that directory. We then used telnet, FTP, or gopher to go directly to that site to investigate it more thoroughly.

Perhaps because of the subject area we chose, ARCHIE and WAIS proved to be relatively ineffective searching tools.

Available Formats of the Guide

Well, you're reading the printed version of our guide. We are both very excited to see our guide and the others in this book sitting in our local bookstore. This guide began as a class project and now we have seen the larger on-line and publishing communities recognize the value of our hard work (fun?).

An on-line version of the guide is available in ASCII/text form.

Eventually (hopefully by the end of July 1994 . . . we're into spring now . . . patience is a virtue) an HTML version of our guide will be available. Announcements about our homepage will be made to the larger on-line community. You can obtain the ASCII guide through FTP or through the University of Michigan Gopher.

Corrections To and Maintenance of This Guide

Corrections: Due to the dynamic and often chaotic nature of the Internet and the time constraints that we all live with, we expect that there will be some errors in this guide. We will gladly correct mistakes that are brought to our attention. If we've really screwed up somewhere, please be tolerant; we are providing a service to the Internet community and are trying to do it in a responsible manner. If you have corrections to make, please send constructive comments to:

Dave Dalquist <dalquist@sils.umich.edu>
or
Christopher Poterala <poterala@ciesin.org>

Maintenance: We (Chris and Dave) both graduated from the University of Michigan in December 1993. Chris is currently working at an honest-to-goodness full-time job for the Consortium for International Earth Science Information Network (CIESIN). He is an information specialist involved in description and access to earth science electronic data. Dave is continuing to interview for full-time positions (know of any? e-mail Dave <wink>). He is currently working at the Michigan Technological University library part-time. He has become the ad-hoc "Net Guru."

Dave has headed back to the Upper Peninsula initially while Chris remains in Ann Arbor. Chris will probably be the easiest person to reach with comments, questions, etc. He will be the main contact for making corrections to the HTML version.

ACKNOWLEDGMENTS

Thanks to Lou Rosenfeld and Joseph Janes who turned surfing the net into a class and guided us along.

A heartfelt thank you to all those who have developed Internet guides over the years. Without their help, we would be lost in space.

Special thanks goes to Diance Kovacs for the many resource guides she provides (the ACAD lists).

Thanks to Scott Yanoff for his regularly updated Special Internet Connections.

Thanks to Maggie Parhamovich at the University of Las Vegas for making available the Internet Resources: U.S. Federal Government Information, 5th edition.

Thanks to all the folks at NASA for all the work they've done in making information available to the public; their sites dominate our list.

We would like to thank Peter Scott for developing HYTELNET and distributing a valuable program at a more than reasonable price (shareware). If you are not familiar with HYTELNET, you really should give it a try. It operates behind your communications program, and, by pressing a key combination, provides Internet addresses, login information, and background information for OPACs and selected databases available on the Internet. New sites can be added easily.

Chris would like to finally thank his wife Lisa Bankey for putting up with his on-line habit, busy phone lines, and trying to seem interested in this project. Chris and Lisa got married on December 18, 1993. Lisa, are you ready for this? As a side note, Lisa is very excited that Chris is now covered by somebody's health insurance and can go to the allergist!

Disclaimer

Because of the dynamic nature of the Internet, some of the information provided in this guide may already be outdated by the time it is issued. If you come across a correction that needs to be made, please notify us so that we can make the necessary changes.

The Electronic Zoo

11

Ken Boschert
Washington University

A List of Animal-Related Computer Resources (Internet/Bitnet Mailing Lists, Gophers, World Wide Web Sites, Mail Servers, Usenet Newsgroups, FTP Archives, Commercial Online Services, and Bulletin Board Systems)Version 3.0 (last revised: May 25, 1994)

Compiled by:

Ken Boschert, DVM
Associate Director
Washington University
Division of Comparative Medicine
Box 8061, 660 South Euclid Ave.
St. Louis, MO 63110
Phone: 314-362-3700
Fax: 314-362-6480
E-mail: ken@wudcm.wustl.edu

INTRODUCTION

There seems to be a list of everything else on the Internet; so I thought, why not a list of animal-related computer systems. Being a veterinarian and a computer nut, I had been net-surfing and cataloging these systems for years for my own use. Noting the spirit of sharing evident all throughout the Internet, I hope this contribution will be helpful to those with similar interests.

As this list will bear witness, animals of all sorts are popular topics of discussion and a number of sites have useful files for downloading. Listservers, Telnet & FTP sites, gophers, dial-up bulletin boards (BBS's)—they're all cataloged here and have a common thread of being related to animals in some form or fashion.

There are other lists around the net with similar, yet different focuses: Wilfred Drew's *not just cows* focuses on agricultural computer themes, including animals and crops; Lee Hancock's *Internet/Bitnet Health Sciences Resources* covers the medical computer field thoroughly; and Una Smith's *A Biologist's Guide to Internet Resources* is a great resource describing flora and fauna computer systems around the world. The *Electronic Zoo* list is cross-checked with these documents and extracts the animal-related computer resources from all three, then combines them with additional resources I have uncovered.

I do not personally subscribe to all of the systems listed below, but have endeavored to insure that they do exist. If you note errors or omissions, please send corrections or additions to me at: <ken@wudcm.wustl.edu>. I would especially appreciate additional sources on network sites containing animal-related materials.

Many of the descriptions below are contributed directly from the list owners, moderators, and sysops around the world who spend their owntime maintaining their respective systems. Collectively, I acknowledge their tremendous efforts and encourage each of you to take the time to pass along a note of thanks when you get a chance.

Internet / Bitnet Mailing Lists (listservs)

AAVI
American Academy of Veterinary Informatics

Internet Subscribe to: ken@wudcm.wustl.edu

Internet Mail to: **aavi@aalas.org**

Description: Discussion and proceedings of the American Academy of Veterinary Informatics. Restricted access to AAVI members only.

List Owner/Contact: Ken Boschert <ken@wudcm.wustl.edu>
Washington University
Division of Comparative Medicine
Box 8061, 660 South Euclid Ave.
St. Louis, MO 63110
Phone: 314-362-3700
Fax: 314-362-6480

AAVLD-L
American Association of Veterinary Laboratory Diagnosticians

Bitnet Subscribe to: `listserv@ucdcvdls`

Internet Subscribe to: **listserv@cvdls.ucdavis.edu**

Bitnet Mail to: **aavld-l@ucdcvdls**

Internet Mail to: **aavld-l@cvdls.ucdavis.edu**

Description: This list has been created to provide a forum for discussion between veterinary diagnostic laboratories and members of the AAVLD. Topics such as test standardization, fees, diagnostic information assistance, animal health surveillance, reports on conferences and symposia are especially welcomed. Discussions related to specific cases should be approached within the limits of diagnostic medicine and restrict discussions of therapy or treatments. The list will be limited to members of the AAVLD.

List Owners/Contact: James T. Case, DVM, Ph.D. <jcase@ucdcvdls.bitnet>
University of California
School of Veterinary Medicine
California Veterinary Diagnostic Laboratory System
P.O. Box 1770
Davis, CA 95617
Phone: 916-752-4408
Bill Cohen <bcohen@ucdcvdls.bitnet>

ABSNET
Animal Behavior Society Newsletter

Internet Subscribe to: jcha@u.washington.edu

Internet Mail to: **jcha@u.washington.edu** (Editor)

Description: An electronic mail system for members of the Animal Behavior Society and anyone interested in its goals to increase communication between animal behaviorists. The system currently includes a directory and an electronic mail newsletter, providing distribution of late-breaking job announcements, requests for information, and news of interest to members of the Animal Behavior Society.

List Owner/Contacts: Dr. James C. Ha <jcha@u.washington.edu>
Regional Primate Research Center, SJ-50
University of Washington
Seattle, WA 98195
Matthew F.S.X. Novak <novak@u.washington.edu>

ACTIV-L
Activists Mailing List

Bitnet Subscribe to: `listserv@mizzou1`

Internet Subscribe to: `listserv@mizzou1.missouri.edu`

Bitnet Mail to: **activ-l@mizzou1**

Internet Mail to: **activ-l@mizzou1.missouri.edu**

Description: Activists for Peace, Empowerment, Human & Animal Rights.

List Owners/Contact: Rich Winkel <`mathrich@mizzou1.missouri.edu`>

AGDG

Animal Genetics Discussion Group

Internet Subscribe to: `listserv@chuck.agsci.colostate.edu`

Internet Mail to: **breeders@chuck.agsci.colostate.edu**

Description: Discussion group for people interested in quantitative animal genetics and animal breeding.

List Owner/Contact: Bruce Golden <`bgolden@cgel.agsci.colostate.edu`>
Phone: 303-491-7128

AGENG-L

Agricultural Engineering & Intelligent Control

Internet Subscribe to: `listserv@ibm.gwdg.de`

Internet Mail to: **ageng-l@ibm.gwdg.de**

Description: Discussion and information on engineering and intelligent control in agriculture.

List Owner/Contact: Johannes grosse Beilage <`jbeilag@gwdg.de`>

AG-EXP-L

Agricultural Production & Management

Bitnet Subscribe to: `listserv@ndsuvm1`

Internet Subscribe to: `listserv@vm1.nodak.edu`

Bitnet Mail to: **ag-exp-l@ndsuvm1**

Internet Mail to: **ag-exp-l@vm1.nodak.edu**

Description: Discussion of the use of expert systems in agricultural production and management. Primary audience is practitioners, extension personnel and experiment station researchers in the land grant system.

List Owners/Contact: Sandy Sprafka <`sprafka@plains.nodak.edu`>
Dave Watt <`watt@vm1.nodak.edu`>

AGRIC-L

Agriculture Discussion Group

Bitnet Subscribe to: `listserv@uga`

Internet Subscribe to: `listserv@uga.cc.uga.edu`

Bitnet Mail to: **agric-l@uga**

Internet Mail to: **agric-l@uga.cc.uga.edu**

Description: Discusses agriculture, including, but not limited to: crop, irrigation and soil science; plant physiology and propagation; grassland husbandry; water resource management; cattle breeding; pig farming; simulation of ecological processes; and crop production and forestry (tropical).

List Owner/Contact: Harold Pritchett <`harold@uga.cc.uga.edu`>

AGRIS-L

Agricultural Information List

Bitnet Subscribe to: `listserv@irmfao01`

Internet Subscribe to: `listserv@irmfao01.bitnet`

Bitnet Mail to: **agris-l@irmfao01**

Internet Mail to: **agris-l@irmfao01.bitnet**

Description: The AGRIS/CARIS Coordinating Centre has established a list for discussion of issues and questions in the field of agricultural information. This list is open to information professionals as well as end users. Among the issues to be included are: bibliographical, current research and numerical databases; information systems, products and services; access to agricultural information, particularly in developing countries; indexing and retrieval systems, and any other relevant topics.

List Owner/Contact: A.I. Lebowitz <gilsn2@irmfao01.bitnet>
Head, AGRIS/CARIS Coordinating Centre
Food and Agriculture Organization of the U.N.
00151 Rome, Italy
Phone: (06) 5797-4993
Fax: (06) 5797-3152

AIDS

Redistribution list for the Usenet `Sci.Med.AIDS` Newsgroup

Bitnet Subscribe to: `listserv@rutvm1`

Internet Subscribe to: `listserv@rutvm1.rutgers.edu`

Bitnet Mail to: **aids@rutvm1**

Internet Mail to: **aids@rutvm1.rutgers.edu**

Description: Information concerning Acquired Immunce Deficiency Syndrome; echoes the Usenet Newsgroup `sci.med.aids`

List Owner/Contact: Dan Greening <dgreen@cs.ucla.edu>

AI-MEDICINE

Artificial Intelligence in Medicine

Internet Subscribe to: `ai-medicine-request@med.stanford.edu`

Internet Mail to: **ai-medicine@med.stanford.edu**

Description: The scope of this mailing list should be limited to "AI in Medicine," which may be defined as "computed-based medical decision support" (or "computer-assisted medical decision making"). This definition may be expanded to include AI-based approaches to computer-assisted medical instruction. According to this definition, topics such as billing systems and hospital/medical office information retrieval systems clearly remain outside the scope of this forum. A medical informatics mailing list exists for the discussion of such topics. There are some borderline topics which cannot readily be classified under AI in Medicine, yet have clear connections to both artificial intelligence and medical practice. Processing and interpretation of medical images and signals are among those subject areas. Subject areas should remain within the scope of the list, as long as the focus lies on the artificial intelligence aspects, and not the detailed engineering principles.

List Owners/Contact: Serdar Uckun <ai-medicine-request@med.stanford.edu>
Knowledge Systems Laboratory
Stanford University
Wanda Pratt <aimed@camis.stanford.edu>

ALTANIM

Alternatives to Animals List

Internet Subscribe to: `listserv@uib.no`

Internet Mail to: **altanim@uib.no**

Description: For exchange of information regarding alternatives to animals.

List Owner/Contact: Richard T. Fosse <richard.fosse@med.uib.no>
Laboratory Animal Veterinary Services
University of Bergen
Armauer Hansens House
Haukeland Hospital
N-5022 Bergen, Norway
Phone: 47-5-97-46-96
Fax: 47-5-97-46-05

ANCHODD
Australian National Clearinghouse on Drug Development

Internet Subscribe to: `listserv@cc.utas.edu.au`

Internet Mail to: **anchodd@cc.utas.edu.au**

Description: Exchanges information between drug scientists. Sponsored by the Centre for Pharmacology, Medicinal Chemistry and Toxicology at the University of Tasmania The Royal Australian Chemical Institute RACI (Division of Medicinal and Agricultural Chemistry), the Australasian Society of Clinical and Experimental Pharmacologists, Toxicologists (ASCEPT) and The Australian Pharmaceutical Sciences Association (APSA).

List Owner/Contact: Stuart McLean <`s.mclean@pharm.utas.edu.au`>

ANEST-L
Anesthesiology Discussion List

Bitnet Subscribe to: `listserv@ubvm`

Internet Subscribe to: `listserv@ubvm.cc.buffalo.edu`

Bitnet Mail to: **anest-l@ubvm**

Internet Mail to: **anest-l@ubvm.cc.buffalo.edu**

Description: This list discusses topics related to anesthesiology, including computer use in anesthesia research.

List Owner/Contact: Andrew M. Sopchak <`sopchaka@vax.cs.hscsyr.edu`>
   Department of Anesthesiology
   SUNY Health Science Center
   750 East Adams Street
   Syracuse, NY 13210

ANSSTDS
Animal, Dairy, & Poultry Science List (Restricted)

Bitnet Subscribe to: `listserv@msu.bitnet`

Internet Subscribe to: `listserv@msu.edu`

Bitnet Mail to: **ansstds@msu.bitnet**

Internet Mail to: **ansstds@msu.edu**

Description: A listserver for undergraduates, graduates and teaching faculty in Department of Animal Science, Dairy Science and Poultry Science at Michigan State University. This listserver is intended to be used by Animal Science Graduate, Undergraduates and Animal Science Teaching Faculty. The discussion list will be used for discussion of curricular information, needs for resources, general discussion about Animal Science topics and various other students activities.

List Owner/Contact: Russel Erickson <`22277rwe@ibm.cl.msu.edu`>
   Department of Animal Science
   Michigan State University
   E. Lansing, MI 48824-1225
   Phone: 517-355-8423

APAARIB
American Psychological Association Animal Research Information Board

Bitnet Subscribe to: `listserv@gwuvm`

Internet Subscribe to: `listserv@gwuvm.bitnet`

Bitnet Mail to: **apaarib@gwuvm**

Internet Mail to: **apaarib@gwuvm.bitnet**

Description: APA's Animal Research Information Board List

   The Animal Research Information Board will have information and items of interest on the use of animals in research. It will include the latest information on: activities in Congress (legislation and hearings), the Federal agencies, and the States; Federal regulations; pro- and anti- animal research groups;

campus activities, and more. This is a moderated board and material for possible posting will be sent to an editor.

List Owners/Contact: Elizabeth Baldwin <apasdeab@gwuvm.bitnet>
Margaret Allen <apasdmaa@gwuvm.bitnet>
Rhonda Fisher <apasdref@gwuvm.bitnet>
American Psychological Association
Science Directorate
1200 17th St. NW
Washington, DC 20036

APPLIED-ETHOLOGY

Applied Animal Ethology Discussion List

Internet Subscribe to: `applied-ethology-request@sask.usask.ca`

Internet Mail to: **`applied-ethology@sask.usask.ca`**

Description: An e-mail network set up for the exchange of information, discussions, announcements, news items, etc., that are of interest to people working and studying in the field of applied animal ethology. This network was the initiative of members from the ISAE (International Society for Applied Ethologist) with the help of computer systems experts from the University of Saskatchewan. Non-ISAE members, with an interest in applied animal ethology, are welcome to participate.

List Owner/Contact: Joseph M. Stookey <stookey@sask.usask.ca>
Western College of Vet. Med.
Department of Herd Medicine and Theriogenology
University of Saskatchewan
Saskatoon, Saskatchewan
CANADA S7N 0W0

AQUA-L

Aquaculture discussion list

Bitnet Subscribe to: `listserv@uoguelph`

Internet Subscribe to: `listserv@vm.uoguelph.ca`

Bitnet Mail to: **`aqua-l@uoguelph`**

Internet Mail to: **`aqua-l@vm.uoguelph.ca`**

Description: The Aquaculture list discusses the science, technology and business of rearing aquatic species. Membership in the list is public and unrestricted. Topics include: Who's doing what and where; problems and solutions rearing aquatic larvae; diseases, parasites and pathology; water quality; recirculation technology and applications; research aquatic systems design and operation; commercial aquatic systems design and operation; site selection and environmental impact; new species under culture; genetics, sex reversal and hormonal manipulation; computers in aquaculture; public perceptions of aquaculture; and aqua-business.

List Owner/Contact: Ted White <zoowhite@vm.uoguelph.ca>

AQUARIUM

Discussion of Home Fish Aquariums

Bitnet Subscribe to: `listserv@emuvm1`

Internet Subscribe to: `listserv@emuvm1.cc.emory.edu`

Bitnet Mail to: **`aquarium@emuvm1`**

Internet Mail to: **`aquarium@emuvm1.cc.emory.edu`**

Description: Aquarium is an open discussion about all things related to the hobby of keeping fish and other aquatic things in an aquarium. If you have questions about how to solve problems with your aquarium or if you have expertise about aquariums and are willing to answer questions, this is the place.

List Owner/Contact: Bert Bruner <osakb@emuvm1.cc.emory.edu>

AR-ALERTS

Animal Rights Alerts

Internet Subscribe to: `listserv@ny.neavs.com`

Internet Mail to: **`ar-alerts@ny.neavs.com`**

Description: The Animal Rights Alerts mailing list has been set up to facilitate communication among Animal Rights groups, activists, and other interested individuals. Its primary purpose is to enable rapid dissemination of important information about Animal Rights issues. This venue, it is hoped, will serve as an important adjunct to periodicals such as Animals Agenda and Animals Voice. Any information pertaining to Animal Rights or to issues that relate to Animal Rights, such as habitat destruction, are welcome.

List Owner/Contact: James Corrigan <james@ny.neavs.com>
New England Anti-Vivisection Society
333 Washington Street, Suite 850
Boston, MA 02108
Phone: 617-523-6020

AR-NEWS

Animal Rights News (Animal Rights Electronic Network)

Internet Subscribe to: `ar-news-request@cygnus.com`

Internet Mail to: **`ar-news@cygnus.com`**

Description: Administered via the Animal Rights Electronic Network (AREN), an organization dedicated to providing mechanisms for the exchange of ideas and information pertaining to the issues of animal rights/welfare. AR-Talk is an open discussion forum and AR-News is a public news wire. The purpose of these lists is to provide open channels where news, ideas, philosophies, and concerns can be exchanged freely. Debates are likely to occur as well as the development of new friendships and associations. The underlying premise behind these mailing lists is that information is fundamental to forming sound beliefs as well as to making sound decisions. These lists are open to anyone who is interested, regardless of his/her opinion(s) on Animal Rights. Here is a list of topics likely to be addressed in these lists; it is, by far, not complete: Animal Rights, Animal Liberation, Vivisection/Dissection, Animals as Research 'Tools', Animals in Laboratories, Animal as Models for Humans, Pet Overpopulation, Animals in Education, Hunting/Trapping/Fishing, Animals in Entertainment, Factory Farming, Fur, Ecology, Environmental Protection, Religious Perspectives, Genetic Engineering, Consumer Product Testing, 'Cruelty-Free' Products, Vegetarianism, and Vegan Lifestyle.

Appropriate postings to AR-News include: posting a news item, requesting information on some event, or responding to a request for information. Discussions on AR-News will NOT be allowed and we ask that any commentary either be taken to AR-Talk or to private E-mail.

List Owners/Contact: Charles S. 'Chip' Roberson <csr@nic.aren.org>
Ian Lance Taylor <ian@cygnus.com>
AREN
P.O. Box 17521
Raleigh, NC 27619-7521

AR-TALK

Animal Rights Talk (Animal Rights Electronic Network)

Internet Subscribe to: `ar-talk-request@cygnus.com`

Internet Mail to: **`ar-talk@cygnus.com`**

Description: See AR-NEWS Description above.

List Owners/Contact: Charles S. 'Chip' Roberson <csr@nic.aren.org>
Ian Lance Taylor <ian@cygnus.com>
AREN
P.O. Box 17521
Raleigh, NC 27619-7521

ASCD-SCI
Alliance for Teaching of Science
Bitnet Subscribe to: `listserv@psuvm`
Internet Subscribe to: `listserv@psuvm.psu.edu`
Bitnet Mail to: **ascd-sci@psuvm**
Internet Mail to: **ascd-sci@psuvm.psu.edu**
List Owner/Contact: Dave Popp <`jdp115@psuvm.psu.edu`>

ASEH-L
American Society of Environmental Historians
Bitnet Subscribe to: `listserv@ttuvm1`
Internet Subscribe to: `listserv@ttuvm1.ttu.edu`
Bitnet Mail to: **aseh-l@ttuvm1**
Internet Mail to: **aseh-l@ttuvm1.ttu.edu**
Description: American Society of Environmental Historians Discussion.
List Owner/Contact: Dennis Williams <`williams.dennis@epamail.epa.gov`>

AVCS Newsletter
American Veterinary Computer Society Newsletter (Restricted)
Internet Subscribe to: **r-smith19@uiuc.edu**
List Owner/Contact: Dr. Ronald Smith <`r-smith19@uiuc.edu`>
University of Illinois
College of Veterinary Medicine
2001 S. Lincoln Avenue
Urbana, IL 61801
Phone: 217-333-3290
Fax: 217-333-4628

AVHIMA-L
American Veterinary Health Information Management Association
Bitnet Subscribe to: `listserv@uiucvmd`
Internet Subscribe to: `listserv@vmd.cso.uiuc.edu`
Bitnet Mail to: **avhima-l@uiucvmd**
Internet Mail to: **avhima-l@vmd.cso.uiuc.edu**
List Owner/Contact: Art Siegel <`siegel@vmd.cso.uiuc.edu`>

AVIFAUNA (BIRDLIFE)
Neotropical Bird Discussion List
Internet Subscribe to: `listasrcp@avifauna.pe`
Internet Mail to: **avifauna@rcp.net.pe**
List Owner/Contact: Roberto Phillips <`phillips@cipa.ec`>

AVSL-L
Australia Vietnam Science Link
Internet Subscribe to: `majordomo@coombs.anu.edu.au`
Internet Mail to: **avsl-l@coombs.anu.edu.au**

Description: This is an e-mail list on science and technology in Vietnam and its vicinity. Discussion topics include: human biology, primatology and forensic science, bu the group is not limited to these areas. Communication is still difficult but Vietnamese scientists are anxious to talk with a post-embargo world. This discussion group should help foreigners contact Vietnamese scientists and soon will be a tool for Vietnamese to communicate to the rest of the world.

List Owner/Contact: Vern Weitzel <vern@coombs.anu.edu.au>
Coombs Computing Unit,
Research School of Social Sciences
Research School of Pacific Studies
Australian National University,
Canberra, ACT 0200 AUSTRALIA
Phone: +61 (6) 283-5845
Fax: +61 (6) 283-5518

BATLINE

Bat Research & Education Discussion Group

Bitnet Subscribe to: `listserv@umnvma`

Internet Subscribe to: `listserv@umnvma.umn.edu`

Bitnet Mail to: **batline@umnvma**

Internet Mail to: **batline@umnvma.umn.edu**

Description: A discussion group to promote the exchange of information, questions, and ideas pertaining to bat research and education.

List Owner/Contact: Mike Balistreri <mikebal@triton.umn.edu>

BEE-L

Discussion of Bee Biology

Bitnet Subscribe to: `listserv@albnyvm1`

Internet Subscribe to: `listserv@uacsc2.albany.edu`

Bitnet Mail to: **bee-l@albnyvm1**

Internet Mail to: **bee-l@uacsc2.albany.edu**

Description: BEE-L discusses the biology of bees, including honey bees, other bees, and wasps, including topics such as: sociobiology, behavior, ecology, adaptation/evolution, genetics, taxonomy, physiology, pollination, and flower nectar and pollen production of bees.

List Owners/Contact: Mary Jo Orzech <mjo@brock1p.bitnet>
Eric Seielstad <eric@brock1p.bitnet>

BEEF-L

Beef Specialists Discussion Group

Bitnet Subscribe to: `listserv@wsuvm1`

Internet Subscribe to: `listserv@wsuvm1.csc.wsu.edu`

Bitnet Mail to: **beef-l@wsuvm1**

Internet Mail to: **beef-l@wsuvm1.csc.wsu.edu**

Description: Discussion group for professionals advising the beef industry and others with an interest in beef cattle management.

List Owners/Contact: Tony Wright <wright@wsuvm1.csc.wsu.edu>

BETTAS

Betta Fish Discussion List

Bitnet Subscribe to: `listserv@arizvm1`

Internet Subscribe to: `listserv@arizvm1.ccit.arizona.edu`

Bitnet Mail to: **bettas@arizvm1**

Internet Mail to: **bettas@arizvm1.ccit.arizona.edu**

Description: A mailing list designed for people interested in the keeping and breeding of Betta splendens (Siamese fighting fish). It is a public, unmoderated list, for the discussion of the above topic. It is NOT for general aquaria information unrelated to Betta splendens.

List Owner/Contact: Jill Firch <jfirch@cnet.shs.arizona.edu>

BIOCIS-L

Biology Curriculum Innovation Study

Bitnet Subscribe to: `listserv@sivm`

Internet Subscribe to: `listserv@sivm.si.edu`

Bitnet Mail to: **`biocis-l@sivm`**

Internet Mail to: **`biocis-l@sivm.si.edu`**

Description: The Biology Curriculum Innovation Study (BIOCIS-L) is a research and development effort between the Smithsonian Institution, IBM, the University of Maryland, UCLA Medical School, and the University of North Carolina.

List Owner/Contact: Mignon Erixon-Stanford <`irmss907@sivm.si.edu`>

BIODIDAC

Electronic Discussion Group for Biology Teachers

Bitnet Subscribe to: `listserv@uottawa`

Internet Subscribe to: `listserv@acadvm1.uottawa.ca`

Bitnet Mail to: **`biodidac@uottawa`**

Internet Mail to: **`biodidac@acadvm1.uottawa.ca`**

List Owner/Contact: Antoine Morin <`jjasb@acadvm1.uottawa.ca`>

BIODIV-L

Biodiversity Networks

Internet Subscribe to: `listserv@bdt.ftpt.br`

Internet Mail to: **`biodiv-l@bdt.ftpt.br`**

Description: The Tropical Data Base manages the discussion list. The intention of this list is to discuss technical opportunities, administrative and economic issues, practical limitations and scientific goals, leading to recommendations for the establishment of a biodiversity network. Individual contributions are requested, not only as to network capabilities, but also as to existing databases of interest to biodiversity.

BIO-GOPHER

Biology Gopher Administrator's List

Internet Subscribe to: **`tim@bch.umontreal.ca`**

Description: The primary function of the Bio-Gopher Administrators list is as a communication forum for all administrators of gopher holes whose primary function is to provide information on the biological sciences through gopher. This list is maintained at the MegaGopher site at the University of Montreal.

List Owner/Contact: Tim Littlejohn <`little@ere.umontreal.ca`>
  tim@bch.umontreal.ca
  Departement de biochimie
  Universite de Montreal
  C.P. 6128, succursale A,
  Montreal (Quebec), H3C 3J7 CANADA
  Phone: 514-343-7936
  Fax: 514-343-2210

BIO-JRNL

BIOSCI Bio-Journals E-conference

Bitnet Subscribe to: `listserv@irlearn`

Internet Subscribe to: `listserv@irlearn.ucd.ie`

Bitnet Mail to: **`bio-jrnl@irlearn`**

Internet Mail to: **`bio-jrnl@irlearn.ucd.ie`**

Description: Postings of Biological Journal tables of contents. Among the journal Table of Contents available in bionet.journals.contents are: Anatomy & Embryology, Applied Microbiology and Biotechnology,

Chromosoma, Current Genetics, EMBO Journal, Environmental Physiology, European Journal of Biochemistry, European Journal of Physiology, Experimental Brain Research, Histochemistry, IEEE Engineering in Medicine and Biology, Immunogenetics Journal of Biological Chemistry, Journal of Comparative Physiology B, Journal of Membrane Biology, Journal of Molecular Evolution, Journal of Virology, MGG—Molecular and General Genetics, Mammalian Genome, Microbial Releases, Molecular Microbiology, Molecular and Cellular Biology, Roux's Archives of Developmental Biology, and Theoretical and Applied Genetics

BIOLOGIA Y EVOLUCION

Biology and Evolution (in Spanish)

Internet Subscribe to: `biologia-request@athena.mit.edu`

Internet Mail to: **`biologia@athena.mit.edu`**

BIOMAT-L

Biomaterials Mailing List

Internet Subscribe to: `listserv@nic.surfnet.nl`

Internet Mail to: **`biomat-l@nic.surfnet.nl`**

Description: This list is intended for members of the Australian, Canadian, European, Japanese, US and other Societies for Biomaterials, and for anyone with an interest in biomaterials. The scope of this list includes the application of all types of materials in medicine and biology. Discussion of all aspects of biomaterials (from materials production and testing to issues of biocompatibility and tissue interactions and specific clinical applications) is encouraged. Also welcome are announcements of meetings and conferences, and discussions of particular technical problems associated with your biomaterials research.

List Owner/Contact: Arthur Brandwood <`a.brandwood@unsw.edu.au`>
　　　　　　　　　Sydney, Australia

BIOMCH-L

Biomechanics Discussion List

Bitnet Subscribe to: `listserv@hearn`

Internet Subscribe to: `listserv@nic.surfnet.nl`

Bitnet Mail to: **`biomch-l@hearn`**

Internet Mail to: **`biomch-l@nic.surfnet.nl`**

Description: E-conference for members of the International, European, American, Canadian and other Societies of Biomechanics, and for others with an interest in the general field of biomechanics and human or animal movement science. For the scope of this e-conference, see, e.g., the Journal of Biomechanics (Pergamon Press), the Journal of Biomechanical Engineering (ASME), and Human Movement Science (North-Holland). Biomch-L is operated under the Patronage of the International Society of Biomechanics.

List Owners/Contact: Krystyna Gielo-Perczak <`kgp@vut.edu.au`>
　　　　　　　　　　Christoph Reinschmidt <`reinschm@acs.ucalgary.ca`>
　　　　　　　　　　Tom van den Bogert <`bogert@acs.ucalgary.ca`>

BIOMED-L

Biomedical Ethics Discussion List

Bitnet Subscribe to: `listserv@ndsuvm1`

Internet Subscribe to: `listserv@vm1.nodak.edu`

Bitnet Mail to: **`biomed-l@ndsuvm1`**

Internet Mail to: **`biomed-l@vm1.nodak.edu`**

Description: Mailing list for discussion of biomedical ethics. Since the field of medicine and medical technology are rapidly changing and the field is so broad, it is difficult to have clearly delineated rules as to what should and should not be discussed, but possible topics might include: paternalism, fetal cell transplant, the right to die, AIDS, suicide, patient autonomy, abortion, drug legalization, euthanasia, respirator withdrawal, transplants, allocation of scarce resources, and many others too numerous to list here. The discussions may be ethical, philosophical, religious, political, social or even, in some cases, personal.

List Owners/Contact: Julie Waters <julie@drycas.club.cc.cmu.edu>
Michelle Francl <mfrancl@cc.brynmawr.edu>

BIOPI-L

Secondary Biology Teacher Enhancement Discussion Group

Bitnet Subscribe to: `listserv@ksuvm`

Internet Subscribe to: `listserv@ksuvm.ksu.edu`

Bitnet Mail to: **biopi-l@ksuvm**

Internet Mail to: **biopi-l@ksuvm.ksu.edu**

Description: A list networking biology teachers and a variety of biologists and science education specialists involved in the teacher enhancement process.

List Owner/Contact: Tom Manney **<tmanney@ksuvm.ksu.edu>**

BIOSPH-L

Biosphere, Ecology, Discussion List

Bitnet Subscribe to: `listserv@ubvm`

Internet Subscribe to: `listserv@ubvm.cc.buffalo.edu`

Bitnet Mail to: **biosph-l@ubvm**

Internet Mail to: **biosph-l@ubvm.cc.buffalo.edu**

Description: Discusses anything related to the biosphere, pollution, CO-2 effect, ecology, habitats, and climate, etc. Also gateway to Usenet Newsgroup bit.listserv.biosph-l.

List Owner/Contact: Dave Phillips <davep@acsu.buffalo.edu>

BIOTECH

Biotechnology Discussion List

Bitnet Subscribe to: `listserv@umdd`

Internet Subscribe to: `listserv@umdd.umd.edu`

Bitnet Mail to: **biotech@umdd**

Internet Mail to: **biotech@umdd.umd.edu**

Description: BIOTECH is an moderated bulletin board dedicated to the free exchange of ideas and data concerning biotechnology. All topics and announcements concerning biotechnology are welcome.

List Owner/Contact: Dan Jacobs <dan@umdd.umd.edu>

BIRDBAND

Bird Bander's Forum

Bitnet Subscribe to: `listserv@arizvm1`

Internet Subscribe to: `listserv@arizvm1.ccit.arizona.edu`

Bitnet Mail to: **birdband@arizvm1**

Internet Mail to: **birdband@arizvm1.ccit.arizona.edu**

Description: Bird Bander's Trade

List Owners/Contact: Charles B. Williamson <chuckw%evax2@arizona.edu>
Norman C. Saunders <nys@cu.nih.gov>

BIRDCHAT

National Birding Hotline Cooperative (Chat Line)

Bitnet Subscribe to: `listserv@arizvm1`

Internet Subscribe to: `listserv@arizvm1.ccit.arizona.edu`

Bitnet Mail to: **birdchat@arizvm1**

Internet Mail to: **birdchat@arizvm1.ccit.arizona.edu**

Description: Discussion of the Birding Hotline Cooperative

List Owners/Contact: Charles B. Williamson <chuckw%evax2@arizona.edu>
   Norman C. Saunders <nys@cu.nih.gov>

BIRDCNTR

National Birding Hotline Cooperative (Central U.S.)

Bitnet Subscribe to: listserv@arizvm1

Internet Subscribe to: listserv@arizvm1.ccit.arizona.edu

Bitnet Mail to: **birdcntr@arizvm1**

Internet Mail to: **birdcntr@arizvm1.ccit.arizona.edu**

List Owners/Contact: Charles B. Williamson <chuckw%evax2@arizona.edu>
   Norman C. Saunders <nys@cu.nih.gov>

BIRDEAST

National Birding Hotline Cooperative (East U.S.)

Bitnet Subscribe to: listserv@arizvm1

Internet Subscribe to: listserv@arizvm1.ccit.arizona.edu

Bitnet Mail to: **birdeast@arizvm1**

Internet Mail to: **birdeast@arizvm1.ccit.arizona.edu**

List Owners/Contact: Charles B. Williamson <chuckw%evax2@arizona.edu>
   Norman C. Saunders <nys@cu.nih.gov>

BIRD_RBA

National Birding Hotline Cooperative

Bitnet Subscribe to: listserv@arizvm1

Internet Subscribe to: listserv@arizvm1.ccit.arizona.edu

Bitnet Mail to: **bird_rba@arizvm1**

Internet Mail to: **bird_rba@arizvm1.ccit.arizona.edu**

Description: National Birding Hotline Cooperative provides a clearing-house for transcribed birding hotlines from around the country.

List Owners/Contact: Charles (Chuck) B. Williamson <chuckw%evax2@arizona.edu>
   4425 E. Pima
   Tucson, AZ 85712
   Phone: 602-323-2955

   Norman (Norm) C. Saunders <nys@cu.nih.gov>
   1261 Cavendish Drive
   Colesville, MD 20905
   Phone: 202-272-5248

BIRDTRIP

Special BIRDCHAT LOGO Project

Bitnet Subscribe to: listserv@arizvm1

Internet Subscribe to: listserv@arizvm1.ccit.arizona.edu

Bitnet Mail to: **birdtrip@arizvm1**

Internet Mail to: **birdtrip@arizvm1.ccit.arizona.edu**

List Owners/Contact: Charles B. Williamson <chuckw%evax2@arizona.edu>
   Norman C. Saunders <nys@cu.nih.gov>

BIRDWEST

National Birding Hotline Cooperative (West U.S.)

Bitnet Subscribe to: listserv@arizvm1

Internet Subscribe to: `listserv@arizvm1.ccit.arizona.edu`

Bitnet Mail to: **`birdwest@arizvm1`**

Internet Mail to: **`birdwest@arizvm1.ccit.arizona.edu`**

List Owners/Contact: Charles B. Williamson <`chuckw%evax2@arizona.edu`>
    Norman C. Saunders <`nys@cu.nih.gov`>

BRINE-L
Brine Shrimp Discussion List

Bitnet Subscribe to: `listserv@uga`

Internet Subscribe to: `listserv@uga.cc.uga.edu`

Bitnet Mail to: **`brine-l@uga`**

Internet Mail to: **`brine-l@uga.cc.uga.edu`**

List Owners/Contact: Lamar Jackson <`ljackson@uga.cc.uga.edu`>
    Mercer University
    Phone: 912-752-4062
    Harold Pritchett <`harold@uga.cc.uga.edu`>

CAMEL-L
Discussion Forum on Camel Research

Bitnet Subscribe to: `listserv@sakfu00`

Internet Subscribe to: `listserv%sakfu00.bitnet@vtvm1.cc.vt.edu`

Bitnet Mail to: **`camel-l@sakfu00`**

Internet Mail to: **`camel-l%sakfu00.bitnet@vtvm1.cc.vt.edu`**

Description: Discusses the field of camel research and studies.

List Owner/Contact: Mustafa Ghazal <`nad@sakfu00.bitnet`>

CANINE-L
Dog Fanciers Discussion List

Bitnet Subscribe to: `listserv@pccvm`

Internet Subscribe to: `listserv@psuvm.psu.edu`

Bitnet Mail to: **`canine-l@pccvm`**

Internet Mail to: **`canine-l@psuvm.psu.edu`**

Description: CANINE-L is a discussion list for and about dogs; all kinds, types and varieties of dogs. Postings ranging from care and feeding of your household 'pooch' to scientific research concerning any aspect of wild or domestic canine populations are welcome. If you wish to discuss training, human-canine psi experiences, dog "ghosts", seek a bit of comfort over the loss of a cherished dog, or find the best way to handle any aspect of dog ownership, you may reasonably expect to be welcome on CANINE-L. Managers and Administrators of any institution maintaining a canine population, such as zoos, game parks or research installations may discuss mutual problems and points of interest here. Graphic discussion of research techniques may be inappropriate for this list and offensive to some subscribers. Use good taste in what you post. Reasonable discussion of conservation and environmental issues, as they specifically relate to canine populations, are welcome here. The same holds true for almost any aspect of canine veterinary care and management. In short, absolutely anything that may reasonably be seen to have a relationship to canines and/or to human-canine interactions may be posted here . . . with one or two exceptions. This is not the place for campaigning for animal rights, debating the ethics of maintaining pets, pleading generalized environmental cases not directly bearing on a canine population, arguing the pros and cons of vegetarianism or any similarly tangential topics. This is, first and foremost, a place for people who love dogs. Any kind of dogs.

List Owner/Contact: W.K. 'Bill' Gorman <`bj496@cleveland.freenet.edu`>

CAYUGABIRDS-L
Birding in Upstate New York Discussion List

Internet Subscribe to: `listserv@cornell.edu`

Internet Mail to: **cayugabirds-l@cornell.edu**

Description: CAYUGABIRDS-L is an informal electronic discussion list for the discussion of topics relevant to wild birds and birding in upstate New York. Goal of the list is to help spread information about about bird sightings in the region, promote local birding events, and provide an effective electronic forum for birders in Ithaca and the finger lakes as well as other regions of Upstate New York. The list is not to be used to discuss pet birds or falconry.

List Owner/Contact: Rob Scott <rs18@cornell.edu>

CBT-GENERAL

Biological timing and circadian rhythms

Internet Subscribe to: cbt-general-request@virginia.edu

Internet Mail to: **cbt-general@virginia.edu**

Description: Mailing list for news and comments of general interest to the biological timing research community. e.g., a forum for discussion of research in biological timing and circadian rhythms, requests for literature pointers, announcements, etc.—anything of general interest.

List Owner/Contact: Tom Breeden <tmb@virginia.edu>
　　　　　　　　　Center for Biological Timing
　　　　　　　　　Phone: 804-982-4513

CLASS-L

Classification, Clustering, and Phylogeny Discussion List

Bitnet Subscribe to: listserv@sbccvm

Internet Subscribe to: listserv@ccvm.sunysb.edu

Bitnet Mail to: **class-l@sbccvm**

Internet Mail to: **class-l@ccvm.sunysb.edu**

Description: Classification, clustering, and phylogeny estimation and related methods of data analysis. The purpose of this list is to enable researchers in classification, clustering, phylogeny estimation, and related methods of data analysis to contact other researchers in that area. The list is not limited to members of particular professional societies.

List Owner/Contact: Jim Rohlf <rohlf@sbbiovm.bitnet>

CNRE

College of Natural Resources and the Environment

Bitnet Subscribe to: listserv@nervm

Internet Subscribe to: listserv@nervm.nerdc.ufl.edu

Bitnet Mail to: **cnre@nervm**

Internet Mail to: **cnre@nervm.nerdc.ufl.edu**

List Owner/Contact: <tsanf@nervm.nerdc.ufl.edu>

COASTNET

Coastal Management Conference

Bitnet Subscribe to: listserv@uriacc

Internet Subscribe to: listserv@uriacc.uri.edu

Bitnet Mail to: **coastnet@uriacc**

Internet Mail to: **coastnet@uriacc.uri.edu**

Description: The COASTNET Listserv list is a forum to discuss National and International Coastal Management issues, and is being facilitated jointly by The Coastal Resources Center and The Department of Marine Affairs at The University of Rhode Island. This forum encourages dialog on coastal management issues from all nations, and is based on the belief that coastal resource planners, managers, researchers, and users from the developed and developing world have much to learn from and contribute to each other. Queries and comments addressed to COASTNET should fall within the realm of coastal management, including, but not limited to: natural resources, research, financial resources, policies and regulations, development, conservation, transfer of science to policy, and management strategies.

List Owner/Contact: Robert H. Puffer <rpuf4584@uriacc.uri.edu>

COGNEURO

Cognitive Neuroscience Mailing List

Internet Subscribe to: **cogneuro-request@ptolemy.arc.nasa.gov**

Description: The Cognitive Neuroscience Mailing List is a way to discuss phenomena at the interface of cognitive science (broadly construed) and biology. The discussion is scientific, multidisciplinary, and academic. Topics include:

- behavioral aspects of neuroanatomy and neurophysiology;
- biological aspects of particular sets of behaviors;
- the neuropsychology of ecology, ethology, genetics,
- ontogeny, endocrinology, info. theory, and pharmacology;
- books, papers, research directions, and new results;
- new imaging, simulation, and measurement techniques;
- curricula, graduate programs, jobs, zeitgeist, and funding.

"Behavior" above is an attempt at a theory-independent, catch-all term for cognition, emotion, volition, and meaningful action in humans and other animals, both normal and abnormal, including subjective reports. Since that is a lot of territory to cover, primary emphasis tends to be:

- on science (measurable phenomena) more than philosophy,
- on the field itself more than its implications, and
- on approaching particular natural phenomena from many
- perspectives rather than approaching many phenomena from a particular
- perspective or technique.

For more details about the Cognitive Neuroscience Mailing List, including how to subscribe, how to get archives, and guidelines, please send email to me at:

cogneuro-request@ptolemy.arc.nasa.gov

with something closely resembling "cogneuro: send info" in the subject line, and I will reply manually with the latest information. (Please use the above cogneuro-request address in correspondence about the list. It will reach me just as quickly, but it helps me organize my mailbox a bit.)

List Owner/Contact: Kimball Collins <kpc@ptolemy.arc.nasa.gov>
Cogneuro participant/administrator/founder
AI Research Branch
NASA Ames Research Ctr.
MS 269-2
Moffett Field, CA 94035
Phone: 415-604-1221

COMPMED

Comparative Medicine Discussion List

Bitnet Subscribe to: **listserv@wuvmd**

Internet Subscribe to: **listserv@wuvmd.wustl.edu**

Bitnet Mail to: **compmed@wuvmd**

Internet Mail to: **compmed@wuvmd.wustl.edu**

Description: COMPMED is a restricted Internet/Bitnet mailing list for discussing the topics of: comparative medicine, laboratory animals (all species), and related topics. This discussion group is primarily intended to provide a forum for information exchange among professionals working in the fields of comparative medicine and biomedical research. Subject matter may range from, but is not limited to: laboratory animal medicine, animal models, news items, meeting announcements, research issues, information requests, veterinary/husbandry topics, job notices, animal exchange information, book reviews, and animal alternatives.

List Owner/Contact: Ken Boschert, DVM <ken@wudcm.wustl.edu>
Washington University
Division of Comparative Medicine
Box 8061, 660 South Euclid Ave.
St. Louis, MO 63110
Phone: 314-362-3700
Fax: 314-362-6480

COMPUMED

Computers in Medicine Discussion List

Bitnet Subscribe to: `listserv@sjuvm`

Internet Subscribe to: `listserv@sjuvm.stjohns.edu`

Bitnet Mail to: **compumed@sjuvm**

Internet Mail to: **compumed@sjuvm.stjohns.edu**

Description: Discusses the role of computers in medicine and software and hardware developments in medicine and medical curriculum.

List Owner/Contact: Dr. Paul S. di Virgilio <virgilio@epas.utoronto.ca>

CONSBIO

Society for Conservation Biology

Bitnet Subscribe to: `listserv@uwavm`

Internet Subscribe to: `listserv@uwavm.u.washington.edu`

Bitnet Mail to: **consbio@uwavm**

Internet Mail to: **consbio@uwavm.u.washington.edu**

Description: Discussion for members of the Society for Conservation Biology (SCB) and others interested in developing the scientific and technical means for the protection, maintenance, and restoration of life on this planet—its species, its ecological and evolutionary processes, and its particular total environment. In the service of this goal, our objectives include: (1) the promotion of research and the maintenance of the highest standards of quality and ethics in this activity; (2) the publication and dissemination of scientific, technical, and management information; (3) the encouragement of communication and collaboration between conservation biology and other disciplines (including other biological and physical sciences, the behavioral and social sciences, economics, law and philosophy) that study and advise on conservation and natural resource issues; (4) the education, at all levels, preparatory and continuing, of the public, of biologists, and of managers, in the principles of conservation biology; (5) the promotion of all of the above through the provision of adequate funding; and (6) the recognition of outstanding contributions made to the field by individuals and organizations. The CONSBIO list is maintained by the University of Washington Chapter of the Society for Conservation Biology. The list will serve to exchange information on SCB activities, job opportunities, education programs, and scholarly research. The list will also serve as a forum for discussion of the multidisciplinary aspects of conservation biology, the interaction of science and society in conservation policy and action, and the relationship between maintaining biodiversity and sustainable development. We encourage anyone interested in conservation biology and the activities of the Society for Conservation Biology to subscribe to the list and publicize it widely to others. Subscription is currently open and unmoderated.

List Owner/Contact: Preston D. Hardison <pdh@u.washington.edu>
University of Washington
Chapter of the Society for Conservation Biology
Department of Psychology NI-25
Seattle, WA 98195

CONSGIS

Biological Conservation and GIS

Bitnet Subscribe to: `listserv@uriacc`

Internet Subscribe to: `listserv@uriacc.uri.edu`

Bitnet Mail to: **consgis@uriacc**

Internet Mail to: **consgis@uriacc.uri.edu**

List Owners/Contact: Pete August <pete@edcserv.edc.uri.edu>

CONSLINK

National Zoological Park, Smithsonian Institution
    Discussion on Biological Conservation

Bitnet Subscribe to: `listserv@sivm`

Internet Subscribe to: `listserv@sivm.si.edu`

Bitnet Mail to: **conslink@sivm**

Internet Mail to: **conslink@sivm.si.edu**

Description: A Bitnet-based electronic conference and bulletin board on all topics of biological conservation. The Smithsonian Institution is involved in conservation related education and research projects worldwide. CONSLINK was established to improve communication between individuals and institutions around the world who are interested in the general topic of biological conservation.

List Owner/Contact: Michael Stuwe <nzpem001@sivm.si.edu>
    Conservation and Research Center
    National Zoological Park
    Smithsonian Institution
    Front Royal, VA 22630, USA

CRUST-L

Crustacean Biology List

Bitnet Subscribe to: `listserv@sivm`

Internet Subscribe to: `listserv@sivm.si.edu`

Bitnet Mail to: **crust-l@sivm**

Internet Mail to: **crust-l@sivm.si.edu**

Description: CRUST-L is an unmoderated discussion list for scholars and students of Crustacean Biology, which, for our present purposes, comprises any matters related to the systematics, distribution, and ecology of members of the arthropod Subphylum Crustacea. Announcements will be made in English and subscribers may use the language of their choice. Translations, however, will not be provided.

List Owners/Contact: Jan Clark <mnhiv002@sivm.si.edu>
    Bill Hart <mnhiv008@sivm.si.edu>
    Jim Thomas <mnhiv040@sivm.si.edu>

    Division of Crustacea
    Department of Invertebrate Zoology
    National Museum of Natural History
    Smithsonian Institution
    Washington, D.C. 20560
    Phone: 202-357-4243
    Fax: 202-786-2687

CSTB

Canadian Society for Theoretical Biology

Internet Subscribe to: `majordomo@biome.bio.ns.ca`

Internet Mail to: **cstbn@biome.bio.ns.ca**

Description: This is the mailing list for the Canadian Society for Theoretical Biology, operated by the Habitat Ecology Division at the Bedford Institute of Oceanography. It is open to CSTB members and anyone else interested in any aspect of Theoretical Biology.

List Owner/Contact: Bill Silvert <silvert@biome.bio.ns.ca>

CTURTLE

Sea Turtle Biology and Conservation List

Bitnet Subscribe to: `listserv@nervm`

Internet Subscribe to: `listserv@nervm.nerdc.ufl.edu`

Bitnet Mail to: **cturtle@nervm**

Internet Mail to: **cturtle@nervm.nerdc.ufl.edu**

List Owner/Contact: <abb@gnv.ifas.ufl.edu>

DAIRY-L

Dairy Cow Discussion List

Bitnet Subscribe to: `listserv@umdd`

Internet Subscribe to: `listserv@umdd.umd.edu`

Bitnet Mail to: **dairy-l@umdd**

Internet Mail to: **dairy-l@umdd.umd.edu**

Description: Discussion group for professional educators and extension workers advising the dairy industry and others with an interest in dairy cattle management. Questions concerning problems or policies faced by dairy producers are encouraged, as are requests for educational tools such as visual aids, computer-aided decision support tools, and outlines of educational programs. Offers to share available educational tools are especially encouraged. Discussions of current problems and controversies facing the dairy industry are also favored.

List Owners/Contact: Mark Varner <varner@umd5.umd.edu>
Phone: 301-405-1396

Roger Cady <cady@wsuvm1.bitnet>
Phone: 206-840-4557

Stephen Emanuele <semanuel@empire.cce.cornaell.edu>

DARWIN-L

History & Theory of the Historical Sciences Discussion Group

Internet Subscribe to: `listserv@ukanaix.cc.ukans.edu`

Internet Mail to: **darwin-l@ukanaix.cc.ukans.edu**

Description: Darwin-L has been established to promote the reintegration of a range of academic fields all of which are concerned with reconstructing the past from evidence in the present, and to encourage communication among professionals in these fields. Darwin-L is not devoted to evolutionary biology nor to the work of Charles Darwin, but instead examines the entire range of historical sciences from an explicitly interdisciplinary perspective. These fields include: evolutionary biology, archeology, historical linguistics, paleontology, textual transmission and stemmatics, historical anthropology, historical geology, cosmology, systematics and phylogeny, and historical geography. Darwin-L is supported by the Center for Critical Inquiry in the Liberal Arts, University of North Carolina at Greensboro, and by the Department of History and the Academic Computing Center, University of Kansas.

List Owner/Contact: Dr. Robert J. O'Hara <darwin@iris.uncg.edu>
Department of Biology
University of North Carolina at Greensboro
Greensboro, North Carolina 27412

DEEPSEA

Deep Sea Biology Discussion List

Bitnet Subscribe to: `listserv@uvvm`

Internet Subscribe to: `listserv@uvvm.uvic.ca`

Bitnet Mail to: **deepsea@uvvm**

Internet Mail to: **deepsea@uvvm.uvic.ca**

Description: Purpose is to serve the world's community of deep sea and hydrothermal vent biologists working in the areas of evolution, ecology, biogeography, paleontology, systematics, phylogenetics, and population genetics.

List Owner/Contact: Andrew McArthur <amcarthu@uvvm.uvic.ca>

DERBY

Horse Racing Discussion List

Internet Subscribe to: derby-request@ekrl.com

Internet Mail to: derby@ekrl.com

Description: To discuss various aspects and strategies of horse racing, primarily dealing with, but not limited to, handicapping. Anyone is free to join.

List Owner/Contact: John Wilkes <wilkes@ekrl.com>
Equine Kinetics Research Laboratories
Box 2230
Aptos, CA 95001-2230

DINOSAUR

Discussion of Dinosaurs and Other Archosaurs

Internet Subscribe to: listproc@lepomis.psych.upenn.edu

Internet Mail to: dinosaur@lepomis.psych.upenn.edu

Description: The Dinosaur list exists to distribute information and foster dialogue amongst people in the electronic community who share an interest in the scientific examination of evidence pertaining to dinosaurs. Also to discuss flying & swimming archosaurs and other animals of that period as well as earlier & later periods. Most participants are not paleontologists but some are extremely well-versed.

List Owner/Contact: Mickey Rowe <rowe@lepomis.psych.upenn.edu>

DIS-L

Drosophila Workers DIS Newsletter

Bitnet Subscribe to: listserv@iubvm

Internet Subscribe to: listserv@iubvm.ucs.indiana.edu

Bitnet Mail to: dis-l@iubvm

Internet Mail to: dis-l@iubvm.ucs.indiana.edu

Description: DIN (Drosophila Information Newsletter) provides a timely forum for informal communication among Drosophila workers. Functions as an edited newsletter, distributed quarterly.

List Owner/Contact: Kathleen Matthews <matthewk@iubvm.bitnet>

DNH-PILOT

Diet, Nutrition, & Health Discussion List

Internet Subscribe to: mailbase@mailbase.ac.uk

Description: The Diet, Nutrition and Health project covers Sociology, Food Science and Technology, Agricultural Economics and Psychology. Researchers in academic institutions across the European Community, hopefully together with industrial partners and with some external funding, are involved.

List Owner/Contact: malcolm hamilton@reading.ac.uk

D-ORAL-L

Oral Microbiology/Immunology Interest Group

Bitnet Subscribe to: listserv@nihlist

Internet Subscribe to: listserv@list.nih.gov

Bitnet Mail to: d-oral-l@nihlist

Internet Mail to: d-oral-l@list.nih.gov

Description: The Oral Microbiology/Immunology Interest Group is an international forum for discussions of problems facing scientists and clinicians that deal with human and mammalian oral microbiota. Microbiology discussions include the prevalence of, and diseases caused by oral microbiota, physiology and genetics of virulence factors, host response to pathogens and virulence factors, autoimmune oral diseases, and the effects of aging on immune response. This forum will also serve as a conduit between members of professional societies that have Oral Microbiology and Immunology interest Sections including the NIDR, IADR/AADR, ASM, FEMS, AAAS and other groups. Announcement of coming events and public pre-meeting organizational communications are encouraged.

List Owners/Contact: Dr. John Spitznagel <jks@giskard.uthscsa.edu>
Cynthia Walczak <caz@cu.nih.gov>

EASTBAYVEGANS

East Bay Vegan Newsletter

Internet Subscribe to: **eastbayvegans@uclink.berkeley.edu**

Description: Grass-roots animal activist group promoting veganism.

List Owner/Contact: East Bay Vegan News <eastbayvegans@uclink.berkeley.edu>
Leor H. Jacobi <veg@uclink.berkeley.edu>
P.O. Box 4353
Berkeley, CA 94704-0353
Phone: 510-843-6343

ECOLOGIA

Ecology Discussion List (in Spanish)

Internet Subscribe to: ecologia-request@athena.mit.edu

Internet Mail to: **ecologia@athena.mit.edu**

Description: La lista de Ecologia tiene como objetivo fomentar el intercambio entre profesionales del area de habla castellana con especial interes en aumentar el flujo de informacion hacia los paises de America Latina.

List Owner/Contact: Ananias A. Escalante <aescalan@darwin.bio.uci.edu>

ECOLOG-L

Ecological Society of America

Bitnet Subscribe to: listserv@umdd

Internet Subscribe to: listserv@umdd.umd.edu

Bitnet Mail to: **ecolog-l@umdd**

Internet Mail to: **ecolog-l@umdd.umd.edu**

Description: This list is a forum for members of the Ecological Society of America and other interested ecologists to exchange information about job opportunities, funding opportunities, and Society activities. It will also serve as a forum for discussion of current (or historical) topics in ecology, about papers from the Society's journals Ecology, Ecological Monographs, and Ecosystem theory and modeling Ecological Applications, and as a resource for people looking for information about research projects. Also gateway to Usenet Newsgroup bit.listserv.ecolog-l

List Owner/Contact: David Inouye <david_w_inouye@umail.umd.edu>

ECOLOGY

Politics and the Environment List

Bitnet Subscribe to: listserv@emuvm1

Internet Subscribe to: listserv@emuvm1.cc.emory.edu

Bitnet Mail to: **ecology@emuvm1**

Internet Mail to: **ecology@emuvm1.cc.emory.edu**

List Owner/Contact: Courtney Brown <polscb@emuvm1.cc.emory.edu>

ECOSYS-L

Ecosystem Theory and Modelling

Bitnet Subscribe to: `listserv@dearn`

Internet Subscribe to: `listserv@vm.gmd.de`

Bitnet Mail to: **ecosys-l@dearn**

Internet Mail to: **ecosys-l@vm.gmd.de**

Description: This mailing list is intended for the discussion in the field of ecosystem theory and modelling. Typically the material will be question-and-answer, where someone wants information on any problem in this field. In addition, contributions are welcome in order to: build up a list of mathematical models, build up an address-list of scientists who are engaged in modelling and to standardize mathematical formulation of ecological processes.

List Owner/Contact: Joachim Benz <`benz@gsf.de`>

ECOTHEOL

Ecological or environmental issues from a theological & ethical perspective

Internet Subscribe to: `mailbase@mailbase.ac.uk`

Internet Mail to: **ecotheol@mailbase.ac.uk**

Description: ECOTHEOL has been established to provide a forum for discussion of ecological or environmental issues from a theological and ethical perspective. Contributions to the list are warmly encouraged. Topics that could be discussed include religious attitudes to the environment, ecofeminist theology, environmental ethics, "deep" ecology, process theology and the works of such people as Matthew Fox, Sallie McFague, Robin Attfield and Jurgen Moltmann. Notifications of forthcoming meetings and conferences of interest to ECOTHEOL members are invited too. The list welcomes contributions from those in other disciplines, including philosophy and the social sciences.

List Owner/Contact: Ian Tilsed <`i.j.tilsed@exeter.ac.uk`>
University of Exeter (UK)

ECOVIS-L

Trends in Ecology of Vision

Bitnet Subscribe to: `listserv@yalevm`

Internet Subscribe to: `listserv@yalevm.cis.yale.edu`

Bitnet Mail to: **ecovis-l@yalevm**

Internet Mail to: **ecovis-l@yalevm.cis.yale.edu**

Description: The purpose of this list is to facilitate electronic discourse among scientists working within Biology, Ecology, and Visual Science.

List Owner/Contact: Adrian Palacios <`palacios@minerva.cis.yale.edu`>

ECS-NEWS

European Cetacean Society News

Internet Subscribe to: `mailbase@mailbase.ac.uk`

Internet Mail to: **ecs-news@mailbase.ac.uk**

Help Info: `ecs-helpdesk-request@mailbase.ac.uk`

Description: Ecs-news is an open list set up to exchange news items within the European Cetacean Society.

List Owner/Contact: `ecs-news-request@mailbase.ac.uk`

EMBINFO

EMBNet (European Molecular Biology Network)

Internet Subscribe to: `listserv@ibacsata.bitnet`

Internet Mail to: **embinfo@ibacsata.bitnet**

List Owner: Sergio Gadaleta <`gadaleta@ibacsata.bitnet`>

ENT-LIST
Entomology Discussion List
Internet Subscribe to: `hcfb@um.cc.umich.edu`
Internet Mail to: **`ent-list@um.cc.umich.edu`**
Contact: Mark O'Brien `<userhcfb@um.cc.umich.edu>`

ENTOMO-L
Entomology Discussion List
Internet Subscribe to: `listserv@uoguelph.ca`
Internet Mail to: **`entomo-l@uoguelph.ca`**

ENV-LINK+
Environmentalists Digest
Internet Subscribe to: `env-link+forms@andrew.cmu.edu`
Internet Mail to: **`env-link@andrew.cmu.edu`**
Description: Provides free information for environmentalists around the world, for the discussion of matters both profound and mundane, which reflects a shared set of core environmental issues.
List Owner/Contact: Josh Knaur `<env-link+@andrew.cmu.edu>`

ENVST-L
Environmental Studies Discussion List
Bitnet Subscribe to: `listserv@brownvm`
Internet Subscribe to: `listserv@brownvm.brown.edu`
Bitnet Mail to: **`envst-l@brownvm`**
Internet Mail to: **`envst-l@brownvm.brown.edu`**
Description: The Environmental Studies list discusses undergraduate and graduate environmental studies and environmental science degree programs.
List Owner/Contact: Harold Ward `<halward@brownvm.brown.edu>`
Steve Trombulak `<trombula@midd.bitnet>`

EQUESTRIANS
Equestrian Activities List
Internet Subscribe to: `majordomo@nda.com`
Internet Mail to: **`equestrians@nda.com`**
Description: Anything and everything related to equestrian activities. This list is gatewayed to the Usenet rec.equestrians newsgroup.
List Owner/Contact: David C. Kovar `<kovar@nda.com>`

EQUINE-D
Equestrian Discussion List
Internet Subscribe to: `listserv@pccvm.bitnet`
Internet Mail to: **`equine-d@pccvm.bitnet`**
Description: The rec.equestrian digest is a redistribution of articles from the USENET `rec.equestrian` newsgroup for persons without USENET access. The list is currently running in read-only mode; no subscriber postings are permitted. EQUINE-D originated as an outgrowth of, and companion list to, EQUINE-L.
List Owner/Contact: W.K. (Bill) Gorman `<34aej7d@cmuvm.csv.cmich.edu>`

EQUINE-L
Horse Fanciers Discussion List
Bitnet Subscribe to: `listserv@pccvm`

Internet Subscribe to: `listserv@psuvm.psu.edu`

Bitnet Mail to: **`equine-l@pccvm`**

Internet Mail to: **`equine-l@psuvm.psu.edu`**

Description: Discussion forum for horse fanciers—all phases of horse ownership, management, use and related concerns for all horse breeds, both hot and cold blood.

List Owner/Contact: W.K. 'Bill' Gorman <`bj496@cleveland.freenet.edu`>

ETHOLOGY

Animal Behaviour and Behavioural Ecology Mailing List

Bitnet Subscribe to: `listserv@searn`

Internet Subscribe to: `listserv@searn.sunet.se`

Bitnet Mail to: **`ethology@searn`**

Internet Mail to: **`ethology@searn.sunet.se`**

Description: Discusses animal behavior and behavioral ecology. Possible topics could be e.g. new or controversial theories, new research methods, and equipment. Announcements of books, papers, conferences, new software for behavioural analysis etc., are also encouraged. Also has a Usenet gateway to `bit.listserv.ethology`

List Owner/Contact: Jarmo Saarikko <`saarikko@helsinki.fi`>
Department of Zoology
Division of Ecology
University of Helsinki

EUROBIRDNET

Information about Birds in Europe

Internet Subscribe to: **`mhe@otax.hut.fi`**

Description: Bird rarity reports and trip reports in Europe.

List Owner/Contact: Martin Helin <`mhe@otax.hut.fi`>

EVOLUTION

Evolutionary Biology Discussion List

Internet Subscribe to: `evolution-request@pogo.cqs.washington.edu`

Internet Mail to: **`evolution@pogo.cqs.washington.edu`**

Description: This group is intended for discussion of all matters pertaining to evolutionary biology. Questions, answers, comments, references, book reviews, even the occasional job opening, are welcome. All posts dealing with creation/evolution controversies, however, will be returned to the authors with the recommendation that they be submitted to the unmoderated Usenet newsgroup talk.origins. The Evolution list is also echoed to the Usenet newsgroup `sci.bio.evolution`.

List Owner/Contact: Josh Hayes <`josh@pogo.cqs.washington.edu`>
Center for Quantitative Sciences
University of Washington
Mail Stop HR-20
Seattle, WA 98195
Phone: 206-543-5004

EXTVET-L

State Extension Veterinarians Mailing List (restricted)

Internet Subscribe to: `listserv@unlvm.unl.edu`

Internet Mail to: **`extvet-l@unlvm.unl.edu`**

Description: This distribution list provides a timely transfer of information to Extension Veterinarians on current issues.

List Owners/Contact: William Sischo <`wms8@psuvm.psu.edu`>

FATFREE

Lowfat Vegetarianism Discussion List

Internet Subscribe to: `fatfree-request@hustle.rahul.net`

Internet Mail to: `fatfree@hustle.rahul.net`

Description: FATFREE, the McDougall/Ornish mailing list, is for discussion about extremely lowfat vegetarianism. For this list, very lowfat indicates diets with less than 15% of calories as fat. Vegetarian includes milk, eggs, and honey, but excludes all meat, fish, and poultry. Two main proponents of this style of diet are John McDougall and Dean Ornish. Members are encouraged to contribute recipes, testimonials, food news, requests, tips on dealing with family and friends, anecdotes, jokes, and questions of any sort at least mildly related to lowfat vegetarianism and living a healthy lifestyle (both McDougall and Ornish emphasize mild exercise and relaxation activities as part of a healthy lifestyle). This is not a moderated list.

List Owner/Contact: Michelle R. Dick <`fatfree-request@hustle.rahul.net`>

FELINE-L

Cat Fanciers Discussion List

Bitnet Subscribe to: `listserv@pccvm`

Internet Subscribe to: `listserv@psuvm.psu.edu`

Bitnet Mail to: `feline-l@pccvm`

Internet Mail to: `feline-l@psuvm.psu.edu`

Description: FELINE-L is a discussion list for and about cats; all kinds, types and varieties of cats. Postings ranging from care and feeding of your household tom or tabby to scientific research concerning any aspect of wild or domestic feline populations are welcome. If you wish to discuss training, human-feline psi experiences, cat "ghosts", seek a bit of comfort over the loss of a cherished cat, or find the best way to handle any aspect of cat ownership, you may reasonably expect to be welcome on FELINE-L. Managers and Administrators of any institution maintaining a feline population, such as zoos, game parks or research installations may discuss mutual problems and points of interest here. Graphic discussion of research techniques may be inappropriate for this list and offensive to some subscribers. Use good taste in what you post. Reasonable discussion of conservation and environmental issues, as they specifically relate to feline populations, are welcome here. The same holds true for almost any aspect of feline veterinary care and management.

List Owner/Contact: W.K. 'Bill' Gorman <`bj496@cleveland.freenet.edu`>

FERRET-LIST

Ferret Discussion List

Internet Subscribe to: `ferret-request@ferret.ocunix.on.ca`

Internet Mail to: `ferret-list@ferret.ocunix.on.ca`

Description: This is a mailing list for people who have or are merely interested in ferrets (Mustela Furo). Discussions are welcome on any subject relating to ferrets—suitability as pets, health information, funny ferret stories, advocacy, etc.

List Owner/Contact: Chris Lewis <`clewis@ferret.ocunix.on.ca`>
Phone: 613-832-0541

FIBROM-L

Fibromyalgia / Fibrositis Discussion Group

Bitnet Subscribe to: `listserv@uiucvmd`

Internet Subscribe to: `listserv@vmd.cso.uiuc.edu`

Bitnet Mail to: `fibrom-l@uiucvmd`

Internet Mail to: `fibrom-l@vmd.cso.uiuc.edu`

Description: FIBROM-L is a discussion forum for the disease/syndrome known as fibromyalgia / fibrositis. It is an opportunity for patients, family and friends of patients, physicians and researchers, and other interested persons to discuss this condition.

List Owners/Contact: Sandra Bott <sbott@vmd.cso.uiuc.edu>
David Ackerman <ackermdj@msuvx1.memst.edu>
Molly Mack <mollym@vmd.cso.uiuc.edu>

FISH-ECOLOGY

Fish and Fisheries Ecology

Bitnet Subscribe to: `listserv@searn`

Internet Subscribe to: `listserv@searn.sunet.se`

Bitnet Mail to: **`fish-ecology@searn`**

Internet Mail to: **`fish-ecology@searn.sunet.se`**

Description: FISH-ECOLOGY is an international computer conference for academic personnel & students involved in empirical and theoretical issues related to fish and fisheries ecology: Evolutionary aspects, population dynamics, modelling, management, conservation, bioeconomics, related software & hardware, reviews, symposium announcements, etc. Membership is open to all interested parties. Commercial announcements are, however, not desired. The list aims to stimulate connections between senior and junior researchers and students on an international and multidisciplinary basis, to exchange views, data and to put forward ideas to approach fisheries ecological issues.

List Owner/Contact: Aldo-Pier Solari <solaris@cicei.ulpgc.es>
Universidad de Las Palmas de G.C.

FISHERIES

Fisheries-related Mailing List

Internet Subscribe to: `majordomo@biome.bio.ns.ca`

Internet Mail to: **`fisheries@biome.bio.ns.ca`**

Description: This is for general discussion of fisheries-related issues, including stock dynamics and fisheries management.

List Owner/Contact: Bill Silvert <silvert@biome.bio.ns.ca>

FISHFOLK

Fisheries Social Science Network

Bitnet Subscribe to: `listserv@mitvma`

Internet Subscribe to: `listserv@mitvma.mit.edu`

Bitnet Mail to: **`fishfolk@mitvma`**

Internet Mail to: **`fishfolk@mitvma.mit.edu`**

List Owner/Contact: Madeleine Hall-Arber <arber@mit.edu>

FISH-JUNIOR

Forum between Marine Scientists and Students

Bitnet Subscribe to: `listserv@searn`

Internet Subscribe to: `listserv@searn.sunet.se`

Bitnet Mail to: **`fish-junior@searn`**

Internet Mail to: **`fish-junior@searn.sunet.se`**

Description: FISH-JUNIOR is a forum for knowledge transfer between marine scientists and children/high school students. The list was initially set up by the Swedish University Network (SUNET) on behalf of a Pilot Project to be conducted by the British Columbia Ministry of Education (Canada). The aim of this forum is to enable juniors of early age to interact with scientists and scientific issues mainly related to Fisheries ecology and related topics. The FISH-ECOLOGY management would like to encourage the participation of scientists, advisors, PhD students and other research personnel who would like to be involved as teachers in FISH-JUNIOR.

List Owner/Contact: Aldo-Pier Solari <solaris@searn.sunet.se>

FROG-NET

Amphibian Researcher Mailing List

Internet Subscribe to: `liaw@rana.usc.edu`

Internet Mail to: **`frog-net@rana.usc.edu`**

Description: This mailing list is set up to facilitate the communication and interactin among researchers interested in the behavior and the underlying neural mechanisms in amphibians.

List Owner/Contact: Jim Liaw `<liaw@rana.usc.edu>`
Center for Neural Engineering
Univ. of Southern California
Los Angeles, CA 90089-2520
Phone: 213-740-6991

FUNDLIST

University Fund Raising Discussion List

Bitnet Subscribe to: `listserv@jhuvm`

Internet Subscribe to: `listserv@jhuvm.hcf.jhu.edu`

Bitnet Mail to: **`fundlist@jhuvm`**

Internet Mail to: **`fundlist@jhuvm.hcf.jhu.edu`**

Description: A forum to exchange information relevant to computer support of fund raising programs at various Universities across the nation.

List Owner/Contact: Joe Meister `<jwm@jhudev.dev.jhu.edu>`

GOLDEN

Golden Retriever Mailing List

Internet Subscribe to: `golden-request@hobbes.ucsd.edu`

Internet Mail to: **`golden@hobbes.ucsd.edu`**

Description: A mailing list for Golden Retriever enthusiasts. Suitable topics include questions and answers regarding the Golden Retriever breed in general, news bits, article summaries, discussions of particular lines and breeders, shows, activities (CCI, therapy dogs, guide dogs), show bragging, summaries of local GR club activities or newsletters, other items which might be too Golden-introverted for rec.pets.dogs, & cooperation on a breed specific FAQ for r.p.d, etc.

List Owner/Contact: Wade Blomgren `<wade@hobbes.ucsd.edu>`

GOPHER JEWELS

Gopher Jewels List

Internet Subscribe to: `listproc@einet.net`

Internet Mail to: **`gopherjewels@einet.net`**

Description: A catalog of gopher sites by category (subject tree). Gopher sites are placed in particular categories as a result of finding related information buried somewhere in their hole. The list was established for the sharing of interesting gopher finds ONLY. This list expects subscribers that are either gopher developers or gopher users.

List Owner/Contact: David Riggins `<david.riggins@tpoint.com>`
Texas Department of Commerce
Office of Advanced Technology
Austin, Texas 78711
Phone: 512-320-9561

GRANT-L

Funding Alert List

Bitnet Subscribe to: `listserv@ua1vm`

Internet Subscribe to: `listserv@ua1vm.ua.edu`

Bitnet Mail to: **`grant-l@ua1vm`**

Internet Mail to: **grant-l@ua1vm.ua.edu**

List Owner/Contact: Bob Wells <sponprog@ua1vm.ua.edu>

GRANTS-L

National Science Foundation Grants & Contracts Bulletin Board

Bitnet Subscribe to: `listserv@jhuvm`

Internet Subscribe to: `listserv@jhuvm.hcf.jhu.edu`

Bitnet Mail to: **grants-l@jhuvm**

Internet Mail to: **grants-l@jhuvm.hcf.jhu.edu**

Description: This list redistributes all materials sent from the National Science Foundation via their Bulletin Board System to Bitnet addresses.

List Owner/Contact: Jim Jones <jimj@jhuvm.hcf.jhu.edu>
Mary Ann Messier <grants-r@nsf.bitnet>
Phone: 202-357-7880

GRNSCH-L

Green School List

Bitnet Subscribe to: `listserv@brownvm`

Internet Subscribe to: `listserv@brownvm.brown.edu`

Bitnet Mail to: **grnsch-l@brownvm**

Internet Mail to: **grnsch-l@brownvm.brown.edu**

List Owner/Contact: Kurt Teichert <kurtt@brownvm.brown.edu>

GSA

Genetic Stock Administrator's Discussion Group

Bitnet Subscribe to: `listserv@iubvm`

Internet Subscribe to: `listserv@iubvm.ucs.indiana.edu`

Bitnet Mail to: **gsa@iubvm**

Internet Mail to: **gsa@iubvm.ucs.indiana.edu**

Description: Welcome to the Genetic Stock Administrator's Discussion Group. The list is open and unmoderated. An archive of GSA discussion is maintained on the IUBio Archive for Biology, available through gopher or by anonymous ftp. IUBio's ftp address is `ftp.bio.indiana.edu`; gsa-archive can be found in `archive/molbio/data`. The GSA list was prompted by stock collection curators' need for information about effective methods of electronic data distribution. We encourage the participation of geneticists, computer scientists, database specialists, and archive administrators, with the hope of providing a useful forum for the exchange of information, ideas, and feedback related to all aspects of the distribution of genetic data.

List Owner/Contact: Kathy Matthews <matthewk@fly.bio.indiana.edu>
Department of Biology
Indiana University
Bloomington, IN 47405

HEEN-LIST

Human Evolution Education Network

Internet Subscribe to: `heen-list-request@uclink.berkeley.edu`

Internet Mail to: **heen-list@uclink.berkeley.edu**

Description: The Human Evolution Education Network, a project of the National Center for Science Education, is starting a maillist for members to share information on working with k-12 schools to educate students on human origins. Heen-list is a forum for professional anthropologists, primatologists, biologists, and others to share information on how they, as professionals, can use their experience and education as a resource for educators and young students in their areas. The list can particularly benefit from having members of different experience levels; some HEEN members have worked extensively in the schools, and others are curious about how they could become involved. Like the HEEN Newsletter _Missing Link_, heen-list is for you to share your ideas, successes, and frustrations. Not only can you be a resource for schools, you can be a resource for your colleagues as well. Heen-list is non-automated; you will not receive immediate confirmation of you subscription, but your name and address will be added to heen-list within a few days of your subscription message. Let us know your name and e-mail address. Since it is non-automated, the format doesn't matter much. Also, please let us know if you would like to be added to the "Missing Link" newsletter mailing list.

List Owner/Contact: Anne Hayes <mayo@uclink.berkeley.edu>
Human Evolution Education Network
National Center for Science Education
Post Office Box 9477
Berkeley, California 94709
Phone: (510) 526-1674
Fax: (510) 526-1675

HERP-L

Herpetology Mailing List

Internet Subscribe to: `listproc@xtal200.harvard.edu`

Internet Mail to: **herp-l@xtal200.harvard.edu**

Description: This mailing list is for disscussion of scientific issues related to herpetology (ecology, evolution, conservation, behavior, systematics, biogeography, etc.) This list cross-posts to the USENET newsgroup `sci.bio.herp`.

Contact: Michael Eisen <eisen@xtal220.harvard.edu>
Program in Biophysics
Harvard University
Phone: 617-495-4091
Fax: 617-495-9613

HMATRIX-L

Online health resources discussion

Internet Subscribe to: `listserv@ukanaix.cc.ukans.edu`

Internet Mail to: **hmatrix-l@ukanaix.cc.ukans.edu**

Description: HMatrix-L is an Internet discussion list concerning online health resources. The primary focus is on Internet/BitNet/UseNet health information, but any electronically accessible service of interest to those involved in health/medical activities, i.e., academic, clinical, research, medical librarians, patients, and interested lay persons, is open for discussion. The intent is to share and document the location, access instructions and quality of information found online. A further purpose is to increase the sharing of resources (i.e., information, search techniques, images, multimedia files, tutorials, etc.) among the health community.

Contact: Lee Hancock <le07144@ukanvm.cc.ukans.edu>
Educational Technologist
University of Kansas Medical Center
Archie R. Dykes Library
3901 Rainbow Blvd.
Kansas City, KS 66160-7181
Phone: 913-588-7144

HOPOS-L

History of the Philosophy of Science Discussion List

Bitnet Subscribe to: `listserv@ukcc`

Internet Subscribe to: `listserv@ukcc.uky.edu`

Bitnet Mail to: **hopos-l@ukcc**

Internet Mail to: **hopos-l@ukcc.uky.edu**

Description: HOPOS-L, the History of Philosophy of Science Discussion List, has been established in conjunction with the new History of Philosophy of Science Working Group (HOPOS) as a forum for the exchange of information, ideas, queries, job notices, course syllabi, conference announcements, and other news of interest to scholars working in areas related to HOPOS's main focus. The discussion list will also be used to distribute occasional HOPOS newsletters.

List Owner/Contact: Don Howard <einphil@ukcc.uky.edu>
Department of Philosophy
University of Kentucky
Lexington, Kentucky 40506-0027
Phone: 606-257-4376
Fax: 606-258-1073

HORSE

Equestrian Discussion List

Internet Subscribe to: `equestrians-request@world.std.com`

Description: Discussion of things equestrian. Horse enthusiasts of all disciplines and levels of experience are welcome. Articles are distributed periodically in digest format, and also appear individually in the Usenet newsgroup "rec.equestrian".

List Owner/Contact: David C. Kovar <equestrians-request@world.std.com>

HPSST-L

History and Philosophy of Science and Science Teaching

Bitnet Subscribe to: `listserv@qucdn`

Internet Subscribe to: `listserv@qucdn.queensu.ca`

Bitnet Mail to: **hpsst-l@qucdn**

Internet Mail to: **hpsst-l@qucdn.queensu.ca**

Description: HPSST-L is an outgrowth of two international conferences on the History and Philosophy of Science and Science Teaching. This group included science teachers, science teacher educators, educational policy makers, scientists, and historians, philosophers, psychologists and sociologists of science. The broad purpose of this group is to foster collaboration in exploring ways in which the 'social studies' of science, including, history, philosophy, psychology and sociology of science has, and can contribute to the preparation of science teachers, the development of curricula, the enhancement of science education, and the development of a more scientifically literate community by making science and technology more accessible and attractive not only to young people but also to the public at large. Discussions to date have ranged over the teaching and learning of science and mathematics from the elementary school to the graduate school. Some possible areas of conversation may be: Science, Technology and Society; Curriculum Reform and Teacher Education; Science Education and the Environment; Scientific Literacy; Exemplary Practice in Science Education and Science Teacher Education; Values and Science Education; Women and Science; Science and Culture; Cognitive Science and Conceptual Change; & Constructivism.

List Owners/Contact: Skip Hills <hillss@qucdn.queensu.ca>
Faculty of Education
Queen's University
Kingston, Ontario, K7L 3N6
Phone: 613-545-6208
Fax: 613-545-6584

Doug Farquhar <farquhad@qucdn.queensu.ca>

HUMBIO-L

Biological Anthropology, Primate Biology & Behavior

Bitnet Subscribe to: `mailserv@fauvax`

Internet Subscribe to: `mailserv@acc.fau.edu`

Bitnet Mail to: **humbio-l@fauvax**

Internet Mail to: `humbio-l@acc.fau.edu`

Description: Deals with biological anthropology, adaptation, environmental stress, biological race, growth, genetics, paleoanthropology, skeletal biology, forensic anthropology, paleodemography, apleopathology, primate biology and behavior.

List Owners/Contact: Ralph P. Carpenter `<ralpho@acc.fau.edu>`
    N.Y. Iscan `<iscan@acc.fau.edu>`
    Florida Atlantic University

HUMEVO

Human Evolutionary Research Discussion List

Bitnet Subscribe to: `listserv@gwuvm`

Internet Subscribe to: `listserv@gwuvm.bitnet`

Bitnet Mail to: `humevo@gwuvm`

Internet Mail to: `humevo@gwuvm.bitnet`

Description: Human evolutionary research discussion examines human biological evolution, adaptation, variation, and evolutionary medicine.

List Owner/Contact: Noel T. Boaz `<boaz@gwuvm.bitnet>`

HUNTING

Hunting Discussion List

Bitnet Subscribe to: `listserv@tamvm1`

Internet Subscribe to: `listserv@tamvm1.tamu.edu`

Bitnet Mail to: `hunting@tamvm1`

Internet Mail to: `hunting@tamvm1.tamu.edu`

Description: This is a reflection of the moderated Usenet group `rec.hunting` for those folks that prefer to read this group via mail instead of a newsreader. `Rec.hunting` (and the LISTSERV list hunting) is a moderated group for the discussion of hunting related issues. These include, but are not limited to, methods, locations, seasons, laws, and hunting ethics. Posts about the morality of hunting will be rejected.

List Owner/Contact: Chris Barnes `<cbarnes@tamvm1.tamu.edu>`
    President—Bryan/College Station Retriever Club
    Phone: 409-845-8300

IAMSLIC

Intl. Assn. of Aquatic & Marine Science Libraries & Information Centers

Internet Subscribe to: `listserv@ucsd.edu`
    In body of the email message, enter: subscribe your E-Mail address IAMSLIC

Internet Mail to: `iamslic@ucsd.edu`

List Owner/Contact: Peter Brueggeman `<pbruggeman@ucsd.edu>`
    Head of Public Services
    Scripps Institution of Oceanography Library
    University of California San Diego

ICAM-L

Integrated Coastal Area Management

Bitnet Subscribe to: `listserv@irmfao01`

Internet Subscribe to: `listserv@irmfao01.bitnet`

Bitnet Mail to: `icam-l@irmfao01`

Internet Mail to: `icam-l@irmfao01.bitnet`

Description: Food and Agriculture Organization of the U.N. Fishery Development Planning Service Integrated Coastal Area Management Discussion List

List Owners/Contact: A.I. Insull `<fippai@irmfao01.bitnet>`
    G. de Manicor `<fidi23@irmfao01.bitnet>`

IRNES

Interdisciplinary Research Network on the Environment & Society

Internet Subscribe to: **mailbase@mailbase.ac.uk**

Description: Communication channel for members of the Interdisciplinary Research Network on the Environment and Society. IRNES is open to all those who have an interest in the interplay between the ecosystem and its sub-unit that we call society. The network is made up of young researchers in this field.

    ListOwner/Contact:<irnes-request@mailbase.ac.uk>

IUBS

International Union of Biological Societies

Internet subscribe to: **listserv@life.anu.edu.au**

Internet Mail to: **iubs@life.anu.edu.au**

List Owner/Contact: Ian Noble <noble@life.anu.edu.au>
    Ecosystem Dynamics Group
    Research School of Biological Sciences
    Australian National University
    GPO Box 475
    Canberra 2601 AUSTRALIA
    Phone: 61-6-249-4020

JAPAN PRIMATE NEWSLETTER

Internet Subscribe to: **yamagiwa@pri.kyoto-u.ac.jp**

Description: The Japan Primate Newsletter is a publication of the Conservation Committee of the Primate Society of Japan.

List Owner/Contact: J. Yamagiwa <yamagiwa@pri.kyoto-u.ac.jp>
    Kyoto University Primate Research Institute
    Inuyama, Aichi 484, Japan
    Phone: 81-568-61-2891
    Fax: 81-568-62-2428

KILLIFISH

Killifish (F. Cyprinodontidae) Mailing List

Internet Subscribe to: **killies-request@mejac.palo-alto.ca.us**

Internet Mail to: **killies@mejac.palo-alto.ca.us**

LACTACID

Lactic Acid Bacteria Forum

Bitnet Subscribe to: **listserv@searn**

Internet Subscribe to: **listserv@searn.sunet.se**

Bitnet Mail to: **lactacid@searn**

Internet Mail to: **lactacid@searn.sunet.se**

Description: Lactic Acid Bacteria Forum discusses and exchanges information on ALL aspects related to the BIOLOGY and USES of lactic acid bacteria e.g., in human beings and animals (e.g., in new-borns, oral cavity, vaginal tract, etc.) in fermented foods (cheese, pickles, sauerkraut, etc) in animal feeds (ensilage), in the production of polysaccharides and other (e.g., idextran).

ListOwner/Contact: Eng-Leong Foo <eng-leong_foo_mircen-ki%micforum@mica.mic.ki.se>
    UNESCO Microbial Resources Center
    Karolinska Institute
    Stockholm, Sweden

LATIN-BIONEWS

Latin-Bionet Electronic Newsletter

Internet Subscribe to: **latinbio@fiocruz.bitnet**

Description: The Latin-Bionet electronic newsletter is published through the Department of Biochemistry and Molecular Biology of the Oswaldo Cruz Foundation at Rio de Janeiro, Brazil. It is distributed through electronic mail to Latin-American scientists and interested researchers in other parts of the world.

List Owners/Contact: Wim Degrave <wim@fiocruz.bitnet>
Carlos Morel <morel@fiocruz.bitnet>
DBBM—Fiocruz
Av. Brasil 4365—Manguinhos
Rio de Janeiro, RJ
21045-900 Brazil
Phone: 55-21-2907549
Fax: 55-21-5903495

LEISH-L

International Leishmaniasis Network

Internet Subscribe to: listserv@bdt.ftpt.br

Internet Mail to: **leish-l@bdt.ftpt.br**

Description: Discusses the various fields of leishmaniasis, such as lists of strains, cryobanks, research workers (fields of interest and contract address), projects, monoclonal antibodies, sequences of specific DNA regions and primers, epidemiology, parasites/vector catalogue, immunology reactions related to infection—experimental and natural, treatment, diagnosis, drug resistance, host resistance, control (methods, countries and responsible governmental body) etc., will either be included in the form of databases that are resident in the Network or indications will be given as to where you might be able to find what you are looking for:

ListOwner/Contact: Jeffrey Show <jeffrey@bdt.ftpt.br>
Phone: 55-91-226-8631
Fax: 55-91-226-6997

L-ETHO

Ethologistes/Ethologists

Bitnet Subscribe to: listserv@uqam

Internet Subscribe to: listserv%uqam.bitnet@cunyvm.cuny.edu

Bitnet Mail to: **l-etho@uqam**

Internet Mail to: **l-etho%uqam.bitnet@cunyvm.cuny.edu**

List Owner/Contact: Jacques Beaugrand <r20370@uqam.bitnet>

LPN-L

Laboratory Primate Newsletter List

Bitnet Subscribe to: listserv@brownvm

Internet Subscribe to: listserv@brownvm.brown.edu

Description: This is a network distribution of the Laboratory Primate Newsletter, which is a central source of information about nonhuman primates and related topics for scientists who use these animals in their research and for those whose work supports such research.

List Owner/Contact: Judith Schrier **<primate@brownvm.brown.edu>**

LYMENET-L

Lyme Disease Newsletter

Internet Subscribe to: listserv@lehigh.edu

Internet Mail to: **lymenet-l@lehigh.edu**

Description: The Lyme Disease Electronic Mail Network publishes the "LymeNet Newsletter" once every 10-15 days. The Newsletter contains timely news about the Lyme disease epidemic. Medical abstracts, treatment protocols, prevention information, and political happenings are all included. In addition, subscribers may ask questions to the patients, doctors and researchers on the net.

List Owner/Contact: Marc Gabriel <mcg2@lehigh.edu>

MAMMALOGISTS ON EMAIL
American Society of Mammalogists

Bitnet Subscribe to: `mnhvz049@sivm`

Internet Subscribe to: **`mnhvz049@sivm.si.edu`** (Editor)

List Owner/Contact: Richard W. Thorington, Jr. <`mnhvz049@sivm.si.edu`>
Department of Vertebrate Zoology
NHB-390, Smithsonian Institution
Washington, DC 20560
Phone: 202-357-2150
Fax: 202-357-4779

MAR-FACIL
Marine Facilities, Aquaculture, Aquaria

Internet Subscribe to: **`mailserv@ac.dal.ca`**

Internet Mail to: **`mar-facil@ac.dal.ca`**

Description: MAR-FACIL is a mailing list for managers and technical staff at marine research facilities, aquaculture operations, public aquaria and other facilities supplying seawater for the support of marine life. The list is intended as a forum for the discussion of technical and business topics, however discussion of other matters is welcome and encouraged. The list is managed by the staff of the Aquatron Laboratory which is situated at Dalhousie University in Halifax, Nova Scotia, Canada. The Aquatron is a specialized marine research facility providing scientists the opportunity to control the environmental variables of large volumes of water. The list will be of primary interest to those individuals who are involved in the operation of similar marine facilities and those who use such facilities for research.

List Owner/Contact: John Stratton <`stratton@ac.dal.ca`>

MARINE-L
Marine Studies/Shipboard Education List

Bitnet Subscribe to: `listserv@uoguelph`

Internet Subscribe to: `listserv@vm.uoguelph.ca`

Bitnet Mail to: **`marine-l@uoguelph`**

Internet Mail to: **`marine-l@vm.uoguelph.ca`**

Description: Marine Studies/Shipboard Education Discussion group addresses the development of Marine-related studies, Semester-at-Sea/Education-at-Sea programs, and the development of e-mail connectivity at sea. Interest areas include: Marine electronic communications/networking/maintenance; Coastal/Marine Database; Marine Parks and Coastal National Parks; General coastal and marine ecosystems; Marine zoology and biology; Aquaculture; Ocean environmental sciences; Ocean and atmospheric sciences; Marine sciences research stations and marine museums; Maritime academies and sail-training; Marine engineering and ship design, shipbuilding, and shipyard management; Fisheries science; Stellar navigation; Satellite oceanography; Blue-water sailing and ship maintenance; History of Sea Education; Traditional navigation methods around the world; Co-operative links between Sea-Education programs; Ocean racing; Marine/maritime publishing and publications; Submersible design; Shipping movements; Ocean research, funding, grants and awards; Oceania and maritime anthropology; International shipboard/port relations; Intercultural communications; Ocean resources management and ocean industries; Weather information transmission and information storage/retrieval; Ham and marine radio communications.

List Owners/Contact: Ted White <`zoowhite@vm.uoguelph.ca`>
Melcir Erskine-Richmond <`globalcp%cue.bc.ca@uvvm.uvic.ca`>

MARINE-TECH
Marine Technology in the U.K.

Internet Subscribe to: `mailbase@mailbase.ac.uk`

Internet Mail to: **`marine-tech@mailbase.ac.uk`**

Description: The aim of this list is to promote contact and discussion amongst the research community of the U.K. who are involved in the field of Marine Technology. This list is open to all people connected with the field of Marine Technology, be their interest in structural analysis, hydrodynamics, marine engineering, optimisation, fishery studies, or oceanography.

List Owner/Contact: <marine-tech-request@mailbase.ac.uk>
Dave Thomas <dave.thomas@newcastle.ac.uk>
Mesut Guner <mesut.guner@newcastle.ac.uk>
Department of Marine Technology
Armstrong Building
Newcastle University
Newcastle upon Tyne
NE1 7RU

MARMAM

Marine Mammal Research & Conservation Discussion List

Bitnet Subscribe to: `listserv@uvvm`

Internet Subscribe to: `listserv@uvvm.uvic.ca`

Bitnet Mail to: **marmam@uvvm**

Internet Mail to: **marmam@uvvm.uvic.ca**

Description: A marine mammal research and conservation e-mail discussion list has been established, using the listserver at the University of Victoria. The purpose of this is to facilitate discussion regarding research and conservation of marine mammals, as well as for posting conference or meeting announcements, volunteer opportunities, new techniques or equipment available, new books published, etc.

List Owners/Contact: David Duffus <ddvffvs@uvvm.uvic.ca>
Robin Baird <rbaird@sfu.ca>

MARVADEL

Mid Atlantic Birders Discussion Group

Internet Subscribe to: `marvadel-request@osi.ncsl.nist.gov`

Internet Mail to: **marvadel@osi.ncsl.nist.gov**

Description: MARVADEL is an electronic discussion group for birders of all descriptions in Maryland, Virginia, Delaware and surrounding areas. The group will concentrate on local birding issues and events, such as interesting sightings, advice on local birding hotspots, announcements of local bird club meetings, events and exhibitions, planning of days out and joint birding expeditions. MARVADEL is open to all individuals with a sense of humor and an interest in wild birds in the mid-Atlantic region.

List Owner/Contact: John Tebbutt <tebbutt@rhino.ncsl.nist.gov>

MEDNETS

Medical Telecommunications Network List

Bitnet Subscribe to: `listserv@ndsuvm1`

Internet Subscribe to: `listserv@vm1.nodak.edu`

Bitnet Mail to: **mednets@ndsuvm1**

Internet Mail to: **mednets@vm1.nodak.edu**

Description: A forum to discuss medical telecommunication networks in the areas of clinical practice, medical research, and administration. The list is intended to be used for ongoing discussions, information searches, contact searches, surveys, and so on.

List Owner/Contact: Marty Hoag <nu021172@vm1.nodak.edu>

MEDNEWS

Health Info-Com Network (HICN) Newsletter

Bitnet Subscribe to: `listserv@asuacad`

Internet Subscribe to: `listserv@asuvm.inre.asu.edu`

Description: The MEDNEWS LISTSERV list is for distribution of the Health Info-Com Network medical newsletter. It is distributed weekly and contains the latest MMWR from the Center for Disease Control, weekly AIDS Statistics, FDA bulletins, medical news from the United Nations, and other assorted medical news items. Submissions for the newsletter are welcomed; please contact the Editor if you have any questions or newsletter submissions. Also gateways to Usenet Newsgroup bit.listserv.mednews

List Owner/Contact: David Dodell <david@stat.com>
FAX: 602-451-6135

MEDSEA-L
Marine Biology of the Adriatic Sea List

Bitnet Subscribe to: `listserv@aearn`

Internet Subscribe to: `listserv@aearn.edvz.univie.ac.at`

Bitnet Mail to: **medsea-l@aearn**

Internet Mail to: **medsea-l@aearn.edvz.univie.ac.at**

Description: The goal of the list is to increase our knowledge on processes controlling life in the Adriatic Sea. Special emphasis is put on the interactions between eutrophication phenomena and foodweb structures. Another main object of research interest are investigations on marine snow and mucilage as mucoid aggregates in the water column of the Northern Adriatic Sea are more abundant than in any other regions of the world's oceans.

List Owner/Contact: Osiander Meixner <meixner@nestroy.wu-wien.ac.at>

MEH2O-L
Middle East Water List

Bitnet Subscribe to: `listserv@taunivm`

Internet Subscribe to: `listserv@vm.tau.ac.il`

Bitnet Mail to: **meh2o-l@taunivm**

Internet Mail to: **meh2o-l@vm.tau.ac.il**

Description: Discussion group for information and research related to water in the Middle East. Possible topics include, but are not limited to: limnology; oceanography; marine biotechnology; aquaculture (marine and freshwater); conservation; reclamation; wetlands development; ecological aspects; shared resource management; notice of upcoming conference and seminars.

List Owner/Contact: Robert Chasan <chasan@hujiagri.huji.ac>
National Center for Mariculture
P.O. Box 1212
Eilat, Israel

METHODS
Biomedical Research Methodology Discussion List

Bitnet Subscribe to: `comserve@rpitsvm`

Internet Subscribe to: `comserve@vm.its.rpi.edu`

Bitnet Mail to: **methods@rpitsvm**

Internet Mail to: **methods@vm.its.rpi.edu**

Description: Discusses issues, share ideas and news items, ask questions, or ask for resources.

List Owner/Contact: Comserve Support Staff <support@vm.its.vpi.edu>

MGI-LIST
Mouse Genome Informatics Group

Internet Subscribe to: `listserver@informatics.jax.org`

Internet Mail to: **mgi-list@informatics.jax.org**

Description: MGI-LIST is for announcements and general discussion of bioinformatics and the mouse genome.

List Owner/Contact: <list-manager@informatics.jax.org>

MINI-JIR
Mini Journal of Irreproducible Results

Bitnet Subscribe to: `listserv@mitvma`

Internet Subscribe to: `listserv@mitvma.mit.edu`

Bitnet Mail to: **`mini-jir@mitvma`**

Internet Mail to: **`mini-jir@mitvma.mit.edu`**

Description: MINI-JIR is the Official Electronic mini-Organ of the Society for Basic Irreproducible Research, produced jointly by The Journal of Irreproducible Results (JIR) and The MIT Museum. The mini-Journal of Irreproducible Results publishes news about overly stimulating research and ideas. Specifically: Haphazardly selected superficial (but advanced!) extracts of research news and satire from the Journal of Irreproducible Results (JIR); News about the annual Ig Nobel Prize ceremony. Ig Nobel Prizes honor "achievements that cannot or should not be reproduced." A public ceremony is held at MIT, in Cambridge Massachusetts, every autumn. The ceremony is sponsored jointly by JIR and by the MIT Museum; and News about other science humor activities conducted by the MIT Museum and JIR.

List Owners/Contact: Marc Abrahams <`jir@mit.edu`>
Marilyn Geller <`mgeller@mit.edu`>

MODEL-HORSE
Model Horse Hobby Discussion List

Internet Subscribe to: `majordomo@qiclab.scn.rain.com`

Internet Mail to: **`model-horse@qiclab.scn.rain.com`**

Description: Discussion of the model horse hobby. All aspects of showing (live and photo), collecting, remaking/repainting for all breeds and makes are discussed. All ages and levels of experience welcome.

List Owner/Contact: Darci L. Chapman <`model-horse-approval@qiclab.scn.rain.com`>

MOLLUSCA
Molluscan Phylogeny & Systematics Discussion List

Internet Subscribe to: `listserv@ucmp1.berkeley.edu`

Internet Mail to: **`mollusca@ucmp1.berkeley.edu`**

Description: Discussion of phylogenetic hypotheses and the construction of classifications within the Mollusca at all taxonomic levels. The list is to foster greater interaction between researchers from different methodological and philosophical backgrounds by welcoming viewpoints from ethology, molecular biology, anatomical and ultrastructural investigations, developmental biology, paleontology, theoretical biology, and any others.

List Owners/Contact: David Lindberg
R. Guralnick
University of California
Museum of Paleontology
Berkeley, CA

MORPHMET
Biological Morphometrics Discussion Group

Bitnet Subscribe to: `listserv@cunyvm`

Internet Subscribe to: `listserv@cunyvm.cuny.edu`

Bitnet Mail to: **`morphmet@cunyvm`**

Internet Mail to: **`morphmet@cunyvm.cuny.edu`**

Description: Biological Morphometrics discuss geometric and new morphometrics, the analysis of size and shape of organisms. For biologists and statisticians.

List Owners/Contact: Leslie F. Marcus <`lamqc@cunyvm.cuny.edu`>
Bill Gruber <`bigcu@cunyvm.cuny.edu`>

MOUNET
Minnesota Ornithologists Union Members

Internet Subscribe to: **wncarols@vax2.winona.msus.edu**

Description: An informal network of Minnesota Ornithologists Union members.

List Owner/Contact: Carol Schumacher <wncarols@vax2.winona.msus.edu>

NATRESLIB-L
Natural Resources Librarians and Information Specialists Discussion Group

Internet Subscribe to: annhed@cc.usu.edu

    Internet Mail to: **natreslib-l@cc.usu.edu**

Description: This new list exists to provide a medium for interaction between Natural Resource Librarians and Information Specialists. All issues, questions, brainstorming, or discussions pertaining to natural resources librarianship are welcome on this unmoderated list.

List Owner/Contact: Anne Hedrich <annhed@cc.usu.edu>
                         Merrill Library
                         Utah State University
                         Logan, Utah 84322-3000

NATURA-L
Ecology and Environmental Protection in Chile

Bitnet Subscribe to: listserv@uchcecvm

Internet Subscribe to: listserv@uchcecvm.cec.uchile.cl

Bitnet Mail to: **natura-l@uchcecvm**

Internet Mail to: **natura-l@uchcecvm.cec.uchile.cl**

Description: (Chile Spanish Language) Ecologia y Proteccion de la Naturaleza en Chile/Latinoamerica. Esta lista pretende abarcar temas sobre todo lo que implica la proteccion de la Naturaleza principalmente en nuestro pais y latinoamerica y tambien en el resto del mundo. La intencion es contar con un medio de difusion y discusion acerca de este tema y en lo posible incentivar al buen uso de nuestros recursos naturales y al respeto por toda forma de vida animal y vegetal.

NEUCHILE
Chile Neurociencias
    Neurosciences in Chile

Bitnet Subscribe to: listserv@yalevm

Internet Subscribe to: listserv@yalevm.cis.yale.edu

Bitnet Mail to: **neuchile@yalevm**

Internet Mail to: **neuchile@yalevm.cis.yale.edu**

Description: (Chile Spanish Language) Esta lista tiene el proposito de ayudar la cooperacion entre cientificos chilenos.

List Owners/Contact: Adrian Palacios <palacios@minerva.cis.yale.edu>
                              Juan Carlos Letelier <letelier@abello.seci.uchile.cl>

NEURO1-L
Neuroscience Information Exchange Forum

Bitnet Subscribe to: listserv@uicvm

Internet Subscribe to: listserv@uicvm.uic.edu

Bitnet Mail to: **neuro1-l@uicvm**

Internet Mail to: **neuro1-l@uicvm.uic.edu**

Description: Neuro1-L has several functions. One is to improve everyday communication and interchange between neuroscientists. The forum promotes ongoing discussions of current issues in Neuroscience. NEURO1-L provides a stimulus for "doing neuroscience" in a more interactive, global way.

List Owner/Contact: E.J. Neafsey <#m01ejn@luccpua.bitnet>
Neuroscience Graduate Program
Department of Cell Biology, Neurobiology & Anatomy
Loyola University Chicago Medical Center
2160 S. First Ave.
Maywood, IL 60153
Phone: 708-216-3355

NEURON-DIGEST
Neural Networks List

Internet Subscribe to: neuron-request@psych.upenn.edu

Internet Mail to: **neuron-request@psych.upenn.edu**

Description: Discussion on all aspects of neural networks. Topics include both artificial neural networks and biological systems: Natural Systems, Software Simulations, Neurobiology, Hardware, Neuroscience, Artifical Systems, Neural Networks, Optical, Algorithms, Cellular Automatons. Any contribution in these areas is accepted. Any of the following types of items are reasonable: Abstracts, Reviews, Lab Descriptions, Research Overviews, Work Planned or in Progress, Half-Baked Ideas, Conference Announcements, Conference Reports, Bibliographies, History Connectionism, Puzzles and Unsolved Problems, Anecdotes, Jokes, and Poems, Queries annd Requests, Address Changes. Also has gateway to Usenet Newsgroup comp.ai.neural-nets.

List Owner/Contact: Peter Marvit <neuron-request@psych.upenn.edu>

NIBNEWS
Biology and Medical Informatics Newsletter

Internet Subscribe to: **listserv@ccsun.unicamp.br**

Description: A biomedical informatics monthly newsletter. Covers Brazilian (and eventually south-american) activities, people, information, events, publications, software, and computer applications in healthcare, medicine and biology.

List Owner/Contact: Renato Sabbatini <sabbatini@ccvax.unicamp.br>
Center for Biomedical Informatics
State University of Campinas
P.O. Box 6005
Campinas, SP 13081—BRAZIL
Phone: +55 192 39-7130
Fax: +55 192 39-4717

NIHDIS-L
NIH Guide Discussion List

Bitnet Subscribe to: listserv@jhuvm

Internet Subscribe to: listserv@jhuvm.hcf.jhu.edu

Bitnet Mail to: **nihdis-l@jhuvm**

Internet Mail to: **nihdis-l@jhuvm.hcf.jhu.edu**

Description: This is a discussion list for institutional hubs who are participating in the E-Guide program and others who are interested in sharing information about how E-Guide material is used at the institutional level to disseminate and make available NIH policy information.

List Owner/Contact: Jim Jones <jimj@jhuvm.hcf.jhu.edu>

NIHGDE-L
NIH Guide Primary Distribution

Bitnet Subscribe to: listserv@jhuvm

Internet Subscribe to: listserv@jhuvm.hcf.jhu.edu

Bitnet Mail to: **nihgde-l@jhuvm**

Internet Mail to: **nihgde-l@jhuvm.hcf.jhu.edu**

Description: This List controls the PRIMARY DISTRIBUTION of the electronic form of the "NIH Guide for Grants & Contracts" from the NIH to institutions participating in this program. As the program is currently defined, each institution on this list will receive one copy of each publication sent and is in turn responsible for "redistributing" or "making available" the publication for others at that institution by whatever means the institution deems appropriate. This list has no formal peers, however some "institutional representatives" on this list are LOCAL List Server lists. These lists may have different list header options than this list and are not managed by the NIH.

List Owners/Contact: Becky Duvall <q2c@nihcu.bitnet>
Institutional Liason Office
National Institutes of Health
Building 31, Room 5B31
9000 Rockville Pike
Bethesda, MD 20892
Phone: 301-496-5366

Bill Jones <wkj@nihcu.bitnet>
John Elrod <jpe@jhuspo.ca.jhu.edu>
Kevin Callahan <kcd@nihcu.bitnet>

NIHTOC-L
NIH Grants Table of Contents List

Bitnet Subscribe to: `listserv@nihlist`

Internet Subscribe to: `listserv@list.nih.gov`

Description: Some users who subscribed to the NIHGDE-L list had problems with the volume of mail that was received each week. They would prefer to see a table of contents, and access the NIH Guide files via Gopher when necessary. For that purpose, the NIHTOC-L list has been established at the NIH. It will contain only the table of contents for each week's NIH Guide.

List Owner/Contact: Myra Brockett <q2c@cu.nih.gov>
Institutional Affairs Office
National Institutes of Health
Building 1, Room 328
Bethesda, MD 20892

OBED-L
Obedience, tracking, agility and schutzhund interests

Internet Subscribe to: `listserver@reepicheep.gcn.uoknor.edu`

Internet Mail to: `obed-l@reepicheep.gcn.uoknor.edu`

Description: This group discusses all issues related to training dogs, particularly for AKC and UKC obedience trials. Canine good citizenship, temperament testing and therapy dog training are also discussed as well as less formal issues.

List Owner/Contact: Mike Richman <richman@reepicheep.gcn.uoknor.edu>

OBOL
Oregon Birders OnLine

Internet Subscribe to: `majordomo@mail.orst.edu`

Internet Mail to: `obol@mail.orst.edu`

Description: A regional mailing list targeted at Birders from Oregon. The purpose of OBOL is to keep its members up-to-date on unusual and rare birds seen recently in Oregon. Rare Bird Alerts should be posted here right away. The Portland Audubon Rare Bird Alert weekly phone message is posted, usually on Thursday. Unusual sightings from the past weekend's birding is welcome. Postings of field trips, bird count announcements, etc. also belong on this list.

List Owner/Contact: Greg Gillson <gregg@tdd.hbo.nec.com>

OCC-ENV-MED-L
Occupational & Environmental Medicine Mailing List

Internet Subcribe to: `mailserv@mc.duke.edu`

Internet Mail to: **occ-env-med-l@mc.duke.edu**

Description: Occupational & Environmental medicine represents a growing clinical and public health discipline, seeking to evaluate and prevent the diseseases and health effects that may be related to exposures at work and from other environments (e.g., pollution). The Occup-Env Med Mail-list provides a moderated forum for announcements, dissemination of text files and academic discussion. The forum is designed to allow presentation of clinical vignettes, synopses of new regulatory issues and reports of interesting items from publications elsewhere (both the medical and the non-medical journals). The Association of Occupational & Environmental Clinics represents the first nucleus of members for the list, and will use the list for announcements. AOEC members are either: A) interested clinics with approved credentials documenting expertise in Occupational & Environmental Medicine or B) individuals interested in sharing this topic, but who have no requirement to show advanced training or expertise Professional affiliations of the Mail-list subscribers will include: Occupational Physicians and Nurses, Industrial Hygienists, Government Public Health officials, University investigators, and regulators in Occupational & Environmental medical diseases.

List Owner/Contact: Gary Greenberg, MD <`green011@mc.duke.edu`>

OCEANTECH
Scripps Institution of Oceanography's Ocean Technology Forum

Internet Subscribe to: `listserv@ucsd.edu`
   In body of the email message, enter: subscribe your E-Mail address OCEANTECH

Internet Mail to: **oceantech@ucsd.edu**

Description: The OCEANTECH conference is an international informal computer conference for discussion of applied technology-related topics in freshwater, marine, and brackishwater environments. Conference membership is open to all interested parties.

Contact: Kevin Hardy <`khardy@ucsd.edu`>
   University of California—San Diego
   Scripps Institution of Oceanography

ONE-L
Organization and the Natural Environment Discussion List

Bitnet Subscribe to: `listserv@clvm`

Internet Subscribe to: `listserv@clvm.clarkson.edu`

Bitnet Mail to: **one-l@clvm**

Internet Mail to: **one-l@clvm.clarkson.edu**

List Owner/Contact: Gary Throop <`throop@clvm.clarkson.edu`>

OTS-L
Organization for Tropical Studies

Bitnet Subscribe to: `listserv@yalevm`

Internet Subscribe to: `listserv@yalevm.ycc.yale.edu`

Bitnet Mail to: **ots-l@yalevm**

Internet Mail to: **ots-l@yalevm.ycc.yale.edu**

Description: Organization for Tropical Studies at Yale University

List Owner/Contact: Phil Sollins <`sollinsp@ccmail.orst.edu`>

OUTDOR-L
Outdoor Discussion List

Bitnet Subscribe to: `listserv@ulkyvm`

Internet Subscribe to: `listserv@ulkyvm.louisville.edu`

Bitnet Mail to: **outdor-l@ulkyvm**

Internet Mail to: **outdor-l@ulkyvm.louisville.edu**

List Owner/Contact: Jim Cocks <jacock01@ulkyvm.louisville.edu>

PARK RANGERS
US National Park Service

Internet Subscribe to: **60157903@wsuvm1.csc.wsu.edu**

Description: This list is primarily for anyone working or interested in working as a ranger (general, interpretive, etc.) for the National Park Service (U.S.A.), but rangers from state and county agencies as well as other countries are also welcome. The group discusses numerous topics related to this profession.

Contact: Cynthia Dorminey <60157903@wsuvm1.csc.wsu.edu>

PATHNET
Armed Forces Institute of Pathology Mailing List

Internet Subscribe to: **pathnet@email.afip.osd.mil**

In the subject header, enter: **subscribe**

Description: An Internet discussion forum for issues related to the art, science and practice of pathology and laboratory medicine, defined broadly as the study of disease as well as whatever pathologists do. Human and animal pathology are included Appropriate topics for discussion include: any pathology—related question, diagnostic questions, laboratory techniques, reimbursement discussions, mechanisms of disease, telepathology, job announcements and searches, announcements of course offerings of interest to pathologists, notices of preprints available by email or FTP, announcements or queries by pathology societies, requests for email addresses, journal contents, announcements of regulatory actions, and guidelines/standards published by NCCLS and others.

List Owner/Contact: Timothy O'Leary <oleary@email.afip.osd.mil>

PETBUNNY
Forum for Owners of Companion Rabbits

Bitnet Subscribe to: **listserv@ukcc**

Internet Subscribe to: **listserv@ukcc.uky.edu**

Bitnet Mail to: **petbunny@ukcc**

Internet Mail to: **petbunny@ukcc.uky.edu**

Description: PetBunny is an open, unmoderated discussion list for owners of pet rabbits. Things such as how to care for a pet rabbit, rabbit diseases and rabbit psychology are likely to be discussed. The list is not intended for rabbit bashing.

List Owner/Contact: Bob Crovo <crovo@ukcc.uky.edu>
University of Kentucky

PETS-L
Domestic Animal Care and Education List

Bitnet Subscribe to: **listserv@itesmvf1**

Internet Subscribe to: **listserv@itesmvf1.rzs.itesm.mx**

Bitnet Mail to: **pets-l@itesmvf1**

Internet Mail to: **pets-l@itesmvf1.rzs.itesm.mx**

List Owner/Contact: Alejandro Kurczyn <akurczyn@itesmvf1.rzs.itesm.mx>

PFERDE
Equine Discussion List (German language)

Bitnet Subscribe to: **listserv@dlrvm**

Internet Subscribe to: **listserv@vm.op.dlr.de**

Bitnet Mail to: **pferde@dlrvm**

Internet Mail to: **pferde@vm.op.dlr.de**

Description: Pferde Diskussionsliste (German language) discusses those things related to horses, riding (competitive or not), owning, breeding, etc. Its intention is to cover Germany and Europe, because show events, legal questions, etc., are country-dependent.

List Owners/Contact: Heike Mueller <rz4p@dlrvmgo.bitnet>
Andreas Landhaeusser <rz5j@dlrvmgo.bitnet>

PHARM

Medical Pharmacy Discussion Group (Restricted)

Internet Subscribe to: pharm-request@dmu.ac.uk

Internet Mail to: **pharm@dmu.ac.uk**

Note: Cross-posts to the Usenet Newsgroup sci.med.pharmacy

Description: To provide pharmacists with a forum for the discussion of issues related to the teaching and practice of the profession. It is expected that sci.med.pharmacy will attract contributions from all the major disciplines including pharmacology and pharmaceutical chemistry as well as areas with more direct professional implications such as pharmacy practice and legislation.

List Owner/Contact: Paul Hodgkinson F.I.Sc.T. <phh@dmu.ac.uk>
Department of Pharmacy
De Montfort University UK

PH-BSG

Biological Sciences Group, STACnet-Philippines

Bitnet Subscribe to: listserv@searn

Internet Subscribe to: listserv@searn.sunet.se

Bitnet Mail to: **ph-bsg@searn**

Internet Mail to: **ph-bsg@searn.sunet.se**

Description: A mailing list for the Biological Sciences Group of STACnet (Philippines Science and Technology Advisory Council Electronic Network) and for individuals who are interested in biosciences and biotechnology in the Philippines. Its scope includes agriculture, medicine, fermentation and food technology, animal husbandry, bioenergy, etc. The purpose of this list is to facilitate information exchange and discussions. The target however, is to enable its subscribers to identify, assist, develop and obtain funding for joint projects with the private and public sectors in the Philippines.

List Owners/Contact: Mr. J. Foo
<eng-leong_foo_mircen-ki%micforum@mica.mic.ki.se>
UNESCO Microbial Resources Center
Karolinska Institute
104 01 Stockholm, Sweden
Fax: 46-8-331547

Joe Lim <joe@credit.erin.utoronto.ca>

PIGFARM

Pig Discussion List

Internet Subscribe to: listserv@ist01.ferris.edu

Internet Mail to: **pigfarm@ist01.ferris.edu**

Description: The PIGFARM list is dedicated to the subject of pigs, their breeding, care, diseases, how to farm them small scale, and other relevant topics.

List Owner/Contact: <jbouman@ist01.ferris.edu>

PLTRYNWS

Commercial Production Poultry Mailing List

Internet Subscribe to: listserv@sdsuvm.sdstate.edu

Internet Mail to: **pltrynws@sdsuvm.sdstate.edu**

Description: PLTRYNWS is an e-mail based newsgroup for those with interest in commercial production poultry, including (but not limited to) broiler chickens, laying chickens, breeding birds, turkeys, gamebirds and waterfowl. Open forum discussions pertaining to issues related to health, management and production of commercial poultry are encouraged. It is anticipated that PLTRYNWS will provide a means to disseminate information rapidly to those with interest in the commercial poultry industry. Examples include information (or inquiries) concerning disease outbreaks, notification of meetings and events, requests for specific information (or service), notification of new products and methodologies, etc. PLTRYNWS will benefit those in commercial companies, academia, government service and/or research organizations and individuals with an interest in poultry.

List Owners/Contacts: Don Reynolds <dlr@iastate.edu>
VMRI / Coll Vet Med
Iowa State University
Ames, IA 50011
Phone: 515-294-0914
Fax: 515-294-1401

Joe Moore <moorej@cc.sdstate.edu>

POP-BIO

Population Ecology & Population Genetics

Bitnet Subscribe to: listserv@irlearn

Internet Subscribe to: listserv@irlearn.ucd.ie

Bitnet Mail to: **pop-bio@irlearn**

Internet Mail to: **pop-bio@irlearn.ucd.ie**

Description: Population Biology is a synthesis of population ecology and population genetics, pursuing a unified theory to explain the structure, functioning and evolution of populations of living beings. Such populations are very complex systems, exhibiting a variety of phenomena that we still do not master. Just to quote a famous example, multiannual density cycles (e.g., in lemmings) have not received a satisfactory explanation, despite of decades of debated studies and speculations. Population Biology is a very active field, encompassing such diverse approaches as tenacious, harsh field work to track long term demographic and genetic fluctuations, or sophisticated conversations with a computer about strange attractors possibly causing chaos in the density fluctuations.

List Owner/Contact: Vincent Bauchau <vincent%bucl1n11.bitnet@vm1.nodak.edu>

PRIMATE-TALK

Primate Discussion List

Internet Subscribe to: primate-talk-request@primate.wisc.edu

Internet Mail to: **primate-talk@primate.wisc.edu**

Description: Primate-Talk is an unmoderated, open forum for the discussion of primatology and related subjects. This list is open to any e-mail user with an interest in primatology. Subject matter may range from, but is not limited to: News items, Meeting announcements, Research issues, Information requests, Veterinary/husbandry topics, Job notices, Animal exchange information, and Book reviews.

List Owner/Contact: Larry Jacobsen <jacobsen@primate.wisc.edu>
Head of Library Services
Wisconsin Regional Primate Research Center Library
1220 Capitol Court
Madison, WI 53715-1299
Phone: 608-263-3512
Fax: 608-263-4031

PRIMATOLOGY

Internet Subscribe to: mailbase@mailbase.ac.uk

Internet Mail to: **primatology@mailbase.ac.uk**

Description: The primatology list provides a discussion forum for issues arising from the study of human and non-human primates. Research news and views across the spectrum of field and laboratory-based work concerned with monkeys, apes and social anthropology are welcome.

List Owner/Contact: Tony Dickinson <tonyd@castle.ed.ac.uk>
Laboratory for Cognitive Neuroscience
Dept. of Psychology
University of Edinburgh

PROTECTION-DOGS

Protection Training Discussion List

Internet Subscribe to: **markwf@kaiwan.com**

Description: The protection-dogs list is for topics of protection training. Topics to be covered in this group include training of sport dogs and or personal protection. Also included is anything that has to do with the protection training field. It is hoped by starting this list will create an atmosphere of interaction with protection enthusiasts the world over. Whether it be for sport or professional training for the public. This group is for the heavy hobbyist or professional in the protection training field. This is a Moderated Mail list. If you think you would like to participate in this group please send E-mail telling a little about yourself and why you want to join the group. In the subject field just put Request Subscription. You will get a reply telling you how to join our group in a few days after you send in your request.

List Owner/Contact: Mark Webb Ferrasci <markwf@kaiwan.com>

PSYC

PSYC: An International Electronic Forum for Scholarly Communication

Bitnet Subscribe to: **listserv@pucc**

Internet Subscribe to: **listserv@pucc.princeton.edu**

PSYCOLOQUY is sponsored by the American Psychological Association (APA) Science Directorate & Office of Publications and Communication and contains announcements of meetings, preprints, employment, journal contents, etc.; discussions pertaining to clinical and professional matters in the field of psychology, and brief reports of recent ideas or findings on which you would like to initiate multiple scholarly discussion.

List Owners/Contact: (scientific discussion)
Stevan Harnad <harnad@clarity.princeton.edu>
Psychology Department
Princeton University

(professional/clinical discussion)
Cary Cherniss (Assoc Ed.)
Graduate School of Applied
Professional Psychology
Rutgers University

Assistant Editor: Colleen Wirth <wirth@clarity.princeton.edu>

Newsletter and Subscriptions: Turgut Kalfaoglu <turgut@trearn.earn>

PSYCHIATRY

Psychiatry Forum

Internet Subscribe to: **mailbase@mailbase.ac.uk**

Internet Mail to: **psychiatry@mailbase.ac.uk**

Description: This mailbase list has been set up with the aim of utilizing the vast resources of the Internet on behalf of everyone interested in issues in psychiatry and abnormal psychology. The forum was judged to be necessary because many of the findings and viewpoints in the fields of psychiatry and abnormal psychology are both controversial and easily misinterpreted, resulting in a lack of empathy and understanding between those pursuing radically different approaches to the aetiology and pathophysiology of mental illness. It is hoped that the forum will act as a bridge between those taking a biomedical viewpoint of the study and treatment of psychopathology, and those taking a more existential or psychodynamic viewpoint. All of those wishing to share personal insights, research findings, philosophical outlooks, clinical case notes, or simple anecdotes on any of the following, are cordially invited to contribute.

List Owner/Contact: Ian Pitchford <i.pitchford@sheffield.ac.uk>
University of Sheffield
Department of Biomedical Science

RESEARCH

Outside Funding Support

Bitnet Subscribe to: `listserv@templevm`

Internet Subscribe to: `listserv@vm.temple.edu`

Bitnet Mail to: **research@templevm**

Internet Mail to: **research@vm.temple.edu**

Description: The RESEARCH list is for those people (primarily at educational institutions) who are interested in applying for outside funding support. That is, support from government agencies, corporations, foundations etc. This list attempts to assist faculty in locating sources of support and also to forward information regarding the latest news from potential sponsors. As an example, National Science Foundation, National Institutes of Health. The list also provides information on upcoming seminars from around the world on various topics from medicine to artificial intelligence.

List Owner/Contact: Eleanor Cicinsky <cicinsky@vm.temple.edu>

QMLIST

Quantitative Morphology List

Internet Subscribe to: `listserver@tbone.biol.scarolina.edu`

Internet Mail to: **qmlist@tbone.biol.scarolina.edu**

Description: This is an open, unmoderated mailing list to support researchers and clinicians in the field of quantitative morphology. This can include (but is not limited to): queries for help with technical or professional problems; pointers to interesting recent publications; summaries and abstracts of your own recent work; news of upcoming meetings; news about job openings or other professional opportunities; and news about granting agencies or programs. We would like to encourage a broad interpretation of "quantitative morphology". We encourage interaction between people working in two- or three-dimensional quantitative analysis of both organic and inorganic structures. Relevant methods include, but are not limited to: serial reconstruction, stereology, geometric modeling, computer graphics, geometric probability, mathematical morphology, pattern analysis, etc. We encourage people from (at least) the following fields to participate: anatomy, biophysics, botany, cell biology, computer vision, forestry, geology, materials sciences, microbiology, pathology, radiology, and zoology.

List Owner/Contact: Dean Pentcheff <dean2@tbone.biol.scarolina.edu>
Department of Biology
University of South Carolina
Columbia, SC 29208
Phone: 803-777-8998

SAFETY

Environmental Health and Safety Discussion List

Bitnet Subscribe to: `listserv@uvmvm`

Internet Subscribe to: `listserv@uvmvm.uvm.edu`

Bitnet Mail to: **safety@uvmvm**

Internet Mail to: **safety@uvmvm.uvm.edu**

Description: E-conference for people interested in the various environmental, health and safety issues and problems on college and university campuses. These can include life safety issues (fire protection, trip and fall and other general safety issues), chemical safety issues (waste disposal, laboratory safety, meeting regulations), biological hazards and radiation safety. Both users of hazardous materials and people administering campus safety programs are welcome on the list.

List Owners/Contact: Ralph Stuart <rstuart@moose.uvm.edu>
Dayna Flath <dmf@uvmvm.uvm.edu>

SBNC-L
Sociedade Brasileira de Neurociencias e Comportamento

Bitnet Subscribe to: `listserv@bruspvm`

Internet Subscribe to: `listserv@bruspvm.bitnet`

Bitnet Mail to: **sbnc-l@bruspvm**

Internet Mail to: **sbnc-l@bruspvm.bitnet**

Description: Discussion list for the Brazilian Society of Neurosciences.

List Owner/Contact: Dora Ventura <dventura@cat.cce.usp.br>

SCIFAQ-L
Frequently Asked Questions from Usenet's `sci.answers` newsgroup

Bitnet Subscribe to: `listserv@yalevm`

Internet Subscribe to: `listserv@yalevm.cis.yale.edu`

Bitnet Mail to: **scifaq-l@yalevm**

Internet Mail to: **scifaq-l@yalevm.cis.yale.edu**

Description: This mailing list is intended primarily to facilitate access to Usenet FAQ documents (documents that address frequently asked questions) by people who have access to local Usenet distributions via NETNEWS or some other medium, but do not have Usenet feeds per se, or who simply want to keep abreast of the latest releases of all Usenet FAQs relating to topics in science. The sci.answers newsgroup is moderated, and therefore the gateway between it and the SCIFAQ-L mailing list has been made one-way, from Usenet into the list. The list itself is not moderated, and may be used for relevant discussion or distribution of FAQ-like documents by e-mail subscribers.

List Owner/Contact: Una Smith <smith-una@yale.edu>
Biology Department
Yale University
New Haven, CT 06511

SCIFRAUD
Discussion of Fraud in Science

Bitnet Subscribe to: `listserv@albnyvm1`

Internet Subscribe to: `listserv@uacsc2.albany.edu`

Bitnet Mail to: **scifraud@albnyvm1**

Internet Mail to: **scifraud@uacsc2.albany.edu**

Description: SCIFRAUD is dedicated to the discussion of fraud in science. Its topics can be easily identified in the last several months with these names: David Baltimore, Stanley Pons and Martin Fleischmann, Shervert Frazier, Viswa Jit Gupta, Philip Berger, Robert Slutsky, and many others. Then, too, there are topics with which the board has been concerned: the prevalence of fraud in science, the use of fraud and dishonesty productively in science, the structure of science, competition in science, Institutionalized Science, and the history of fraud in science.

List Owners/Contact: Al Higgins <ach13@albnyvms.bitnet>
Mike Ramundo <sysmrr@albnyvm1.bitnet>

SCIMAT-L
Arkansas Science and Math Education

Bitnet Subscribe to: `listserv@uafsysb`

Internet Subscribe to: `listserv@uafsysb.uark.edu`

Bitnet Mail to: **scimat-l@uafsysb**

Internet Mail to: **scimat-l@uafsysb.uark.edu**

List Owner/Contact: William L. Fulton <wlfulton@uafsysb.uark.edu>

SCUBA
Discussion of Scuba Diving

Bitnet Subscribe to: `listserv@tritu`

Internet Subscribe to: `listserv@cc.itu.edu.tr`

Bitnet Mail to: **scuba@tritu**

Internet Mail to: **scuba@cc.itu.edu.tr**

Description: SCUBA is a discussion list featuring SCUBA and skin diving. Topics include illnesses of a diver, dangers under water, equipment of diving, diving sites all around the world, wonderful feeling of breathing under water, magical and mysterious world under water, etc. Either English or Turkish languages may be used on this list.

List Owner/Contact: Gokhan Boybek <gokhan@cc.itu.edu.tr>

SCUBA-D
Digest of the Usenet rec.scuba newsgroup

Bitnet Subscribe to: `listserv@brownvm`

Internet Subscribe to: `listserv@brownvm.brown.edu`

Bitnet Mail to: **scuba-d@brownvm**

Internet Mail to: **scuba-d@brownvm.brown.edu**

List Owners/Contact: Catherine Yang <cyang@brownvm.brown.edu>
    Nick Simicich <njs@watson.ibm.com>

SCUBA-L
Scuba Diving Mailing List

Bitnet Subscribe to: `listserv@brownvm`

Internet Subscribe to: `listserv@brownvm.brown.edu`

Bitnet Mail to: **scuba-l@brownvm**

Internet Mail to: **scuba-l@brownvm.brown.edu**

Description: Mailing list for discussion of all aspects of SCUBA diving. Any articles, views, ideas, and opinions relating to SCUBA diving are welcome. Areas discussed will include, but are not limited to: Safety/first aid; places to dive; decompression; computation; decompression tables; history; new equipment; dive shops; new technologies; mail order shopping; diving science & technology; travel; computers; tropical diving; underwater photography; underwater animal life; underwater vehicles; questions/quizzes; PADI certifications; NAUI certifications; & YMCA certifications. Also gateways to Usenet Newsgroup `bit.listserv.scuba-l`.

List Owner/Contact: Catherine Yang <cyang@brownvm.brown.edu>

SEABIRD
International Marine Ornithologists' Network

Internet Subscribe to: **seabird@zoo.uct.ac.za**

Note: In the SUBJECT FIELD of an email letter, enter: SUBSCRIBE SEABIRD and in the body of the email letter your full name and postal, telephone and fax addresses as you would like them listed in the network's address list. Leaving these out will mean that you will only appear in the address list under your e-mail address. If you so desire you may also list your research interests as well for inclusion with the address list.

Description: Membership of this network is not restricted in any way. The network has been initiated to help marine ornithologists exchange information and keep in contact on a worldwide basis. Examples of its use are requests for and offers of information, ideas, data and collected material (such as skeletal and soft-tissue samples), advertising employment, bursary, fellowship and volunteer opportunities, notices of meetings, availability of written materials (e.g., expedition reports, books, proceedings, reprints), etc.

Contact: John Cooper <jcooper@zoo.uct.ac.za>
    UCT Senior Research/SANAP Antarctic Officer
    Room 2.06, John Day Zoology Building

University Avenue, Upper Campus
Percy FitzPatrick Institute of African Ornithology
University of Cape Town
Rondebosch 7700
South Africa
Phone: 27-21-650-3294
Fax: 27-21-650-3295

SEASHEPHERD

Sea Shepherd Electronic Mailing List

Internet Subscribe to: `dcasmedic@aol.com`

Description: The Sea Shepherd is involved in several campaigns, including the fight against whaling, dolphin slaughter, drift nets and seal killing. This is a volunteer, information collection and distribution service, for the Sea Shepherd Conservation Society and related issues.

List Owner/Contact: Nick Voth <`dcasmedic@aol.com`>
3725 Westland Pl.
Lawrence, KS 66049
Sea Shepherd Conservation Society
1314 2nd Street
Santa Monica, CA 90401
Phone: 310-394-3198

SFER-L

South Florida Environmental Reader

Bitnet Subscribe to: `listserv@ucf1vm`

Internet Subscribe to: `listserv@ucf1vm.cc.ucf.edu`

Bitnet Mail to: **sfer-l@ucf1vm**

Internet Mail to: **sfer-l@ucf1vm.cc.ucf.edu**

Description: The South Florida Environmental Reader is a electronic newsletter covering topics concerning the South Florida environment. The newsletter is published on a monthly basis.

Contact: Andrew Mossberg <`aem@miavax.ir.miami.edu`>

SIERRA CLUB

Sierra Club Mailing List

Internet Subscribe to: **sierra-request@pc.f1.n136.z1.fidonet.org**

SKEPTIC

Skeptic Discussion Group

Bitnet Subscribe to: `listserv@jhuvm`

Internet Subscribe to: `listserv@jhuvm.hcf.jhu.edu`

Bitnet Mail to: **skeptic@jhuvm**

Internet Mail to: **skeptic@jhuvm.hcf.jhu.edu**

Description: SKEPTIC is a mailing list devoted to critical discussion of extraordinary claims. Among the paranormal topics that are commonly examined are parapsychology and psychic claims, creationism, cult archaeology, UFO's, cryptozoology, reincarnation/survival, quackery, the occult and divination; but the discussion is not limited to any predetermined set of magical beliefs or alleged pseudosciences. In connection with paranormal claims, issues involving science and philosophy in general are often raised. There is no policy of excluding any topic from consideration. While the common point of view expressed is skepticism about claims that go against current scientific pictures, critical approaches to science itself are also encouraged.

List Owner/Contact: Taner Edis <`edis@eta.pha.jhu.edu`>

SMBNET
Society for Mathematical Biology Digest
Internet Subscribe to: `listserv@fconvx.ncifcrf.gov`
Internet Mail to: **smbnet@fconvx.ncifcrf.gov**
List Owner/Contact: Ray Mejia

SOCETH-L
The Social Ethics Discussion List
Bitnet Subscribe to: `listserv@uscvm`
Internet Subscribe to: `listserv@vm.usc.edu`
Bitnet Mail to: **soceth-l@uscvm**
Internet Mail to: **soceth-l@vm.usc.edu**

Description: SOCETH-L is an electronic discussion group for Social Ethics and is primarily a forum for interdisciplinary approaches to ethics. General topics of discussion include major traditions of ethical thought, the place of values and moral norms in culture, the construction of moral and ethical meaning, analysis of modern moral issues, professional ethics, and public policy. Members are invited to engage in conversations such as you might encounter in a university lounge—considered but informal. You are encouraged to pose queries, ask leading questions, report on conferences, informally review books and articles, ask for collaborators, invite contructive criticism of new ideas, discuss each other's work, gossip, and so on.

List Owners/Contact: Aditi Gowri <gowri@scf.usc.edu>
David Edward Armstrong <dearms@scf.usc.edu>

SOCINSCT
Social Insect Biology Research List
Bitnet Subscribe to: `listserv@albanyvm1`
Internet Subscribe to: `listserv@vacsc2.albany.edu`
Bitnet Mail to: **socinsct@albanyvm1**
Internet Mail to: **socinsct@vacsc2.albany.edu**

Description: SOCINSCT is dedicated to communication among investigators active in the discipline of social insect biology. It is restricted to discussions of research at the university level. Eusocial insects (bees, wasps, ants and termites) are the main interest but information to be shared could include any area of sociobiology, or solitary bees and wasps. Such areas could include orientation, navigation, adaptation/selection/evolution, superorganism concept, behavior, physiology and biochemistry, pheromones, flight and energetics, taxonomy and systematics, ecology, genetics, pollination and nectar/pollen biology. Announcements of meetings and professional opportunities, requests for research help, sharing of literature references, sharing research topics and discussion of ideas are welcome.

List Owner/Contact: Erik Seielstad <erik@acspr1.acs.brockport.edu>

STARNET
Echinoderm Newsletter
Internet Subscribe to: whide@matrix.bchs.uh.edu
Internet Mail to: **star@matrix.bchs.uh.edu**
Description: The STARNET echhindoerm electronic newsletter is distributed quarterly.
List Owner/Contact: Win Hide <whide@matrix.bchs.uh.edu>

STLHE-L
Forum for Teaching & Learning in Higher Education
Bitnet Subscribe to: `listserv@unbvm1`
Internet Subscribe to: `listserv@unb.ca`
Bitnet Mail to: **stlhe-l@unbvm1**

Internet Mail to: **stlhe-l@unb.ca**

Description: The Society of Teaching and Learning in Higher Education (STHLE), Canada, Forum is to exchange ideas, views and experiences of importance to STLHE members and others who are interested in the subject of teaching and learning in higher education.

List Owner/Contact: Esam Hussein <hussein@unb.ca>

SUER-WG

Sustainable Use of Ecosystem Resources Working Group of The Wildlife Society

Internet Subscribe to: suer-req@ncatfyv.uark.edu

Intenet Mail to: **suer-wg@ncatfyv.uark.edu**

Description: SUER-WG is a moderated list for those members of The Wildlife Society that wish to participate in the Sustainable Use of Ecosystem Resources Working Group. This working group will provide a forum for TWS members to investigate the related issues of multiple use and sustainable development of natural resources. The topics investigated will depend upon the interests of Working Group members and might include the impacts of grazing, timber harvest, agriculture, water allocation, mining, tourism, industrial development, and other activities. Both domestic and international policies and programs will be considered. The emphasis will be on identifying approaches that use natural resources in ways which are compatable with the maintenance of viable wildlife populations.

List Owner/Contact: Bob Wilson <bobw@ncatfyv.uark.edu>

SUSTAG-L

Discussions about Sustainable Agriculture

Bitnet Subscribe to: listserv@wsuvm1

Internet Subscribe to: listserv@wsuvm1.csc.wsu.edu

Bitnet Mail to: **sustag-l@wsuvm1**

Internet Mail to: **sustag-l@wsuvm1.csc.wsu.edu**

List Owner/Contact: Tony Wright <wright@wsuvm1.csc.wsu.edu>

SVHP-L

Veterinary Pharmacy Issues (restricted membership)

Bitnet Subscribe to: listserv@uga

Internet Subscribe to: listserv@uga.cc.uga.edu

Bitnet Mail to: **svhp-l@uga**

Internet Mail to: **svhp-l@uga.cc.uga.edu**

List Owner/Contact: Doug Kemp <vetpharm@uga.cc.uga.edu>

TAXACOM

Biological Systematics Discussion List

Bitnet Subscribe to: listserv@harvarda

Internet Subscribe to: listserv@harvarda.harvard.edu

Bitnet Mail to: **taxacom@harvarda**

Internet Mail to: **taxacom@harvarda.harvard.edu**

List Owner/Contact: James H. Beach <beach@huh.harvard.edu>

TDR-SCIENTISTS

Tropical Disease Research Scientists Network

Internet Subscribe to: tdr-scientists-REQUEST@who.ch

Internet Mail to: **tdr-Scientists@who.ch**

Description: The List is a cost-free media for the World Health Organization TDR Communications Unit to propagate important public information texts to any e-mail users connected to the Internet, with interest in TDR. The List may also serve as an informal Forum among TDR scientists to exchange ideas/information which may be helpful to each other.

List Owner/Contact: Bob Hata <hata@who.ch>
UNDP/WorldBank/WHO Special Programme
Tropical Diseases Research (TDR)
WHO, 1211 Geneva 27, Switzerland

TITNET

Paridae and Hole-nesting Bird Discussion List

Bitnet Subscribe to: **jhailman@wiscmacc**

Internet Subscribe to: **jhailman@macc.wisc.edu**

Note: Send (1) full name, (2) mailing address, which is forwarded to Dr. Ficken for PARUS INTERNATIONAL, (3) email address(es), (4) species studied, and (5) types of studies (population dynamics, general ecology, vocalizations, nesting, behavior, etc.).

Description: Promotes communication among scientists working on tits (Paridae) and other hole-nesting birds. TITNET is a publication listing e-mail addresses of conference members. TITNEWS contains announcements and discussions of activities such as bibliographic systems, and hence serves as the email newsletter. TITNOTES contains material on the biology of the birds, and hence serves as a kind of email journal.

List Owner/Contact: Jack P. Hailman <jhailman@macc.wisc.edu>

TWEETERS

Washington State Birding List

Internet Subscribe to: **dvictor@u.washington.edu**

Description: Tweeters is a mailing list covering birding topics in Washington State.

List Owner/Contact: Dan Victor <dvictor@u.washington.edu>

TWSGIS-L

GIS/Remote Sensing/Landscape Ecology Working Group of The Wildlife Society

Bitnet Subscribe to: **listserv@ndsuvm1**

Internet Subscribe to: **listserv@vm1.nodak.edu**

Bitnet Mail to: **twsgis-l@ndsuvm1**

Internet Mail to: **twsgis-l@vm1.nodak.edu**

Description: TWSGIS-L is a list for the GIS/Remote Sensing/Landscape Ecology working group of The Wildlife Society. It is intended as a clearing house of information for biological use and abuse of GIS and Remote Sensing Technology.

List Owner/Contact: Tom Sklebar <sklebart@mail.fws.gov>
Northern Prairie Wildlife Research Center
US Fish and Wildlife Service
Jamestown, ND 58401
Phone: 701-252-5363
David Bergman <dbergman@vm1.nodak.edu>

VEGCMTE

Vegetarian Resource Committee

Bitnet Subscribe to: **listserv@vtvm1**

Internet Subscribe to: **listserv@vtvm1.cc.vt.edu**

Bitnet Mail to: **vegcmte@vtvm1**

Internet Mail to: **vegcmte@vtvm1.cc.vt.edu**

List Owners/Contact: Chuck Goelzer Lyons <cgl1@cornell.edu>
Darrell A. Early <paddy@cadserv.cadlab.vt.edu>

VEGCNY-L
Vegetarians in Central New York area

Internet Subscribe to: `listserv@cornell.edu`

Internet Mail to: **`vegcny-l@cornell.edu`**

Description: VegCNY-L is an open discussion list intended to serve those people living in the Central New York area who are vegetarians and those who, while not yet vegetarian, are interested in vegetarianism. Our goal is to promote vegetarianism, which we define as the practice of living without the use of flesh, fowl or fish. We encourage a sense of inquiry, openness, and tolerance about all matters related to vegetarianism. Topics may include but are not limited to: discussing co-operative and natural food markets; finding a place to dine out; raising a vegetarian child; eating in a college dining hall; shopping animal-free; attending local vegetarian cooking classes; and starting a VegCNY conference.

List Owner/Contact: Chuck Goelzer Lyons <`cgl1@cornell.edu`>

VEGLIFE (formerly GRANOLA)
Vegetarian Life List

Bitnet Subscribe to: `listserv@vtvm1`

Internet Subscribe to: `listserv@vtvm1.cc.vt.edu`

Bitnet Mail to: **`veglife@vtvm1`**

Internet Mail to: **`veglife@vtvm1.cc.vt.edu`**

Description: Welcome to VegLife! VegLife provides a supportive atmosphere for the discussion of issues related to the vegetarian lifestyle. We define vegetarianism as the quality of living without the use of meat, poultry, or fish, and the ideal of living independent of using animals. Not all our active members are vegetarian; we welcome vegetarians of all degrees as well as non-vegetarians. Discussion topics include, but are not limited to: various types of vegetarianism (lacto, ovo, pesco, vegan, etc.); nutritional information; ideas/support for shifting to a vegetarian diet; diet and the environment; diet and human health; cookbooks, books, magazines, and newsletters on vegetarianism; dining out vegetarian; vegetarian eating while on a college meal plan; vegetarian recipes; organic and natural foods; starting a local vegetarian group; encouraging institutions to become vegetarian-friendly; herbal remedies; animal rights; and your other interests related to vegetarianism.

List Owners/Contact: Darrell A. Early <`bestuur@vtvm1.cc.vt.edu`>
Charles Goelzer Lyons <`cgl1@cornell.edu`>

VETADM-L
Veterinary Hospital Administration List

Bitnet Subscribe to: `listserv@tamvm1`

Internet Subscribe to: `listserv@tamvm1.tamu.edu`

Bitnet Mail to: **`vetadm-l@tamvm1`**

Internet Mail to: **`vetadm-l@tamvm1.tamu.edu`**

Description: Discussion group for veterinary hospital administration.

List Owner/Contact: Joel Hammond <`joel@tamvet.bitnet`>

VETCAI-L
Veterinary Medicine Computer Assisted Instruction

Bitnet Subscribe to: `listserv@ksuvm`

Internet Subscribe to: `listserv@ksuvm.ksu.edu`

Bitnet Mail to: **`vetcai-l@ksuvm`**

Internet Mail to: **`vetcai-l@ksuvm.ksu.edu`**

Description: Veterinary medicine computer-assisted instruction discussion.

List Owner/Contact: Pat Oblander <`oblandr@ksuvm.ksu.edu`>

VETHIS-L
Veterinary Hospital Information Systems

Bitnet Subscribe to: `listserv@uiucvmd`

Internet Subscribe to: `listserv@vmd.cso.uiuc.edu`

Bitnet Mail to: **vethis-l@uiucvmd**

Internet Mail to: **vethis-l@vmd.cso.uiuc.edu**

Description: In light of heightened interest in veterinary hospital information systems (HIS), a discussion group devoted to veterinary HIS has been created. VETHIS-L is intended to serve as a forum for the exchange of information on veterinary hospital information systems. Because of the interrelationship between veterinary hospitals and diagnostic laboratories, topics of mutual interest can be discussed here as well. The forum was created in response to initiatives by members of the American Association of Veterinary Medical Colleges (AAVMC) and the American Academy of Veterinary Informatics (AAVI).

List Owner/Contact: Ron Smith <r-smith19@uiuc.edu>
University of Illinois
College of Veterinary Medicine
2001 S. Lincoln Ave.
Urbana, IL 60801

VETIMM-L

Veterinary Immunology Discussion Group

Bitnet Subscribe to: `listserv@ucdcvdls`

Internet Subscribe to: `listserv@cvdls.ucdavis.edu`

Bitnet Mail to: **vetimm-l@ucdcvdls**

Internet Mail to: **vetimm-l@cvdls.ucdavis.edu**

List Owners/Contact: James T. Case, DVM, Ph.D. <jcase@ucdcvdls.bitnet>
University of California
School of Veterinary Medicine
California Veterinary Diagnostic Laboratory System
P.O. Box 1770
Davis, CA 95617
Phone: 916-752-4408

Bill Cohen <bcohen@ucdcvdls.bitnet>

VETINFO

Discussion of Veterinary Informatics

Bitnet Subscribe to: `listserv@ucdcvdls`

Internet Subscribe to: `listserv@cvdls.ucdavis.edu`

Bitnet Mail to: **vetinfo@ucdcvdls**

Internet Mail to: **vetinfo@cvdls.ucdavis.edu**

Description: This list has been created to stimulate discussion in the area of Informatics, with special reference to the field of Veterinary Medicine. Related topics include Clinical decision support systems, laboratory information management, imaging, disease nomenclature and coding systems, expert systems, knowledge bases, etc. Discussions related to specific hardware and software implementations are welcome as well as approaches to specific approaches to challenges in veterinary informatics.

List Owners/Contact: James T. Case, DVM, Ph.D. <jcase@ucdcvdls.bitnet>
University of California
School of Veterinary Medicine
California Veterinary Diagnostic Laboratory System
P.O. Box 1770
Davis, CA 95617
Phone: 916-752-4408

Bill Cohen <bcohen@ucdcvdls.bitnet>

VETLIB-L
Veterinary Medicine Librarians List

Bitnet Subscribe to: `listserv@vtvm1`

Internet Subscribe to: `listserv@vtvm1.cc.vt.edu`

Bitnet Mail to: **`vetlib-l@vtvm1`**

Internet Mail to: **`vetlib-l@vtvm1.cc.vt.edu`**

Description: VETLIB-L is an e-mail discussion group for librarians in schools and colleges of veterinary medicine world-wide. It is made available by Virginia Polytechnic Institute and State University (VPI or Virginia Tech), Blacksburg, Virginia.

List Owners/Contact: Victoria T. Kok `<kok@vtvm1.cc.vt.edu>`
Veterinary Medicine Librarian
Veterinary Medical Library
Virginia Polytechnic Institute & State University
Blacksburg, VA 24061-0422
Phone: 703-231-6610
Fax: 703-231-7367

James Powell `<jpowell@vtvm1.cc.vt.edu>`

VETMED-L
Veterinary Medicine Discussion List

Bitnet Subscribe to: `listserv@uga`

Internet Subscribe to: `listserv@uga.cc.uga.edu`

Bitnet Mail to: **`vetmed-l@uga`**

Internet Mail to: **`vetmed-l@uga.cc.uga.edu`**

Description: Discussion group for students, professionals and others employed in or interested in the veterinary profession.

List Owners/Contact: Doug Kemp `<vetpharm@uga.cc.uga.edu>`
Jean Snow `<jean@uga.cc.uga.edu>`
Harold Pritchett `<harold@uga.cc.uga.edu`

VETMICRO
Veterinary Microbiology Discussion List

Bitnet Subscribe to: `listserv@ucdcvdls`

Internet Subscribe to: `listserv@cvdls.ucdavis.edu`

Bitnet Mail to: **`vetmicro@ucdcvdls`**

Internet Mail to: **`vetmicro@cvdls.ucdavis.edu`**

Description: Discussion group for veterinary microbiology

List Owners/Contact: James T. Case, DVM, Ph.D. `<jcase@ucdcvdls.bitnet>`
University of California
School of Veterinary Medicine
California Veterinary Diagnostic Laboratory System
P.O. Box 1770
Davis, CA 95617
Phone: 916-752-4408

Bill Cohen `<bcohen@ucdcvdls.bitnet>`

VETMYCOP
Veterinary Mycoplasma Discussion Group

Bitnet Subscribe to: `listserv@ucdcvdls`

Internet Subscribe to: `listserv@cvdls.ucdavis.edu`

Bitnet Mail to: **`vetmycop@ucdcvdls`**

Internet Mail to: **vetmycop@cvdls.ucdavis.edu**

List Owners/Contact: James T. Case, DVM, Ph.D. <jcase@ucdcvdls.bitnet>
University of California
School of Veterinary Medicine
California Veterinary Diagnostic Laboratory System
P.O. Box 1770
Davis, CA 95617
Phone: 916-752-4408

Bill Cohen <bcohen@ucdcvdls.bitnet>

VETSTU-L

Veterinary Student Discussion List

Bitnet Subscribe to: `listserv@uga`

Internet Subscribe to: `listserv@uga.cc.uga.edu`

Bitnet Mail to: **vetstu-l@uga**

Internet Mail to: **vetstu-l@uga.cc.uga.edu**

Description: This list is for Veterinary Students to use as a general discussion list of vet student concerns and discuss career opportunities.

List Owner/Contact: Fred Smith <smith.f@calc.vet.uga.edu>
Anne Swagler <ars95@calc.vet.uga.edu>

VETTOX-L

Veterinary Toxicology Discussion List (restricted)

Bitnet Subscribe to: `listserv@ucdcvdls`

Internet Subscribe to: `listserv@cvdls.ucdavis.edu`

Bitnet Mail to: **vettox-l@ucdcvdls**

Internet Mail to: **vettox-l@cvdls.ucdavis.edu**

Description: A list dedicated to diagnostic toxicology has been established at the University of California. This list will be restricted to those in the practice of diagnostic toxicology, although it will not be an edited list. We hope to provide an atmosphere of cooperation amongst those in the field of diagnostic toxicology to seek solutions to the many challenges that arise during the course of a disease investigation. Subscription is restricted.

List Owners/Contact: James T. Case, DVM, Ph.D. <jcase@ucdcvdls.bitnet>
University of California
School of Veterinary Medicine
California Veterinary Diagnostic Laboratory System
P.O. Box 1770
Davis, CA 95617
Phone: 916-752-4408

Bill Cohen <bcohen@ucdcvdls.bitnet>

WILDNET

Computing and Statistics in Fisheries & Wildlife Biology

Internet Subscribe to: `wildnet-request@tribune.usask.ca`

Internet Mail to: **wildnet@tribune.usask.ca**

Description: The Wildnet mailing list was established for the exchange of ideas, questions, and solutions in the area of fisheries and wildlife computing and statistics. Possibilities include reviews of literature, reports on conferences, questions on experimental design, field techniques, relevant hardware, software, databases, etc.

List Owner/Contact: Eric Woodsworth <woodsworth@sask.usask.ca>
Canadian Wildlife Service
Saskatoon, Canada
Phone: 306-975-4023

WISENET
Women In Science and Engineering Network
Bitnet Subscribe to: `listserv@uicvm`
Internet Subscribe to: `listserv@uicvm.uic.edu`
Bitnet Mail to: **`wisenet@uicvm`**
Internet Mail to: **`wisenet@uicvm.uic.edu`**

Description: Women in science, mathematics or engineering and students interested in those disciplines are encouraged to join a newly established network to help them progress in their careers. WISENET/Midwest is a Midwest network that promotes women and girls of diverse backgrounds in science, mathematics and engineering. Its objectives include: to improve access tto careers and advancement in science and engineering for girls and women of diverse backgrounds.

List Owner/Contact: Dr. Alice Dan `<u35049@uicvm.uic.edu>`

YSN
Young Scientists' Network
Internet Subscribe to: `ysnadm@ren.sdsc.edu`
Internet Mail to: **`ysn@ren.sdsc.edu`**

Description: YSN is a loose-knit organization of young PhD scientists, science graduate students, and many other people who observe and participate in a discussion of issues involving the employment of scientists. There is no governing board, no membership fees, and no requirements for joining the electronic mailing lists. The following three general goals which are intended to guide the discussion and to stimulate members to work together for the benefit of all young scientists.

1. to inform government officials, the press, and the general public that despite widely publicized forecasts of an impending shortage of scientists, there is in reality an oversupply of young scientists.
2. to find and develop traditional and non-traditional employment opportunities for scientists in response to this oversupply of young scientists.
3. to confront the organizations which have created and continue to exacerbate this problem of oversupply of scientists in order to encourage them to change their policies and operations.

List Owners/Contact: Kevin Aylesworth, Ph.D `<kda@pinet.aip.org>`
1600 Massachusetts Ave. Apt. #208,
Cambridge, MA 02138
Phone: 617-354-9931

John Quackenbush `<ysnadm@ren.sdsc.edu>`
Jennifer Cohen `<jenc@aip.org>`

INTERNET MAILSERVERS & DATABASES

AGRALIN
Agricultural Bibliographic Information System of the Netherlands
Internet: Telnet to 137.224.140.15
    At the prompt, enter: `hello opac.bas`
URL: **`telnet://137.224.140.15`**

Description: AGRALIN is a system is maintained by the joint efforts of the Wageningen Agricultural University and the Dutch Ministry of Agriculture, Nature Conservation and Fisheries. Part of this system is the Union Catalogue of Agricultural Books and Periodicals containing bibliographic data on the collections of the Wageningen Agricultural University Library and some 70 other Dutch libraries with large collections on agriculture.

Contact: B.F.M. Leemreize `<leemreize@jka.wau.nl>`
Phone: 31-837083602
Fax: 31-837084761

AGRICULTURAL INFORMATION

Internet: telnet to idea.ag.uiuc.edu or 128.174.134.152

    At the login prompt, enter: `flood`

URL: `telnet://idea.ag.uiuc.edu`

Description: Agricultural info (livestock reports, current market prices, etc.)

ALMANAC

USDA Extension Service Mail Server

Mail to: `almanac@esusda.gov`

    In body of letter, enter: `send guide`

Note: Almanac is a tool for storing information which can be requested by sending an e-mail message to the Almanac. Messages consist of very basic commands. Responses are provided via e-mail messages back to the user. Among the USDA Extension Service mailing lists are the following:

List: `USDA.DVM`

Type: Server

Description: The purpose of this newsletter is to provide information relating to veterinary medicine, science and agriculture which may include: grants from USDA-ES; FDA/EPA/USDA regulations and changes; industry news; food safety and quality updates; meetings; employment opportunities and scientific news.

List: `USDA Dairy Update`

Type: Server

Description: Postings of USDA information affecting policy decisions that affect the dairy community.

List Owner: Basil Eastwood <`beastwood@esusda.gov`>

List: `USDA.RRDB`

Type: Server

Description: The U.S. Department of Agriculture (USDA) Extension Service offers the Research Results Database (RRDB), containing brief summaries of recent research from the USDA's Agricultural Research Service (ARS) and Economic Research Service (ERS).

    Extension's Other Almanac Sites

Location	Internet Address
Auburn University	almanac@acenet.auburn.edu
Cornell University	almanac@cce.cornell.edu
Extension Service-USDA	almanac@ace.esusda.gov
National Ag Library/ES-USDA	almanac@cyfer.esusda.gov
North Carolina State University	almanac@ces.ncsu.edu
Oregon State University	almanac@oes.orst.edu
Purdue University	almanac@ecn.purdue.edu
University of California	almanac@silo.ucdavis.edu
University of Missouri	almanac@ext.missouri.edu
University of Wisconsin	almanac@joe.uwex.edu
	almanac@wisplan.uwex.edu

Description: Offer USDA market news, articles about use of computer in agricultural science, and Extension Computing Technology Newsletters.

    To find what is in an Almanac server, send an email message one of the almanac server addresses listed above, since each site maintains a subject catalog for that location. In the body of your message, enter: `send catalog`

    To get the Almanac Users Guide, send an email message to `almanac@esusda.gov` or any other almanac and in the body of the message, enter: `send guide`

To subscribe to an Almanac Mailing Group, send an email message to to the almanac site where the mailing group you wish to join is located. In the body of your message type the command: subscribe mailing group name.

AQUATIC CONSERVATION NETWORK
National Capital Freenet

Internet: telnet to `freenet.carleton.ca`

At the login prompt, enter: `guest` then enter: `go acn` and follow the menus to the list.

URL: `telnet://freenet.carleton.ca`

Description: Aquarists Dedicated to the Preservation of Aquatic Life—maintains IUCN list of Fishes Section of the Red List of Threatened Animals and an International Directory of Aquarist Organizations.

Contact: Rob Huntley <`ag508@freenet.carleton.ca`>
Aquatic Conservation Network
540 Roosevelt Avenue
Ottawa, Ontario, Canada K2A 1Z8
phone: 613-729-4670
fax: 613-729-5613

ATCC RECOMBINANT COLLECTIONS
NIH/ATCC Repository of human and mouse DNA probes and libraries

Internet: telnet to `atcc.nih.gov` or `156.40.144.248`

URL: `telnet://atcc.nih.gov`

username: `search`

password: `common`

Contact: email to <`help@atcc.nih.gov`>
phone: 301-231-5586 (Donna Maglott)

Requests for materials from the ATCC: email to <`request@atcc.nih.gov`>
phone: 800-638-6597
local: 301-881-2600
fax: 301-231-5826

ATI-NET
California State University-Fresno
Agricultural Information

Internet: telnet to `caticsuf.csufresno.edu` or `129.8.100.15`

At the login prompt, enter: `public`

URL: `telnet://caticsuf.csufresno.edu`

Description: ATI-Net is a full service information source designed to assist several markets within California. Individual systems provide information for the agricultural market, the educational community (CSUPER-Net), Automated Trade Library Service (ATLS), Biotechnology Information (CSUPERB).

BIOETHICS ONLINE SERVICE
Medical College of Wisconsin

Internet: telnet to `min.lib.mcw.edu` or `141.106.32.20`

URL: `telnet://min.lib.mcw.edu`

Modem: 414-266-5777

Help Line: 414-257-8700

— If you do not have a post account at MCW, at the login prompt, enter: `c min`

— If you do have a post account at MCW, at the login prompt, enter: `c post`, then at the prompt (`post>`), enter: `biomenu`

Description: The Bioethics Online Service is an information resource of the Center for the Study of Bioethics and the Health Information Technology Center (HITC) of the Medical College of Wisconsin (MCW). The Bioethics Online Service consists of: (1) The Bioethics Database; (2) The Bioethics Center and Wisconsin Ethics Committee; Network (WECN) News and Announcements section; and (3) The Bioethics Online E-mail Service. The Bioethics Database is an update service providing information on current bioethics topics, including news reports, abstracts of pertinent journal articles, legislative actions and court decisions, with intermittent commentary. The information is searchable by key words. The Bioethics Center and Wisconsin Ethics Committee Network (WECN) News and Announcements section posts news from the Bioethics Center, including speakers, conferences, journal clubs, and other presentations. It also posts news of the Wisconsin Ethics Committee Network, and information about its Speakers Bureau. A second feature of this section is a case discussion area.

Contact: Arthur R. Derse, MD, JD
Bioethics Online Service <biohelp@its.mcw.edu>
Information Technology Services
Medical College of Wisconsin
8701 Watertown Plank Road
Milwaukee, WI 53226

BIOMOO

Internet: telnet to `bioinfo.weizmann.ac.il` or `132.76.55.12`, port `8888`
   At the login prompt, enter: `guest`

URL: `telnet://bioinfo.weizmann.ac.il`

Description: BioMOO is a virtual meeting place for biologists, connected to the Globewide Network Academy. The main physical part of the BioMOO is located at the BioInformatics Unit of the Weizmann Institute of Science, Israel. BioMOO is a professional community of Biology researchers. It is a place to come meet colleagues in Biology studies and related fields and brainstorm, to hold colloquia and conferences, to explore the serious side of this new medium. MOO stands for MUD, Object Oriented. MUD stands for Multiple User Dimension. This means, that MOO is an object-oriented computer program that allows many users to log in at the same time, and interact among themselves, and with the program.

Contact: Gustavo Glusman <bmgustav@bioinformatics.weizmann.ac.il>

BIOSCI ELECTRONIC NEWSGROUP NETWORK

Biological Scientists Electronic Discussion Groups (Animal-related portions)

This is a very rich and complex resource.

The first thing you should do is send email to: `biosci@net.bio.net`
   In the body of the message, enter: `help`

This will send you the very latest instructions on how to proceed. The following is generally how you will proceed from there.

Internet Subscribe to: `biosci-server@net.bio.net`
   In the body of the message, enter: `lists`

to obtain a listing of all current BIOSCI mailing lists.

After obtaining the names of the mailing lists using the "lists" command, send e-mail to: `biosci-server@net.bio.net`
   In the body of the message, enter: `subscribe listname`

to add your address to the appropriate mailing lists. Please substitute "`listname`" above with the appropriate name of the list that you want to join/cancel. These are listed below.

Note: Please note that if you have access to Usenet News, you do not need an e-mail subscription! Simply read and post to the newsgroups in the "`bionet`" newsgroup hierarchy using your USENET news software.

Description: The BIOSCI newsgroup network was developed to allow easy worldwide communications between biological scientists who work on a variety of computer networks. By having distribution sites or "nodes" on each major network, BIOSCI allows its users to contact people around the world without having to learn a variety of computer addressing tricks. Any user can simply post a message to his/her regional BIOSCI node and copies of that message will be distributed automatically to all other subscribers on all of the participating networks, including the Internet, Usenet, Bitnet, EARN, NetNorth, Heanrt, and JANET.

If you get lost, send email to: <biosci-help@net.bio.net> to request manual help.

Contact: Dave Kristofferson <kristoff@net.bio.net>
BIOSCI/bionet Manager

List of BIOSCI Newsgroup Topics

MAILING LIST NAME	*TOPIC*
ACEDB-SOFT	Discussions by users and developers of genome databases using the ACEDB software
AGEING	Discussions on ageing research
AGROFORESTRY	Discussions about agroforestry research
ARABIDOPSIS	Newsgroup for the Arabidopsis Genome Project
BIOFORUM	Discussions about biological topics for which there is not yet a dedicated newsgroup
BIOLOGICAL-INFORMATION-THEORY-AND-CHOWDER-SOCIETY	Applications of information theory to biology; this group is not for general information or for discussion of theories in general
BIONAUTS	Question/answer forum for help using electronic networks, locating e-mail addresses, etc.
BIONEWS **	General announcements of widespread interest to biologists
BIO-JOURNALS **	Tables of Contents of biological journals
BIO-MATRIX	Applications of computers to biological databases
BIOPHYSICAL-SOCIETY **	Official announcements/information from the Biophysical Society
BIOPHYSICS	Discussion of issues related to the science and profession of biophysics
BIO-SOFTWARE	Information on software for the biological sciences
BIOTHERMOKINETICS	Discussions about the kinetics, thermodynamics and control of biological processes at the cellular level
CELL-BIOLOGY	Discussions about cell biology including cancer research at the cellular level
CHLAMYDOMONAS	Discussions about the biology of the green alga Chlamydomonas and related genera
CHROMOSOMES	Discussions about mapping and sequencing of eucaryote chromosomes
COMPUTATIONAL-BIOLOGY **	Mathematical and computer applications in biology
CYTONET	Discussions about research on the cytoskeleton, plasma membrane, and cell wall
DROSOPHILA	Discussions about biological research on Drosophila
EMBL-DATABANK	Messages to and from the EMBL database staff
EMPLOYMENT	Job opportunities in biology (see BIOSCI FAQ *before* posting commercial job openings)
GDB	Messages to and from the Genome Data Bank staff
GENBANK-BB	Messages to and from the GenBank database staff
GENETIC-LINKAGE	Newsgroup for genetic linkage analysis
HIV-MOLECULAR-BIOLOGY	Discussions about the molecular biology of HIV
HUMAN-GENOME-PROGRAM	NIH-sponsored newsgroup on human genome issues
IMMUNOLOGY	Discussions about research in immunology
INFO-GCG	Discussions about the GCG sequence analysis software
JOURNAL-NOTES	Practical advice on dealing with professional journals
METHODS-AND-REAGENTS	Requests for information and lab reagents
MOLECULAR-EVOLUTION	Discussions about research in molecular evolution

MYCOLOGY	Discussions about research on filamentous fungi
NEUROSCIENCE	Discussions about research in the neurosciences
N2-FIXATION	Discussion about biological nitrogen fixation
PARASITOLOGY	Discussions about research in parasitology
PHOTOSYNTHESIS	Discussions about photosynthesis research
PLANT-BIOLOGY	Discussions about research in plant biology
POPULATION-BIOLOGY	Discussions about research in population biology
PROTEIN-ANALYSIS	Discussions about research on proteins and messages for the PIR and SWISS-PROT databank staffs
PROTEIN-CRYSTALLOGRAPHY	Discussion about crystallography of macromolecules and messages for the PDB staff
PROTISTA	Discussions about research on ciliates and other protists
RAPD	Discussions about Randomly Amplified Polymorphic DNA
SCIENCE-RESOURCES **	Information from/about scientific funding agencies
STRUCTURAL-NMR	Discussions about the use of NMR for macromolecular structure determination
TROPICAL-BIOLOGY	Discussions about research in tropical biology
VIROLOGY	Discussions about research in virology
WOMEN-IN-BIOLOGY	Discussions about issues concerning women biologists
YEAST	Discussions about the molecular biology and genetics of yeast

** Note that newsgroups flagged with ** are moderated, i.e., postings are directed to a moderator (editor) who later forwards messages (possibly edited or condensed) to the newsgroup.

Those who use e-mail to post messages should send their mail to the following Internet addresses in the USA and Pacific Rim. In Europe, Africa, and Central Asia, use `biosci@daresbury.ac.uk`

MAILING LIST NAME	Mailing Address
ACEDB-SOFT	acedb@net.bio.net
AGEING	ageing@net.bio.net
AGROFORESTRY	ag-forst@net.bio.net
ARABIDOPSIS	arab-gen@net.bio.net
BIOFORUM	bioforum@net.bio.net
BIO-INFORMATION-THEORY +	bio-info@net.bio.net
BIONAUTS	bio-naut@net.bio.net
BIONEWS **	bionews@net.bio.net
BIO-JOURNALS **	bio-jrnl@net.bio.net
BIO-MATRIX	biomatrx@net.bio.net
BIOPHYSICAL-SOCIETY **	bphyssoc@net.bio.net
BIOPHYSICS	biophys@net.bio.net
BIO-SOFTWARE	bio-soft@net.bio.net
BIOTHERMOKINETICS	btk-mca@net.bio.net
CELL-BIOLOGY	cellbiol@net.bio.net
CHLAMYDOMONAS	chlamy@net.bio.net
CHROMOSOMES	biochrom@net.bio.net
COMPUTATIONAL-BIOLOGY **	comp-bio@net.bio.net
CYTONET	cytonet@net.bio.net
DROSOPHILA	dros@net.bio.net
EMBL-DATABANK	embl-db@net.bio.net
EMPLOYMENT	biojobs@net.bio.net

GDB	gdb@net.bio.net
GENBANK-BB	genbankb@net.bio.net
GENETIC-LINKAGE	gen-link@net.bio.net
HIV-MOLECULAR-BIOLOGY	hiv-biol@net.bio.net
HUMAN-GENOME-PROGRAM	gnome-pr@net.bio.net
IMMUNOLOGY	immuno@net.bio.net
INFO-GCG	info-gcg@net.bio.net
JOURNAL-NOTES	jrnlnote@net.bio.net
METHODS-AND-REAGENTS	methods@net.bio.net
MOLECULAR-EVOLUTION	mol-evol@net.bio.net
MYCOLOGY	mycology@net.bio.net
NEUROSCIENCE	neur-sci@net.bio.net
N2-FIXATION	n2fix@net.bio.net
PARASITOLOGY	parasite@net.bio.net
PHOTOSYNTHESIS	photosyn@net.bio.net
PLANT-BIOLOGY	plantbio@net.bio.net
POPULATION-BIOLOGY	pop-bio@net.bio.net
PROTEIN-ANALYSIS	proteins@net.bio.net
PROTEIN-CRYSTALLOGRAPHY	xtal-log@net.bio.net
PROTISTA	protista@net.bio.net
RAPD	rapd@net.bio.net
SCIENCE-RESOURCES **	sci-res@net.bio.net
STRUCTURAL-NMR	str-nmr@net.bio.net
TROPICAL-BIOLOGY	trop-bio@net.bio.net
VIROLOGY	virology@net.bio.net
WOMEN-IN-BIOLOGY	womenbio@net.bio.net
YEAST	yeast@net.bio.net

BIOSCI "PROTOTYPE" NEWSGROUPS

To assist areas of research in developing their own electronic communication forums, BIOSCI at net.bio.net will set up, on request, a mailing list *without* an associated USENET newsgroup. The mailing list is created only at net.bio.net, the U.S. BIOSCI node, and all subscription requests must be sent to the e-mail server at `biosci-server@net.bio.net` regardless of one's geographical location. The prototype newsgroup has six months to build up its readership after which time it is put out for a vote for full newsgroup status (i.e., to have both a mailing list *and* parallel USENET newsgroup created at both BIOSCI nodes in the U.S. and U.K.). The current prototype newsgroups are listed below. Please send subscription requests to `biosci-server@net.bio.net` and NOT to the newsgroup posting addresses. Prototype newsgroups may *not* be fully archived, so please be sure to save any messages that you may want to refer to again.

Posting Address	*Purpose*
`biocan@net.bio.net`	An unmoderated forum established by the Canadian Federation of Biological Societies (CFBS) to serve as a multidisciplinary forum for the exchange of information within the Canadian biological and biomedical science community.
`biogopher@net.bio.net`	A communication forum for all Bio-Gopher administrators.
`emf-bio@net.bio.net`	Discussions on the electromagnetic field interactions with biological systems.
`grasses@net.bio.net`	Scientific discussions/questions regarding grasses, especially cereal, forage, and turf species.
`nmr-str@net.bio.net`	A forum for all those interested in studying three dimensional structure of macromolecules using Nuclear Magnetic Resonance Spectroscopy (NMR).

`rna@net.bio.net`	Discussions about RNA editing, RNA splicing, and ribozyme activities of RNA.
`staden-users@net.bio.net`	Discussions about the Staden Package for molecular sequence analysis.
`urodeles@net.bio.net`	Discussions among research scientists using urodele amphibians (axolotls, salamanders, and newts) in any biological field.
`yac@net.bio.net`	Dicussions about yeast artificial chromosomes

BYTE ANIMAL CLINIC
Cleveland Academy of Veterinary Medicine

Internet: telnet to: `freenet-in-a.cwru.edu` or `129.22.8.51`
`freenet-in-b.cwru.edu` or `129.22.8.32`
`freenet-in-c.cwru.edu` or `129.22.8.51`

    At the login prompt, enter: `visitor`

URL: `telnet://freenet-in-a.cwru.edu`
`telnet://freenet-in-b.cwru.edu`
`telnet://freenet-in-c.cwru.edu`

Description: The Byte Animal Clinic is an electronic veterinary clinic on the Cleveland Freenet and sponsored by the Cleveland Academy of Veterinary Medicine. Freenets offer services like Telnet, full email, USA Today news and weather, and are typically set up like 'cities'. Registration is (as the name implies) free, but usually requires a snail-mailed form. The Cleveland Freenet is the first Freenet and by far the largest. Lots of other features.

Contact: D.B. Cameron, DVM <`aa266@cleveland.freenet.edu`>

CAMIS
Center for Advanced Medical Informatics at Stanford

Internet: telnet to `camis.stanford.edu` or `36.44.0.7`

    At the login prompt, enter: `gopher`

URL: `gopher://camis.Stanford.edu:70`

CANCERNET
National Cancer Institute Cancer Information Network

Mail to: `cancernet@icicb.nci.nih.gov`

    Leave Subject line blank

    In body of letter, enter: `help`

Help Line: 301-486-7403

Description: CancerNet is a quick and easy way to obtain, through electronic mail, recommended treatment guidelines in English or Spanish from the National Cancer Institute's Physician Data Query (PDQ) system. CancerNet also lets you request information about PDQ, PDQ distributors, and other products and services from the NCI, including a list of patient publications available from the Office of Cancer Communications. You can access CancerNet through a number of different networks including BITNET and Internet. There is no charge for the service unless your local computer center charges for use of e-mail. The CancerNet Contents List may change as new statements and other information is included.

Contact: Cheryl Burg <`cheryl@icicb.nci.nih.gov`>
    Building 82, Room 103A
    Bethesda, Maryland 20892
    Phone: (301) 496-8880
    Fax: (301) 480-8105

CARL System
Colorado Alliance of Research Libraries

Internet: telnet to `database.carl.org` or `192.54.81.76`

URL: `telnet://database.carl.org`

Description: A collection of library catalogs, business databases, and includes more than 14,000 titles, and more than 4 million articles. over 750,000 articles are added annually. In addition to being able to search by keyword, you can search by author and you can browse by journal title. Many biological holdings are indexed.

CENET
Cornell Cooperative Extension Network

Internet: telnet to `empire.cce.cornell.edu` or `132.236.89.2`

    At the login prompt, enter: `guest`

URL: `telnet://empire.cce.cornell.edu`

Description: Educational resources in agriculture, natural resources, pest management, etc.

Contact: Henry DeVries <`eetg@cce.cornell.edu`>
    Phone: 607-225-8127

CENTERS FOR DISEASE CONTROL AND PREVENTION
WONDER Database

Help Line: 404-332-4569

Description: CDC has a wide variety of databases—including mortality data, hospital discharge, SEER cancer sets, etc.— available through WONDER, a free package that provides a pc based graphical front end to format and analyze requests for data and communication software allowing connection to the CDC.

Contact: Dan Rosen <`dhr0@opsirm8.em.cdc.gov`>
    Centers for Disease Control and Prevention
    1600 Clifton Rd., MS F-51
    Atlanta, GA 30333
    Phone: 404-488-7521

CUFAN
Clemson University Forestry & Agriculture Network, South Carolina

Internet: telnet to `eureka.clemson.edu` or `130.127.8.2`

    At the login prompt, enter: `PUBLIC`

URL: `telnet://eureka.clemson.edu`

Description: VTX (Videotex) Information Base, Electronic mail, and conference system. Subject Scope: Information on weather, agricultural economics, plant and animal science, agricultural engineering, home food preparation and preservation, & agricultural news.

Contact: Ray Holliday <`rhlldy@clust1.clemson.edu`>
    210 Barre Hall
    Clemson University
    Clemson, SC 29634-0310
    Phone: 803-656-3383

DATA ZOO
Center for Coastal Studies
Scripps Institution of Oceanography

Internet: telnet to `coast.ucsd.edu` or `128.54.21.56`

    At the login prompt, enter: `gopher`

URL: `telnet://coast.ucsd.edu`

Description: The Data Zoo is brought to you by the Center for Coastal Studies at the Scripps Institution of Oceanography, University of California, San Diego with funding generously provided by the Mineral Management Service, Bureau of Land Management, Department of the Interior. The Data Zoo contains data collected by various California coastal data collection programs and studies and organized synoptically by experiment, instrument type and geographical region. These data were procured by the Center for Coastal Studies for inclusion in the Data Zoo and have been checked for consistency and validity to the best of our ability using Data reports and documentation provided by the source organization/individuals for each data set.

Contact: <zookeeper@coast.ucsd.edu>

ECOSYSTEMS
University of Virginia

Internet: telnet to ecosys.drdr.virginia.edu or 128.143.96.10

    At the login prompt, enter: gopher or lynx or echochat

URL: **telnet://ecosys.drdr.virginia.edu**

Description: A recycling and environmental information server. It provides and connects users to local, regional, national, and international environmental info.

ENVIRONMENTAL HEALTH & SAFETY BBS
University of Illinois

Internet: telnet to romulus.ehs.uiuc.edu or 128.174.74.24

URL: **telnet://romulus.ehs.uiuc.edu**

Description: The University of Illinois Division of EnvironmentalHealth and Safety maintains a large collection of Material Safety Datasheets. Part of the collection (approximately 26,000 MSDS's) is maintained in paper files at the Division headquarters located at 101 South Gregory St., Urbana, Illinois. The paper collection is constantly updated as new or more current MSDS's are received from manufacturers and suppliers. Each MSDS, is assigned a unique serial number upon arrival. These numbers are referred to as DEHS ID numbers or DEHSID's. A file listing the dehsid, the chemical name and the supplier for each of these MSDS's is maintained on-line. It is accessible through this BBS at the MSDS MENU. In addition to the paper file, the Division also maintains a file containing approximately 86,000 MSDS in the form of a database which is also directly accessible through this BBS. This database consists of a collection which is distributed quarterly by the Canadian Centre for Occupational Health and Safety (CCOHS). The CCOHS is a non-profit organization dedicated to promoting a safe and healthy environment by providing information about occupational health and safety. The information contained in the CCOHS database is contributed directly to CCOHS by manufacturers and suppliers of chemical products. The MSDS's in the CCOHS database are in English and/or French, as supplied by the contributors. They contain basic information on the properties and potential hazards of chemical products, how to use them safely, and what to do if there is an emergency. The MSDS MENU allows you to simultaneously search the index of all of the paper MSDS's contained in our files as well as the MSDS's obtained on a quarterly basis from CCOHS. As you search the index, you will notice that some of the dehsid's start with the letter "T". These represent MSDS which you may directly look at in their entirety on-line. This program will eventually be used for accessing many information sources in the Division of Environmental Health and Safety. It is currently being developed, so please keep in mind that some things will not work correctly.

Contact: Hector Mandel <mandel@romulus.ehs.uiuc.edu>

EPA ONLINE LIBRARY SYSTEM
Environmental Protection Agency

Internet: telnet to epaibm.rtpnc.epa.gov or 134.67.180.1

    At the login prompt, enter: public

URL: **telnet://epaibm.rtpnc.epa.gov**

Description: Searchable databases with citations, hazardous wastes, clean lakes, environmental financing, and Access EPA

FDA BBS
Food and Drug Administration Bulletin Board System

Internet: telnet to fdabbs.fda.gov or 150.148.8.48

    At the login prompt, enter: bbs

URL: **telnet://fdabbs.fda.gov**

Description: The FDA's online information service includes information on topics such as, FDA news releases, Drug and Device product approvals list, current information on AIDS, Veterinary Medicine news, import alerts, and many other FDA related subjects.

FEDIX
Federal Information Exchange

Internet: telnet to `fedix.fie.com` or `192.111.228.33`

    At the login prompt, enter: `fedix`

URL: **telnet://fedix.fie.com**

Description: FEDIX is an on-line information service that links thehigher education community and the federal government to facilitate research, education, and services. The system provides accurate and timely federal agency information to colleges, universities, and other research organizations. FEDIX provides daily information updates on: Federal education and research programs (including descriptions, eligibility, funding, deadlines); scholarships, fellowships, and grants; available used government research equipment; new funding for specific research and education activities from the Commerce Business Daily, Federal Register, and other sources; minority assistance research and education programs; news & current events within participating agencies; general information such as agency history, budget, organizational structure, and mission statements.

Contact: <comments@fedix.fie.com>

Help Line: 301-975-0103

FEDWORLD
National Technical Information Service
    Federal Information Gateway

Internet: telnet to `fedworld.gov` or `192.239.92.201`

    At the Login prompt, enter: `new`

URL: **telnet://fedworld.gov**

Help Line: 703-487-4608

Description: Access to more than 100 U.S. government computer bulletin boards, many of them previously accessible only by modem. Also includes full text of select U.S. government publications, statistical files, federal job lists, satellite images and more.

Contact: Ken Royer
    Phone: 703-487-4850

4-H YOUTH PROJECTS
University of California-Davis

Almanac: Send e-mail to `almanac@ucdavis.edu`

    In the body of the message, enter: send extension 4h-youth catalog

Description: 4-H project manuals in several different project areas. This is a joint experimental project between University of California Cooperative Extension and the Tennessee State 4-H Program.

Contacts: Penny Risdon <plrisdon@ucdavis.edu>
    Mina Ostergard <mostergard@ucdavis.edu>

GBASE
Genomic Database of the Mouse
    Jackson Laboratory

Internet: telnet to `morgan.jax.org` or `192.233.41.26`

    At the login prompt, enter: `guest`

URL: **telnet://morgan.jax.org**

Description: GBASE is the genomic database of the mouse at the Jackson Laboratory, and consists of: genetic linkage maps, all known literature on locus mapping, lists of all locus symbols, locus names, chromosomal locations, and references; information about alleles at polymorphic loci for over 1100 inbred mouse strains; & descriptions of genes and loci.

Contact: Alan Hillyard, Ph.D. <alh@morgan.jax.org>
The Jackson Laboratory
600 Main St.
Bar Harbour, ME 04609-0800
Phone: 207-288-3371
FAX: 207-288-5079

GENETICS BANK
Genetic Database & Nucleic Acid/Protein Sequences

Mail to: gene-server@bchs.uh.edu
retrieve@ncbi.nlm.nih.gov
blast@ncbi.nlm.nih.gov

In subject of letter, enter: help

GENOME CENTER GENETIC MAP OF THE MOUSE
Massachusetts Institute of Technology

Mail to: genome_database@genome.wi.mit.edu

In subject of letter, enter: help

Description: Using this service you can obtain locus and assay names of mapped SSLPs, the forward and reverse primer sequences, the genotypes of the loci on the mapping cross, the sizes of the PCR products on selected standard inbred strains, and other useful information. The database can be queried for markers meeting a number of different criteria. For example, you can ask for markers by name, by chromosome, or by position on the map. You can even request a list of markers that are polymorphic between two mouse strains. This project is an ongoing one. As new markers are added to the map they will be released on a quarterly basis on approximately the following schedule: 1 January 1994, 1 April 1994, 1 July 1994, 1 October 1994, etc. Release five of the Whitehead Institute/MIT Genome Center Genetic Map of the Mouse is now available. This map consists of randomly-chosen simple sequence length polymorphisms (microsatellites) that can be analyzed using the polymerase chain reaction, as described in Dietrich, W., et al., Genetics 131:423-447 (1992). Currently the released map contains 3011 markers. The markers fall into 20 linkage groups spanning approximately 1400 cM with an average spacing of less than 0.5 cM. To obtain copies of the most current query forms, send a message to "genome_database@genome.wi.mit.edu" with either a subject line or body text of "help". You will receive instructions and a query form by return mail. Just fill out the form, send it to "genome_database@genome.wi.mit.edu", and the answer to your query will be mailed back automatically.

Contact: Ert Dredge <ert@genomewi.mit.edu>
Whitehead Institute's Center for Genome Research
One Kendall Sq, Bldg 300, 5th floor
Cambridge, MA 02139
Phone: 617-252-1922
Fax: 617-252-1902

LOCIS
Library of Congress Information System

Internet: telnet to locis.loc.gov or 140.147.254.3

URL: telnet://locis.loc.gov

Description: The world's most extensive card catalog and search through and read pending legislation from as far back as the 1970's. Directory of more than 12,000 organizations qualified and willing to answer questions and provide information on many topics in science, technology and the social sciences.

MEDLINE
National Library of Medicine

Internet: telnet to `medlars.nlm.nih.gov` or `130.14.10.200`

URL: **telnet://medlars.nlm.nih.gov**

Modem: Access via Grateful Med software

Help Line: 800-638-8480; NLM Customer Service: 703-555-1212

Grateful Med BBS: 800-525-5756

E-mail contact: `gmhelp@gmedserv.nlm.nih.gov`

Notes: Account needed to access MEDLINE.

Databases include:
- AIDSDRUGS
- AIDSLINE (AIDS Information online)
- AIDSTRIALS (AIDS Clinical TRIALS)
- ALERTS (Clinical Alerts)
- AVLINE
- BIOETHICSLINE
- CANCERLIT
- CATLINE (CATalog online)
- CHEMID (CHEMical Identification)
- TELNET MEDLARS.NLM.NIH.GOVCHEMLINE (CHEMical dictionary onLINE)
- DIRLINE (DIRectory of Information Resources onLINE)
- HEALTH (Health planning & administration)
- MEDLINE (MEDlars onLINE)
- - MED86
- - MED80
- - MED77
- - MED72
- - MED66
- PDQ (Physician Data Query)
- SDILINE (Selective Dissemination of Information onLINE)
- SERLINE (SERials onLINE)
- TOXLINE (TOXicology Information onLINE)
- - TOXLINE65
- TOXLIT (TOXicology LITerature)
- CCRIS (Chemical Carcinogenesis Research Information System)
- HSDB (Hazardous Substances Data Bank)
- RTECS (Registry of Toxic Effects of Chemical Substances)
- TRI (Toxic chemical Release Inventory)
- - TRI87
- - TRI90

MIGRATORY BIRD COLLECTION
University of Puget Sound

Description: The catalog from the University of Puget Sound bird collection is available over Internet. This catalog consists of 18,500+ records of "core data" which includes the museum number, species name, sex, plumage, country, state (or other geopolitical entity), county/other, date, and preparation. Initially, the catalog is only accessible by obtaining a password from Gary Shugart or Dennis Paulson at "`slater@ups.edu`". The University of Puget Sound has the largest computerized bird collection in the northwest USA.

Contact: Gary Shugart or Dennis Paulson <`slater@ups.edu`>
Slater Museum of Natural History
University of Puget Sound
Tacoma, WA 98416
Phone: 206-756-3798

NATIONAL AGRICULTURAL LIBRARY
Reference Services
Send email to: agref@nalusda.gov

NATIONAL LIBRARY OF MEDICINE EDUCATIONAL TECHNOLOGY NETWORK
Internet: telnet to etnet.nlm.nih.gov or 130.14.10.123

    At the login prompt, enter: etnet

URL: `telnet://etnet.nlm.nih.gov`

NEWTON
U.S. Government bulletin board for those teaching and studying science.

Internet: telnet to newton.dep.anl.gov or 146.139.100.50

    At the login prompt, enter: bbs

URL: `telnet://newton.dep.anl.gov`

NIH GRANT LINE
National Institutes of Health

Internet: telnet to wylbur.cu.nih.gov or 128.231.64.82

    When a message has been received that the connection is open, type ,GEN1 (the comma is mandatory). At the INITIALS? prompt, type BB5 and at the

ACCOUNT? prompt, type CCS2. This should put the user into the DRGLINE Bulletin Board (also known as NIH Grant Line at NIH).

URL: `telnet://wylbur.cu.nih.gov`

Description: The purpose of NIH Grant Line is to make program and policy information of the Public Health Service (PHS) agencies rapidly available to the biomedical research community. Most of the research opportunity information available on this bulletin board is derived from the weekly publication, "NIH Guide for Grants and Contracts", consisting of Notices, RFAs, RFPs (announcements of availability), Numbered Program Announcements, and statements of PHS policy. The electronic version known as E-Guide is available for electronic transmission each week, sometimes a day or two in advance of the nominal Friday publication dates. The material consists predominantly of statements about the research interests of the PHS Agencies, Institutes, and National Centers that have funds to support research in the extramural community. The information found on the NIH Grant Line is grouped into three main sections: (1) short News Flashes that appear without any prompting shortly after you have logged on; (2) Bulletins that are for reading; and (3) Files that are intended mainly for downloading.

OCEANIC INFORMATION CENTER
University of Delaware

Internet: telnet to delocn.udel.edu or 128.175.24.1

    At the login prompt, enter: oceanic

URL: `telnet://delocn.udel.edu`

Description: The Oceanic Information Center is maintained by the University of Delaware College of Marine Studies.

PENPAGES
Agricultural Information

Internet: telnet to psupen.psu.edu or 128.118.36.4

    At the login prompt, enter: your two-letter state abbreviation

URL: `telnet://psupen.psu.edu`

Description: PENpages is a full-text information service containing thousands of research-based fact sheets, news articles, newsletters, and reports. Information is entered by faculty and staff of Penn State University, the Pennsylvania Department of Agriculture, USDA and many cooperators nationwide. Information is agricultural-based and consumer-oriented. Topics include: 4-H and youth development, agricultural education, agronomy; dairy and animal science, engineering, entomology, family life and resource management, food safety, forest resources, gerontology, horticulture, human nutrition, pesticide education, plant pathology, poultry science, rural development, veterinary science, water quality, and many others.

Contact: Diann Leri <dleri@psupen.psu.edu>
405 Ag Admin.
College of Agricultural Sciences
University Park, PA 16802
Phone: 814-863-3449

PRAiRIE FALCON NEWSLETTER
Northern Flint Hills Audubon Society

Internet: telnet to `ksuvm.ksu.edu` or `129.130.12.1`
    At the login prompt, enter: `UNICORN`

URL: `telnet://ksuvm.ksu.edu`

Description: The Northern Flint Hills Audobon Society newsletter is available in the Kansas State University Information system in the subdirectory News and Announcements.

Contact: David A. Rintoul <drintoul@ksu.ksu.edu>

PRIMATE TALK ALMANAC
Primate-Talk Information Mail Server

Mail to: `almanac@primate.wisc.edu`
    Leave subject line blank
    In the body of the message, enter: `send primate-talk <request>`

The <request> part indicates the information you would like to receive.

Currently the Primate-Talk almanac knows about the following:

`help`	(this file)
`index`	(what is available)
`calendar`	(calendar of events)
`directory`	(directory of Primate-Talk recipients)
`etiquette`	(e-mail etiquette for the Primate-Talk mailing list) archive <year> <month> (past messages from the Primate-Talk list)

Contact: `primate-talk-request@primate.wisc.edu`

QUERRI
Questions on University Extension Regional Resource Information

Internet: telnet to `exnet.iastate.edu` or `129.186.20.200`
    At the login prompt, enter: `querri`

URL: `telnet://exnet.iastate.edu`

Description: Database of bibliographic info. of over 12,000 educational resources produced by Extension specialists in the north central states. Covers all Extension subject areas.

STIS
National Science Foundation
    Science & Technology Information System

Internet: telnet to `stis.nsf.gov` or `128.150.195.40`
    At the login prompt, enter: `public`

URL: `telnet://stis.nsf.gov`

Modem: 202-357-0359 or 202-357-0360
    12/24/9600 baud, E-7-1
Help Line: 202-357-7555
    When connected, press enter. At the login prompt, enter: `public`.
Description: Provides access to grant information, NSF directories and phone books, press releases, full text of select NSF publications and more.

THE SCIENTIST NEWSLETTER
Internet: telnet to `ds.internic.net` or `192.20.225.200`
    At the login prompt, enter: `guest`
URL: `telnet://ds.internic.net`

Description: THE SCIENTIST is a biweekly newspaper for scientists and the research community. It is circulated internationally to researchers, administrators, and policy makers in academia, industry, and government and covers current issues and events that impact the professional research environment. News includes funding legislation, new grants, employment and salary trends, career advancement opportunities, ethics and conflicts of interest, representation of women and minorities in science, and the interplay of industrial, academic, and governmental research.

To request The Scientist from its email server, send a message to:

`mailserv@ds.internic.net`

with the following line in the body (not the subject) of the message:

`file /ftp/pub/the-scientist/the-scientist-yymmdd`

change "yymmdd" to the issue date you want

USDA Statistical Data
Cornell Mann Library

Internet: telnet to `usda.mannlib.cornell.edu` or `128.253.78.240`
    At the login prompt, enter: `usda`
URL: `gopher://oldal.mannlib.cornell.edu:70`

Description: Computer users worldwide now have access to statistical data gathered by the USDA. Cornell's Mann Library became the host for more than 140 free agricultural data sets, available to anyone with Internet access. The system is easy to search. Data are formatted for importing into existing computer analysis programs. Each data set is accompanied by an explanatory document, and all text documents are indexed for electronic searching.

Contact: Oya Y. Rieger <`oyr1@cornell.edu`>
    Numeric Files Librarian
    Mann Library
    Cornell University
    Ithaca, NY 14853
    Phone: 607-255-7960

U.S. GOVERNMENT PRINTING OFFICE (GPO)
Federal Bulletin Board

Internet: telnet to `federal.bbs.gpo.gov` or `162.140.64.8`, port 3001
URL: `telnet://federal.bbs.gpo.gov`

Description: The Federal Bulletin Board is a service of the U.S. Government Printing Office (GPO). This bulletin board service enables Federal agencies to provide the public with immediate, self-service access to Government information in electronic form at reasonable rates.

VEGETARIAN
World Guide to Vegetarians

Mail to: `mail-server@rtfm.mit.edu`

In the body of the message, enter any combination of the following:

```
send usenet/news.answers/vegetarian/guide/canada1
send usenet/news.answers/vegetarian/guide/canada2
send usenet/news.answers/vegetarian/guide/california1
send usenet/news.answers/vegetarian/guide/california2
send usenet/news.answers/vegetarian/guide/usa1
send usenet/news.answers/vegetarian/guide/usa2
send usenet/news.answers/vegetarian/guide/usa3
send usenet/news.answers/vegetarian/guide/europe
send usenet/news.answers/vegetarian/guide/other
send usenet/news.answers/vegetarian/faq
```

Description: The rec.food.veg World Guide to Vegetarianism_ lists restaurants, stores, organizations, and travel info of interest to vegetarians.

WHITE HOUSE ELECTRONIC PUBLICATIONS

Mail to: `clinton-info@campaign92.org`
  In subject of letter, enter: help
Bill Clinton E-mail: `president@whitehouse.gov`
Al Gore E-Mail: `vice.president@whitehouse.gov`

USENET NEWSGROUPS

Below are those USENET newsgroups which have some connection to animal topics.

Inclusion here of the `alt.` hierarchy is "to be complete," as they say. A few of the "`alt`" newsgroups and their subject matter may be offensive to some of you. You have been warned. I didn't make up the descriptions either. They come from the official Usenet list of newsgroups and excerpted mostly verbatim.

`alt.activism`	Activities for activists.
`alt.activism.d`	Discussion of activist newsgroup.
`alt.agriculture.misc`	Discussion on farming and raising animals.
`alt.animals.badgers`	From the cheese state.
`alt.animals.dolphins`	Flipper and friends.
`alt.animals.foxes`	Foxes, real or imagined.
`alt.animals.humans`	Guess we can't leave these out.
`alt.animals.lampreys`	They're eel-like, and they suck.
`alt.aquaria`	Aquariums as hobbies.
`alt.bigfoot`	Pushing it, but this is the alt category.
`alt.binaries.pictures.furry`	Originaly funny animal art.
`alt.bio.hackers`	Those interested in biohacking.
`alt.bitch.pork`	Complaints about pork.
`alt.chinchilla`	The smooth-furred rodent.
`alt.cows.moo.moo.moo`	Ostensibly, cows.
`alt.devilbunnies`	Stopping the deadly devilbunnies.
`alt.fan.furry`	Fans of funny animals.
`alt.fan.lemurs`	Fans of the big-eyed primates.
`alt.fan.lemurs.cooked`	Not so big fans of the big-eyed primates.
`alt.fishing`	Fishing as a hobby and sport.
`alt.kill.the.whales`	Takeoff on the "Save the Whales" mentality.
`alt.lemmings`	Rodents with a death-wish.
`alt.mythic.animals`	Animals that just don't exist.
`alt.pets.chia`	Stoneware with hair, the famous chia pets.
`alt.pets.rabbits`	Discussions on pet rabbits.
`alt.save.the.earth`	Environmentalist causes.
`alt.skunks`	Enthusiasts of skunks and other mustelidae.
`alt.sport.falconry`	Discuss the age old sport of falconry.
`alt.sustainable.agriculture`	Sustainable agriculture.

`alt.swine.oink.oink.oink`	See alt.cows.moo.moo.moo.
`alt.wolves`	Discussion on wolves and wolf-mix dogs.
`bionet.software.acedb`	Discussion of genome dbase ACEDB software.
`bionet.molbio.ageing`	Discussions about ageing research.
`bionet.agroforestry`	Discussions about agroforestry research.
`bionet.genome.arabidopsis`	The Arabidopsis Genome Project.
`bionet.general`	Discussions about general biological topics.
`bionet.info-theory`	Applications of information theory to biology.
`bionet.users.addresses`	Help on network use & locating addresses, etc.
`bionet.announce`	Announcements of interest to biologists.
`bionet.journals.contents`	Tables of Contents of biological journals.
`bionet.molbio.bio-matrix`	Computers & biological databases.
`bionet.prof-society.biophysics`	Official information from Biophysical Society.
`bionet.biophysics`	Discussion of biophysics.
`bionet.software`	Discussion of software for biological science.
`bionet.metabolic-reg`	Kinetics & control of cellular bioprocesses.
`bionet.cellbiol`	Biological processes at the cellular level.
`bionet.chlamydomonas`	Discussions on biology of green algae.
`bionet.genome.chromosomes`	Discussions about eucaryote chromosomes.
`bionet.biology.computational`	Math & computer applications in biology.
`bionet.cellbiol.cytonet`	Research on plasma membrane & cell wall.
`bionet.drosophila`	Discussions about research on Drosophila.
`bionet.molbio.embldatabank`	Messages to and from the EMBL database staff.
`bionet.jobs`	Job opportunities in biology.
`bionet.molbio.gdb`	Messages to & from the Genome Data Bank staff.
`bionet.molbio.genbank`	Messages to & from the GenBank database staff.
`bionet.molbio.gene-linkage`	Newsgroup for genetic linkage analysis.
`bionet.molbio.hiv`	Discussions about molecular biology of HIV.
`bionet.molbio.genome-program`	NIH newsgroup on human genome issues.
`bionet.immunology`	Discussions about research in immunology.
`bionet.software.gcg`	Discussions on GCG sequence analysis software.
`bionet.journals.note`	Advice on dealing with professional journals.
`bionet.molbio.methds-reagnts`	Requests for information and lab reagents.
`bionet.molbio.evolution`	Research in molecular evolution.
`bionet.mycology`	Research on filamentous fungi.
`bionet.neuroscience`	Research in the neurosciences.
`bionet.biology.n2-fixation`	Discussions on biological nitrogen fixation.
`bionet.parasitology`	Discussions about research in parasitology.
`bionet.photosynthesis`	Discussions about photosynthesis research.
`bionet.plants`	Discussions about research in plant biology.
`bionet.population-biology`	Research in population biology.
`bionet.molbio.proteins`	Research on proteins & PIR & SWISS-PROT dbase.
`bionet.xtallography`	Crystallography of macromolecules & PDB staff.
`bionet.protista`	Research on ciliates and other protists.
`bionet.molbio.rapd`	Randomly Amplified Polymorphic DNA.
`bionet.sci-resources`	Information on scientific funding agencies.
`bionet.structural-nmr`	NMR for macromolecular structure determination.
`bionet.biology.tropical`	Discussions about research in tropical biology.
`bionet.virology`	Discussions about research in virology.
`bionet.women-in-biology`	Issues concerning women biologists.
`bionet.molbio.yeast`	Molecular biology and genetics of yeast.
`bit.listserv.biosph-l`	Discussion on the Biosphere & ecology.
`bit.listserv.ecolog-l`	Ecological Society of America.
`bit.listserv.ethology`	Animal behavior and behavioral ecology.
`bit.listserv.mednews`	Health InfoCom Newsletter.
`bit.listserv.scuba-l`	Scuba diving discussion.

chile.science	Information exchange bet. Chile and the World.
clari.living.animals	(Clarinet) Animals in the news.
clari.tw.health	Disease, medicine, health care.
clari.tw.science	General science stories.
comp.ai.neural-nets	Artificial & Biological neural networks.
comp.ai.philosophy	Consciousness in Computers, Humans & Animals.
comp.simulation	Simualtion methods and problems.
info.nsf.grants	National Science Foundation grant notes.
k12.ed.science	Science education.
misc.activism.progressive	Progressive activism.
rec.aquaria	Keeping fish and aquaria as a hobby.
rec.birds	Hobbyists interested in bird watching.
rec.equestrian	Discussion of things equestrian.
rec.flyfish	Discussion of flyfish.
rec.food.veg	Vegetarians.
rec.hunting	Discussions about hunting.
rec.outdoors.fishing	All aspects of sport and commercial fishing.
rec.pets	Pets, pet care & household animals in general.
rec.pets.birds	The culture and care of indoor birds.
rec.pets.cats	Discussion about domestic cats.
rec.pets.dogs	Any and all subjects relating to dogs as pets.
rec.pets.herp	Reptile, amphibian, & exotic vivarium pets.
rec.pets.rabbits	Discussion about pet rabbits.
rec.scuba	Hobbyists interested in scuba diving.
sci.agriculture	Farming, agriculture and related topics.
sci.agriculture.beekeeping	Bees, beekeeping, and hive products.
sci.answers	Frequently Asked Questions about SCI groups.
sci.anthropology.paleo	Evolution of man and other primates.
sci.aquaria	Only science-oriented posts about aquaria.
sci.bio	Biology and related sciences.
sci.bio.ecology	Ecological research (sponsored by ESA).
sci.bio.ethology	Animal behavior and behavioral ecology.
sci.bio.evolution	Discussions of evolutionary biology.
sci.bio.herp	Biology of amphibians and reptiles.
sci.bio.technology	Any topic relating to biotechnology.
sci.eng.biomed	Discussions on biomedical engineering.
sci.environment	Science and its relation to the environment.
sci.image.processing	Imaging and image processing.
sci.med	Medicine and its related products and regs.
sci.med.aids	AIDS: treatment, path./biol., HIV prevention.
sci.med.psychobiology	Dialog & news in psychiatry and psychobiology.
sci.med.radiologyq	All aspects of radiology.
sci.philosophy	Genl. Discussion on the philosophy of science.
sci.philosophy.tech	Various Topics,including animal consciousness.
sci.psychology.digest	Psycoloquy—APA Electronic Newsletter
sci.research	Research methods, funding, ethics, & misc.
sci.research.careers	Information relevant to careers in science.
sci.research.postdoc	Anything about postdoctoral studies.
sci.techniques.microscopy	Information and techniques with microscopes.
sci.virtual-worlds	Modelling the Universe.
sci.virtual-worlds.apps	Virtual reality technology and applications.
soc.culture.scientists	The social enviroment of science.
talk.environment	Discussions about environmental issues.
talk.politics.animals	The use and/or abuse of animals.

Anonymous FTP Sites

Archival FTP sites containing animal-related text files and software programs are not well documented on the Internet. Help in locating more sites is appreciated.

ANIMAL RIGHTS
FTP: think.com or 131.239.2.1

Directory: /pub/animal-rights

URL: **ftp://think.com/pub/animal-rights/**

AQUARIA
FTP: camel.scubed.com or 192.31.63.74

Directory: /aquaria

URL: **ftp://camel.scubed.com/aquaria/**

AQUARIA
FTP: jerico.usc.edu or 128.125.51.47

Directory: /pub/aquaria

URL: **ftp://jerico.usc.edu/pub/aquaria/**

Description: The FAQ for sci.aquaria, rec.aquaria and alt.aquaria is posted monthly on the first on of the month.

Contact: Tony Li <tli@cisco.com>
    Patti Beadles <patti@hosehead.hf.intel.com>

BIODIVERSITY
Brazil

FTP: bdt.ftpt.br or 192.207.195.1

URL: **ftp://bdt.ftpt.br/**

BIOINFORMATICS
Australian National University

FTP: 150.203.38.74

URL: **ftp://150.203.38.74/**

Description: ANU's Bioinformatics Facility provides information on Internet under a number of themes. At present the major themes include: biodiversity; bioinformatics & biocomputing; biomathematics and biostatistics; complex systems; general interest; landscape ecology and the environment; molecular biology; neurosciences; viruses; and weather and global monitoring.

Contact: David Green <david.green@anu.edu.au>

BIOLOGY—INTRODUCTION
FTP: ics.uci.edu or 128.195.1.1

Directory: /pub/bvickers/origins

URL: **ftp://ics.uci.edu/pub/bvickers/origins/**

BIOLOGY SOFTWARE AND DATA—Indiana University
(Molecular Biology)

FTP: ftp.bio.indiana.edu or 129.79.224.25

URL: **ftp://ftp.bio.indiana.edu/**

BIOSCI/bionet Info
FTP: net.bio.net or 134.172.2.69

Directory: /pub/BIOSCI/

URL: **ftp://net.bio.net/pub/BIOSCI/**

Description: The BIOSCI newsgroup network was developed to allow easy worldwide communications between biological scientists who work on a variety of computer networks. BIOSCI is supported by the National Science Foundation, Department of Energy, and National Institutes of Health in the U.S.A. and by the Science and Engineering Research Council Daresbury Laboratory in the United Kingdom. BIOSCI services are available to users free of charge. New users of BIOSCI/bionet may want to read the "Frequently Asked Questions" or "FAQ" sheet for BIOSCI. The FAQ provides details on how to participate in these forums and is available in pub/BIOSCI/doc/biosci.FAQ.

Contact: Dave Kristofferson <kristoff@net.bio.net>
BIOSCI/bionet Manager

BIOTECHNOLOGY INFORMATION CENTER
US Department of Agriculture

FTP: inform.umd.edu or 128.8.10.29

URL: **ftp://inform.umd.edu/**

Description: Agricultural biotechnology information, including bioethics, current gene mapping projects, patenting issues, legislation and regulation, and much more. Developed by the Biotechnology Information Center, an information center of the National Agricultural Library (USDA). Files include bibliographies primarily composed of peer-reviewed scientific journal citations, with abstracts, on subjects ranging from bovine somatotropin to gene expression in algae and fungi.

Contact: Daniel Cabirac <biotech@nalusda.gov>
Biotechnology Information Center
NAL/USDA
10301 Baltimore Blvd.
Beltsville, MD 20705-2351
Phone: 301-504-5947
Fax: 301-504-7098

CANCERNET
FTP: ftp.nus.sg or 137.132.9.11

URL: **ftp://ftp.nus.sg/**

Description: The National University of Singapore has been designated by the National Cancer Institute (NCI), National Institutes of Health, USA as a distribution site for its highly popular cancer information database known as CancerNet.

CENTER FOR BIOMEDICAL INFORMATICS—(State University of Campinas, Brazil)
FTP: ftp.unicamp.br or 143.106.10.54

Directory: /pub/medicine/conferences

URL: **ftp://ftp.unicamp.br/pub/medicine/conferences/**

Description: This site contains conferences announcements, calls for papers, and preliminary programs to conferences devoted to Medical Informatics and Biomedical Engineering.

Contact: Renato Sabbatini <sabbatini@ccvax.unicamp.br>
Center for Biomedical Informatics
State University of Campinas
P.O. Box 6005
Campinas, SP 13081—BRAZIL
Phone: +55 192 39-7130
Fax: +55 192 39-4717

CLEARINGHOUSE FOR SUBJECT-ORIENTED INTERNET RESOURCE GUIDES

FTP: una.hh.lib.umich.edu or 141.211.190.102

Directory: /inetdirsstacks

URL: **ftp://una.hh.lib.umich.edu/inetdirsstacks/**

Description: The Clearinghouse for Subject-Oriented Internet Resource Guides is jointly sponsored by the University Library and the School of Information and Library Studies at the University of Michigan, the Clearinghouse provides access to subject-oriented resource guides created by members of the Internet community. There are currently over 60 guides available via anonymous FTP, Gopher, and WorldWideWeb/Mosaic. Titles and authors of animal-related resource guides include:

> Agriculture; W. Drew
> Animals; K. Boschert
> Biological Sciences; D. Kovacs
> Conservation; D. Wendling, J. Christianson
> Diversity; L. Heise
> Environment; T. Murphy, C. Briggs-Erickson
> Health Sciences; L. Hancock
> Health Sciences; N. Martin, P. Redman, G. Oren
> Math & Science Education; T.C. O'Haver
> Multiple Subjects (Gopher Jewels); D. Riggins
> Neurosciences; S. Bonario, S. Cormicle

Contact: Louis Rosenfeld <lou@umich.edu>
> School of Information and Library Studies
> University of Michigan
> 403B West Engineering
> Ann Arbor, MI 48109-1092
> Phone: 313-747-3581
> Fax: 313-764-2475

COGNITIVE NEUROSCIENCE

FTP: ego.psych.mcgill.ca or 132.206.106.211

Directory: /pub/cogneuro/

URL: **ftp://ego.psych.mcgill.ca/pub/cogneuro/**

Description: Cogneuro Mailing List Archives

Contact: Kimball Collins <kpc@ptolemy.arc.nasa.gov>
> AI Research Branch
> NASA Ames Research Ctr
> MS 269-2, Moffett Field, CA 94035
> Phone: 415-604-1221

COMPMED

Washington University Comparative Medicine

FTP: wuarchive.wustl.edu or 128.252.135.4

Directory: /doc/techreports/wustl.edu/compmed

URL: **ftp://wuarchive.wustl.edu/doc/techreports/wustl.edu/compmed/**

Contact: Ken Boschert <ken@wudcm.wustl.edu>
> Washington University
> Division of Comparative Medicine
> Box 8061, 660 South Euclid Ave.
> St. Louis, MO 63110
> Phone: 314-362-3700
> Fax: 314-362-6480

DAIRY CATTLE
FTP: yorick.umd.edu or 128.8.10.37
Directory: pub/dairy-l
URL: **ftp://yorick.umd.edu/pub/dairy-l/**

DATA ZOO
Center for Coastal Studies
    Scripps Institution of Oceanography

FTP: coast.ucsd.edu or 128.54.21.56
Directory: /zoo
URL: **ftp://coast.ucsd.edu/zoo/**

Description: The Data Zoo is brought to you by the Center for Coastal Studies at the Scripps Institution of Oceanography, University of California, San Diego with funding generously provided by the Mineral Management Service, Bureau of Land Management, Department of the Interior. The Data Zoo contains data collected by various California coastal data collection programs and studies and organized synoptically by experiment, instrument type and geographical region. These data were procured by the Center for Coastal Studies for inclusion in the Data Zoo and have been checked for consistency and validity to the best of our ability using Data reports and documentation provided by the source organization/individuals for each data set.

Contact: <zookeeper@coast.ucsd.edu>

DOGS—Usenet's rec.pets.dogs newsgroup Frequently Asked Questions (FAQ)
FTP: rtfm.mit.edu or 18.70.0.209
Directory: /pub/usenet/news.answers/dogs-faq
URL: **ftp://rtfm.mit.edu/pub/usenet/news.answers/dogs-faq/**

Description: Files are: introduction, getting-a-dog, new-puppy, new-dog, health-care, medical-info, training, behavior, working, service, AKC-titles, misc/part1, misc/part2, publications and resources. To obtain the files, first try ftp to rtfm.mit.edu and look under that directory. If ftp does not work from your site, then try the mail server. Send email to mail-server@rtfm.mit.edu with:

```
send usenet/news.answers/dogs-faq/introduction
send usenet/news.answers/dogs-faq/getting-a-dog
send usenet/news.answers/dogs-faq/new-puppy
send usenet/news.answers/dogs-faq/new-dog
send usenet/news.answers/dogs-faq/health-care
send usenet/news.answers/dogs-faq/medical-info
send usenet/news.answers/dogs-faq/training
send usenet/news.answers/dogs-faq/behavior
send usenet/news.answers/dogs-faq/working
send usenet/news.answers/dogs-faq/service
send usenet/news.answers/dogs-faq/AKC-titles
send usenet/news.answers/dogs-faq/misc/part1
send usenet/news.answers/dogs-faq/misc/part2
send usenet/news.answers/dogs-faq/publications
send usenet/news.answers/dogs-faq/resources
send usenet/news.answers/dogs-faq/rescue/part1
send usenet/news.answers/dogs-faq/rescue/part2
```

in the body of the message (leave the subject line empty). If you don't want all of them, include only the lines of the ones you want. You do have to repeat the path information for each file.

Also, there are some breed specific faqs kept in the dogs-faq/breeds directory. Just as with the files above, you can ftp and look for them. The existing faqs are: bloodhounds (Bloodhounds), cavaliers (Cavalier King Charles Spaniels), chessies (Chesapeake Bay Retrievers), chows (the Chow

Chow), `collies` (Rough and Smooth Collies), `greyhounds` (Greyhounds), `havanese` (Havanese), `huskies` (Siberian Huskies), `labradors` (Labrador Retrievers), `malamutes` (Alaskan Malamutes), `ridgebacks` (Rhodesian Ridgebacks), and `tollers` (Nova Scotia Duck Tolling Retrievers).

These are all the breeds currently covered; new ones are added from time to time as readers contribute them. You can obtain any or all of them from the mail server (as above) with the following commands:

```
send usenet/news.answers/dogs-faq/breeds/bloodhounds
send usenet/news.answers/dogs-faq/breeds/cavaliers
send usenet/news.answers/dogs-faq/breeds/chessies
send usenet/news.answers/dogs-faq/breeds/chows
send usenet/news.answers/dogs-faq/breeds/collies
send usenet/news.answers/dogs-faq/breeds/greyhounds
send usenet/news.answers/dogs-faq/breeds/havanese
send usenet/news.answers/dogs-faq/breeds/huskies
send usenet/news.answers/dogs-faq/breeds/labradors
send usenet/news.answers/dogs-faq/breeds/malamutes
send usenet/news.answers/dogs-faq/breeds/ridgebacks
send usenet/news.answers/dogs-faq/breeds/tollers
```

These faqs are written by different readers of rec.pets.dogs who have experience with the breed in question. You are encouraged to volunteer to write new breed faqs, please contact `tittle@netcom.com` for details.

Finally, there is a FAQ on fleas and ticks. It is not included with the dog FAQs because it is generalized for dogs AND cats. However, it is archived in the same spot, under:

`/pub/usenet/news.answers/fleas-ticks for ftp,` or
`"send usenet/news.answers/fleas-ticks"` to the mail-server.

DOGS

FTP: `bietel.uia.ac.be` or `143.169.1.9`

Directory: `/pub/Dogs`

URL: **`ftp://bietel.uia.ac.be/pub/Dogs/`**

Description: contains information from those subscribed to the canine-l mailing list.

Contact: Marc Gemis `<makke@wins.uia.ac.be>`
University of Antwerp, Belgium

ECONET

Institute for Global Communications

FTP: `igc.org` or `192.82.108.1`

Directory: `/pub`

URL: **`ftp://igc.org/pub/`**

Description: Commercial online service for ecological and environmental databases. Subscription fees. Several hundred email conferences available. The FTP site is a public.

Contact: Institute for Global Communications
18 De Boom Street
San Francisco, CA 94107
Phone: 415-442-0220

ENDANGERED SPECIES

FTP: `wiretap.spies.com` or `130.43.43.43`

Directory: `/Gov/Treaties/Treaties/endanger.un`

URL: **`ftp://wiretap.spies.com/Gov/Treaties/Treaties/endanger.un/`**

Description: United Nations Treaty with text on the international trade in endangered species of wild fauna and flora.

ENTOMOLOGY
Australia
FTP: spider.ento.csiro.au or 138.44.23.1
URL: **ftp://spider.ento.csiro.au/**

ENVIROFTP
The EnviroLink Network
FTP: envirolink.hss.cmu.edu or 128.2.19.92
URL: **ftp://envirolink.hss.cmu.edu/**

Contact: The EnviroLink Network <env-link@andrew.cmu.edu>
       4551 Forbes Avenue—Third Floor
       Pittsburgh, PA 15213
       Voice: (412) 681-8300
       Fax: (412) 681-6707

ENVIRONMENTAL PROTECTION AGENCY LIBRARY
FTP: epaibm.rtpnc.epa.gov or 134.67.180.1
Directory: /public
URL: **ftp://epaibm.rtpnc.epa.gov/public/**

ERIN
Environmental Resources Information Network (ERIN) Newsletter (Australia)
FTP: huh.harvard.edu or 128.103.108.123
URL: **ftp://huh.harvard.edu/**

EQUESTRIAN ARCHIVE
FTP: ucssun1.sdsu.edu or 130.191.1.100
Directory: /pub/equestrian
URL: **ftp://ucssun1.sdsu.edu/pub/equestrian/**

FLEAS & TICKS
FTP: pit-manager.mit.edu or 18.70.0.209
Directory: /pub/usenet/news.answers/fleas-ticks
URL: **ftp://pit-manager.mit.edu/pub/usenet/news.answers/fleas-ticks/**

FLYBASE (Drosophila Melanogaster)
FTP: ftp.bio.indiana.edu or 129.79.224.25
Directory: /flybase
URL: **ftp://ftp.bio.indiana.edu/flybase/**

Contact: <flybase@morgan.harvard.edu>

GENOME CENTER GENETIC MAP OF THE MOUSE
Massachusetts Institute of Technology
FTP: genome.wi.mit.edu or 18.157.0.135
Directory: /distribution/mouse_sslp_release/jan94
URL: **ftp://genome.wi.mit.edu/distribution/mouse_ssllp_releases/jan94/**

Description: Release five of the Whitehead Institute/MIT Genome Center Genetic Map of the Mouse is now available. This map consists of randomly-chosen simple sequence length polymorphisms (microsatellites) that can be analyzed using the polymerase chain reaction, as described in Dietrich, W., et al., Genetics 131:423-447 (1992). Currently the released map contains 3011 markers. The markers fall into 20 linkage groups spanning approximately 1400 cM with an average spacing of less than 0.5 cM.

Contact: Ert Dredge <ert@genomewi.mit.edu>
Whitehead Institute's Center for Genome Research
One Kendall Sq, Bldg 300, 5th floor
Cambridge, MA 02139
Phone: 617-252-1922
Fax: 617-252-1902

2. Via internet e-mail using a database e-mail server. Using this service you can obtain locus and assay names of mapped SSLPs, the forward and reverse primer sequences, the genotypes of the loci on the mapping cross, the sizes of the PCR products on selected standard inbred strains, and other useful information. The database can be queried for markers meeting a number of different criteria. For example, you can ask for markers by name, by chromosome, or by position on the map. You can even request a list of markers that are polymorphic between two mouse strains.

To obtain copies of the most current query forms, send a message to "genome_database@genome.wi.mit.edu" with either a subject line or body text of "help". You will receive instructions and a query form by return mail. Just fill out the form, send it to "genome_database@genome.wi.mit.edu", and the answer to your query will be mailed back automatically.

GREENDISK PAPERLESS ENVIRONMENTAL JOURNAL

FTP: csus.edu or 130.86.90.1

Directory: /pub/greendisk

URL: ftp://csus.edu/pub/greendisk/

Description: The Greendisk Paperless Environmental Journal is a forum for the publication of research reports, press releases, action alerts, and news summaries from the world's environmental groups and governmental agencies. Samples are available. Subscribers must pay a subscription fee.

Contact: <greendisk@igc.apc.org>
P.O. Box 32224
Washington, DC 20007
Phone: 800-484-7616

GUIDE DOGS

FTP: handicap.shel.isc-br.com or 129.189.4.184

Directory: /pub/dogs

URL: ftp://handicap.shel.isc-br.com/pub/dogs/

Description: Guide dog information, newsletters, and laws.

HEALTH SCIENCES RESOURCES

FTP: ftp.sura.net or 128.167.254.179

Directory: /pub/nic

URL: ftp://ftp.sura.net/pub/nic/

Description: A comprehensive list of on-line resources available to people interested in the Health Sciences. The list is compiled by Lee Hancock. Please send any comments, suggestions, corrections, additions, deletions to Le07144@Ukanvm or Le07144@Ukanvm.cc.ukans.edu.

HORSE RACING

FTP: simpatico.inslab.uky.edu

URL: ftp://simpatico.inslab.uky.edu/

Contact: Steve McNatton <stevem@inslab.uky.edu>

JACKSON LABORATORY
Mouse Genome Database

FTP: `hobbes.jax.org`

URL: **`ftp://hobbes.jax.org/`**

Contact: Alexander G. Smith <`ags@zappa.jax.org`>

JACKSON LABORATORY
Bioinformatics Archives

FTP: `ftp.informatics.jax.org` or `192.233.41.22`

Directory: `/pub/informatics/mailing-lists`

URL: **`ftp://ftp.informatics.jax.org/pub/informatics/mailing-lists/`**

Description: All messages posted to lists maintained by the BioInformatics ListServer are archived.

Contact: `list-manager@informatics.jax.org`

LOCIS
Library of Congress Information System

FTP: `ftp.loc.gov`

Directory: `/pub/lc.online`

URL: **`ftp://ftp.loc.gov/pub/lc.online/`**

Description: Several databases, including the LC Catalog of books.

LYMENET
Lyme Disease Newsletters

FTP: `ftp.lehigh.edu` or `128.180.63.4`

Directory: `/pub/listserv/lymenet-l/Newsletters`

URL: **`ftp://ftp.lehigh.edu/pub/listserv/lymenet-l/Newsletters/`**

Description: The Lyme Disease Electronic Mail Network publishes the "LymeNet Newsletter" once every 10-15 days. The Newsletter contains timely news about the Lyme disease epidemic. Medical abstracts, treatment protocols, prevention information, and political happenings are all included. In addition, subscribers may ask questions to the patients, doctors and researchers on the net.

Contact: Marc Gabriel <`mcg2@lehigh.edu`>

MARINE SCIENCE SOFTWARE

FTP: `biome.bio.dfo.ca` or `142.2.20.2`

Directory: `/pub`

URL: **`ftp://biome.bio.dfo.ca/pub/`**

MATHEMATICAL BIOLOGY

FTP: `fconvx.ncifcrf.gov` or `129.43.52.4`

URL: **`ftp://fconvx.ncifcrf.gov/`**

NATIONAL BIOLOGICAL IMPACT ASSESSMENT PROGRAM (NBIAP)

FTP: `ftp.vt.edu` or `128.173.4.49`

Directory: `/pub/biotechnology`

URL: **`ftp://ftp.vt.edu/pub/biotechnology/`**

Description: NBIAP mission is to facilitate and assess the safe application of new techniques for genetically modifying plants, animals, and microorganisms to benefit agriculture and the environment. Subjects include: advancing research and monitoring techniques, and expediting the flow of biotechnology information. Databases include companies involved in biotechnology R&D; State research and development centers; State biotech regulatory agencies and contacts; publications relating to biotechnology; International biotech researchers; Research sites; International biotech field test approvals; Institutional Biosafety Committees and contacts; APHIS field test approvals; and Scientific references.

Contact: Daniel Cabirac <biotech@nalusda.gov>
Biotechnology Information Center
NAL/USDA
10301 Baltimore Blvd.
Beltsville, MD 20705-2351
Phone: 301-504-5947
Fax: 301-504-7098

Doug King <nbiap@vt.edu>
120 Engel Hall
Virginia Tech
Blacksburg, VA 24061
Phone: 703-231-3747
Bulletin Board: 800-NBIAPBD

NATIONAL INSTITUTES OF HEALTH

FTP: ftp.cu.nih.gov or 128.231.64.7

Password: guest

Directory: /nih-eguide

URL: ftp://ftp.cu.nih.gov/nih-eguide/

Description: Various items related to medical research, grants, and other government agencies.

NATIONAL SCIENCE FOUNDATION

STIS—Science & Technology Information System

FTP: stis.nsf.gov or 128.150.195.40

URL: ftp://stis.nsf.gov/

NEURON Newsletter

FTP: psych.upenn.edu or 130.91.68.31

Directory: /pub

URL: ftp://psych.upenn.edu/pub/

Description: Archives of the Neuron Digest Newsletter—discusses neural networks. Neuron-Digest is also posted to the Usenet newsgroup comp.ai.neural-networks.

Contact: Peter Marvit <neuron-request@psych.upenn.edu>

NEXTSTEP BIOLOGY APPLICATIONS

FTP: ftp.alleg.edu or 141.195.5.3

Directory: /pub/ESDG/Biology

URL: ftp://ftp.alleg.edu/pub/ESDG/Biology/

NORINA

Norwegian Inventory of Audiovisuals

FTP: wuarchive.wustl.edu or 128.252.135.4

Directory: /doc/techreports/wustl.edu/compmed/mac

URL: ftp://wuarchive.wustl.edu/doc/techreports/wustl.edu/compmed/mac/

Description: NORINA—NORWEGIAN INVENTORY OF AUDIOVISUALS—The Laboratory Animal Unit, Norwegian College of Veterinary Medicine, Oslo, has compiled an English-language database of audiovisuals for use in the biological sciences. The primary purpose of the database is to offer an overview of possible alternatives or supplements to the use of animals in student teaching, at all levels from schools to university. The database consists at present of around 1300 entries, including computer programs, interactive video, films and more traditional teaching aids such as slide series, 3-D models and classroom charts. There is also a section for Contact Persons who are developing and/or using audiovisuals at their institution, and for suppliers of audiovisuals. NORINA has been written in Filemaker Pro, originally for Macintosh, but now also available for IBM Windows. NORINA is also available as a "stand-alone" IBM version that will run on any PC with harddisc, with no additional software. NORINA is a non-profit venture (none of the developers receive any commission on sales) and income from sales is used purely to offset wage expenses. Three files available by FTP are the demo version for machines with Filemaker Pro (`norina.bin`), a text file with information on NORINA (`norina.txt`) and a tab-delimited version of the demo version (`norina.tab`).

Contact: Adrian Smith <adrian.smith@veths.no>
Laboratory Animal Unit
Norwegian College of Veterinary Medicine
P.O. Box 8146 Dep., 0033 Oslo 1, Norway
Phone: +47 22 96 45 74
Fax: +47 22 96 45 35

OCEAN ENVIRONMENT
FTP: `ariel.unm.edu` or `129.24.8.1`
Directory: `/pub/MAC/HYPERCARD/Museum`
URL: **ftp://ariel.unm.edu/pub/MAC/HYPERCARD/Museum/**

PARASITOLOGY
FTP: `net.bio.net` or `134.172.2.69`
Directory: `/pub/BIOSCI/PARASITOLOGY`
URL: **ftp://net.bio.net/pub/BIOSCI/PARASITOLOGY/**

PENPAGES
FTP: `psupen.psu.edu` or `128.118.36.4`
URL: **ftp://psupen.psu.edu/**
Login: U.S. state abbreviation or "`world`" if outside
Description: U.S. agricultural database administered by Pennsylvania State University which contains information on agriculture and weather.

PRIMATE
FTP: `ftp.primate.wisc.edu` or `144.92.43.11`
URL: **ftp://ftp.primate.wisc.edu/**
Description: Archive provides distribution point for software developed at the Wisconsin Regional Primate Research Center at the University of Wisconsin-Madison.

RACHEL'S HAZARDOUS WASTE NEWS
FTP: `world.std.com` or `192.74.137.5`
Directory: `/periodicals/rachel`
URL: **ftp://world.std.com/periodicals/rachel/**
Contact: Environmental Research Foundation <erf@igc.apc.org>
P.O. Box 5036
Annapolis, MD 21403
Fax: 410-263-8944

SOCIETY FOR MATHEMATICAL BIOLOGY
Society for Mathematical Biology Digest
FTP: `fconvx.ncifcrf.gov` or `129.43.52.4`

Directory: /smb/digest
URL: ftp://fconvx.ncifcrf.gov/smb/digest/
Description: Back issues of the Digest
Contact: Ray Mejia

SOFTWARE
SunSITE Archives
FTP: sunsite.unc.edu or 198.86.40.81
Directory: /pub/academic
URL: ftp://sunsite.unc.edu/pub/academic/
Description: This archive at the University of North Carolina contains a huge amount of information and files written by researchers in a number of disciplines, including: agriculture, biology, and medicine.
Contact: <ftpkeeper@sunsite.unc.edu>

SUPREME COURT RULINGS
FTP: ftp.cwru.edu or 129.22.4.2
Directory: /hermes
URL: ftp://ftp.cwru.edu/hermes/

THE SCIENTIST Newsletter
FTP: ds.internic.net or 192.20.239.132
Directory: /pub/the-scientist
URL: ftp://ds.internic.net/pub/the-scientist/
Description: THE SCIENTIST is a biweekly newspaper for scientists and the research community. It is circulated internationally to researchers, administrators, and policy makers in academia, industry, and government and covers current issues and events that impact the professional research environment. News includes funding legislation, new grants, employment and salary trends, career advancement opportunities, ethics and conflicts of interest, representation of women and minorities in science, and the interplay of industrial, academic, and governmental research.

SMITHSONIAN INSTITUTE
FTP: simsc.si.edu or 160.111.64.1
URL: ftp://simc.si.edu/
FTP: photo1.si.edu or 160.111.16.2
URL: ftp://photo1.si.edu/
Description: Located in the Smithsonian Institution's Office of Printing & Photographic Services in Washington, D.C. and is designed to make a variety of Smithsonian photographs available as electronic image files.
Contact: <psdmx@sivm.si.edu>
Smithsonian Institution
Office of Printing & Photographic Services
MAH CB-054
Washington, DC 20560

TAXACOM—Archive for Systematic Biology and Biological Collections Computing
FTP: huh.harvard.edu or 128.103.108.123
Directory: /pub
URL: ftp://huh.harvard.edu/pub/

US SENATE
FTP: ftp.senate.gov or 198.22.59.23

Directories for Senator's offices are structured as follows:

    /member/state_abbrev./senator's_name/releases/filename

or

    /member/state_abbrev./senator's_name/general/filename

URL: **ftp://ftp.senate.gov/member/state_abbrev./senator's_name/releases/filename/**

or

ftp://ftp.senate.gob/memnber/state_abbrev./senator's_name/general/filename/

The "releases" subdirectories contain press releases and related materials, and "general" subdirectories contain information of long-term interest such as office contacts.

Description: This service is provided by the Office of the U.S. Senate Sergeant at Arms and the Senate Committee on Rules and Administration. This server contains general information files about the United States Senate in the directory "general". Directories are also provided for specific Senators' offices, in alphabetical order by two-letter state abbreviations, and for Senate committees and other Senate offices. If an office is not included in the directory, this indicates no files have been posted by that office. No files can be uploaded to this system. Please direct questions about a specific Senate office's use of this service to the Senate office in question.

Contact: `<ftpadmin@scc.senate.gov>`—for general information

USDA Statistical Data
Cornell Mann Library

FTP: `usda.mannlib.cornell.edu` or `128.253.78.240`

Directory: `/usda`

URL: **ftp://usda.mannlib.cornell.edu/usda/**

Description: Computer users worldwide now have access to statistical data gathered by the USDA. Cornell's Mann Library became the host for more than 140 free agricultural data sets, available to anyone with Internet access. The system is easy to search. Data are formatted for importing into existing computer analysis programs. Each data set is accompanied by an explanatory document, and all text documents are indexed for electronic searching.

Contact: Oya Y. Rieger `<oyr1@cornell.edu>`
Numeric Files Librarian
Mann Library
Cornell University
Ithaca, NY 14853
Phone: 607-255-7960

VEGETARIAN

FTP: `rtfm.mit.edu` or `18.70.0.209`

Directory: `/pub/usenet/news.answers/vegetarian/guide`

URL: **ftp://rtfm.mit.edu/pub/usenet/news.answers/vegetarian/guide/**

FTP: `ftp.geod.emr.ca` or `132.156.28.3`

Directory: `/pub/Vegetarian/Articles/`

URL: **ftp://ftp.geod.emr.ca/pub/Vegetarian/Articles/**

Description: The `rec.food.veg` World Guide to Vegetarianism_ lists restaurants, stores, organizations, and travel info of interest to vegetarians.

VIROLOGY bionet.virology archives
Institute for Molecular Virology
Robert M. Bock Laboratories
University of Wisconsin-Madison

FTP: `rhino.bocklabs.wisc.edu` or `144.92.19.130`

URL: **ftp://rhino.bocklabs.wisc.edu/**

VIRUS Database
Australian National University Bioinformatics Facility

FTP: `life.anu.edu.au` or `150.203.38.74`

Directory: /pub/viruses

URL: **ftp://life.anu.edu.au/pub/viruses/**

Description: The approved names of virus families/groups and members are now available on-line from the Australian National University's Bioinformatics Facility. This folder will soon contain hold databases about viruses, which are currently being compiled under the Virus Identification Data Exchange.

Contact: Dr Cornelia Buchen-Osmond <`buchen@life.anu.edu.au`>
Research School of Biological Research
Australian National University
GPO Box 475
Canberra ACT 2601 AUSTRALIA
Phone: 61-6-249-4842
Fax: 61-6-249-0758

WORLD HEALTH ORGANIZATION
FTP: `ftp.who.ch` or `158.232.17.1`

URL: **ftp://ftp.who.ch/**

Contact: WHO Internet Anonymous FTP Root Server Administrator
Information Technology Office (ITO)
World Health Organization (WHO)
CH-1211 Geneva 27
Switzerland
Phone: +41 22 791 2434
FAX: +41 22 791 0746
E-mail: <`ftp-admin@who.ch`> or <`akazawa@who.ch`>

Gopher Sites

ACADEME THIS WEEK
The Chronicle of Higher Education Gopher

Internet: gopher to `chronicle.merit.edu` or `35.1.1.98`

URL: **gopher://chronicle.merit.edu**

Contact: E-mail to: `chronicle-help@chronicle.merit.edu`
Call Judith Turner or Ed Piou at The Chronicle of Higher Education
Phone: 202-466-1000

Description: The Chronicle of Higher Education sponsors "ACADEME THIS WEEK," a free electronic service on the Internet. "ACADEME THIS WEEK" will include: 1. A guide to the news in the current week's issue of The Chronicle of Higher Education. 2. A calendar of the week's events in academe. 3. A schedule of the week's events in Washington, D.C., of interest to the men and women of academe. 4. The week's important deadlines for fellowships, grant applications, exchange programs, and more. 5. A listing of hundreds of job openings at colleges, universities, and other non-profit institutions worldwide. The job announcements come from The Chronicle's "Bulletin Board" section—the world's largest academic-job marketplace. New edition available every Tuesday at noon, Eastern time (US).

AGRICULTURE & BIOLOGY
North Carolina State University

Internet: gopher to `dewey.lib.ncsu.edu` or `152.1.24.90`

URL: **gopher://dewey.lib.ncsu.edu**

AMERICAN PHYSIOLOGICAL SOCIETY

Internet: gopher to gopher.uth.tmc.edu or 129.106.30.1

URL: **gopher://gopher.uth.tmc.edu**

Description: The American Physiological Society (APS) Information Server provides for the electronic distribution of APS information, documents and publications via the National Research and Education Network (NREN)/Internet. The American Physiological Society offers Tables of Contents for the following journals: Advances in Physiology Education, American Journal of Physiology (6 consolidated journals), Journal of Applied Physiology, Journal of Neurophysiology News in Physiological Sciences, Physiological Reviews, and The Physiologist.

AMERICAN TYPE CULTURE COLLECTION (ATCC) DATABASES

NIH

Internet: gopher to atcc.nih.gov or 156.40.144.248

URL: **gopher://atcc.nih.gov**

AQUANAUT

Scuba Diving Forum

Internet: WWW client at http://www.opal.com/aquanaut

URL: **http://www.opal.com/aquanaut**

Description: Contains: rec.scuba newsgroup archive, TechDiver mailing list archive, Wreck Database—a database of diveable shipwrecks, reviews of Dive Gear and Equipment, reviews of popular dive destinations, information about training agencies, worldwide fish pictures, marketplace for diving products and much more.

AVES ARCHIVE

Bird Related Information

Internet: gopher to vitruvius.cecer.army.mil or 129.229.21.78

URL: **gopher://vitruvius.cecer.army.mil**

Contact: rglaser@vitruvius.cecer.army.mil

Description: An anonymous FTP archive which contains bird images and sound and text files.

BIODIVERSITY GOPHER

Brazil

Internet: gopher to bdt.ftpt.br or 192.207.195.1

URL: **gopher://bdt.ftpt.br**

BIODIVERSITY & BIOLOGICAL COLLECTIONS

Harvard University

Internet: gopher to huh.harvard.edu or 128.103.108.123

URL: **gopher://huh.harvard.edu**

Description: Contains biological collections catalogs (Harvard and Cornell), taxonomic authority files, directories of biologists, journals (Flora On-line, The Bean Bag, Florida Entomologist), and information about biodiversity projects.

BIOETHICS ONLINE SERVICE GOPHER

Medical College of Wisconsin

Internet: gopher to post.its.mcw.edu or 141.106.32.10

URL: **gopher://post.its.mcw.edu**

Description: The Bioethics Online Service is an information resource of the Center for the Study of Bioethics and the Health Information Technology Center (HITC) of the Medical College of Wisconsin (MCW).

Contact: Arthur R. Derse, MD, JD
Bioethics Online Service <biohelp@its.mcw.edu>
Information Technology Services
Medical College of Wisconsin
8701 Watertown Plank Road
Milwaukee, WI 53226

BIOINFORMATICS

Australian National University

Internet: gopher to `life.anu.edu.au` or `150.203.38.74`

URL: `gopher://life.anu.edu.au`

Description: ANU's Bioinformatics Facility provides information on Internet under a number of themes. At present the major themes include: biodiversity; bioinformatics & biocomputing; biomathematics and biostatistics; complex systems; general interest; landscape ecology and the environment; molecular biology; neurosciences; viruses; and weather and global monitoring.

BIOLINE PUBLICATIONS GOPHER

Online publication and delivery of full text and graphics for the bioscience community.
Campinas, Brasil

Internet: gopher to `bdt.ftpt.br` or `192.207.195.1`

URL: `gopher://bdt.ftpt.br`

Description: BIOLINE PUBLICATIONS has been set up to help make information more easily available online to the vast community of scientists in universities, institutes and industry, government and regulatory people via the Internet. Focuses on the biosciences (biotechnology, biodiversity, biopolicy, bioinformatics) Using the Internet network, 'readers' may browse and search without cost through large quantities of abstracts, summaries and contents lists, using simple menus, or keywords and phrases to search across the whole system. Full text and associated graphics of material of interest can be ordered online and e-mailed to the reader's computer. Access to Journal abstracts, report summaries and contents lists is available free to all; readers must subscribe to Bioline Publications in order to receive the full text/graphics of documents of interest. Additional registration with the publishers of commercial journals is necessary if full text and graphics of scientific papers are required. Information on registration is available from the main menu of Bioline Publications. The cost of commercial journals is considerably less than the printed version.

Contact: Bioline Publications <bio@biostrat.demon.co.uk>
Stainfield House
Stainfield, Bourne, Lincs
PE10 0RS, UK
Phone: +44 778 570618
FAX: +44 778 570175

BIOLOGICAL COMPUTING

Oregon State University

Internet: gopher to `gopher.bcc.orst.edu` or `128.193.86.4`

URL: `gopher://gopher.bcc.orst.edu`

BIOLOGY

University of California—Santa Barbara

Internet: gopher to `ucsbuxa.ucsb.edu` or `128.111.122.5`, port 3001

URL: `gopher://ucsbuxa.ucsb.edu`

BIOLOGY

University of Missouri—St. Louis

Internet: `gopher to umslvma.umsl.edu` or `134.124.1.2`

URL: `gopher://umslvma.umsl.edu:70/11/library/subjects/biology`

BIOLOGY
Internet: gopher to `gopher.fragrans.riken.go.jp` or `134.160.52.5`
URL: **`gopher://gopher.fragrans.riken.go.jp`**

BIOLOGY
Internet: gopher to `gopher.dna.cedb.uwf.edu` or `143.88.10.3`
URL: **`gopher://gopher.dna.cedb.uwf.edu/`**

BIOSCI/bionet
Indiana University
Internet: gopher to `ftp.bio.indiana.edu` or `129.79.224.25`
URL: **`gopher://ftp.bio.indiana.edu`**

BIOTECHNOLOGY INFORMATION CENTER
US Department of Agriculture
Internet: gopher to `inform.umd.edu` or `128.8.10.29`
URL: **`gopher://inform.umd.edu`**

Description: Agricultural biotechnology information, including bioethics, current gene mapping projects, patenting issues, legislation and regulation, and much more. Developed by the Biotechnology Information Center, an information center of the National Agricultural Library (USDA). Files include bibliographies primarily composed of peer-reviewed scientific journal citations, with abstracts, on subjects ranging from bovine somatotropin to gene expression in algae and fungi.

Contact: Daniel Cabirac <`biotech@nalusda.gov`>
Biotechnology Information Center
NAL/USDA
10301 Baltimore Blvd.
Beltsville, MD 20705-2351
Phone: 301-504-5947

BIRD THINGS
Internet: gopher to: `simon.wharton.upenn.edu` or `165.123.8.108`
URL: **`gopher://simon.wharton.upenn.edu:70/11/birding`**

Description: A birdgopher with newsletters, checklists, and access to the AVES GIF/Sound archive.
Contact: Jack Siler <`siler@wharton.upenn.edu`>

BOING
Bio Oriented INternet Gophers
Internet: gopher to `merlot.welch.jhu.edu` or `192.239.77.4`
URL: **`gopher://merlot.welch.jhu.edu`**

Description: Search through the titles of items in Bio-Gopher space and access the items returned. This Bio-veronica style database is called: BOING—Bio Oriented INternet Gophers. Search for your topic of interest. You can use booleans (and, or, not) and wildcards (*) to restrict or broaden your searches. Searchable directories of scientists and research projects currently funded by the U.S. National Institutes of Health (NIH), National Science Foundation (NSF), Department of Agriculture (USDA), and genome researchers funded by several other departments, together with several topical directories, are available.

BUBL
News & Announcements in the Biomedical field
Internet: gopher to `bubl.bath.ac.uk` or `138.38.32.45`, Port 7070
URL: **`gopher://bubl.bath.ac.uk`**

CAMIS

Center for Advanced Medical Informatics at Stanford University

Internet: gopher to `camis.stanford.edu` or `36.44.0.7`

URL: `gopher://camis.stanford.edu`

Description: The CAMIS gopher features much of the usual and the following: (1) technical report abstracts from the last 10 years from the Knowledge Systems Laboratory (which includes the Section on Medical Informatics and the Heuristic Programming Project); (2) an extensive collection of Mac documentation (including Word 5, Canvas and other applications); and (3) a search test directory, originally designed for testing the NeXT's Digital Librarian indexing) that now can be used to test the searching capabilities of Don Gilbert's WAIS enhancements (in the About the CAMIS Gopher directory). It's simple, but especially useful for novices like myself to figure out what you will get with a particular search on a small, well-defined database.

CANCERNET PDQ

Internet: gopher to `gopher.nih.gov` or `128.231.2.5`
URL: `gopher://gopher.nih.gov`

Internet: gopher to `biomed.nus.sg` or `137.132.9.61`
URL: `gopher://biomed.nus.sg`

Description: CancerNet is a quick and easy way to obtain, through electronic mail, recommended treatment guidelines in English or Spanish from the National Cancer Institute's Physician Data Query (PDQ) system. CancerNet also lets you request information about PDQ, PDQ distributors, and other products and services from the NCI, including a list of patient publications available from the Office of Cancer Communications. There is also a collaboration between the National University of Singapore and the National Cancer Institute, Bethesda, MD, a secondary site for the NCI CancerNet files in Singapore.

Contact: Cheryl Burg <cheryl@icicb.nci.nih.gov>
Building 82, Room 103A
Bethesda, Maryland 20892
Phone: (301) 496-8880
Fax: (301) 480-8105

Tan Tin Wee, PhD <bchtantw@leonis.nus.sg>
Department of Biochemistry,
and Biocomputing Research and User Support (BRUS)
National University of Singapore
Kent Ridge
Singapore 0511
Phone: 65-772-3678
Fax: 65-779-1453

CAUZ Gopher

Consortium of Aquariums, Universities, and Zoos

Internet: telnet to `vax.csun.edu`
    At the USERNAME prompt, enter: `INFO`

URL: `telnet://vax.csun.edu`

Description: The Consortium of Aquariums, Universities and Zoos goals are to bring scientists and educators at universities into closer working relations with their counterparts at zoos and aquariums. C.A.U.Z. has now grown into an international network of some 650 people in 332 institutions in 19 countries. These people submit information about their interests and professional focus—as well as their current research projects—and this information is published each summer in the annual C.A.U.Z. Directories. Most of the directory is now available on our campus Gopher.

Contact: Donna FitzRoy Hardy <dhardy@vax.csun.edu>
Professor of Psychology
California State University, Northridge
18111 Nordhoff Street

Northridge, California 91330 USA
Phone: 818-885-4970 [2827 for messages]
FAX: 818-885-2829

CENTER FOR THE INTEGRATIVE STUDY OF ANIMAL BEHAVIOR

Internet: gopher to `gopher.cisab.indiana.edu` or `129.79.80.14`

URL: **`gopher://gopher.cisab.indiana.edu`**

Contact: Shan Duncan <`duncan@loris.cisab.indiana.edu`>

CICNET

Committee on Institutional Cooperation Network

Internet: gopher to `gopher.cic.net` or `192.131.22.5`

URL: **`gopher://gopher.cic.net`**

Description: Attempts to put in one place all the public domain electronic journals currently available on the Internet.

Contact: CICNET, Inc. <`holbrook@cic.net`>
2901 Hubbard Road
Ann Arbor, MI 48105
Phone: 313-998-6103
Fax: 313-998-6105

CLEARINGHOUSE FOR SUBJECT-ORIENTED INTERNET RESOURCE GUIDES

University of Michigan

Internet: gopher to: `gopher.lib.umich.edu` or `141.211.73.100`

URL: **`gopher://una.hh.lib.umich.edu:70/11/inetdirs`**

Description: The Clearinghouse for Subject-Oriented Internet Resource Guides is jointly sponsored by the University Library and the School of Information and Library Studies at the University of Michigan, the Clearinghouse provides access to subject-oriented resource guides created by members of the Internet community. There are currently over 75 guides available via anonymous FTP, Gopher, and WorldWideWeb/Mosaic. Titles and authors of animal-related resource guides include:

- Agriculture; W. Drew
- Animals; K. Boschert
- Biological Sciences; D. Kovacs
- Conservation; D. Wendling, J. Christianson
- Diversity; L. Heise
- Environment; T. Murphy, C. Briggs-Erickson
- Health Sciences; L. Hancock
- Health Sciences; N. Martin, P. Redman, G. Oren
- Math & Science Education; T.C. O'Haver
- Multiple Subjects (Gopher Jewels); D. Riggins
- Neurosciences; S. Bonario, S. Cormicle

Contact: Louis Rosenfeld <`lou@umich.edu`>
School of Information and Library Studies
University of Michigan
403B West Engineering
Ann Arbor, MI 48109-1092
Phone: 313-747-3581
Fax: 313-764-2475

CRIS—Current Research Information System

North Carolina State University Cooperative Extension Gopher

Internet: gopher to `gopher.ces.ncsu.edu` or `152.1.45.21`

URL: **gopher://gopher.ces.ncsu.edu**

Description: WAIS-based information on agricultural and forestry research projects in the USDA and at land-grant institutions, State Agricultural Experiment Stations, Schools of Forestry, and cooperating Schools of Veterinary Medicine.

CYFER-NET
USDA Extension Service Gopher

Internet: gopher to `cyfer.esusda.gov` or `192.73.224.110`

URL: **gopher://cyfer.esudsda.gov**

Description: This server is set up to provide access to the information from the USDA Extension Service and the National Agriculture Library. This gopher server is maintained by the USDA Extension Service.

Contact: <almanac-admin@esusda.gov>

COMPUTATIONAL BIOLOGY
Johns Hopkins University

Internet: gopher to `merlot.welch.jhu.edu` or `192.239.77.4`

URL: **gopher://merlot.welch.jhu.edu**

CONSORTIUM FOR INTERNATIONAL EARCH SCIENCE (CIESIN)

Internet: gopher to `gopher.ciesin.org` or `160.39.8.201`

URL: **gopher://gopher.ciesin.org**

Description: Addresses environmental data management issues raised by the United States Congress, the Administration and the advisory arms of the federal policy community.

CTI CENTRE FOR BIOLOGY GOPHER

Internet: gopher to `gopher.csc.liv.ac.uk` or `138.253.42.174`

URL: **gopher://gopher.csc.liv.ac.uk/11/ctibiol**

Description: Educational software for biology catalog.

Contact: CTI Centre for Biology <ctibiol@liverpool.ac.uk>
Donnan Labs
University of Liverpool
P.O. Box 147
Liverpool L69 3BX, UK
Phone: 051-794-5118
Fax: 051-794-3588

DANA-FARBER CANCER INSTITUTE
Boston, MA

Internet: gopher to `dfci.harvard.edu` or `134.174.51.100`

URL: **gopher://dfci.harvard.edu**

DATA ZOO
Center for Coastal Studies
Scripps Institution of Oceanography

Internet: gopher to `coast.ucsd.edu` or `128.54.21.56`

URL: **gopher://coast.ucsd.edu**

Description: The Data Zoo is brought to you by the Center for Coastal Studies at the Scripps Institution of Oceanography, University of California, San Diego with funding generously provided by the Mineral Management Service, Bureau of Land Management, Department of the Interior. The Data Zoo contains data collected by various California coastal data collection programs and studies and organized synoptically by experiment, instrument type and geographical region. These data were procured by the Center for Coastal Studies for inclusion in the Data Zoo and have been checked for consistency and validity to the best of our ability using Data reports and documentation provided by the source organization/individuals for each data set.

Contact: <zookeeper@coast.ucsd.edu>

DOGS
CNS, Inc.

Internet: gopher to `ftp.win.tue.nl` or `131.155.70.100`

Description: USENET FAQ on pet dogs

URL: **gopher://gopher.win.tue.nl:70/11/internet/archives/usenet/news.answers**

ECOSYSTEMS
University of Virginia

Internet: gopher to `ecosys.drdr.virginia.edu` or `128.143.96.10`

URL: **gopher://ecosys.drdr.virginia.edu**

Description: A recycling and environmental information server. It provides and connects users to local, regional, national, and international environmental info.

ENTOMOLOGY GOPHER
University of Delaware

Internet: gopher to `bluehen.ags.udel.edu` or `128.175.73.132`

URL: **gopher://bluehen.ags.udel.edu**

ENVIROGOPHER
Environmental Gopher

Internet: telnet to `envirolink.org` or `128.2.19.119`

   At the login prompt, enter: gopher

URL: **telnet://envirolink.org**

Contact: The EnviroLink Network <env-link@andrew.cmu.edu>
   4551 Forbes Avenue—Third Floor
   Pittsburgh, PA 15213
   Voice: (412) 681-8300
   Fax: (412) 681-6707

ENVIRONMENT
Victoria Freenet Association

Internet: gopher to `freenet.victoria.bc.ca` or `134.87.16.100`

URL: **gopher://freenet.victoria.bc.ca**

Description: The Environment Menus are a source of up-to-date information about the global, national, provincial and local

ENVIRONMENTAL PROTECTION AGENCY
Internet: gopher to `futures.wic.epa.gov` or `134.67.112.42`

URL: **gopher://futures.wic.epa.gov**

Description: Covers agriculture, air, water, land, and related environmental topics.

Contact: Michael Manning <manning.michael@epamail.epa.gov>

ERIN
Environmental Resources Information Network (ERIN) Newsletter (Australia)

Internet: gopher to `kaos.erin.gov.au` or `155.187.2.2`

URL: `gopher://kaos.erin.gov.au`

Description: Covers endangered species, vegetation, international agreements, legislation, and conference information.

EXPERIMENTAL BIOLOGY
Worcester Foundation
Internet: gopher to `sci.wfeb.edu` or `192.190.14.2`
URL: `gopher://sci.wfeb.edu`

EXTENSION SERVICE GOPHER
US Department of Agriculture
Internet: gopher to `zeus.esusda.gov` or `192.73.224.100`
URL: `gopher://zeus.esusda.gov`

Description: To Advance Science and Technology in Support of Agriculture, Forestry, People and Communities. Other Extension Gopher Sites:

Location	Host Address
Extension Service, USDA	`esusda.gov` or `192.73.224.110`
Michigan State University	`gopher.msu.edu` or `35.8.2.61`
North Carolina State University	`gopher.ces.ncsu.edu` or `152.1.45.21`
North Dakota State University	`ndsuext.nodak.edu` or `134.129.48.1`
Oregon State University	`gopher.oes.orst.edu` or `128.193.124.3`
Purdue University	`hermes.ecn.purdue.edu` or `128.46.157.183`
Texas A&M University	`taex-gopher1.tamu.edu` or `128.194.44.70`
Texas A&M University	`leviathan.tamu.edu` or `128.194.44.200`
University of California-Davis	`gopher.ucdavis.edu` or `128.120.8.149`
University of Delaware	`bluehen.ags.udel.edu` or `128.175.73.132`
University of Illinois	`ilces.ag.uiuc.edu` or `128.174.134.150`
University of Kentucky	`gopher.ca.uky.edu` or `128.163.192.5`
University of Minnesota	`tinman.mes.umn.edu` or `134.84.162.9`
University of Missouri	`bigcat.missouri.edu` or `128.206.1.3`
University of Nebraska-Lincoln	`ianrvm.unl.edu` or `129.93.200.1`
University of Wisconsin	`wissago.uwex.edu` or `144.92.121.13`
Virginia Tech	`gopher.ext.vt.edu` or `128.173.55.112`
Utah State University	`extsparc.agsci.usu.edu` or `129.123.13.55`
Washington State University	`cru1.cahe.wsu.edu` or `134.121.80.31`

FDA (Food and Drug Administration)
Database of Pharmaceutical Products & Ingredients
Internet: gopher to `gopher.austin.unimelb.edu.au` or `128.250.186.4`
URL: `gopher://gopher.austin.unimelb.edu.au`

Description: This gopher is located at Austin Hospital, Heidelberg, Victoria, Australia. The databasse is the Food and Drug Administration (USA)'s database of pharmaceutical products and their ingredients. The database is searchable by keyword. The fields in the results files are: Trade_name, Doc_no, App_date, Applicant, Dose_form, Ingredients, and Bioequivalence rating.

Contact: Doug Kemp <vetpharm@uga.cc.uga.edu>

FEDIX
Federal Information Exchange
Internet: gopher to `fedix.fie.com` or `192.111.228.33`
URL: `gopher://fedix.fie.com`

FISH-ECOLOGY
Fish-Ecology Archives

Internet: gopher to `searn.sunet.se` or `192.36.125.4`

URL: `gopher://searn.sunet.se`

FOOD & AGRICULTURE
United Nations

Internet: gopher to `gopher.fao.org` or `192.156.137.25`, port 2070

URL: `gopher://gopher.fao.org:2070`

Contact: Ken Novak <`k.novak@cgnet.com`>

GBASE (ENCYCLOPEDIA OF THE MOUSE GENOME)
Mouse Chromosome Genetic Maps

Internet: gopher to `merlot.welch.jhu.edu` or `192.239.77.4`

URL: `gopher://merlot.welch.jhu.edu`

Description: View the genetic maps of each mouse chromosome, search for specific loci on these maps as well as search for references and notes associated with each locus on the map. In addition you can search the Mouse Locus Catalog which contains detailed information on mouse loci. The Encyclopedia of the Mouse Genome is built and maintained at The Jackson Laboratory in Bar Harbor Maine. For further information about the Encyclopedia contact `davidnaman@jax.org` at the Jackson Laboratory. The Gopher version of the Encyclopedia has been created by Dan Jacobson at Johns Hopkins University.

Contact: e-mail to Dan Jacobson <`danj@welchgate.welch.jhu.edu`>

GOPHER JEWELS

Internet: gopher to `cwis.usc.edu` or `128.125.1.11`

URL: `gopher://cwis.usc.edu:70/11/Other_Gophers_and_Information_Resources/Gophers_by_Subject/Gopher_Jewels`

Description: a catalog of gopher sites by category (subject tree). Among the topics include: Agriculture and Forestry, Biology and Biosciences, Environment, Federal Agency and Related Gopher Sites, Geology and Oceanography, Grants, & Medical Related Gophers.

Contact: David Riggins <`david.riggins@tpis.cactus.org`>
Texas Department of Commerce
Office of Advanced Technology
Austin, TX 78711
Phone: 512-320-9561

GRANTS
Grants information, University of Idaho

Internet: gopher to `gopher.uidaho.edu` or `129.101.119.223`

URL: `gopher://gopher.uidaho.edu:70/11/science_research_grant`

GREAT LAKES INFORMATION NETWORK

Internet: gopher to `gopher.cic.net` or `192.131.22.5`

URL: `gopher://gopher.cic.net`

Description: Information about the environment, habitats and ecosystems of the Great Lakes Region of the United States.

GRIN
National Genetic Resources Program
USDA Agricultural Research Service

Internet: gopher to `gopher.ars-grin.gov` or `192.100.146.3`

URL: `gopher://gopher.ars-grin.gov`

HEALTHLINE
University of Montana Student Health Services

Internet: gopher to `selway.umt.edu:700` or `150.131.14.2`, port 700

URL: `gopher://selway.umt.edu:700/`

IUBIO BIOLOGY ARCHIVE
Indiana University

Internet: gopher to `ftp.bio.indiana.edu` or `129.79.224.25`

URL: `gopher://ftp.bio.indiana.edu/11`

JACKSON LABORATORY
Mouse Genome Database

Internet: gopher to `hobbes.jax.org` or `192.233.41.22`

URL: `gopher://hobbes.jax.org`

Contact: Alexander G. Smith <ags@zappa.jax.org>

LIBRARY OF CONGRESS MARVEL

Internet: gopher to `marvel.loc.gov` or `140.147.2.69`

URL: `gopher://marvel.loc.gov`

Description: Marvel contains congressional information, census data, White House documents, crime statistics, State Department reports, the Global Electronic Library, copyright information and U.S. Federal Government Information.

Contact: <lcmarvel@seq1.loc.gov>

LISTGOPHER

Internet: gopher to `dewey.lib.ncsu.edu` or `152.1.24.90`

URL: `gopher://dewey.lib.ncsu.edu`

Description: The purpose of LISTGopher is to search LISTSERV archives. It uses a Gopher interface, and performs LISTSERV commands in the background, making the search easier. Results are sent to your E-mail account. Currently the system only searches library-related lists.

MATERIAL SAFETY DATA SHEETS

Internet: gopher to `isumvs.iastate.edu` or `129.186.1.1`

URL: `gopher://isumvs.iastate.edu`

Description: Though not technically government information, material safety data sheets are produced by chemical manufacturers to comply with a variety of government regulations. They provide safety data on hundreds of chemicals.

MORBIDITY AND MORTALITY WEEKLY REPORT (MMWR)

Internet: gopher to `odie.niaid.nih.gov` or `128.231.240.12`

URL: `gopher://odie.niaid.nih.gov`

Description: Full text of the Centers for Disease Control and Prevention weekly journal, available long before libraries receive the paper edition.

NATIONAL AGRICULTURAL LIBRARY
U.S. Department of Agriculture

Internet: gopher to `locus.nalusda.gov` or `192.54.138.46`

URL: `gopher://locus.nalusda.gov`

NATIONAL ENVIRONMENTAL DATA REFERRAL SERVICE
National Oceanic and Atmospheric Administration

Internet: gopher to scilibx.ucsc.edu or 128.114.143.4

URL: **gopher://scilibx.ucsc.edu**

NATIONAL INSTITUTE OF ALLERGY & INFECTIOUS DISEASE (NIAID) GOPHER
Internet: gopher to gopher.niaid.nih.gov or 128.231.240.12

URL: **gopher://gopher.niaid.nih.gov**

Description: Full text of NIAID press releases, AIDS information publications, institute directories and more.

NATIONAL INSTITUTE OF ENVIRONMENTAL HEALTH SCIENCES (NIEHS) GOPHER
Internet: gopher to jeeves.niehs.nih.gov or 157.98.8.9

URL: **gopher://jeeves.niehs.nih.gov**

NATIONAL INSTITUTE OF MENTAL HEALTH (NIMH) GOPHER
Internet: gopher to gopher.nimh.nih.gov or 156.40.186.8

URL: **gopher://gopher.nimh.nih.gov**

NATIONAL INSTITUTES OF HEALTH GOPHER
Division of Computer Research and Technology

Internet: telnet to gopher.nih.gov or 128.231.2.5

    At the login prompt, enter: gopher

URL: **gopher://gopher.nih.gov**

Questions/comments to: gopher@gopher.nih.gov

Description: Provides access to a broad range of NIH resources, including institute phone books and calendars, library catalogs, molecular biology databases, full text of the NIH Guide for Grants and Contracts, files containing AIDS and cancer information and more.

NATIONAL LIBRARY OF MEDICINE GOPHER
Internet: gopher to gopher.nlm.nih.gov or 130.14.70.3

URL: **gopher://gopher.nlm.nih.gov**

Description: The National Library of Medicine's Gopher contains information about the Library and selected references materials. It also provides access to Locator, NLM's online catalog system, and to MEDLARS and TOXNET (for those with access codes). The NLM Gopher does not provide direct access to the contents of journal articles or books.

Contact: <admin@gopher.nlm.nih.gov>

NATIONAL INSTITUTE OF STANDARDS AND TECHNOLOGY (NIST)
Internet: Web client at www.nist.gov

URL: **http://www.nist.gov/**

Description: News releases, announcements, and newsletters from the National Institute of Standards and Technology such as the biweekly NIST UPDATE, and "Science Beat", a tip sheet for science journalists.

NATIONAL OCEANIC & ATMOSPHERIC ADMINISTRATION (NOAA)
National Environmental Information Services Gopher

Internet: gopher to gopher.esdim.noaa.gov or 140.90.235.168

URL: **gopher://gopher.esdim.noaa.gov**

Description: NOAA catalog provides keyword access to sources of environmental information nationwide.

NATIONAL OCEANOGRAPHIC DATA CENTER (NODC)
National Oceanic and Atmospheric Administration (NOAA)

Internet: gopher to `nodc.noaa.gov` or `140.90.235.171`

URL: `gopher://nodc.noaa.gov`

Description: Internet access to information about NODC ocean data holdings, products, and services. The NODC is one of the national environmental data centers operated by the National Oceanic and Atmospheric Administration (NOAA) of the U.S. Department of Commerce. The primary mission of the NODC is to maintain a growing archive of historical oceanographic data and to make its data resources easily accessible to users in the United States and around the world. The NODC's global holdings of physical, chemical, and biological oceanographic data currently total over 60 gigabytes, making it the world's largest publicly available ocean data archive. Information already installed on the NODC Gopher server includes: NODC telephone numbers and e-mail addresses, how to obtain NODC data products, detailed descriptions of the NODC's major oceanographic databases, a complete list and descriptions of the NODC's CD-ROM data products, and reports on NODC's international oceanographic data management and data exchange activities.

Contact: Parmesh Dwivedi <pdwivedi@nodc.noaa.gov>
Bruce C. Douglas <bdouglas@nodc.noaa.gov>
National Oceanographic Data Center
DOC/NOAA/NESDIS E/OC
1825 Connecticut Avenue, NW
Washington, DC 20235
Phone: 202-606-4594
Fax: 202-606-4586

NATIONAL SCIENCE FOUNDATION
Science and Technology Information System (STIS)

Internet: gopher to `stis.nsf.gov` or `128.150.195.40`

URL: `gopher://stis.nsf.gov`

Description: Provides a wide variety of government information including easy access to many U.S. government gophers. Includes indexes to National Science Foundation (NSF) Award Abstracts and NSF Publications, NSF Phone Directory, and program guidelines for biological sciences; computer and information science and engineering; education and human resource; engineering; geosciences; math and physical sciences; social, behavioral and economic sciences.

Contact: <stis@nsf.gov>

NATIONAL SCIENCE FOUNDATION
Center for Biological Timing

Internet: gopher to `gopher.virginia.edu` or `128.143.22.36`

URL: `gopher://gopher.virginia.edu`

NETVET
Veterinary Resources Gopher

Internet: gopher to `netvet.wustl.edu` or `128.252.235.17`

URL: `gopher://netvet.wustl.edu:70/11n%3a/vet`

Description: The NetVet Veterinary Resources Gopher is provided as a resource for the Internet Community by the Washington University Division of Comparative Medicine and acts as as a central pointer to all known resources related to veterinary medicine. Contains the following services: archives of veterinary Internet/Bitnet listservs, pointers to veterinary school gophers, pointers to veterinary conference proceedings, pointers to FDA animal drug database, pointers to AVMA Network of Animal Health (NOAH), archives of USDA Animal Welfare Information Center documents, American Academy of Veterinary Informatics information, American Veterinary Computer Society newsletters, the Electronic Zoo animal-related computer resource document, American Association for Lab Animal Science information, miscellaneous animal species-specific information, and pointers to most major Internet resources in agriculture, biology, medicine, ecology, and government.

Contact: Ken Boschert, DVM <ken@wudcm.wustl.edu>
Washington University
Division of Comparative Medicine
Box 8061, 660 S. Euclid Ave.
St. Louis, MO 63110
Phone: 314-362-3700
Fax: 314-362-6480

NOT JUST COWS
Internet/BITNET Resources in Agriculture

Internet: gopher to `snymorvb.cs.snymor.edu` or `136.204.1.2`

URL: `gopher://snymorvb.cs.snymor.edu`

Description: NOT JUST COWS—A Guide to INTERNET/Bitnet Resources in Agriculture and Related Sciences; The purpose of this Guide is to list Agricultural and Related Sciences information resources available through the INTERNET. Agricultural information resources listed include; an index of over 40 libraries with extensive collections in agriculture; INTERNET BBS such as Advanced Technology Information Network and CENET; a collection of mail based services such as Almanac Servers and over 60 Listserve Discussion Groups; other miscellaneous information resources such as WAIS and FEDIX. In addition to the above; now includes gopher, a larger number of libraries, many more Almanac servers, NEWS Groups, and new electronic bulletin boards.

Contact: Wilfred Drew <drewwe@snymorva.cs.snymor.edu>
SUNY at Morrisville
College of Agriculture and Technology
Serials/Reference/Systems Librarian
P.O. Box 902
Morrisville, NY 13408-0902
Phone: 315-684-6055
Fax: 315-684-6115

ONCOLINK
University of Pennsylvania Multimedia Oncology Resource

Internet: gopher to `cancer.med.upenn.edu`, port 80

URL: `gopher://cancer.med.upenn.edu`

Description: Subjects include: medical oncology, radiation oncology, pediatric oncology, surgical oncology, medical physics, psychosocial support for oncology patients & families, and links to other oncology centers in the world.

Contact: Dr. E. Loren Buhle, Jr. <buhle@xrt.upenn.edu>
University of Pennsylvania School of Medicine
Rm. 440A, 3401 Walnut St.
Philadelphia, PA 19104-6228
Phone: 215-662-3084
Fax: 215-349-5978

PENPAGES
Agricultural Information
    Pennsylvania State University

Internet: gopher to `penpages.psu.edu` or `128.118.36.4`

URL: `gopher://penpages.psu.edu`

Description: PENpages is a full-text information service containing thousands of research-based fact sheets, news articles, newsletters, and reports. Information is entered by faculty and staff of Penn State University, the Pennsylvania Department of Agriculture, USDA and many cooperators nationwide. Information is agricultural-based and consumer-oriented. Topics include: 4-H and youth development, agricultural education, agronomy; dairy and animal science, engineering, entomology, family life aand resource management, food safety, forest resources, gerontology, horticulture, human nutrition, pesticide education, plant pathology, poultry science, rural development, veterinary science, water quality, and many others.

Contact: Kirk Barbieri <kirk@psupen.psu.edu>

PRIMATE INFORMATION NETWORK
Wisconsin Regional Primate Research Center

Internet: gopher to gopher.primate.wisc.edu or 144.92.43.15

URL: **gopher://gopher.primate.wisc.edu**

Internet: telnet to telnet.wiscinfo.wisc.edu or 144.92.104.37

URL: **telnet://telnet.wiscinfo.wisc.edu**

At the login prompt, enter: wiscinfo
Choose: UW-Madison Information Servers Wisconsin Primate Research Center Server

Questions/Comments to: jacobsen@primate.wisc.edu

Help Line: 608-263-3512

RACHEL'S HAZARDOUS WASTE NEWS

Internet: gopher to world.std.com or 192.74.137.5

URL: **gopher://world.std.com**

Contact: Environmental Research Foundation <erf@igc.apc.org>
P.O. Box 5036
Annapolis, MD 21403
Fax: 410-263-8944

SAFETY
Safety Information Resources on the InterNet, Vermont

Internet: gopher to siri.uvm.edu or 132.198.205.92

URL: **gopher://siri.uvm.edu**

SMITHSONIAN INSTITUTION
Natural History Gopher

Internet: gopher to nmnhgoph.si.edu or 160.111.64.84

URL: **gopher://nmnhgoph.si.edu**

Description: The Smithsonian Institution's National Museum of Natural History is pleased to announce the Smithsonian Natural History Gopher Server. With over 120 million collections and 135 professional scientists, the National Museum of Natural History is one of the world's largest museums devoted to natural history and anthropology. This server will provide access to data associated with the collections, and information and tools for the study of the natural world. The Department of Vertebrate Zoology includes checklists of known species names. Currently the Mammal Species of the World have been posted. We plan to expand this to include Amphibians, Fishes, etc.

Contact: Don Gourley <don@smithson.si.edu>
Smithsonian Institution
Washington, D.C.

SOCIETY FOR NEUROSCIENCE CENTRAL OFFICE

Internet: gopher to gopher.sfn.org or 198.6.70.2

URL: **gopher://gopher.sfn.org**

Contact: R. Cliff Young <gopher-admin@sfn.org>
Phone: 202-462-6688

SUPREME COURT DECISIONS

Internet: gopher to `info.umd.edu` or `128.8.10.29`

URL: **gopher://info.umd.edu**

Description: Full text of Supreme Court decisions issued since 1989. Also includes brief biographies of Court justices.

THE SCIENTIST Newsletter

Internet: gopher to `internic.net` or `198.41.0.5`

URL: **gopher://internic.net**

Description: THE SCIENTIST is a biweekly newspaper for scientists and the research community. It is circulated internationally to researchers, administrators, and policy makers in academia, industry, and government and covers current issues and events that impact the professional research environment. News includes funding legislation, new grants, employment and salary trends, career advancement opportunities, ethics and conflicts of interest, representation of women and minorities in science, and the interplay of industrial, academic, and governmental research.

UNITED NATIONS

Internet: gopher to `nywork1.undp.org` or `165.65.6.4`

URL: **gopher://nywork1.undp.org**

Description: Full text of U.N press releases, U.N. Conference on Environment and Development reports, United Nations Development Programme documents, U.N. telephone directories and more.

USDA AGRICULTURAL EXTENSION SERVICE

Internet: gopher to `cyfer.esusda.gov` or `192.73.224.110`

URL: **gopher://cyfer.esusda.gov**

Description: Includes information from the USDA Extension Service, National Agriculture Library and Americans Communicating Electronically

(ACE)

USDA Statistical Data

Cornell Mann Library

Internet: gopher to `usda.mannlib.cornell.edu` or `128.253.78.240`

URL: **gopher://usda.mannlib.cornell.edu**

Description: Computer users worldwide now have access to statistical data gathered by the USDA. Cornell's Mann Library became the host for more than 140 free agricultural data sets, available to anyone with Internet access. The system is easy to search. Data are formatted for importing into existing computer analysis programs. Each data set is accompanied by an explanatory document, and all text documents are indexed for electronic searching.

Contact: Oya Y. Rieger <oyr1@cornell.edu>
Numeric Files Librarian
Mann Library
Cornell University
Ithaca, NY 14853
Phone: 607-255-7960

U.S. CONGRESS

Internet: gopher to `marvel.loc.gov`

URL: **gopher://marvel.loc.gov:70/11/congress**

   or

Internet: gopher to `info.umd.edu`, port 901

URL: **gopher://info.umd.edu:901/11/inforM/Educational_Resources/Government/United_States/Congress**

U.S. HOUSE OF REPRESENTATIVES
Internet: gopher to `gopher.house.gov` or `143.231.252.207`
URL: **gopher://gopher.house.gov/**

U.S. SENATE
Internet: gopher to `gopher.senate.gov`
URL: **gopher://gopher.senate.gov**

U.S. SUPREME COURT
Internet: gopher to `info.umd.edu`, port 901
URL: **gopher://info.umd.edu:901/11/inforM/Educational_Resources/AcademicResourcesByTopic/UnitedStates/SupremeCt**

VERTEBRATE MUSEUM
University of California-Berkeley
Internet: gopher to `ucmp1.berkeley.edu` or `128.32.146.30`
URL: **gopher://ucmp1.berkeley.edu**

VERTEBRATE WORLD GOPHER SERVER
Colorado State University
Internet: gopher to `neptune.rrb.colostate.edu` or `129.82.125.6`
URL: **gopher://neptune.rrb.colostate.edu**

VIRUS GOPHER SERVER
Australian National University Bioinformatics Facility
Internet: gopher to `life.anu.edu.au` or `150.203.38.74`
URL: **gopher://life.anu.edu.au**

Description: The approved names of virus families/groups and members are now available on-line from the Australian National University's Bioinformatics Facility.

Contact: Dr Cornelia Buchen-Osmond <`buchen@life.anu.edu.au`>
Research School of Biological Research
Australian National University
GPO Box 475
Canberra ACT 2601 AUSTRALIA
Phone: 61-6-249-4842
Fax: 61-6-249-0758

WELCH MEDICAL LIBRARY
The Johns Hopkins University
Internet: gopher to `welchlink.welch.jhu.edu` or `128.220.59.78`
URL: **gopher://welchlink.welch.jhu.edu**

Description: Unique task oriented biomedical information gopher

Contact: Karla Hahn <`khahn@welchlink.welch.jhu.edu`>
Welch Medical Library
Johns Hopkins University

WHITE HOUSE INFORMATION
Internet: gopher to `sunsite.unc.edu` or `198.86.40.81`

URL: `gopher://sunsite.unc.edu`
   or
Internet: gopher to `gopher.tamu.edu`
URL: `gopher://gopher.tamu.edu:70/11/.dir/president.dir`

Description: Full text of major policy statements, daily press briefings, speeches, proclamations, the president's daily schedule and more.

WOODS HOLE OCEANOGRAPHIC INSTITUITION

Internet: gopher to `gopher.whoi.edu` or `128.128.16.114`
URL: `gopher://gopher.whoi.edu`

Description: This gopher server is intended to be used to make information about the Woods Hole Oceanographic Institution and oceanographic databases available for both public and internal use.

Contact: Julie Allen <`jallen@whoi.edu`>
Information Systems Center
W.H.O.I.
Woods Hole, MA 02543
Phone: 508-457-2000, ext. 2357
Fax: 508-457-2174

WORLD HEALTH ORGANIZATION

Internet: gopher to `gopher.who.ch` or `158.232.17.1`
URL: `gopher://gopher.who.ch`

Contact: WHO Internet Gopher Root Server Administrator
Information Technology Office (ITO)
World Health Organization (WHO) Headquarters
CH-1211 Geneva 27
Switzerland
Phone: +41 22 791 2434
FAX: +41 22 791 0746
E-mail: <`gopher@who.ch`> or <`akazawa@who.ch`>

WORLD WIDE WEB (WWW) SITES

AGRICULTURAL ENGINEERING
Texas A&M University
URL: `http://ageninfo.tamu.edu`

Description: This server features mainly departmental information, but also has pointers to information relevant to agriculture, earth science, GIS, remote sensing, and GPS.

BIOCATALOGUE
Catalog of Bio Software
   GENETHON—Human Genome Research Centre
URL: English version—`http://www.genethon.fr/genethon_en.html`
   French version—`http://www.genethon.fr/genethon_fr.html`
Contact: Patricai Rodriguez-Tome <`pat@genethon.fr`>

BIOINFORMATICS
Johns Hopkins University
URL: `http://www.gdb.org/hopkins.html`

Description: The Johns Hopkins University BioInformatics Web Server is a Web server for biology, with some interesting biological databases (which have hot links to each other as well as to other databases around the world), electronic publications for biology, software, links to other Web servers.

Contact: Dan Jacobson <danj@gdb.org>

BIOLOGY & MEDICINE
WWW Virtual Library

URL: `http://golgi.harvard.edu/biopages/all.html`

Description: List of biological and medical WWW resources.

BIRDS

URL: `http://compstat.wharton.upenn.edu:8001/`

Description: Bird newsletters, checklists, and access to the AVES GIF/Sound archive.

Contact: Jack Siler <siler@wharton.upenn.edu>

CANCERNET

URL: `http://biomed.nus.sg:80/`

Description: A collaboration between the National University of Singapore and the National Cancer Institute, Bethesda, MA, is a secondary site for the NCI CancerNet files.

Contact: Tan Tin Wee, PhD <bchtantw@leonis.nus.sg>
Department of Biochemistry,
and Biocomputing Research and User Support (BRUS)
National University of Singapore
Kent Ridge
Singapore 0511
Phone: 65-772-3678
Fax: 65-779-1453

CLEARINGHOUSE FOR SUBJECT-ORIENTED INTERNET RESOURCE GUIDES
University of Michigan

URL: `http://http2.sils.umich.edu/~lou/chhome.html` or
`http://www.lib.umich.edu/chhome.html` or
`gopher://una.hh.lib.umich.edu/11/inetdirs`

Description: The Clearinghouse for Subject-Oriented Internet Resource Guides is jointly sponsored by the University Library and the School of Information and Library Studies at the University of Michigan, the Clearinghouse provides access to subject-oriented resource guides created by members of the Internet community. There are currently over 60 guides available via anonymous FTP, Gopher, and WorldWideWeb/Mosaic. Titles and authors of animal-related resource guides include:

>   Agriculture; W. Drew
>   Animals; K. Boschert
>   Biological Sciences; D. Kovacs
>   Conservation; D. Wendling, J. Christianson
>   Diversity; L. Heise
>   Environment; T. Murphy, C. Briggs-Erickson
>   Health Sciences; L. Hancock
>   Health Sciences; N. Martin, P. Redman, G. Oren
>   Math & Science Education; T.C. O'Haver
>   Multiple Subjects (Gopher Jewels); D. Riggins
>   Neurosciences; S. Bonario, S. Cormicle

Contact: Louis Rosenfeld <lou@umich.edu>
School of Information and Library Studies
University of Michigan
403B West Engineering
Ann Arbor, MI 48109-1092
Phone: 313-747-3581
Fax: 313-764-2475

ECOSYSTEMS
University of Virginia

Internet: gopher to `ecosys.drdr.virginia.edu`

URL: `http://ecosys.drdr.virginia.edu/EcoWeb.html`

Description: A recycling and environmental information server. It provides and connects users to local, regional, national, and international environmental info.

telnet: `EcoSys.drdr.Virginia.EDU` login as `gopher`, `lynx`, or `ecochat`

ENTOMOLOGY
Colorado State University

URL: `http://www.colostate.edu/Depts/Entomology/ent.html`

Description: The Entomology Department at Colorado State University has resources that pertain to insects and related organisms.

Contact: Lou Bjostad <lbjostad@lamar.colostate.edu>

ENTOMOLOGY
Iowa State University

URL: `http://www.public.iastate.edu/~entomology/homepage.html`

ERIN
Environmental Resources Information Network (ERIN) Newsletter (Australia)

URL: `http://kaos.erin.gov.au/erin.html`

Description: The Australian Environmental Resources Information Network (ERIN) enhanced World Wide Web Server containing information and data on Australia's environment, and including links to ERIN's ORACLE database. Covers endangered species, vegetation, international agreements, legislation, and conference information.

FDA
Approved Animal Drug Database

URL: `http://scholar.lib.vt.edu/ejournals/vetfda.html`

Contact: Richard Talbot <rtalbot@vt.edu>

FINS
Fish Information Service

URL: `http://www.actwin.com/fish/index.html`

Description: Contains information about keeping aquariums, both marine and freshwater.

GOPHER JEWELS
Gopher Jewels List

URL: `http://galaxy.einet.net/galaxy.html`

Description: A catalog of gopher sites by category (subject tree). Gopher sites are placed in particular categories as a result of finding related information buried somewhere in their hole. The list was established for the sharing of interesting gopher finds ONLY. This list expects subscribers that are either gopher developers or gopher users.

List Owner/Contact: David Riggins <david.riggins@tpoint.com>
Texas Department of Commerce
Office of Advanced Technology
Austin, Texas 78711
Phone: 512-320-9561

IUBIO BIOLOGY ARCHIVE
Indiana University
URL: `gopher://ftp.bio.indiana.edu/11%09%2Btext/html`

JACKSON LABORATORY
Mouse Genome Informatics Group
URL: `http://www.informatics.jax.org/`

MEDNEWS
URL: `http://biomed.nus.sg:80`

Description: MEDNEWS is for distribution of the Health Info-Com Network medical newsletter. It is distributed weekly and contains the latest MMWR from the Center for Disease Control, weekly AIDS Statistics, FDA bulletins, medical news from the United Nations, and other assorted medical news items.

Contact: Dr. KC Lun <coflunkc@leonis.nus.sg>
Dept of Community Medicine
National University Hospital
Lower Kent Ridge Road, Singapore 0511
Phone: +65-772-4296
Fax: +65-779-1489

NATIONAL OCEANOGRAPHIC DATA CENTER (NODC)
National Oceanic and Atmospheric Administration (NOAA)
URL: `http://www.nodc.noaa.gov/`

Description: Internet access to information about NODC ocean data holdings, products, and services. The NODC is one of the national environmental data centers operated by the National Oceanic and Atmospheric Administration (NOAA) of the U.S. Department of Commerce. The primary mission of the NODC is to maintain a growing archive of historical oceanographic data and to make its data resources easily accessible to users in the United States and around the world. The NODC's global holdings of physical, chemical, and biological oceanographic data currently total over 60 gigabytes, making it the world's largest publicly available ocean data archive. Information already installed on the NODC Gopher server includes: NODC telephone numbers and e-mail addresses, how to obtain NODC data products, detailed descriptions of the NODC's major oceanographic databases, a complete list and descriptions of the NODC's CD-ROM data products, and reports on NODC's international oceanographic data management and data exchange activities.

Contact: Parmesh Dwivedi <pdwivedi@nodc.noaa.gov>
Bruce C. Douglas <bdouglas@nodc.noaa.gov>
National Oceanographic Data Center
DOC/NOAA/NESDIS E/OC
1825 Connecticut Avenue, NW
Washington, DC 20235
Phone: 202-606-4594
Fax: 202-606-4586

NIH
National Institutes of Health
URL: `http://www.nih.gov/`

Description: The NIH WWW server of the Division of Computer Research and Technology contains biomedical info generated or pertaining to the NIH campus. Hypertext links exist for the following: Biomedical—health issues and clinical protocols; "NIH Grants and Contracts"; Research opportunities at the NIH campus; Molecular biology and modeling topics; NIH computer and network resources; NIH calendar; NIH phone directory; NIH Bethesda Campus info; NIH Library; & Other NIH info services.

Contact: <gopher@gopher.nih.gov>

NOT JUST COWS
Internet/BITNET Resources in Agriculture

URL: `gopher://dewey.lib.ncsu.edu/0ftp%3adewey.lib.ncsu.edu%40/pub/stacks/guides/not-just-cows`

Description: NOT JUST COWS—A Guide to INTERNET/Bitnet Resources in Agriculture and Related Sciences; The purpose of this Guide is to list Agricultural and Related Sciences information resources available through the INTERNET. Agricultural information resources listed include; an index of over 40 libraries with extensive collections in agriculture; INTERNET BBS such as Advanced Technology Information Network and CENET; a collection of mail based services such as Almanac Servers and over 60 Listserve Discussion Groups; other miscellaneous information resources such as WAIS and FEDIX. In addition to the above; now includes gopher, a larger number of libraries, many more Almanac servers, NEWS Groups, and new electronic bulletin boards.

Contact: Wilfred Drew <drewwe@snymorva.cs.snymor.edu>
SUNY at Morrisville
College of Agriculture and Technology
Serials/Reference/Systems Librarian
P.O. Box 902
Morrisville, NY 13408-0902
Phone: 315-684-6055
Fax: 315-684-6115

PATHOLOGY
University of Washington

URL: `http://www.pathology.washington.edu`

Description: The server includes access to human and mouse chromosome idiograms and photomicrograph scans; the Genome Machine: a simple graphical interface experiment; a pathology gallery; and information about the UW Medical Scientists Training Program (MSTP).

Contact: David A. Adler <dadler@u.washington.edu>
Pathology SM-30
University of Washington
Seattle, WA 98195
Phone: 206-543-0716
Fax: 206-543-3644

PRIMATE INFO NET
Wisconsin Regional Primate Research Center

URL: `http://www.primate.wisc.edu`

PUBLIC HEALTH
Boston University School of Public Health

URL: `http://www-busph.bu.edu`

Description: Boston University School of Public Health (BUSPH) offers the School's entire 1994/95 bulletin, current schedule of Public Health Forums (including a campus map to help get you there), and more.

US FISH & WILDLIFE SERVICE
U.S. Department of the Interior

URL: **http://bluegoose.arw.r9.fws.gov/**(Division of Refuges)
     http://ash.lab.r1.fws.gov/(Division of Law Enforcement, Forensic Lab)
Contact: John Clark <**clarkj@mail.fws.gov**>
    US Fish & Wildlife Service
    Systems Analyst
    Division of Refuges

MISCELLANEOUS INTERNET RESOURCES

UNC BBS
University of North Carolina Bulletin Board System
    Access to Library of Congress & nationwide libraries
Internet: telnet to `launchpad.unc.edu` or `152.2.22.80`
    At the login prompt, enter: `launch`

WAISTATION
Wide Area Information Service
Internet: telnet to `quake.think.com` or `192.31.181.1`
      `swais.cwis.uci.edu` or `128.200.15.2`
      `sunsite.unc.edu` or `198.86.40.81`
    At the login prompt, enter: swais

WHITE HOUSE PRESS RELEASES
News, Speeches
Mail to: `Clinton-Info@Campaign92.Org`
    In the subject of the letter, enter: `help`
URL: `gopher://calypso-2.oit.unc.edu:70/11/../.pub/Politics/whitehouse-papers`

WORLD WINDOW
Washington University Internet Services
    Access to Gopher & other Internet Services
Internet: telnet to `library.wustl.edu` or `128.252.173.4`
    At the login prompt, enter your terminal type, then bypass username prompt with another carriage return.

DIALUP BULLETIN BOARD SYSTEMS (NON-INTERNET)

NOTE
The computer systems (BBS's) listed in this section are NOT accessible via the Internet unless otherwise stated. In other words, you need a modem to dial in and connect to these systems. In most instances, I have included both the phone number of the system and a voice line in case you need help. Modem speeds range from 1200—16800 baud and the modem settings (i.e., N-8-1) stands for No Parity, 8 data bits, and 1 stop bit.

AFIP BBS
Armed Forces Institute of Pathology Bulletin Board System
Modem: 202-576-2911
Help Line: 202-576-2453
12/2400 baud, N-8-1

AG-BBS
California State University-Fresno
Modem: 209-294-4819
Help line: 209-294-2547
12/2400 baud, N-8-1

AFEBB
Agricultural Electronic Bulletin Board
 University of Missouri
Modem: 314-882-8289
Help line: 314-882-4827
12/2400 baud, N-8-1

Description: Information on Farm Management and computer technology to and among Missouri Farmers and Extension Specialists. The basic goal of the bulletin board is to provide the University of Missouri with a technologically current tool to distrte information on management, marketing, production and computer technology to and among Missouri farmers, Extension specialists and University faculty.

AGRICULTURAL LIBRARY FORUM (ALF) BBS
USDA National Agricultural Library Bulletin Board System
Modem: 301-504-8510 / 301-504-5111 / 301-504-5496 / 301-504-5497
Help Line: 301-504-5113
12/24/96/144/16800 baud, N-8-1
Note: Also available via Telnet to FEDWORLD

Internet: telnet to `fedworld.gov` or `192.239.92.201`

Login to FedWorld for the first time requires a user to register on FedWorld, then access the Gateway system via the "D" command from the main conference. Entry of another "D" brings up the list of federal systems for selection. Enter "2" to select ALF. After the first registration, a user may enter "D D 2" to make an immediate l ink to ALF from the main FedWorld menu.

Description: ALF is a convenient, economical tool for electronically accessing information about NAL'S programs, projects, products and services. It provides a forum for exchanging information among agricultural libraries, information centers and others in the agricultural field. This BBS contains extensive up-to-date bibliographies on many topics related to agriculture and other areas. These are updated on a regular basis. These are from searches on AGRICOLA. ALF is open to anyone. The board is accessible 24 hours a day, 7 days a week.

AMERICA ONLINE

VIN
Veterinary Information Network

Description: National Communications Network for Veterinarians. There are 4 bulletin boards within the VIN area: VIN Information, Vet Industry Connection, Associations and Foundations, and the vet-to-vet board. VIN represents an electronic community of veterinary specialists that spans the country—there are no geographic or structural boundaries. A university of personalized information. Current subscription fees are: $250 per year, $150 per 6 months, or $30 per month. A subscription to VIN entitles use of all areas. There are no limits to the general use bulletin boards or libraries. Included in this fee is the unlimited right to request "public" case consults in the appropriate VIN folder. The appropriate specialists will be constantly monitoring their folders and will turn answers around within 24 hours. Certain conferences, most CE courses, private consultations, individual literature searches, and other "one-to-one" services will cost extra.

VIN provides an extended services database. VIN's Extended Services allow you to find information from past and current VIN boards. VIN's EXTENDED SERVICES also provide access to the veterinary literature (the Quarterly Index and author abstracts from the current literature).

FEES FOR VIN'S EXTENDED SERVICES DATABASE
One year access to non-VIN members: $250
6 month access for VIN members and non-members: $150
One month access for VIN members and non-members: $30
One year access for VIN members: $449 (including one year VIN subscription)

Contact: Duncan Ferguson, DVM <duncanf@aol.com>
Paul Pion <pdp1@aol.com>
VINgram <vingram@aol.com>
Veterinary Information Network, Inc.
1411 W. Corvell Blvd., Suite 106-131
Davis, CA 95616
Phone: 800-700-4636
FAX: 916-756-6035

AMNET ON-LINE
Animal Rights Bulletin Board System
Modem 1: 303-364-2257 (TBBS)
Modem 2: 303-680-7791
Modem 3: 212-724-6826
Help Line: 303-680-9011
12/24/9600 baud, N-8-1
SysOp: James Cherry <james.cherry@f539.n104.f1.fido.org>

ANIMAL HOUSE BBS
Modem: 609-488-4527
12/24/96/19200 baud, N-8-1

ATI-NET
California State University-Fresno
    Agricultural Information
Modem: 209-294-4265
Help Line: 209-278-4819
    12/2400 baud, N-8-1

Description: ATI-Net is a full service information source designed to assist several markets within California. Individual systems provide information for the agricultural market, the educational community (CSUPER-Net), Automated Trade Library Service (ATLS), Biotechnology Information (CSUPERB).

BEENET INTERNATIONAL HEADQUARTERS
The BEE Bulletin Board System
    Amsterdam, Holland
Modem: 31-20-6764105

Description: Disseminates bee-software and text files all over Europe. Aims for the Beenet include: making (scientific and other) knowledge available to the common beekeeper of rope. The only requirement is utethe ownership or availability of a computer, modem, a telephone line, and communication software.

Contact: Hugo Veerkamp
THE BEE BBS
P.O. BOX 51008
1007EA AMSTERDAM
the NETHERLANDS

Other BEENET SYSTEMS

Name	Location	System Operator	Modem Number
WILDBEES BBS	California USA	Andy Nachbaur	209-826-8107
APIMO BBS	Mariager Denmark	Jorn Johanesson	45-98-583997
ECONNECT BBS	Prague CSR	Vojtech Kment	42-2-802908
AMIGABEE BBS	London UK	Steven Turner	44-81-695-5328
EXCALIBUR BBS	Luebeck Germany	Dirk Benemann	49-451-46093
CUCUMBER CITY BBS	Vasteras Sweden	John Haglof	46-21-333282

BIOSIS
Taxononmic Reference File

Modem: 215-972-6759

Description: Online bacterial taxmic databases, conferences on IOSbiology & life sciences. Sponsored by BIOSIS—producers of Biological Abstracts.

BIOTRON
American Foundation for Biological Sciences
   The Biologist's Electronic Network (BioScience)

Modem: 202-628-2427

Help Line: 202-628-1500

(TBBS) 12/2400 baud, N-8-1

Description: E-mail, job listings, organization news, & the AIBS Forum.

Contact: American Foundation for Biological Sciences
   730 11th Street, NW
   Washington, DC 20001-4521

BIRD INFO NETWORK BBS
Modem: 303-423-9775

12/2400 baud, N-8-1

BLACK BAG BBS
Medical Information Bulletin Board

Modem: 302-994-3772

Fidonet Address: 1:150/140

12/24/9600 baud, N-8-1

BRS
AFTER DARK & COLLEAGUE and SEARCH SERVICE

Modem: Access is through Sprintnet, Tymenet, or Datapac local access phone numbers.

Description: Commercial online database

Contact: BRS Information Technologies
   Division of Maxwell Online, Inc.
   8000 Westpark Drive
   McLean, VA 22102
   Phone: 800-955-0906

Notes: Animal-related databases on BRS include:

   AGRICOLA—1970-present
   CAB Abstracts—1980-present
   Current Contents: Agriculture, Biology, & Environment—last 12 months
   Wilson Biological and Agricultural Index—1983-present
   BIOSIS—1970-present
   Cambridge Scientific Abstracts Life Science—1981-present

Current Contents: Life Sciences—last 12 months
TOXLINE—1965-present
Zoological Record Online—1978-present
Federal Register Abstracts—1986-present
Disclosure/Health—current
Health Industry Research Reports—1982-present

CARL
Colorado Alliance of Research Libraries

Modem: 303-758-1551

12/2400 baud, N-8-1

Description: A collection of library catalogs, business databases, and includes more than 14,000 titles, and more than 4 million articles. Over 750,000 articles are added annually. In addition to being able to search by keyword, you can search by author and you can browse by journal title. Many biological holdings are indexed.

COLORADO CONNECTION BBS
Bird Info Network & Birdnet

Modem: 303-423-9775

Help Line: 303-422-6529 (Fax)

12/24/9600 baud, N-8-1

P.O. Box 632

Arvada, CO 80001

COMPU-FARM BBS
Alberta Agriculture
    Farm Business Management Information Network

Modem: 403-556-4104 (Maximus)

Help line: 403-556-4243

12/24/96/144/19200 baud, N-8-1

Fidonet Node 1:134/4001

Description: A joint project of the Canadian Farm Business Management Council and Alberta Agriculture Farm Business Management Branch.

COMPUSERVE

Internet: telnet to compuserve.com or 194.4.8.1

CompuServe Incorporated has become a leading provider of computer-based information, software and communications services to businesses and personal computer owners. In total, the CompuServe Information Service provides access to more than 1,700 databases covering hundreds of subject areas.

For Information on Compuserve, Phone: 800-524-3388

PETS (Pets/Animal Forum)
Access: GO PETS

Description: The PETS/ANIMAL Forum provides information exchange on a variety of animals and discussions about animal issues, and is a place to chat with other people interested in animals. Many animal-related files can be found the library section, including articles, technical reports, product information, species guides, & graphics. Message Sections include: Using This Forum; Health Professional (private); Dogs' World; Cat's Meow; Caged Birds; Reptiles/Exotic; Ask-A-Vet; Horse Management; Cat Breeders' World; The Support Group; Small Mammals; Horse Training; The Watering Hole; Issues/News/Laws; Livestock; NAIA; and PETS University (private). Library Sections include: Using this Forum; Veterinary; Dog Library; Cat Library; Caged Bird Library; Reptiles/Exotic; Software/Programs; Horse Library; Pet Products; Support Library; Small Mammals; Graphics Library; Community Library; News/Issues/Laws; Livestock Library; and NAIA Library.

Contact: John Benn [76703,4256]—Forum Director
    Martha Ashley [76702,1760]—Operations Manager
Voice Help Phone: 205-383-3009 from 6pm to 10pm (ET)
Fax Help Phone: 205-386-7615

PETPRO (Pet Products/Reference Forum)

Access: GO PETPRO

Description: The PET PRODUCTS/REFERENCE FORUM is a customer support forum for businesses with products or services for pet owners and professionals who care for animals and aquatic life. Also it includes reference files of interest to aquarists, pet owners, scientists, and others. Message Sections include: PETPRO Info Center; Allerpet; Aquarium Pharm; Aquatic Book Shop; Champion Supply Co.; Kent Marine; Kordon; Mardel; Marineland; Oasis Products; Other Companies; Pet Warehouse; SeaClear/Biologic; Thiel Aqua Tech; Ultramarine; Wardley; and Man's Best Friend. Library sections include: CS-Products Lib; Gov't Pubs/Fish; Monographs/Fish-Inv; Monographs/Plants; Aquarium Fish Mag.; Drum & Croaker; J. of Aquariculture; Marine Reef/SRAB; Today's Aquar & TAQ; PIJAC Library; Pictures/All; and Internet List Lib.

Contact: John Benn [76703,4256]—Forum Director
    Pat Gatlin [76711,1040]—Operations Manager

FISHNET (Aquaria/Fish Forum)

Access: GO FISHNET

Description: Aquarium hobbyists can find information and others interested in fish on FISHNET. Along withrs ongoing educational effortFISHNET offers a Duty Team which will assist with any aquarium problems you may encounter. Library Sections include: Your First Aquarium; Equipment/Products; Freshwater Aquaria; Disease/Treatment; Marine/Reef; Aquaria Community Library; ACN/CMDB/Conserv.; FISHNET Archives; Koi/Fish Ponds; Aquaculture/Fishery; Graphics Library; Law Library; FPE Volumes & Suppl; and Software/Programs.

Contact: John Benn [76703,4256]—Forum Director
    Deb Tanaka [76702,1467]—Operations Manager

HSUS Forum (Humane Society of the United States)

Access: GO HSUS

Description: Discussions ranging from environmental protection to humane education of children to experimentation on animals. Message Sections include: General Information; Animal Experiments; ShelterNet; Wildlife Rehab; Into the Maelstrom; Animal Ethics; Wildlife Protection; and Action Alert.

Contact: P.E. Preston [76702,2013]—SysOp

EARTH Forum

Access: GO EARTH

Description: The Earth Forum is for individuals and organizations concerned about the earth and its environment. Library sections include: Earth Graphics/GIFs; General Air/Climate; Water; Lands & Forests; Wetlands; Recycle; Wildlife; Energy; Population; Professional Corner; Wastes/Toxics; Eco-philosophy; Animal Rights; and Greenpeace.

Contact: Joe Reynolds [76704,37]—SysOp

NATIONAL AUDUBON Forum

Description: The National Audubon Forum is a Private Forum on Compuserve. It is only accessible by special CompuServe ID obtained from the National Audubon Society. Coverage includes national and international conservation issues, legislative alerts and updates, information about upcoming conferences, newsletter exchange materials, and a variety of other activities.

Contact: Connie Mahan
    </PN=Connie.MAHAN/OU=AUDUBON-DC/O=SMTCN/PRMD=LANG-
    ATE/ADMD=TELEMAIL/C=US/@sprint.com>

OUTDOORS Forum

Access: GO OUTDOORS

Description: The Outdoors Forum is a place to discuss a topics such as fishing, hunting, camping, scouting, cycling, birding, climbing, skiing, boating, environment, photography, shooting sports and other outdoor activities.

OUTNEWS News Clips
Access: GO OUTNEWS

Description: OUTNEWS is comprised of news stories related to topics and issues found in the Outdoors Forum. Stories are clipped from various news sources.

ENVIRO BBS
Environmental Bulletin Board System
Modem: 703-524-1837
Help Line: 703-522-5427
12/24/96/14400 baud, N-8-1

Description: Exchange of information on environmental protection, ecology, wildlife, endangered species, natural resources and other topics generally related thereto.

EPA BBS
Environmental Protection Agency
Modem: 919-541-5742
Help Line: 202-260-6523
12/24/9600 baud, N-8-1
Note: This number is the master gateway to 10 different EPA BBSes, most of which are only available through this number.
Contact: Dave Rejeski <rejeski.dave@epamail.epa.gov>

FDA BBS
Food and Drug Administration Bulletin Board System
Modem: 800-222-0185
Help Line: 301-443-3285
12/24/9600 baud, E-7-1
   At the login prompt, enter: bbs

Description: The FDA's online information service includes information on topics such as, FDA news releases, Drug and Device product approvals list, current information on AIDS, Veterinary Medicine news, import alerts, and many other FDA related subjects.

FEDIX
Federal Information Exchange
Modem: 800-783-3349 or 301-258-0953
Help Line: 301-975-0103
12/24/9600 baud, N-8-1
Note: Previously discussed under TELNET services. At login prompt, logon as FEDIX.

FEDWORLD GATEWAY BBS
National Technical Information Service
   Federal Information Gateway
Modem: 703-321-8020
Help Line: 703-487-4608
12/24/9600 baud, N-8-1
Help Line: 703-487-4608

Description: Access to more than 100 U.S. government computer bulletin boards, many of them previously accessible only by modem. Also includes full text of select U.S. government publications, statistical files, federal job lists, satellite images and more.

Contact: Ken Royer
Phone: 703-487-4850

FLORIDA FISHLINE

Florida Game and Fresh Water Fish Commission

Modem: 904-488-3773

Help Line: 904-488-4066

12/2400 baud, N-8-1

Fidonet address: 1:3605/32

Description: For anyone interested in fishing or in the fresh water fish of Florida. It contains general and scientific message areas, GFC (Game and Fish Commission) literature, news releases, abstracts, and more.

GOVERNMENT PRINTING OFFICE BBS

The Federal Bulletin Board

Modem: 202-512-1387

Help Line: 202-512-1524

12/24/9600 baud, N-8-1

Description: Provides access to Federal information in electronic form. Some fees apply, but access is free.

GREENPEACE ENVIRONET

Greenpeace Bulletin Board System

Modem: 415-512-9108

Description: Press releases and position papers, Rachel's Hazardous Waste News, and several conferences.

HERPNET BBS

Herpetology Online Network

Modem: 215-464-3562 or 215-698-1905

Help Line: 215-464-3561

(TBBS) 12/24/9600 baud, N-8-1

SysOp: Mark F. Miller <iei036g@tjuvm.tju.edu>

Description: National forum for the exchange of information and ideas relating to all aspects of herpetology. Anyone with an interest in the study or conservation of reptiles or amphibians is welcome to participate. The BBS includes message and file areas, as well as the Herp Society Database, and a calendar of conferences, meetings and events.

KNOWLEDGE INDEX

Dialog Information Services

Modem: Access is through Sprintnet, Tymenet, or Datapac local access phone numbers and through CompuServe.

Description: Online Commercial Database; there are over 100 different databases available.

Note: Animal-related databases on Knowledge Index include:

AGRICOLA: Worldwide information on agriculture. 1970 to present. Bibliographic database. AGRI1

AIDSLINE(TM): Provides complete access to the medical literature related to AIDS. 1980 to present. Bibliographic database. MEDI17

CAB ABSTRACTS 1984-present: Detailed summaries of worldwide agricultural and biological research. Bibliographic database. AGRI3

CAB ABSTRACTS 1972-1983: Detail summaries of worldwide agricultural and biological research. Bibliographic database. AGRI4

CANCERLIT(r): Wide coverage of cancer research. 1963 to present. Bibliographic database. MEDI10

CURRENT BIOTECHNOLGY ABSTRACTS: Covers all aspects of biotechnology, including genetic manipulation, monoclonal antibodies, and fermentation technology. 1983 to present. Bibliographic database. BIOL2

DISSERTATION ABSTRACTS ONLINE: Abstracts of all U.S.dissertations since 1861 and citations for some Canadian dissertations. Also includes selected Master theses since 1962. 1861 to present. Bibliographic database. REFR5

DRUG INFORMATION FULLTEXT: Complete text of the American Hospital Formulary Service and the Handbook on Injectable Drugs. Current. Fulltext, directory database. DRUG2

EMBASE: One of the leading sources for searching biomedical literature. June 1974 to present. Bibliographic database. MEDI3

FOOD SCIENCE AND TECHNOLOGY ABSTRACTS: Provides access to research and new development literature in the areas related to food science and technology. 1969 to present. Bibliographic database. FOOD1

INTERNATIONAL PHARMACEUTICAL ABSTRACTS: Research and current health-related drug literature. 1970 to present. Bibliographic database. DRUG1

LIFE SCIENCES COLLECTION: Worldwide coverage of research in biology, medicine, biochemistry, ecology, and microbiology. 1978 to present. Bibliographic database. BIOL1

MEDLINE(r) 1983-present: Biomedical literature and research. Bibliographic database. MEDI1

MEDLINE(r) 1966-present: Biomedical literature and research. Bibliographic database. MEDI2

MERCK INDEX ONLINE(sm): Updated and expanded version of the Merck Index, an internationally recognized encyclopedia of chemicals, drugs, and biologicals. Late 19th century to present. Fulltext database. DRUG4

PsycINFO(r): Leading source of published research in psychology and behavioral sciences. 1967 to present. Bibliographic database. PSYC1

Contact: Dialog Information Services, Inc.
3460 Hillview Avenue
Palo Alto, CA 94303
Phone: 800-334-2564

LABBS

American Association for Laboratory Animal Science (AALAS)
Lab Animal Bulletin Board System

Modem: 901-758-0401/901-758-0402

Help Line: 901-754-8620

12/24/96/144/16800 baud, N-8-1 (PCBoard)

Contact: Ken Boschert, DVM <ken.boschert@aalas.org>
Paul Merz <paul.merz@aalas.org>
Enrique Morales <enrique.morales@aalas.org>
AALAS
70 Timber Creek Drive, Suite 5
Cordova, TN 38018

MARTA BBS

Middle Atlantic Reproduction and Teratology Association

Modem: 215-594-8524

12/24/96/14400, N-8-1 (Wildcat)

Description: The Middle Atlantic Reproduction and Teratology Association (MARTA) is a professional society that was established in 1968 and is dedicated to encouraging proficiency and knowledge in the field of animal reproduction and developmental toxicology. MARTA encourages the frank exchange of ideas and information in areas such as historical control data, testing procedures, laboratory problems, and employment oppurtunities.

Contact: Robert Veneziale
  750 Chessie Court
  West Chester, PA 19380

NATIONAL BIOLOGICAL IMPACT ASSESSMENT PROGRAM BBS

Virginia Polytechnic Institute and State University

Modem: 800-624-2723 or 703-231-3858

12/2400 baud, N-8-1 (PCBoard)

Description: Safe performance evaluation of genetically modified organisms in the environment.

NEWSNET

Modem: Access is through Sprintnet, Tymenet, or Datapac local access phone numbers.

Description: Online Commercial Database; full text of over 600 specialty newsletters and other news sources.

Contact: NewsNet, Inc.
  945 Haverford Road
  Bryn Mawr, PA 19010
  Phone: 800-345-1301

Note: Animal-related newsletters on NewsNet include:

  Applied Genetics News
  Biotech Business
  Biotechnology Investment Opportunities
  Biotechnology Newswatch
  Comline Japan Daily: Biotechnology
  Food Channel
  Food Chemical News
  Food & Drink Daily
  Genetic Technology News
  Hazardous Waste News
  Industrial Bioprocessing
  State Environment Report
  Toxic Materials News

NIH GRANT LINE

National Institutes of Health

Modem: 301-402-2221

12/2400 baud, E-7-1

Note: When you get a response indicating that you have been connected, then type ,GEN1 (the comma is mandatory) and press ENTER; you will be prompted by the NIH system for "INITIALS?". Type BB5 and press ENTER. You will then be prompted for "ACCOUNT?". Type CCS2 and press ENTER.

Description: The purpose of NIH Grant Line is to make program and policy information of the Public Health Service (PHS) agencies rapidly available to the biomedical research community. Most of the research opportunity information available on this bulletin board is derived from the weekly publication, "NIH Guide for Grants and Contracts", consisting of Notices, RFAs, RFPs (announcements of availability), Numbered Program Announcements, and statements of PHS policy. The electronic version known as E-Guide is available for electronic transmission each week, sometimes a day or two in advance of the nominal Friday publication dates. The material consists predominantly of statements about the research interests of the PHS Agencies, Institutes, and National Centers that have funds to support research in the extramural community. The information found on the NIH Grant Line is grouped into three main sections: (1) short News Flashes that appear without any prompting shortly after you have logged on; (2) Bulletins that are for reading; and (3) Files that are intended mainly for downloading.

NOAH (Network of Animal Health)
American Veterinary Medical Association (AVMA Network)

Description: National electronic communications network for AVMA members and affiliated groups. NOAH exists to bring communications services and informational resources to the entire veterinary medical profession and associated organizations and individuals. The mission of NOAH is to improve and enhance cunication among those persons t ocommitted to advancing the science and art of veterinary medicine, and the health of human beings and animals. NOAH is a private information service on CompuServe. NOAH has five primary forums: Clinical and Specialty Medicine, Organizations, Professional Issues, and Industry. Each of the forums has 18 sections covering special interest subjects. NOAH has regular updates from the AVMA's Governmental Relations Division, animal regulatory information (such as current import/export and interstate transport regulations), disease incidence and diagnostic lab reporting (such as Dx Monitor), and sections devoted to computer usage and practice management. Other medical and clinical databases and applications are available through an Internet gateway. Additional forums will be developed as needed to expand and enhance the network. NOAH basic services will also include: an online searchable database of the AVMA membership directory; a cumulative index of JAVMA and AJVR articles; and associated abstracts or interpretive summaries from the journals. Other searchable databases will be added to further enhance the NOAH basic services area.

Contact: Karl Wise <72662.3434@compuserve.com>
Jim Brewer <72662.3435@compuserve.com>
American Veterinary Medical Association
1931 North Meacham Road, Suite 100
Schaumburg, IL 60173-4360
Phone: 708-925-8070
Fax: 708-925-1329

ORBIT
Orbit Search Service

Description: Bibliographic retrieval service for science researchers.
Contact: Orbit Search Service
Division of Maxwell Online, Inc.
8000 Westpark Drive
McLean, VA 22102
Phone: 703-442-0900
Note: Service contains the following animal-related databases:

Biotechnology Abstracts—1982-present
Current Patents Evaluations—1990-present
Current Patents Fast Alert—1989-present
Drug Patents International—current
PESTDOC—1968-present
Pharmaceutical News Index—1974-present
Tropical Agriculture—1975-present
US Classifications—1790-present
US Patents—1970-present
VETDOC—1968-present
World Patents Index—1963-present

OSPREY'S NEST BBS
Birders Bulletin Board System
Modem: 301-989-9036
(ROBBS) 12/24/9600 baud, N-8-1
Description: BBS for birders, naturalists, and conservationists in the Washington, DC Metropolitan area. Associated with the National Birding Hotline Cooperative.
Contact: Norm Saunders <nys@cu.nih.gov>

PENPAGES
Agricultural Information
Modem: 814-863-4820
    At the login prompt, enter: your two-letter state abbreviation
Description: PENpages is a full-text information service containing thousands of research-based fact sheets, news articles, newsletters, and reports. Information is entered by faculty and staff of Penn State University, the Pennsylvania Department of Agriculture, USDA and many cooperators nationwide. Information is agricultural-based and consumer-oriented. Topics include: 4-H and youth development, agricultural education, agronomy; dairy and animal science, engineering, entomology, family life and resource management, food safety, forest resources, gerontology, horticulture, human nutrition, pesticide education, plant pathology, poultry science, rural development, veterinary science, water quality, and many others.
Contact: Diann Leri <dleri@psupen.psu.edu>
    405 Ag Admin.
    College of Agricultural Sciences
    University Park, PA 16802
    Phone: 814-863-3449

RABBIT CONNECTION BBS
House Rabbit Society
Modem: 508-777-0648
Help Line: 508-750-8447
12/2400 baud, N-8-1

RUTGERS COOPERATIVE EXTENSION BBS
Modem: 800-722-0335 or 201-383-8041
12/24/9600 baud, N-8-1 (PCBoard)
Contact: Bruce Barbour
    County Agricultural Agent
    Rutgers Cooperative Extension
    Everex 3000, 150 MB

SOUTH ARIZONA BIRDING BBS
Modem: 602-881-4280
Help Line: 602-323-2955

STIS
National Science Foundation
    Science & Technology Information System
Modem: 202-357-0359 or 202-357-0360
12/24/9600 baud, N-8-1
Help Line: 202-357-7555
    When connected, press enter. At the login prompt, Enter: public.

Description: Provides access to grant information, NSF directories and phone books, press releases, full text of select NSF publications and more.

TAXACOM BULLETIN BOARD SYSTEM
An Electronic Service for Biosystematics
Modem: 716-896-7581
Help Line: 716-896-5200
1200/2400 baud, N-8-1
Description: An electronic journal, data bank and symposium for collections-oriented biosystematists and biogeographers. Unique features are the electronic journal Flora Online and the Latin Translation Service.

THE WELL
The Whole Earth 'Lectronic Link
Internet: telnet to `well.sf.ca.us` or `198.93.4.10`
Modem: 415-332-6106
Help Line: 415-332-4335
Notes: Commercial network sponsored by the Whole Earth Catalog and Whole Earth Review. This network's specialty is online conversations; network live chat and files are also available. There are 14 major conference sections with several sub-conferences contained within each.

>   Animal Related Conferences
>   Agriculture
>   Access: `g agri`
>   Description: Discussions among producers and consumers of food.
>
>   Bioinfo
>   Access: `g bioinfo`
>   Description: Discussions of links between biological and information sciences.
>
>   Wildlife
>   Access: `g wild`
>   Description: Discussions on flora and fauna.

WILDBEES BBS
Bee Bulletin Board System
   California, USA
Modem: 209-826-8107
Contact: Andy Nachbaur

ACKNOWLEDGEMENTS AND REFERENCES

The world is divided into lumpers and splitters. In addition to my own scouring of the Net, the following individuals have made enormous contributions to the collective Internet community in their respective arenas. I gratefully acknowledge their efforts and recommend you obtain the following documents from their respective FTP sites.

1. *Not Just Cows*
   A Guide to Internet/Bitnet Resources in Agriculture and Related Sciences
   Compiled by: Wilfred Drew
   FTP to `ftp.sura.net` or `128.167.254.179` in `/pub/nic/agricultural.list`
2. *Internet/bitnet Health Sciences Resources*
   Compiled by: Lee Hancock <1e07144@ukanvm.cc.ukans.edu>
   FTP to `ftp.sura.net` or `128.167.254.179` in `/pub/nic/medical.resources.2-23`

3. *A Biologist's Guide to Internet Resources*
   Compiled by: Una R. Smith
   FTP to `rtfm.mit.edu` or `18.70.0.226` in `/pub/usenet/news.answers/biology/guide`
4. *Special Internet Connections*
   Compiled by: Scott Yanoff
   FTP to `csd4.csd.uwm.edu` in `/pub/inet.services.txt`
5. *Gopher Jewels*
   Compiled by: David Riggins <`riggins_dw@dir.texas.gov`>
   Gopher to: `cwis.usc.edu`
   `Path=1/Other_Gophers_and_Information_Resources/Gophers_by_Subject/Gopher_Jewels`
   URL: `gopher://cwis.usc.edu/11/Other_Gophers_and_Information_Resources/Gophers_by_Subject/Gopher_Jewels`
6. *Aim Related Internet Resources* Compiled by: David Tong
   <`tong@sones.vahsc.uokhsc.edu`>
7. *Directory of Scholarly Electronic Conferences* (7th REVISION)
   Compiled by: Diane Kovacs <`dkovacs@kentvm.kent.edu`>
   FTP to `ksuvxa.kent.edu` in `/library/acadlist.*`
8. *Internet Sources of Government Information*
   Compiled by: Blake Gumprecht <`gumpbw@vm.temple.edu`>
9. *Whole Earth Online Almanac* by Don Rittner, Brady Publishing, New York, 1993, ISBN: 1-56686-090-3
10. *The Internet Directory* by Eric Braun, Ballantine Books, New York, 1993, ISBN: 0-449-90898-4

Individuals who sent me additional resources include: Doug Kemp, D.B. Cameron, Jon Shiroma, Doug Hart, Joseph Stookey, Rob Scott, Anj Petto, and Ron Smith.

Thanks!

Aquatic Biology Information Resources on the Internet

12

Barry N. Brown
(barry@selway.umt.edu)
Science Librarian & Access Services Coordinator
Mansfield Library
University of Montana

Version 2 (revised quarterly; last revision 14 July 1994)
Initially prepared on 5/17/94 for the North American Benthological Society, Computer Information Committee.
Corrections, additions, suggestions, comments, questions, etc. are welcomed!
Descriptive Keywords: aquatic, freshwater, marine, limnology, benthos, biology, ecology.
Intended audience: aquatic (freshwater & marine) biologists, botanists, and ecologists (and everyone else researching those fields).

TABLE OF CONTENTS

I. Taxonomy of Information Resources Available on the Internet
II. Gopher
III. World Wide Web
IV. WAIS
V. Library Catalogs
VI. Databases and Special Collections
VII. Specimen Collections
VIII. Electronic Journals and Newsletters
IX. Publicly Accessible Files
X. Computer Conferences, Newsgroups, Listservs, and Mailing Lists

I. Taxonomy of Information Resources Available On The Internet
    a. Computer Mediated Communication (e-mail, talk, internet relay chat)
    b. Directory Services: White Pages, etc.
    c. Computer Conferences, Newsgroups, Listservs, and Mailing Lists
    d. Electronic Books & Journals & Newspapers
    e. Library Catalogs and Databases
    f. Commercial Databases (e.g., Dialog, STN, etc.)
    g. Publicly Accessible Files (textual, numeric, image, software)
    h. Specimen Collections
    i. BBSs, Freenets, CWISs
    j. Information Servers: Gopher, WAIS, World Wide Web
    k. Super Computers
    l. Simulation Environments (e.g., MUDs, MOOs, MUSEs, MUSHs, etc.)

II. GOPHERS

Aquanaut—Scuba Diving
URL: **gopher://gopher.opal.com**

Aquanic—Aquaculture Network Information Center
URL: gopher://thorplus.lib.purdue.edu

Australian National University, Bioinformatics
URL: gopher://life.anu.edu.au

Australian Oceanographic Data Centre
URL: gopher://dir.ic.ac.uk

Bedford Institute of Oceanography
URL: gopher://biome.bio.dfo.ca

Biodiversity and Biological Collections at Harvard
URL: gopher://huh.harvard.edu

CIESIN, Global Ecology and the Environment
URL: gopher://gopher.ciesin.org

Deep-Sea and Hydrothermal Vent Info.
URL: gopher://info.uvic.ca/11/academic/biology/deep

EcoGopher at U. VA
URL: gopher://ecosys.drdr.virginia.edu

Ecological Data Exchange at Yale
URL: gopher://gopher.yale.edu

Econet
URL: gopher://gopher.igc.apc.org/11/environment

Entomology Gopher—Australia
URL: gopher://spider.ento.csiro.au

Entomology Gopher—Iowa State Univ.
URL: gopher://gopher.ent.iastate.edu

Entomology Gopher—Univ. of Deleware
URL: gopher://bluehen.ags.udel.edu

Envirogopher
URL: gopher://envirolink.hss.cmu.edu

Environmental Resources Info. Network
URL: gopher://kaos.erin.gov.au

Forestry Gopher—Univ. of Minn.
URL: gopher://minerva.forestry.umn.edu

Great Lakes Info. Network
URL: gopher://gopher.great-lakes.net:2200/11/

Harvard Gray Herbarium Index of New World Plants
URL: gopher://huh.harvard.edu

IUBio Biology Archive, Indiana University
URL: gopher://fly.bio.indiana.edu

Long Term Ecological Research (LTER) Network
URL: gopher://lternet.edu

Marine Biological Lab—Woods Hole
URL: gopher://hoh.mbl.edu

National Oceanographic Data Center—NODC
URL: **gopher://gopher.nodc.noaa.gov**

National Science Foundation Gopher, database of current awards
URL: gopher://stis.nsf.gov/77/.index/wais-sources/nsf-awards

NABS Biblio.& Info.
URL: gopher://gopher.nd.edu:70/00/Notre Dame Academic and Research Data/Aquatic Biology/About NABS Bibliographies Searchable Databases

NEODAT Fish Biodiversity Gopher
URL: gopher://fowler.acnatsci.org

NOAA—Environmental Information
URL: gopher://gopher.esdim.noaa.gov

NOAA—Great Lakes Env. Res. Lab
URL: gopher://gopher.glerl.noaa.gov

NODC—National Oceanographic Data Center
URL: gopher://ariel.nodc.noaa.gov

Scripps Institution of Oceanography
URL: gopher://sio.ucsd.edu

Smithsonian Instutition's—Natural History Gopher
URL: gopher://nmnhgoph.si.edu

UNC Sunsite, Collection of ecology and evolution materials
URL: gopher://sunsite.unc.edu/11/../.pub/academic/biology/ecology%2bevolution

Universities Water Information Network
URL: gopher://gopher.c-wr.siu.edu

Univ. of California, Berkeley, Museum of Paleontology
URL: gopher://ucmp1.berkeley.edu

Univ. of California, InfoSlug
lots of biology,ecology,etc.
URL: gopher://scilibx.ucsc.edu

Univ. of California, Santa Barbara—Marine Biology Library
URL: gopher://gopher.lscf.ucsb.edu/1

USGS—Atlantic Marine Geology
URL: gopher://bramble.er.usgs.gov

Virginia Institute of Marine Science
URL: gopher://gopher.vims.edu

Woods Hole Oceanographic Institution
URL: gopher://bramble.er.usgs.gov/11/etc/woodshole

III. World Wide Web (WWW)

Aquanaut—scuba diving related information
URL: **http://www.opal.com/aquanaut**

Australian Environmental Resources Information Network
URL: **http://kaos.erin.gov.au/erin.html**

Australian National University Biodiversity
URL: http://life.anu.edu.au/biodiversity.html

CSU Stanislaus—Biology Department
URL: http://lead.csustan.edu/home.html

Colorado State University—Entomology
URL: http://www.colostate.edu/Depts/Entomology/ent.html

CYAMUS
regional group of IAMSLIC = Marine Libraries
URL: http://scilibx.ucsc.edu/iamslic/cyamus.html

Earth Observing System Project
URL: http://spso2.gsfc.nasa.gov/spso_homepage.html

Iowa State Univ.—Entomology
URL: http://www.public.iastate.edu/~entomology/

Institute of Oceanographic Sciences, Deacon Laboratory, Wormley
URL: http://wocomms.nwo.ac.uk/pub/www/welcome.html

Lamont-Doherty Earth Observatory, Columbia University
URL: http://www.ldeo.columbia.edu/

NATO SACLANT—Undersea Research Centre
URL: http://www.saclantc.nato.int/

Nauticus—National Maritime Center
URL: http://www.nauticus.org/Nauticus/nauticus.html

NCDC—US National Climatic Data Center
URL: http://www.ncdc.noaa.gov/ncdc.html

NGDC—US National Geophysical Data Center
URL: http://web.ngdc.noaa.gov

NMFS—US National Marine Fisheries Service
URL: http://kingfish.ssp.nmfs.gov/home-page.html

NOAA—US National Oceanic & Atmospheric Administration
URL: http://www.noaa.gov/

NOAA—Environmental Info Services
URL: http://www.esdim.noaa.gov/

NODC—US National Oceanographic Data Center
URL: http://www.nodc.noaa.gov/

Oceanic, Ocean Information Center
URL: http://diu.cms.udel.edu/

The Oceanography Society's Distributed Ocean Data System project
URL: http://lake.mit.edu/jgofs/index

Rosenstiel School of Marine and Atmospheric Sciences
URL: http://www.rsmas.miami.edu/

Scripps Institution of Oceanography
URL: http://sio.ucsd.edu/

Scripps Institution of Oceanography Library
URL: http://orpheus.ucsd.edu/sio/

SeaWIFS Project
URL: `http://seawifs.gsfc.nasa.gov/SEAWIFS.html`

Unidata Program
URL: `http://www.unidata.ucar.edu/`

University of Hawaii, School of Ocean & Earth Science & Technology
URL: `http://www.soest.hawaii.edu/`

US Fish & Wildlife Service—Division of Law Enforcement
URL: `http://ash.lab.r1.fws.gov/`

US Fish & Wildlife Service—Division of Refuges
URL: `http://bluegoose.arw.r9.fws.gov/`

USGS Global Change and Climate History Program
URL: `http://geochange.er.usgs.gov/gch.html`

Woods Hole Oceanographic Institution
URL: `http://www.whoi.edu/`

IV. WAIS

The following "sources" are from a public WAIS server.

- Biology Journal Contents, #239
- Biosci (Usenet Bionet Newsgroups), #240
- Coastal, #271
- DOE Climate Data, #76
- Environment Newsgroups, #350
- Global Change Data Directory, #83
- Invertebrate Paleontology Database, #106
- NOAA Environmental Services, #127
- NOAA National Environmental Referral Service, #128
- The Scientist, #562
- Smithsonian Pictures, #530
- USDA CRIS (Current Research Information Service), #575
- U.S. Fish & Wildlife Service (Region 9), #197
- Water Quality Database, #590

V. LIBRARY CATALOGS

Catalogs of particular interest to aquatic biologists include the EPA Library, the University of California Library System (Melvyl) with over 10 million records, Harvard, Yale, the Library of Congress, University of Michigan, University of Washington, Illinet (the union catalog for Illinois), among others. Generally those institutions with strong programs in a discipline have good library collections in those areas.

Other criteria for selecting a library catalog to search might include: geographical location, size of the collection, and consulting a reference guide (e.g., "Subject Collections").

Most catalogs provide a variety of search options such as browsing an exact title, author or subject heading, or using keywords to search those indexes. Productive words to input for a "subject browse" include: aquatic (e.g., aquatic biology, aquatic botany, aquatic ecology, aquatic invertebrates, etc.), freshwater, marine, stream, lake, limnology, etc.

VI. DATABASES & SPECIAL COLLECTIONs

There are a variety of databases available through telnet or a gopher or email.

- The Archie Carr Sea Turtle Bibliographic Database. It consists of allaspects of sea turtle biology. Log on as LUIS.
  URL: `telnet://luis.nerdc.ufl.edu`

- Aquaculture Information Center at the National Agricultural Library. Reference questions answered via email. Send messages to: `aic@nalusda.gov`
- AquaNIC—Aquaculture Network Information Center.
  URL: `telnet://thorplus.lib.purdue.edu` (login: `cwis`)
- Bibliography of Attractants of Blood-Feeding Arthropods.
  URL: `gopher://minerva.forestry.umn.edu`
- CARL Uncover—over 14,000 journals, with 3 million citations, indexed for the last 5 years, accessed by keyword (W) or by table of contents (B). Document delivery also available.
  URL: `telnet://database.carl.org`
- Center for the Great Lakes Information Service.
  URL: `gopher://gopher.great-lakes.net:2200/11/`
- Crayfish Bibliography. Gopher path: `/Invert. Zool. at the Smith. /Crustaceans /Crayfish`
  URL: `gopher://nmnh.goph.si.edu`
- Entomology Database, University of Colorado. Gopher path: `/Online Library Catalogs..... /Univ. of CO. Ent. Dat.`
  URL: `gopher://gopher.colorado.edu/11/Online%20Library%20Catalogs%2c%20 Electronic%20Books%20and%20Reference%20Databases/University%20of%20 Colorado%20Entomology%20Database`
- Fisheries Technical Reports, British Columbia. Gopher path: `/Environ. & Sci. Info /Biodiv. Info. /Fish, Wildlife and Endang... /BC Environ. Fish. Tech. Reports`
  URL: `gopher://freenet.victoria.bc.ca/11/environment/biodiversity/F.W`
- Galveston Bay Bibliography. (login: `GBAY`)
  URL: `telnet://tamug.tamu.edu`
- Marine and Aquatic Sciences Serials Lists. Gopher path: `/Library /Other Libraries.`
  URL: `gopher://gopher.ucsc.edu/11/The%20Library/Other%20Libraries/Marine%20 and%20Aquatic%20Sciences%20Serials%20Lists`
- Marine Organism Images. (`/Biology Dept./Delta Project`).
  URL: `http://lead.csustan.edu/home.html`
- New England Algae Database (freshwater and marine). Gopher path: `/MBL Databases/Algae.`
  URL: `gopher://hoh.mbl.edu`
- North American Benthological Society (NABS), Information & Bibliography. The bibliography is available for keyword searching, and there are several other text files available. Gopher path: `/Notre Dame Acad. & Res. Data/Aquatic Biology/NABS.`
  URL: `gopher://gopher.nd.edu:70/00/Notre Dame Academic and Research Data/Aquatic Biology/About NABS Bibliographies Searchable Databases`
- NOAA National Environmental Referral Service. Gopher path: `/Researcher /Sci. & Eng. /Biol. & Life Sci. /Worldwide Biol. Gopher Serv. /Env. Sci.`
  URL: `gopher://gopher.ucsc.edu/11/The%20Researcher/Science%20and%20Engineering/ Environmental%20Science/NOAA%20National%20Environmental%20Referral%20 Service`
- Nudibranch Bibliography. Gopher path: `/Researchers/Science/Earth & Marine.`
  URL: `gopher://gopher.ucsc.edu/7waissrc%3a/.WAIS/Nudibranch-bib.src`
- Ocean Network Information Center. (login: `info`)
  URL: `telnet://delocn.udel.edu`
- Periphyton Images. Gopher path: `/Info. Organized by Coll. & Dept/Biology/Algae.`
  URL: `gopher://gopher.bgsu.edu/11/Departments/biol/algae`

- Sea Grant documents. Documents are retrieved via a mail program. To request information—send email to almanac@oes.orst.edu, leave the subject blank and in the body of the message type the desired command:
    - `send ext seagrant abstracts help` List of Sea Grant abstracts topics
    - `send ext seagrant index` List of Sea Grant information
    - `end guide` Information on using the Almanac program
- University of Idaho—Aquaculture Databases. (login: `fish`)
  URL: `telnet://129.101.14.18`
- U.S. National Fungus Collection.(access with `login user and user`)
  URL: `telnet://fungi.ars-grin.gov`
- Water Quality Data Directory. Gopher path: /Researcher /Sci. & Eng. /Biol. & Life Sci./Worldwide Biol. Gopher Serv. /Env. Sci.
  URL: `gopher://scilibx.ucsc.edu`

VII. SPECIMEN COLLECTIONS

Museum and laboratory specimen collections are often little used data repositories that contain a wealth of potential information. Automation of these collections and global access through the Internet can greatly assist researchers. There are currently over 2 million plant and animal specimens online from a variety of institutions.

The following are available via gopher at: `huh.harvard.edu` (URL: `gopher://huh.harvard.edu/`)

- Museum, Herbarium & Arboretum Collection Catalogs.
- California Academy Invertebrate Zoology & Geology Type Catalog
- Cornell Fish Collection
- Farlow Herbarium Diatom Catalog
- Harvard MCZ (Museum of Comparative Zoology) Entomology Type Catalog
- Harvard MCZ (Museum of Comparative Zoology) Fish Type Catalog
- Texas Natural History Collection, Fishes
- University of Colorado Entomology Database

The following is available via gopher at: `fowler.acnatsci.org` (URL: `gopher://fowler.acnatsci.org`)

- Neotropical Database of Fish Biodiversity

VIII. ELECTRONIC JOURNALS AND NEWSLETTERS

There are several hundred e-journals and e-newsletters currently available on the Internet. Some are peer reviewed and some are fee based, but most are neither. They can be accessed by sending a subscription request via email to the editor, or through gophers. A main archive is at the Cicnet gopher (gopher.cic.net).

Aquatic Conservation Notes
A publication of the Aquatic Conservation Network—to receive a copy email Rob Huntley (rob@pinetree.org).

Aquatic Survival
A newsletter of the Aquatic Conservation Network—to receive a copy email Rob Huntley (rob@pinetree.org).

Environmental Resources Information Network (ERIN) Newsletter, Australia.
URL: `ftp://huh.harvard.edu`

URL: `gopher://huh.harvard.edu`

Climate/Ecosystem Dynamics (CED).
URL: `gopher://lternet.edu`

E-mail subscriptions are available from Daniel Pomme `daniel@lternet.washington.edu`

Conservation Ecology
URL: `gopher://journal.biology.carleton.ca`

Directory of Phycologists.
To receive this directory email a request to `MARK@IMB.LAN.NRC.CA`

Env-Link (Student EnviroLink)
URL: `gopher://gopher.cic.net/11/e-serials/alphabetic/e/env-link`

Florida Entomological Society's Electronic Publication Project
URL: `gopher://sally.fcla.ufl.edu/11/fla_entomologist`

LTER Data Management Bulletin (DATABITS).
URL: `gopher://lternet.edu`

The Scientist
URL: `ftp://nnsc.nsf.net`
Made available by The Institute for Scientific Information and the NSF Network Service Center.

STARNET Echinoderm Newsletter.
E-mail subscriptions are available from Win Hide (`whide@matrix.bchs.uh.edu`)

Today's Aquarist
The leading publication for professionals at public aquariums—to receive a copy of this publication email Don S. Johnson (`71631.42@Compuserve.com`).

IX. PUBLICLY ACCESSIBLE FILES (TEXT, DATA, SOFTWARE, IMAGES, SOUND)
To identify a general source for biological files consult *A Biologist's Guide to Internet Resources*.

Bibliographic research guides—includes: freshwater ecology and dolphins.
URL: `ftp://ftp.loc.gov/pub/reference.guides`

Environment of the seas.
URL: `ftp://ariel.unm.edu/pub/MAC/HYPERCARD/Museum`

Programs and data by and for marine scientists.
URL: `ftp://biome.bio.dfo.ca`

Tide Program (calculates tides for all of the coastal U.S.)
URL: `ftp://biome.bio.ns.ca` (`/dfo/habitat/dan`)

X. COMPUTER CONFERENCES, NEWSGROUPS, LISTSERVS, MAILING LISTS

Internet Listservs

`aqua-l@vm.uoguelph.ca`	aquaculture & aquariums
`aquifer@ibacsata.bitnet`	pollution and groundwater recharge
`biocontrol-l@ftpt.br`	entomological biological control
`biodiv-l@bdt.ftpt.ansp.br`	biodiversity networks
`biosph-l@ubvm.cc.buffalo.edu`	biosphere, ecology, discussion list
`bmdp-l@vm1.mcgill.ca`	bmdp software users
`brine-l@uga.cc.uga.edu`	brine shrimp discussion list
`bugnet@wsuvm1.csc.wsu`	entomology for teachers and bug enthusiasts
`coastnet@uriacc.uri.edu`	coastal managment and resources
`consbio@uwavm.u.washington.edu`	conservation biology list
`conslink@sivm.si.edu`	discussion on biological conservation
`crust-l@sivm.si.edu`	crustacean biology
`cturtle@nervm.nerdc.ufl.edu`	sea turtle biology and conservation list
`cyan-tox@grearn.csi.forth.gr`	toxic cyanobacteria
`deepsea@uvvm.uvic.ca`	deep sea and vent news
`diatom-l@iubvm.ucs.indiana.edu`	research on the diatom algae `ecolog-l@umdd.umd.edu` ecological society of america
`ecosys-l@vm.gmd.de`	list for ecosystem theory and modeling
`ecs-news@mailbase.ac.uk`	european cetacean society news

AQUATIC BIOLOGY

`edstat-l@jse.stat.ncsu.edu`	journal of statistics education list
`entomo-l@vm.uoguelph.ca`	entomology discussion list
`envst-l@brownvm.brown.edu`	environmental studies discussion list
`ethology@finhutc.hut.fi`	ethology
`fishfolk@mitvma.mit.edu`	socioeconomics & anthro. of fisheries
`fish-junior@searn.sunet.se`	marine science and children/youth
`hypbar-l@technion.technion.ac.il`	hyperbaric & diving medicine list `iamslic@-ucsd.edu` marine science library info.service.
`iapwild@vm1.nodak.edu`	international arctic project wildlife
`marman@uvvm.uvic.ca`	mammal research and cons.
`marine-l@vm.uoguelph.ca`	marine studies/shipboard education
`meh2o-l@taunivm.tau.ac.il`	middle east water (including limnology)
`micronet@vm.uoguelph.ca`	fungus and root interaction
`molluska@uvvm.uvic.ca`	molluscan taxonomy
`oceantech@ucsd.edu`	applied tech.—freshwater, marine
`odp-l@tamvm1.tamu.edu`	ocean drilling program open discussion
`ots-l@yalevm.cis.yale.edu`	organization for tropical studies
`polpal-l@vm.uoguelph.ca`	pollination and palynology list
`pstat-l@irlearn.ucd.ie`	discussion of stats and programming
`sas-l@uga.cc.uga.edu`	sas discussion (peered)
`saspac-l@umslvma.umsl.edu`	sas public access consortium
`scuba@cc.itu.edu.tr`	scuba and skin diving
`spssx-l@uga.cc.uga.edu`	spssx discussion (peered)
`stat-l@vm1.mcgill.ca`	statistical consulting
`thphysio@frmop11.cnusc.fr`	thermal physiology
`water@gibbs.oit.unc.edu`	water science network
`water-l@wsuvm1.csc.wsu.edu`	water quality

Internet Conferences
with special subscription instructions

`ent-list@um.cc.umich.edu`	entomology (contact Mark O'Brien: mfobrien@umich.edu)
`env.seashepherd (reposted)`	Sea Sheperd Conservation Society (send a subscription request containing your full name, real address and e-mail address to Nick Voth: `dcasmedic@aol.com`)
`fish-ecology@biome.bio.ns.ca`	fish and fisheries ecology (send email to: `majordomo@biome.bio.ns.ca` with the message "subscribe fish-ecology")
`fisheries@biome.bio.ns.ca`	fisheries management (send email to: `majordomo@biome.bio.ns.ca` with the message subscribe fisheries)
`killie@mejac.palo-alto.ca.us`	killifish, Cyprinodontidae (send email to: `killie-request@mejac.palo-alto.ca.us`)
`mar-facil@ac.dal.ca`	marine facilities & aquaria, etc. (send email to: `mailserv@ac.dal.ca` with the message subscribe mar-facil)
`nia-net@archive.orst.edu`	neotropical fish (send email to: `nia-net-request@archive.orst.edu` with the message sub nia-net)
`wildnet@access.usask.ca`	fish and wildlife biology (send email to: `wildnet-request@access.usask.ca`)

Sea Grant "Mailing List" Conferences:
To generate a list of discussion groups and procedures for how to subscribe send email to: `almanac@oes.orst.edu` with the message send mail-catalog. To subscribe to any of the following groups send email to `almanac@oes.orst.edu` with the message subscribe mailing-list (where mailing list is the name of the desired list). To send mail to all members of a particular group, address your message to the appropriate address listed below.

`oesg-mg@oes.orst.edu`	Oregon Sea Grant staff, leader, director
`aesg-mg@oes.orst.edu`	Oregon Sea Grant agents and prog. leader
`masldr-mg@oes.orst.edu`	All Sea Grant MAS leaders
`sg-comm-mg@oes.orst.edu`	All Sea Grant Communicators
`opac-mg@oes.orst.edu`	Oregon's Ocean Policy Advisory Council
`crt-mg@oes.orst.edu`	Sea Grant Coastal Rec. and Tourism staff
`global-mg@oes.orst.edu`	Oregon Global Issues Mailing Group
`sgglobal-mg@oes.orst.edu`	Sea Grant National Global Initiative
`aexcomm-mg@oes.orst.edu`	MAS Assembly Executive Committee

Usenet Newsgroups

`bionet.biology.computational`	comp. and math applications in biology
`bionet.biology.tropical`	tropical biology and ecology
`bionet.jobs`	job opportunities in biology
`bionet.journals.contents`	biological journals table of contents
`bionet.metabolic.-reg`	metabolic reg. and thermodynamics
`bionet.photosynthesis`	photosynthesis research
`bionet.population-bio`	population biology
`bionet.sci-resources`	information about funding agencies
`bionet.software`	software for biology
`bit.listserv.biosph-l`	biosphere, ecology, discussion list
`bit.listserv.ethology`	ethology
`sci.bio.ecology`	ecological research (ESA)

Some Chemistry Resources on the Internet

13

Gary Wiggins
Indiana University Chemistry Library

Originally compiled: October 20, 1993
Latest revision: #7b, June 11, 1994
Added or revised entries are preceded by:
Gopher port numbers are assumed to be port 70 unless specified.
For WWW resources, the URL for the home page is listed.

Agricola records
All of the records in the U.S. National Agricultural database Agricola are available via WWW.
The generic URL is: `http://probe.nalusda.gov:8300/cgi-bin/getagr.sh?number` where **number** is the accession number, e.g., `ind20356956`.

AMBER mail reflector
To subscribe, send a request to:
       `amber-request@cgl.ucsf.edu` or
       `amber-request@ucsfcgl.bitnet`.
Messages are sent to `amber@cgl.ucsf.edu` or `amber@ucsfcgl.bitnet`.

American Chemical Society Gopher
The ACS Gopher contains Supplementary Material pages from the Journal of the American Chemical Society, beginning 1993 (Page images as TIFF with Group 4 fax compression and as GIF files), Copyright Transfer Form (same format), and Instructions for Authors for ACS journals (ASCII file). Among other resources, there are the ACS Books Catalog, ACS information numbers, and links to other chemistry gophers.
URL: `gopher://acsinfo.acs.org` or `134.243.230.66`

American Chemical Society Division of Computers in Chemistry (COMP) Newsletter
URL: `ftp://kekule.osc.edu/pub/chemistry/comp_news directory`

American Chemical Society Publications
Direct access to ACS publication information.
URL: `gopher://infx.infor.com:4500`

American Institute of Physics (AIP) Gopher
URL: `gopher://pinet.aip.org`

Analytical Chemistry Center, University of Texas, Houston Health Sciences Center
URL: `gopher://oac.hsc.uth.tmc.edu/11/hsc_info/Support%20Services/anal_chem`

ANCHODD, Medicinal Chemistry/Pharmacy List
Send the message: `SUBSCRIBE ANCHODD FIRSTNAME LASTNAME` to:
`listserv@cc.utas.edu.au`

ASCHIN-LIST, Asia Pacific Chemical Information List.

Send the message `subscribe aschin-list firstname lastname` to:
`listserver@nuscc.nus.sg`

Australian Chemistry Network Server
Located on the WWW Server at the Chemistry Department, University College (UNSW) at the Australian Defence Force Academy in Canberra.
URL: `http://apamac.ch.adfa.oz.au/ChemDept/Chem.html`

Biochemistry Journals: Tables of Contents
Coverage of some titles is not up to date, but Journal of Biological Chemistry and others may be.
URL: `gopher://gopher.genethon.fr/11/Biblio/Journaux/Biological%20Chemistry`

BioNet Electronic Newsgroup Network
This network was developed to allow easy worldwide communications between biological scientists who use a variety of computer networks. Newsgroup topics can be distributed to sites on Internet, USENET, BITNET, EARN, NETNORTH, HEANET, and JANET. Unix computers access the newsgroups via software like rn (read news) or nn (nonews).

BioQUEST.
BioQUEST is a set of simulations and related material for biology instruction (genetics, biometrics, molecular biology, etc.). It's a cooperative effort of several academic institutions. Write to `asdg@umdd.umd.edu` for information. An introduction to the project can be obtained from:
URL: `ftp://cs.beloit.edu/MathDeptQuadra/Public/BioQuest`

Biosciences File Server
Send the message HELP to: `bioserve@umdc.umd.edu` or `bioserve@umdc`

BIOSYM Users Group
Send a request to join to: `dibug-request@comp.bioz.unibas.ch`

BOING, Bio Oriented INternet Gophers
Search Databases at Hopkins (Vectors, etc....) > Search BOING (Bio Oriented INternet Gophers) <?>
URL: `gopher://merlot.welch.jhu.edu:3005/7`

Brown University Chemical Physics Preprint Database
URL: `http://www.chem.brown.edu/chem-ph.html`
BRS's Internet address: `brs.com`

Bucky News Service (Buckminster Fullerene mailer)
Bucky is a weekly list of the latest titles on C-60 and related fullerenes, fullerites, and molecular/solid state derivatives. Each week the latest 50 titles is electronically mailed to subscribers.

Send the message: INTRO or HELP to: `bucky@sol1.lrsm.upenn.edu`. To get the bibliography, send the keyword BIBLIO to the same address. The service is maintained by Jack Fischer's group at the University of Pennsylvania.

Buckyball database
This fullerene database is accessible from the site listed below. The site has a program called PCBIB that allows searches of the database by keywords. The resource is based on materials from Professor Richard E. Smalley's Bucky-Ball Bibliography. It can also be searched by telnetting to: `sabio1.arizona.edu` Choose `Other databases` from the menu, then `BuckyBall Database`.
URL: **ftp://physics.arizona.edu/afc/ibmpc**

Buckyballs
See also: fullerene

Cambridge Structural Database
See: University of Cambridge Crystallographic Data Centre

CancerNet, National Cancer Institute's Mail Server
CancerNet is available on the NIH gopher server. Select #3 `Health and Clinical Information` and #1 `CancerNet information`.
Send the message: `HELP` to: **cancernet@icicb.nci.nih.gov**
URL: **gopher://gopher.nih.gov**

CARL
See: UnCover

CCL, Computational Chemistry List
Send the message: `send help from chemistry` to: **OSCPOST@ohstpy** or **OSCPOST@oscsunb.osc.edu**

Ceramics
See: Material Database

CHARMM Users Group
Send a request to join to: **charmm-bbs-sysop@emperor.harvard.edu**

CHEM-COMP, Computational Chemistry
Send the message: `join chem-comp firstname lastname` to: **mailbase@mailbase.ac.uk**

CHEMCONF, the Online Computer Conference.
The first online computer conference took place June 14-August 20, 1993 on the topic "Applications of Technology in Teaching Chemistry." The proceedings can be accessed by sending the e-mail message: `GET CHEMCONF WELCOME` to: **listserv@umdd** OR **listserv@umdd.umd.edu**

CHEMCORD, the General Chemistry Coordinators' Discussion Group
Send the message: `subscribe chemcord firstname lastname` to: **listserv@umdd** or **listserv@umdd.umd.edu**

CHEME-L, the Chemical Engineering List
Send the message: `subscribe cheme-l firstname lastname` to: **listserv@psuvm** or **listserv@psuvm.psu.edu**

CHEMED-L, Chemistry Education Discussion List
Send the message: `subscribe chemed-l firstname lastname` to: **listserv@uwf.bitnet**

Chemical Communications
See: Imperial College, London

Chemical Engineering Digest; ChE Electronic Newsletter
URL: `ftp://cc.curtin.edu.au`

Login: anonymous and Password: chemeng
To subscribe, send a request to Dr. Martyn S. Ray: **TRAYM@CC.CURTIN.EDU.AU**

Chemical Resources
See: Chemistry Information

Chemistry and Materials (NASA SCAN)
URL: `gopher://netsrv.casi.sti.nasa.gov/11/scan/current/23`
References taken from the NASA database.

Chemistry at NISS (National Information Services & Systems, U.K.)
URL: `gopher://gopher.niss.ac.uk:71/11/N/3`

Chemistry Gopher at Yale
The Chemistry Gopher at Yale is an excellent example of a resource that leads through Gopherspace for topics such as chemical software, funding information, directories of scientists, etc.
URL: `gopher://yaleinfo.yale.edu:7000/11/Chemistry`

Chemistry Gopher server in Finland
URL: `gopher://gopher.csc.fi/11/tiede/kemia`

Chemistry Information. San Diego State University
"Chemistry Information" is an electronic reference source covering such topics as nomenclature, compound identification, properties, structure determination, toxicity, synthesis, registry numbers, and synthesis. It also provides definition of terms, meanings of acronyms, etc.
URL: `ftp://ucssun1.sdsu.edu/pub/chemras` (use binary and the mget *.* command to transfer all files to an IBM DOS-compatible PC).

Chemistry Information on the Internet (Northern Illinois University)
Steven Bachrach's list of WWW and gopher sites.
URL: `http://hackberry.chem.niu.edu:70/0/cheminf.html`

Chemistry Resources on the Internet
URL: `gopher://gopher.micro.umn.edu`

Remote Gopher Resources via University of Minnesota/Internet file Center/InterNIC Information Services (General Atomics)/Internet Information for Everybody/Things to Do on the Internet/Chemistry. This Gopher path leads you to an extensive listing of chemistry-related newsgroups, software archives, and information about resources on the Internet that may be of interest to chemists. See also: InterNIC Chemistry Directory in this listing for direct access.

Chemistry Textbooks in Print Archive
The archive covers chemistry textbooks from freshman level through graduate school. High school texts may be added later. Bibliographic information, price, and references to reviews are included, as are the addresses and telephone numbers of publishers.
URL: `gopher://slvaxa.umsl.edu/11gopher_root_chem%3a%5bbooks%5d`

CHEM-MOD, Modeling Aspects of Computational Chemistry
Send the message: join chem-mod firstname lastname to: **mailbase@mailbase.ac.uk**.

ChemViz (Chemical Visualization Project)
ChemViz is an NSF funded grant project to use high-powered computing and communications to help high school students better visualize abstract concepts of chemistry. Images and animations of calculated atomic and molecular orbitals can be made on Macintoshes. Contact Todd Veltman (tveltman@ncsa.uiuc.edu) for details.
URL: `ftp://zaphod.ncsa.uiuc.edu/Education/ChemViz`

CHMINF-L, the Chemical Information Sources Discussion List
CHMINF-L covers all information sources that can be used to answer questions a chemist might have. Send the message: subscribe chminf-l firstname lastname to: `listserv@iubvm` or `listserv@iubvm.ucs.indiana.edu`. A gopher archive of chminf-l is available from the chemistry gopher at the University of California, Davis
URL: `gopher://gopher-chem.ucdavis.edu/11/Email_Archive/ChmInf-L`

Clay
See: Material Database

Clearinghouse for Chemical Information Instructional Materials (CCIIM)
The CCIIM is jointly sponsored by the Special Libraries Association Chemistry Division and the American Chemical Society Division of Chemical Information. It includes items that have been developed by chemistry or science librarians, chemists, and others for instruction in the use of chemical information sources. Paper copies of most materials in the CCIIM are available for the cost of reproduction, but many of the titles are also available as ASCII or other files in the FTP archives of the Indiana University Center for Innovative Computer Applications. The complete list of holdings is found in the file: `cciimlst.xxx`, where xxx represents the date of the latest version. The ASCII files are also accessible on the Indiana University Chemistry Library Gopher.
URL: `gopher://gopher.cica.indiana.edu:72/11/chem`
URL: `gopher://lib-gopher.lib.indiana.edu:7050/1`

CMTS-L, the Chemical Management and Tracking Systems List
CMTS-L serves as a forum for the exchange of ideas on the establishment of computerized systems to manage chemical inventories. Send the message:
```
subscribe CMTS-L firstname lastname to: listserv@cornell.edu
```

Computational Chemistry Newsletter
URL: `_gopher://gopher.tc.cornell.edu:70/11/Forefronts/Computational.Chemistry.News`

Computer Center of the Institute for Molecular Science
Okazaki National Research Institute, Japan.
URL: `http://ccinfo.ims.ac.jpccims.html`

CORROS-L, The Corrosion Special Interest List
Send the message: subscribe corros-l firstname lastname to: `listserv@ib.rl.ac.uk`

Crystallography
URL: `gopher://concise.level-7.co.uk/Special Interest Groups/Crystallography`

Crystallography in Europe
URL: `http://www.unige.ch/crystal/crystal_index.html`
These WWW pages are maintained on the server at the University of Geneva.

CZE-ITP, Discussion on Problems of Capillary Electrophoretic Methods
The list covers Capillary zone electrophoresis (CZE) and Isotachophoresis (ITP).
Send the message: subscribe cze-itp firstname lastname to:
LISTSERV@CSBRMU11.BITNET or **LISTSERV@VM.ICS.MUNI.CZ**

Derwent International Patents Copy Service
e-mail address: **patents@derwent.co.uk**

DIALOG's Internet address: **DIALOG.COM** or **192.132.3.254**

DIALOG Online Chemistry Search Manual
URL: **ftp://oavax.csuchico.edu/chemistry**

DIMDI's Internet address: **129.143.3.20**

DISCUS's Internet address: **DISCUS.dante.net**

Engineering International Internet Services (EiNet)
This is the producer of Engineering Index and the COMPENDEX database.
URL: **telnet://MACK.EINET.COM**
   login: guest

European Synchrotron Radiation Facility
URL: **gopher://fox.esrf.fr:3600/h/GET/**

FORENS-L, Forensic Sciences Discussion Group
Send the message: subscribe firstname lastname to: **FORENS-REQUEST@FAUVAX** or **FORENS-REQUEST@ACC.FAU.EDU**

Fullerene Contents Alert (Elsevier)
Once a month subscribers receive an ASCII file with information on fullerene papers from various Elsevier journals. Address: **c-alert.fullerene@elsevier.nl** Contact: Dr. Egbert van Wezenbeek (**e.wezenbeek@elsevier.nl**) for details.

Fullerenes
See also: Buckyball

Genetic Algorithms Users Group
Send a request to: **ga-molecule-request@tammy.harvard.edu**

Genome Data Base
Send a message to: **help@gdb.org** A password and loginid will be issued.
URL: **ftp://ftp.gdb.org**
URL: **gopher://gopher.gdb.org**
URL: **WAIS://wais.gdb.org**

hep-th@xxx.lanl.gov
Bulletin Board for String/Conformal/Field Theory Preprints.
This includes a preprint file on Condensed Matter Theory.
Send the message: HELP on the subject line to: **hep-th@xxx.lanl.gov**

HIRIS-L, High Resolution IR Spectroscopy List
Send the message SUB HIRIS-L firstname lastname to: **listserv@iveuncc**

HyperChem Users' E-Mail Group
Send a request to: **hyperchem-request@autodesk.com**

ICS-L, International Chemometrics Society
Send the message: subscribe ICS-L firstname lastname to: **listserv@umdd** or **listserv@umdd.umd.edu**

IFPHEN-L, the Interfacial Phenomena Discussion Group
Send the message: subscribe ifphen-l firstname lastname to: **listserv@wsuvm1** or **listserv@wsuvm1.csc.wsu.edu**

Imperial College, London Gopher Server
Posted here are Quicktime movies, playable on either Macintosh or Microsoft Windows using appropriate software, e.g., TurboGopher for the Macintosh.
URL: **gopher://argon.ch.ic.ac.uk**

Quicktime movies are also archived on the Gopher+ server:
gopher://argon-fddi.ch.ic.ac.uk

Files which reside in the directory `Royal_Society_of_Chemistry/Chemical_Communications/3-02351F` are from the Journal of the Chemical Society: Chemical Communications.

Indiana University Chemistry Library Gopher
Text files of various handouts and user guides to reference tools (e.g., Beilstein) as well as the text files of the Clearinghouse for Chemical Information Instructional Materials are found on this gopher.
URL: **gopher://lib-gopher.lib.indiana.edu:7050/1**

Information Retrieval in Chemistry
URL: **ftp://leon.nrcps.ariadne-t.gr/pub/chemistry**

URL: **ftp://ftp-chem.ucdavis.edu/go_chem/Index/ChemSites_ac/leon.nrcps.ariadne-t.gr**

URL: **gopher://gopher-chem.ucdavis.edu/Index/ChemSites_ac/leon.nrcps.ariadne-t-gr**

URL: **www-chem.ucdavis.edu/Information Retrieval in Chemistry** (mirror)

Institut fuer Physikalische und Theoretische Chemie, Regensburg
Besides links to chemistry-related gophers, it contains compilations of some mailing lists which are of interest to theoretical chemists.
URL: **gopher://rchs1.chemie.uni-regensburg.de**

Interface-L
To encourage and facilitate the spread of information about the connection and control af any laboratory equipment by computer. To subscribe, send the message: subscribe interface-l to: **maiser@fs4.in.umist.ac.uk**

Internet Patent News Service
You may sign up for a weekly mailing list of US patents in the Mechanical, Chemical, and Electrical categories. Requests to subscribe should include the desired file format (ASCII or UUZIP) and be sent to:
patents-request@world.std.com

For further information, contact Gregory Aharonian at: **patents@world.std.com** with the message: help or call 617-489-3727.

Internet Resources for Mathematics and Science Education
Version 1.2, October 19, 1993, Compiled by T. C. O'Haver.
This is a very good comilation of resources in all areas of math and science education.
URL: **file://inform.umd.edu/inforM/Computing_Resources/NetInfo/ReadingRoom/InternetResources/math-science-edu**

InterNIC (Internet Network Information Center) Chemistry Directory
There are listings of FTP sites, mailing lists, newsgroups, online databases, etc.
URL: `gopher://is.internic.net/11/infoguide/resources/chemistry`

IUBIO Archive for Molecular Biology
This is Don Gilbert's archive at Indiana University.
URL: `ftp://fly.bio.indiana.edu/molbio/ibmpc`
URL: `ftp://fly.bio.indiana.edu/molbio/mac`

JCPExpress
This is a free trial service for electronic distribution of preprints of manuscripts between acceptance and publication in the Journal of Chemical Physics. Format is PostScript and the original TeX, WordPerfect, or Microsoft Word format if available.

To access by e-mail, send a message to: `express@jcp.uchicago.edu`

Put in the Subject line: `help` and an instruction file will be returned.

For instructions on obtaining FTP copies, put the word: `ftpinfo` on the Subject line of your message.

Journal of Chemical Education Gopher
The site lists such things as the JCE: Software offerings.
URL: `gopher://jchemed.chem.wisc.edu`

Journal of Chemical Physics
See: JCPExpress

Journal of the American Chemical Society (JACS) Supplementary Material
See: American Chemical Society Gopher

Laboratory Safety
URL: `gopher://gizmo.ehs.cornell.edu/1Gizmo%3aCornell%20OEH%20Gopher%3a Laboratory%20Safety%3aInternet%20Chem.%20Resoures%3a`

LiMB; Listing of Molecular Biology Databases. 3.0 ed.
LiMB lists over 100 databases in molecular biology. Copies of LiMB in hardcopy or floppy disk are available from: Christian Burks, LiMB, Theoretical Biology and Biophysics Group, T-10, K710, Los Alamos National Laboratory, Los Alamos, NM 87545 (505-667-7510)

Internet: `limb@life.lanl.gov`. To obtain the LiMB file, send the message: `limb-data` to: `bioserve@t10.Lanl.GOV`

List of Molecular Science Applications for Digital Platforms.
URL: `file://gatekeeper.dec.com/pub/DEC/DECNEWS/news0409.txt`

Listservs in Chemistry and Chemical Engineering
Compiled by Amey Park (`apark@kentvm` or `apark@kentvm.kent.edu`). Includes a few listservs not listed in this compilation plus information about the listowner, archives, etc.
URL: `gopher://ucsbuxa.ucsb.edu:3001/00/.Sciences/.Chemistry/.chem-lists`

Macintosh Chemistry Tutorials
URL: `ftp://archive.umich.edu/mac/misc/chemistry`

Macintosh Science Software
URL: `ftp://ra.nrl.navy.mil/MacSciTech/chem`

Material Database, San Diego State University
This is a factual database on clays, ceramics, feldspar, etc. It has such data as MW, Molecular Analysis, and Percentage Analysis.

URL: `gopher://Gopher.SDSU.Edu/11/SDSU%20Campus%20Topics/Departmental%20Information/Art%20Department/The%20Ceramics%20Gopher/Material%20Database`

Corrections or additions should be sent to: rburkett@ucssun1.sdsu.edu

Material Safety Data Sheets
See: MSDS

Medlars Internet address: `medlars.nlm.nih.gov`

MMODINFO, MacroModel Users Group
Send the message SUBSCRIBE MMODINFO to: mmodinfo-request@uoft02.utoledo.edu Archives of the MMODINFO list are available at the following site (NB: This is a VAX VMS machine.):

URL: `ftp://ftp.utoledo.edu`
    [.MMOD] for mail;
    [.CHEMISTRY] for others.

MOPAC 93 Network Forum
MOPAC 93 is distributed through QCPE. Fujitsu has set up a MOPAC 93 Network Forum to provide a communications link with those who have access to Internet. This service is not free. It is scheduled to begin February 1, 1994. Contact Ms. Miyoko Murakami (`kumikoi@fsba.com`).

MOSSBA, Mossbauer Spectroscopy, Software & Forum
Send the message: subscribe mossba firstname lastname to: `listserv@usachvm1`

MSDS (Material Safety Data Sheets) at the University of Utah
URL: `gopher://atlas.chem.utah.edu:70/11/MSDS`

National
See: U.S. National ...

Northern Illinois University Chemical Gopher
This is an experimental site that includes among other things American Chemical Society Meeting times and sites, Journal submission guidelines, and a "Quantum Chemistry Acronyms" database.

URL: `gopher://hackberry.chem.niu.edu`

Nucleic Acid Database (NDB) Archive
URL: `gopher://ndb.rutgers.edu`

ORBIT's Internet address: `orbit.com`

ORGCHEM, Organic Chemistry Discussion Group BBS
For the latest information on this list, contact Curt Breneman: breneman@xray.chem.rpi.edu

The BBS address is: orgchem@extreme.chem.rpi.edu

All of orgchem's mail messages are archived and can be retrieved from the following site:

URL: `ftp://extreme.chem.rpi.edu/pub/orgchem`

ORG-GEOCHEM
Send the message: `join org-geochem firstname lastname` to: **mailbase@mailbase.ac.uk**

PACS, Physics and Astronomy Classification System
PACS is the thesaurus used in Physics Abstracts.
URL: **file://aps.org/pub/pacs/pacs_94.asc**
The alphabetical index is also there as `index_94.asc`

Patents
See: Derwent Internet Patent News Service U.S. Patents

Periodic Table at the University of California, Berkeley
Contains in addition to the Periodic Table, movies of some of the interesting vibrational modes of benzene, movies of some interesting chemical reactions, and software goodies. This is a true periodic table with data supplied by Mark Winter at the Department of Chemistry, University of Sheffield.
URL: **http://www.cchem.berkeley.edu**

Periodic Table at the University of California, Santa Barbara
An alphabetic listing of the elements with physical properties taken from the CRC Handbook of Chemistry and Physics and Lange's Handbook of Chemistry.
URL: **gopher://ucsbuxa.ucsb.edu:3001/11/.Sciences/.Chemistry/.periodic.table**

Periodic Table
See also: WebElements

POLYMERP, the Polymer Physics Discussion List
Send the message: `subscribe polymerp firstname lastname` to: **listserv@rutvm1.rutgers.edu** or **listserv@rutvm1.bitnet**

POSTDOC INTERNATIONAL
To get information on available postdoc positions or to advertise positions, send the message: GET INDEX to: **POST@DOCSERV.SACLAY.CEA.FR**

Process-L
To discuss the problems associated with the sampling and subsequent analysis of any chemical process, with special reference to industrial scale processing. To subscribe, send the message: `subscribe process-l` to: **maiser@fs4.in.umist.ac.uk**

QCPE Catalog (Quantum Chemistry Program Exchange)
URL: **ftp://qcpe6.chem.indiana.edu**
   login: `anonymous`
   password: `guest`

If you then enter: ls you will find a directory of files with names like 1,2,3, etc. corresponding to the sections into which the QCPE Catalog is divided. To find out the contents of each file, refer to the file CAT_MENU. There is also a file SEARCH.EXE which can be downloaded as a binary file to a PC and used to search the contents of the sections. Also at this site is the QCPE fee schedule and a general information file. QCPE's Internet address is: qcpe@ucs.indiana.edu

Quantum Chemistry Acronyms database
See: Northern Illinois Chemical Gopher

RADCH-L, Radiochemistry Discussion List
Send the message: `sub RADCH-L firstname lastname` to: `LISTSERV@FRCPN11.BITNET`
The discussions are devoted to research in radiochemistry, nuclear chemistry, and nuclear analytical sciences.

REACTIVE
This list is for discussion and exchange of information about air sampling and monitoring of short-lived reactive pollutants.
Send the message: `subscribe reactive firstname lastname` to: `LISTSERV@MCGILL1.BITNET`

Retrieve server (genetics databases)
Send the message `HELP` to: `retrieve@ncbi.nlm.nih.gov`

Rutgers University Department of Chemistry Gopher Server
Found here are entries such as "Chemistry Software and Information Archives" and the "Nucleic Acid Database Archive," as well as links to other chemistry software archives and data.
URL: `gopher://ndb.rutgers.edu`

SAFETY, The Laboratory Safety List
Send the message: `subscribe safety firstname lastname` to: `listserv@uvmvm` OR `listserv@uvmvm.uvm.edu`

Safety Information Resources on the InterNet (SIRI) Gopher
URL: `gopher://SIRI.UVM.EDU`

SCODAE, a communications network for pharmacy schools
Send the message: `subscribe scodae firstname lastname` to: `listserv@umab`

SHARE-L, Spectroscopic Happenings on Actinides and Rare Earths List
Send the message: `subscribe share-l firstname lastname` to: `listserv@frors12`

Silicon Graphics, Inc.
URL: `http://www.sgi.com`

STN Database Summary Sheets
Either ASCII or PostScript versions of more than 160 STN Database Summary Sheets are available.
URL: `ftp://infor.cas.org`

STN International's Columbus Internet address: `stnc.cas.org` or `134.243.5.32`.

STN Karlsruhe's Internet address: `stn.fiz-karlsruhe.de` or `141.66.16.150`.

SVJPS, Springer Journals Preview Service, and SVSERV
Tables of contents, titles (article heads), and summaries (abstracts) of papers from 90 Springer journals are available 3 to 6 weeks before the appearance of the printed version. There is an annual fee for the abstract information, but the other data can be had at no cost. Send the message: `help` to:

   `svjps@vax.ntp.springer.de`

or point your gopher at: `trick.ntp.springer.de` (192.129.24.12).
Available via WWW, the server also has demonstrations of Springer's software and CD-ROM products, TeX macro packages, and indexes of various book series.

Sybyl Users Group
Send a request to join to: `sybylreq@quant.chem.rpi.edu`

Training Program at the Chemistry-Biology Interface (TCBI)
URL: `gopher://cwis.usc.edu/11/University_Information/Academic_Departments/Natural_Sciences/Chemistry/TCBI%20Chemistry%20Biology`

UnCover's Internet address: `database.carl.org` or `192.54.81.76`.
UnCover has tables of contents of many journals of interest to chemists. In addition, copies of articles can be ordered from the source. To exit from the system, enter: `//exit`

University of Alabama Crystallographic Gopher
URL: `gopher://xtal.cmc.uab.edu/11%5b._cmc%5d`

University of California, Davis Chem_Guide
This is an interesting site because of the unique menu arrangement.
URL: `gopher://gopher-chem.ucdavis.edu`

University of Cambridge Crystallographic Data Centre
There are brief descriptions and bassic search guides for QUEST, VISTA, PLUTO, and GSTAT, as well as information on how to obtain the Cambridge Structural Database AND Mr. Bucketheads alternative section.
URL: `http://csdvx2.ccdc.cam.ac.uk`

University of Genoa Biophysical Institute Labs Gopher
Also accessible via WWW, it includes a copy of the Protein Data Bank and an archive of free software.
URL: `gopher://gopher.unige.it`

University of London Imperial College, CCS
URL: `http://diapason.cc.ic.ac.uk`

University of Sheffield WWW Server
This links to other chemistry WWW sites and features WebElements: includes a periodic table database, an interactive isotope pattern calculator, and an interactive element percentage calculator.
URL: `http://www2.shef.ac.uk/`

For further information contact: Dr. Mark J. Winter (`M.Winter@sheffield.ac.uk`).

University of Waterloo Library
URL: `gopher://watserv2.uwaterloo.ca/11/facilities/University%20of%20Waterloo%20Library/finding/discipline/Chemistry` (which some interesting entries, e.g., "Doing Research in Chemistry," which has a "Beginner's Guide to Chemical Abstracts")

U.S. Defense Technical Information Center Information Analysis Center (IAC) Directory
A description of the IACs, including High Temperature Materials Information Analysis Center, Nondestructive Testing Information Analysis Center, Metals Information Analysis Center and others.
URL: `gopher://asc.dtic.dla.mil/11/DTIC%20Services/iac`

U.S. Environmental Protection Agency
Among other items is the EPA National Online Library System (found in the EPA Information Locators path) and Other Environmental Gophers (found in the Other Environmental Information path).
URL: `gopher://gopher.epa.gov`

U.S. National Aeronautics and Space Administration (NASA) Scientific and Technical Information Program Internet Server
URL: `ftp://ftp.sti.nasa.gov`

URL: `gopher://gopher.sti.nasa.gov`

URL: `http://www.sti.nasa.gov/STI-homepage.html`

For additional information, contact: `postmaster@sti.nasa.gov`

You will find WAIS access to the NASA RECON database 1990-92, the NASA thesaurus, and SCAN (Selected Current Aerospace Notices). Some SCAN topics: Chemistry and Materials, Life Sciences, Physics.

U.S. National Institute for Standards and Technology
The Laboratory Programs link includes descriptions of the NIST Chemical Science and Technology and the NIST Materials Science and Engineering Laboratories, among others.

URL: `http://www.nist.gov/`

URL: `gopher://zserve.nist.gov:76/1/.pubmenu/NIST%20Laboratory%20Programs`

U.S. National Institute of Environmental Health Sciences
This site includes information on the National Toxicology Program and NIEHS Bibliographies from 1990 on.

URL: `gopher://gopher.niehs.nih.gov`

U.S. National Institutes of Health
URL: `gopher://gopher.nih.gov`

U.S. National Library of Medicine Gopher
The NLM gopher contains information about the library and selected reference materials. It also provides access to Locator, NLM's online catalog system and to MEDLARS and TOXNET (for those with access codes).

URL: `gopher://gopher.nlm.nih.gov`

U.S. National Library of Medicine Educational Technology Branch
The ETB conducts R & D in computer and multimedia technologies. There are texts of monographs on "Authoring Systems" and "Guidelines for Designing Effective and Healthy Learning Environments for Interactive Technologies."

URL: `http://wwwetb.nlm.nih.gov`

U.S. National Library of Medicine Publications
Access to items such as NLM Current Bibliographies in Medicine, AIDS Bibliography, NLM Fact Sheets, chapters of the Online Services Reference Manual, Toxicology Information Program publications and others in both ASCII and PostScript formats.

URL: `ftp://nlmpubs.nlm.nih.gov`

    login: `nlmpubs`

U.S. National Science Foundation Science & Technology Information System
URL: `telnet://stis.nsf.gov`

    login: `public`

    personal ID of up to eight characters

URL: `gopher://stis.nsf.gov`

U.S. Patent and Trademark Office Bulletin Board System
This provides limited patent searching, viewing, and downloading of files. Descriptions of services and products, the current week's Official Gazette notice for patents, a list of recently expired patents, and the bibliographic data

of the current month's issue of patents are found here. There are also files for downloading from the previous week's issue of patents, the previous week's Official Gazette notices, and other files. Also has a telephone directory for PTO and depository libraries, where the PTO's Automated Patent System can be accessed. Internet access is through FedWorld:

URL: `telnet://fedworld.gov (192.239.92.201)`.

U.S. Patent and Trademark Office database 1994-

This database comes from Internet Town Hall.

URL: `gopher://town.hall.org`

USENET News Groups:
```
sci.chem
sci.chem.organomet
sci.engr.chem
sci.polymers.
```

WAIS, Inc.

URL: `http://www.wais.com`

Water Science Network (WSN): Physics, Chemistry, and Biology of Water and Aqueous Systems

Send the message: `subscribe water firstname lastname` to: `listserv@gibbs.oit.unc.edu`

WATOC, World Association of Theoretical Organic Chemists

This is a mail exploder which can be joined by sending the message: `subscribe watoc firstname lastname` to: `listserver@ic.ac.uk`

There is also an associated World-Wide Web server.

URL: `http://www.ch.ic.ac.uk/watoc.html`

WebElements

URL: `http://www2.shef.ac.uk/chemistry/web-elements/web-elements-home.html`

This includes the Periodic Table database, an Isotope Pattern Calculator, and an Element percentage calculator.

On-line Resources for Earth Scientists (ORES)

14

Bill Thoen

June, 1994
This is a list of on-line resources available through the Internet and other networks that may be useful to those who have an interest in the earth sciences. These resources consist of digital documents, news sources, software, data sets and other on-line services that are available to the public.

Table of Contents

1. Table of Contents
2. Resource References, Indexes and Pointers
3. Resources by Subject

1.1. Copyright Notice

This document is copyright (c) 1994 by Bill Thoen. It may be freely distributed in electronic and printed form for noncommercial purposes provided this entire copyright notice is included intact.

The information in this article is provided as-is, with no warranties or assurances as to its accuracy or suitability. If you find errors or omissions, please send a message to Bill Thoen at bthoen@gisnet.com.

1.2. Introduction

The rapid growth and expansion of the on-line web of information is really challenging our best efforts to manage it. Various new software tools have appeared such as World Wide Web's Mosaic and Lynx browsers, Gopher, and WAIS, in addition to e-mail and FTP and telnet. There are new services appearing that serve mainly as gateways to other resources, and explosion of FAQ (Frequently Asked Questions) documents, resource documents (like this one) and books on navigating the Internet. Efforts like the Interpedia project are attempting to index the entire matrix, and diversions like the monthly Internet Hunt explore the ways people can find obscure information from the matrix, and to test its limits. New experiments in developing network "scavengers" such as automatic news filters and "knowbots" are becoming more common.

This is a guide for earth scientists who would like to get to know this cyberspace world better. The first section covers methods and resources that you can use to explore on your own, and the last part is a fairly exhaustive list of known resources that are related to the earth sciences.

There are many different services that can be used to retrieve electronic documents from the Internet. Each service is designed to serve different needs and is usually accessed through different software or methods. The resources section of this article is organized by subject, and so you will often see several methods listed that can be used to access resources on a subject. In this article we use the proposed Universal Resource Locator (URL) convention so that each resource can be presented in a standard way.

2. Resource References, Indexes and Pointers

Due to the dynamic nature of the internet, any "list of resources" is out of date almost as soon as it is published or distributed. It would be incomplete if it did not also provide the reader with methods for extending his or her knowledge as the Matrix evolves. The following section provides a list of resources that are themselves continually updated pointers to resources.

2.1. Online Documents

These are files that are relatively static. They are updated occasionally, but generally they are designed to be a summary of the current state of things in the are they attempt to cover.

2.1.1. Online Resources for Earth Scientists (ORES)

This is what you are reading now. It is updated only as I get time (about every two years it seems). An appropriate reference would be:

Thoen, Bill (1994), "Online Resources for Earth Scientists", digital text file, June 1994 version. Available via ftp from ftp.csn.org in the COGS directory, 100K

URL: `ftp://ftp.csn.org/COGS/ores.txt`

Contact: `bthoen@gisnet.com` (Bill Thoen)

2.1.2. List of Mailing Lists

This list describes many mailing lists; not just those related to earth sciences.

URL: `ftp://rtfm.mit.edu/pub/usenet/news.answers/mail/mailing-lists`

2.1.3. The Clearinghouse for Subject-Oriented Internet Resource Guides (UMich)

The Clearinghouse for Subject-Oriented Internet Resource Guides is a joint effort of the University of Michigan's University Library and the School of Information and Library Studies (SILS). Its goal is to collect and make widely available guides to Internet resources which are subject-oriented. These guides are produced by members of the Internet community, and by SILS students who participate in the Internet Resource Discovery project.

URL: `ftp://una.hh.lib.umich.edu/inetdirs`

URL: `gopher://una.hh.lib.umich.edu:70/11/inetdirs`

URL: `http://http2.sils.umich.edu/~lou/chhome.html`

Contact: Lou Rosenfeld (`lou@umich.edu`)

2.1.4. Manual of Federal Geographic Data Products

The Federal Geographic Data Committee (FGDC) has compiled the Manual of Federal Geographic Data Products to promote the coordinated development, use, sharing, and dissemination of surveying, mapping, and related spatial data. The manual describes Federal geographic data products that are national in scope and commonly distributed to the public. Geographic data products include maps, digital data, aerial photography and multispectral imagery, earth science, and other geographically-referenced data sets. Federal agencies were encouraged to list only those geographic data products that are supported by an office to which the public could make inquiries and place orders. Data products are described in a standard format and grouped by producing agency. A cross-reference matrix is provided to help readers find products by data type.

Federal Geographic Data Committee Secretariat
U.S. Geological Survey
590 National Center
Reston, VA 22092
Tel: 703-648-4533
Fax: 703-648-5755

However, the supply of printed copies of the "Manual of Federal Geographic Data Products" has been exhausted. The following options are available to obtain the information from the manual:

(1) black-and-white reproductions of the manual are being sold by the NTIS. Paper copies are sold for $44.50; microfiche for $17.50. In addition, there is a $3 fee for handling (US/Canada/Mexico). Telephone orders can be paid for by VISA, MasterCard, American Express, or NTIS Deposit Account. Be sure to mention stock number PB 93236503 in correspondence with NTIS.

National Technical Information Service
5285 Port Royal Road
Springfield, Virginia 22161

Attention: Order Desk
Tel: 703-487-4650

The FGDC manual is also available via the World Wide Web Service on the Internet. The text of the manual, and some of the illustrations, are available from:

URL: `http://info.er.usgs.gov/fgdc-catalog/title.html`

2.1.5. GPS Information Sources

Langley, Richard B., 1994, "GPS Information Sources", digital text file, updated periodically, Apr 1994 version, 20747 bytes

URL: `ftp://unbmvs1.csd.unb.ca/PUB.CANSPACE.GPS.INFO.SOURCES`

2.1.6. World Wide Elevation Data Sources

Gittings, Bruce (1994) "Catalogue of Digital Elevation Data", Usenet `comp.infosystems.gis`; periodic posting

URL: `mailto:geoinfo@geovax.edinburgh.ac.uk`

Contact: `bruce@geovax.ed.ac.uk` (Bruce Gittings)

2.2. Frequently Asked Questions (FAQ) Files

These are files that are created to provide answers to the most often asked questions in their particular area of interest. If you have any questions about a particular subject, you should first see if there is a "FAQ" on it, and read it first if there is.

2.2.1. Data Standards

Lutz, Dale (1994), "SAIF Frequently Asked Questions", Usenet `comp.infosystems.gis`, digital text file.

Contact: `infosafe@safe.com` (Dale Lutz)

2.2.2. GIS

Nyman, Lisa and Virgil Sealy, (1994) "Frequently Asked Questions with Answers about Geographic Information Systems", Usenet comp.infosystems.gis, updated monthly, 117K.

URL: `ftp://abraxas.adelphi.edu/pub/gis/FAQ`
URL: `ftp://ftp.census.gov/pub/geo/gis-faq.txt`

Contact: `panda@syrinx.umd.edu` (Lisa Nyman)

2.2.2.1. IDRISI

Morgan, Jay, 1994, "IDRISI-L Frequently Asked Questions (FAQ) List (Version 1.3)", digital text file, 27K.

URL: `ftp://midget.towson.edu/`

Contact: `E7G4MOR@TOE.TOWSON.EDU` (Jay Morgan)

2.2.2.2. MapInfo

McCombs, John (1994), "MapInfo Frequently Asked Questions", Windows Help file, updated monthly, 139K.

URL: `ftp://ftp.csn.org/mapinfo/mi_faq.zip`

Contact: `john@inmap.co.nz` (John McCombs)

2.2.3. Geology

Ramshaw, R. Spencer (1994) "FAQ sci.geo.geology", Usenet `sci.geo.geology`, digital text file. updated monthly

Contact: `rsr@amthyst.dweomer.org` (R. Spencer Ramshaw)

2.2.4. Biology
Smith, Una R. (1993), "A Biologist's Guide to Internet Resources", Usenet sci.answers. Available via gopher, anonymous FTP and e-mail from various archives. For a free copy via e-mail, send the text send `pub/usenet/sci.answers/biology/guide/*` to the e-mail address `mail-server@rtfm.mit.edu`. ~45 pages.
Contact: `smith-una@yale.edu` (Una Smith)

2.2.5. Meteorology
Stern, Illana (1994), "Sources of Meteorological Data Frequently Asked Questions (FAQ)". Usenet news.answers (bi-monthly). digital text file, 68K

To recieve this document via e-mail, send a message to `mail-server@rtfm.mit.edu` with the line:

send `/pub/usenet/news.answers/weather/data/part1`

in the body. Other sources are listed below.

URL: `ftp://rtfm.mit.edu/pub/usenet/news/answers/weather/data/part1`
URL: `ftp://vmd.cso.uiuc.edu/wx/sources.doc`
URL: `http://www.cis.ohio-state.edu/hypertext/faq/usenet/weather/top.html`
Contact: `ilana@ncar.ucar.edu` (Ilana Stern)

2.3. Online Catalogs and Resource Pointers

As the Internet grows we are beginning to see an explosion of growth in "pointer to resources" like WWW pages and gopher sites. These are great to find out the latest resources, but they tend to be overly-redundant, and some are not organized as long lists of pointers without much help on where to find anything specific.

2.3.1. Information Sources: the Internet and Computer-Mediated Communication
URL: `file://ftp.rpi.edu/pub/communications/internet-cmc.html`

This points to just about every Internet reference guide around!

2.3.2. Michael McDermott's GIS Resources Pointers
URL: `ftp://gis.queensu.ca/pub/gis/docs/gissites.txt`
URL: `ftp://gis.queensu.ca/pub/gis/docs/gissites.html`
IP: 130.15.94.1
Contact: `mcdermom@gisdog.gis.queensu.ca` (Michael J. McDermott)

2.3.3. Roland Stahl's GIS Resource Pointers
URL: `http://www.laum.uni-hannover.de/gis/gisnet/gisnet.html`

2.3.4. A GIS User Guide to Tools
Murnion, Shane and George Munroe (1994?) "A GIS User Guide to Tools", Html text file.
This guide provides a good overview of some of the software tools that can be used to find GIS information on the Internet.

URL: `file://jupiter.qub.ac.uk/pub/GIS/GIS.html`

2.3.5. United States Geological Survey Home Page
This is the main starting point for on-line information about the USGS, its programs and missions. It also has lists of other pointers to resources not specifically run by the USGS.

URL: `http://info.er.usgs.gov/`

2.3.6. CERN—WWW Virtual Library on the subject of Geography
URL: `http://info.cern.ch/hypertext/DataSources/bySubject/Geography/Overview.html`

2.3.7. Annotated Scientific Visualization URL Bibliography
This is a collection of pointers to weblets on the subject of scientific visualisaztion. It looks well-maintained.

URL: `http://www.nas.nasa.gov/RNR/Visualization/annotatedURLs.html`

2.3.8. EINet Galaxy's Pointers to Geosciences Resources
Large list of pointers to earth science resources.

URL: `http://galaxy.einet.net/galaxy/Science/Geosciences.html`

2.3.9. Software Support Laboratory for Space and Earth Scientists
Software tools for Space and Earth Scientists

URL: `http://sslab.colorado.edu:2222/ssl_homepage.html`

2.3.10. National Geophysical Data Center
This is the main starting point for information on NGDC programs and activities.

URL: `gopher://gopher.ngdc.noaa.gov`

URL: `http://www.ngdc.noaa.gov/ngdc.html`

2.3.11. MIT Earth Resources Laboratory—Home Page
URL: `http://www-erl.mit.edu/`

2.3.12. CIESIN—Information Gateway
The Consortium for International Earth Science Information Network (CIESIN) is cataloging metadata on the human dimensions of global environmental change, also in the Directory Interchange Format (DIF).

URL: `telnet://gopher@gopher.ciesin.org`

Contact: MDUSO@NSSDCA.GSFC.NASA.GOV

2.3.13. ERIN—Environmental Resources Information Network
Environmental Resources Information Network (ERIN) has been established in Australia to draw together and distribute any information on the environment.

URL: `http://kaos.erin.gov.au:80/erin.html`

URL: `gopher://kaos.erin.gov.au`

2.3.14. GCMD—The Global Change Master Directory
The Global Change Master Directory (GCMD) is a multidisciplinary on-line information system containing descriptions of Earth and space science data holdings available to the science community. These include data from NASA, NOAA, NCAR, USGS, DOE (CDIAC), EPA, NSF and other U.S. agencies, universities, research centers as well as international agencies. For assistance, you may contact:

URL: `telnet://NSSDC@128.183.36.23:` (U.S.A.)

URL: `telnet://GCNET@132.156.47.218:` (Canada)

URL: `telnet://ESAPID@192.106.252.160:` (Europe)

URL: `telnet://NASDADIR@133.56.72.1:` (Japan)

Contact: mduso@nssdca.gsfc.nasa.gov

2.3.15. GLIS—Global Land Information System
TELNET hypertext system about land information databases. You can order data through here as well as download direct to PC.

URL: `telnet://glis.cr.usgs.gov`

IP: `152.62.192.54` (unofficial)

2.3.16. NASA Information by Subject
URL: `http://hypatia.gsfc.nasa.gov/nasa_subjects/nasa_subjectpage.html`

2.3.17. NASA Master Directory of Earth Science Data Sets
To find high-level information about any science data from earth satellites or planetary missions, including land observations, ocean data, meteorology, astronomy, earth/sun science, etc., use the NASA Master Directory. Also available are data/observations made from earth or of earth. Navigate the menus and you'll find out where to get the information you want on any satellite or instrument on a satellite.

Once you locate interesting data sets through the MD, it's often possible to link to the specific system that holds the data and order it online. From NSI/DECNet, SET HOST NSSDCA.

URL: `ftp://nssdca.gsfc.nasa.gov`

Contact: mduso@nssdca.gsfc.nasa.gov

2.3.18. NSSDC— National Space Science Data Center On-Line Data
The National Space Science Data Center (NSSDC) On-Line Data and Information Service (NODIS) is a menu-driven interactive system which provides information on services and data supported by NSSDC. Includes *NASA Master Directory*—an online search system providing brief overview information about NASA and many important non-NASA space and earth science data, and data information systems. In some cases, the directory offers automatic network connections to catalogs or other systems. Some topics: Nimbus-7 GRID TOMS Data, Geophysical Models, Standards and Technology Information System.

URL: `telnet://NSSDC@nssdca.gsfc.nasa.gov`

IP: 128.183.36.23

2.3.19. Naval Observatory Automated Data Service
URL: `telnet://ads@tycho.usno.navy.mil`

IP: 192.5.41.239

2.3.20. NCAR—National Center for Atmospheric Research data support archive
URL: `ftp://ncardata.ucar.edu`

IP: 128.117.8.111

2.3.21. STIS—Science & Technology Information Service
Science & technology Information Service STIS is maintained by the National Science Foundation.

URL: `telnet://public@stis.nsf.gov`

IP: 128.150.195.40

2.3.22. NCSU Library—Earth and Geography gophers
URL: `gopher://dewey.lib.ncsu.edu:70/11/library/disciplines/earth`

URL: `gopher://dewey.lib.ncsu.edu:70/11/library/disciplines/geography/gis`

2.3.23. UCSC— University of California—Santa Cruz Earth and Marine Science Gopher
URL: `gopher://scilibx.ucsc.edu:70/11/The Researcher/Science and Engineering/Earth and Marine Sciences`

2.3.24. Rice University
URL: `gopher://chico.rice.edu:70/11/Subject/Geology`

2.3.25. UTEP—University of Texas at El Paso GeoGopher
This is one of the better subject-oriented lists of resource pointers for Geology interests.

URL: `gopher://dillon.geo.ep.utexas.edu:70/11/EarthScienceRes`

2.3.26. Oklahoma Geological Survey gopher
URL: `gopher://wealaka.okgeosurvey1.gov`

2.3.27. UCSB—University of California—Santa Barbara Geological Sciences Gopher
URL: `gopher://gopher.geol.ucsb.edu`

2.3.28. Northwestern University, Dept. of Geological Sciences gopher
URL: `gopher://gopher.earth.nwu.edu`

2.4. Newsletters

2.4.1. Electronic Atlas Newsletter
This is a hard copy newsletter "dedicated to information about 'real-life' and professional applications of Geographic Information Systems (GIS)". To receive a free sample copy of the newsletter contact:

> Brian J. Matuschak
> c/o Electronic Atlas Newsletter
> 1414 N Northgate #101
> Seattle, WA 98133
> Tel: 206-525-7155

Contact: `bjm@hebron.connected.com` (Brian Matuschak)

2.4.2. HOTLINE Climate Change Newsletter
HOTLINE is an occasional newsletter from the US Climate Action Network dedicated to updates and information on climate change science and policy. HOTLINE will include information on climate change science, as well as updates on current events: from local initiatives in the United States, to international treaty negotiations. HOTLINE is intended to inform scientists, local activists and organizations about the science surrounding the potential threat of climate change, and current policy efforts to avoid this threat.

URL: `ftp://igc.apc.org/pub/ECIX/hotlineMMYY`
  (MMYY = month/year, e.g., 0194=Jan 94)
IP: `192.82.108.1`
Contact: `uscan@igc.org`
> US Climate Action Network
> 1350 New York Ave.
> NW Suite 300
> Washington, D.C. 20005

2.4.3. GPS Digest
The GPS Digest is a forum for the discussion of topics related to the USAF Global Positioning System (GPS) and other satellite navigation positioning systems. The GPS Digest is moderated and is not presently available via USENET newsgroup. Submissions should be made to `gps@tws4.si.com` Administrative requests should be made to `gps-request@tws4.si.com`
   Past issues of the GPS Digest can be found in the file archives of the Canadian Space Geodesy Forum are at:

URL: `ftp://unbmvs1.csd.unb.ca/PUB.CANSPACE.GPS.DIGEST.V1`
URL: `ftp://unbmvs1.csd.unb.ca/PUB.CANSPACE.GPS.DIGEST.V2`
IP: `131.202.1.2`
Contact: `lang@unb.ca` (Richard Langley)

2.5. Usenet Newsgroups

2.5.1. `comp.infosystems.gis`
Discussion of Geographic Information Systems (GIS) topics. This is the main GIS newsgroup.

2.5.2. `sci.geo.fluids`
Discussion of geophysical fluid dynamics.

2.5.3. `sci.geo.geology`
Discussion of general interest geological topics. This is the main newsgroup for geology.

2.5.4. `sci.geo.meteorology`
Discussion of general interest meteorological topics. This is the main newsgroup for meteorology.

2.5.5. `sci.techniques.spectroscopy`
The main aim of sci.techniques.spectroscopy is to provide an open forum for the discussion of spectroscopy and related fields on the Internet and to provide a catalyst for improved dissemination of information between those working with spectroscopy.

2.5.6. `sci.geo.hydrology`
The objective of this newsgroup is to provide a forum for discussion on issues pertaining to surface and groundwater hydrology, their relation to climate, water quality issues and water resource management and policy issues.

2.6. Mailing Lists

2.6.1. `ACDGIS-L`   GIS Discussions for German-speaking Countries
Topics include GIS, Cartography, Remote Sensing and Image Processing as related to GIS, Geo-Statistics. This list aims at improving local/regional communication and is viewed as complementary to GIS-L.

Server: `listserv@awiimc12.bitnet`
List: `ACDGIS-L@awiimc12.bitnet`
Contact: `wigeoarn@awiwuw11.bitnet` (Zoltan Daroczy)

2.6.2. `AQUIFER`   Pollution and Groundwater Recharge
Server: `listserv@ibacsata.bitnet`
List: `AQUIFER@ibacsata.bitnet`

2.6.3. `CANSPACE`   Canadian Space Geodesy Forum
Any topic related to the space geodetic techniques of GPS, Transit, VLBI, SLR, satellite altimetry, etc., may be discussed. Information concerning satellite launches and orbital elements may be posted. Questions are particularly encouraged. GPS Constellation daily status reports and ionospheric disturbance warnings are posted.

Server: `listserv@unbvm1.bitnet`
List: `CANSPACE@unbvm1.bitnet`
Contact: `lang@unb.ca` (Richard B. Langley)

2.6.4. `CLIMLIST`   Climatology Information and News
Server: `listserv@ohstvma.bitnet`
List: `CLIMLIST@ohstvma.bitnet`

2.6.5. `COASTGIS`   Coastal GIS Mailing List
This is set up to discuss issues relating to Coastal Applications of GIS.

Server: `listserv@irlearn.ucd.ie`
List: `COASTGIS@irlearn.bitnet`
Contact: `STGG8004@iruccvax.ucc.ie` (Darius Bartlett)

2.6.6. `COASTNET`   Coastal Management and Resources
This discussion list covers topics related to Coastal Management and Resources.

Server: `Listserv@uriacc.uri.edu`
`listserv@uriacc.bitnet`
List: `COASTNET@uriacc.uri.edu`
`COASTNET@uriacc.bitnet`
Contact: `rpuf4584@uriacc.uri.edu` or `puf4584@uriacc.bitnet` (Robert H. Puffer)

2.6.7. **CONSGIS** Conservation Biology And GIS
Server: `listserv@uriacc.bitnet`
List: `CONSGIS@uriacc.bitnet`

2.6.8. **ENERGY-L** Energy Discussion List
Server: `listserv@taunivm.bitnet`
List: `ENERGY-L@taunivm.bitnet`

2.6.9. **ESRI-L** Arc/Info Support List
The purpose of this list is to provide users of ESRI software with a forum to ask questions of each other and exchange technical information and expertise. It is not seen as a competitor to our CompuServe forum which serves a different clientele and is primarily to support ESRI's PC based products.

Server: `listserv@esri.com`
List: `ESRI-L@esri.com`
Contact: `esrilhuman@esri.com`

2.6.10. **GEOCAL** Geography, Geology, Town and Regional Planning, Meteorology
The CTI Centre for Geography has established a discussion list on Computer Assisted Learning at the University of Leicester. This moderated list will discuss all aspects of CAL/CBT/CAI/CML within the Centre's 'community' of Geography, Geology, Town and Regional Planning and Meteorology. from outside UK:

Server: `mailbase@mailbase.ac.uk`
List: `GEOCAL@mailbase.ac.uk`

Server: `mailbase@uk.ac.mailbase`
List: `GEOCAL@uk.ac.mailbase`
Contact: `cti@uk.ac.leicester` (John Castleford)

2.6.11. **GEOGRAPH** Geography discussion list
GEOGRAPHy is an experimental BULLETIN BOARD and DISCUSSION FORUM for academic geography—faculty, students and other persons having interests in the field of modern geographic research.

Server: `listserv@searn.sunset.se`
List: `GEOGRAPH@searn.sunset.se`

2.6.12. **GEOLOGY** Geology discussion list
Discussion of Geology topics

Server: `listserv@ptearn.bitnet`
List: `GEOLOGY@ptearn.bitnet`
Contact: `AMORIM@PTEARN.bitnet` (Pedro Amorim)

2.6.13. **GEONET-L** Geoscience Librarians & Information Specialists
Server: `listserv@iubvm.bitnet`
List: `GEONET-L@iubvm.bitnet`

2.6.14. **GIS-L**   Geographic Information Systems Topics
This discussion group focuses on all aspects of GIS and digital cartography and analysis. This is generally considered to be the main list for GIS. It is also available as a Usenet newsgroup as `comp.infosystems.gis`

Server: `listserv@ubvm.cc.buffalo.edu`
         `listserv@ubvm.bitnet`
List: `GIS-L@ubvm.cc.buffalo.edu`
      `GIS-L@ubvm.bitnet`
Contact: `GISLRequest@ubvm.cc.buffalo.edu`

2.6.15. **GIST-L**   GIS Transport Discussion Group
Server: `listserv@ukacrl.bitnet`
List: `GIST-L@ukacrl.bitnet`

2.6.16. **GPS-L**   Globally Positioned Satellite Topics
Server: `gps-request@tws4.si.com`
List: `GPS-L@tws4.si.com`

2.6.17. **GRASS** lists
Sending mail to either server address with `SUB Your Name` in the subject line or in the text (left-justified, no quotes) will sign you up for the list and you will begin receiving mail from others. To quit, just replace `SUB` above with `UNSUB`.

GRASS Users' list
Server: `grassu-request@moon.cecer.army.mil`
List: `grassu-list@moon.cecer.army.mil`

GRASS Programmers List
Server: `grassp-request@moon.cecer.army.mil`
List: `grassp-list@moon.cecer.army.mil`
Contact: `grass-lists-owner@moon.cecer.army.mil`

2.6.18. **HYDROLOGY**   Hydrology Topics
Monash University in Australia has a Hydrology Mailing List set up for general open discussion on all matters concerning hydrology.

Server: `listserv@eng.monash.edu.au`
List: `HYDROLOGY@eng.monash.edu.au`

2.6.19. **IDRISI-L**   Idrisi Support List
IDRISI-L is an Internet and Bitnet discussion group for users of the IDRISI software package developed by the Graduate School of Geography at Clark University. The purposes of IDRISI-L are: 1) to foster communication among the community of IDRISI users; 2) to encourage the application of IDRISI to real world problems; and 3) to provide user feedback regarding IDRISI to the Graduate School of Geography at Clark University. IDRISI-L is supported by the Department of Geography and Environmental Planning at Towson State University.

Server: `mailserv@towsonvx.bitnet` or `mailserv@toe.towson.edu`
List: `IDRISI-L@towsonvx.bitnet` or `IDRISI-L@toe.towson.edu`
Contact: `e7g4mor@toe.towson.edu` (Dr. John M. Morgan, III).

2.6.20. **IMGRS-L**   Digital Image Processing of Remotely Sensed Data
Server: `listserv@csearn.bitnet`
List: `IMAGRS-L@csearn.bitnet` or `IMAGRS-L@csearn.earn`

2.6.21. MAPHIST — Historical Maps Topics

MAPHIST-L is a discussion group whose primary focus is historical maps, atlases, globes and other cartographic formats. This listserv is open to all persons interested in the history of cartography and discussion is encouraged on all aspects of this broad subject.

The primary purpose of MAPHIST-L is to encourage individuals to communicate current research; evaluate methods and tools of analysis; announce important acquisitions and news; announce position vacancies; announce new publications (direct advertising, however, is discouraged); investigate library holdings; and to share information between conferences and the appearance of relevant journals.

Server: `listserv@harvarda.harvard.edu`
List: `MAPHIST@harvarda.harvard.edu`
Contact: `cobb@widener1.mhs.harvard.edu` (David Cobb)

2.6.22. MAPINFO-L — MapInfo Discussion Group

The purpose of the MAPINFO-L mailing list is to provide a world-wide E-mail forum for discussing issues of interest to users, dealers, and developers of MapInfo software, applications and data sets. Topics can range from narrow technical details of using MapInfo to broad issues about GIS and Mapping.

To join, send e-mail to the server, and put

`SUBSCRIBE MAPINFO-L`

On the first line of the message. You will receive a confirmation message with additional information once you are successfully signed up. Note that this list does not use 'listserv' software, so do not put your name on the subscribe line!. Also the word 'subscribe' must be spelled out completely, but it can be in either upper or lower case text.

Server: `majordomo@csn.org`
List: `MAPINFO-L@csn.org`
Contact: `MAPINFOLOwner@gisnet.com` (Bill Thoen)

2.6.23. MAPS-L — Maps and Air Photos Systems Forum

This list is strongly oriented towards issues involved in map librarianship; such as storing, cataloging, preserving, classification, etc. of maps and air photos. Also good source for information on ancient sites and maps, and hard-to-answer geography questions.

Server: `listserv@uga.bitnet`
List: `MAPS-L@uga.bitnet` or `MAPS-L@uga.cc.uga.edu`
Contact: `jsuther1@uga.cc.uga.edu` (Johnnie D. Sutherland)

2.6.24. MDGIS-L — Discussion list for Maryland GIS users

Server: `mailserv@towsonvx.bitnet` or `mailserv@toe.towson.edu`
List: `MDGIS-L@towsonvx.bitnet` or `MDGIS-L@toe.towson.edu`

2.6.25. NSDI-L — US National Spatial Data Infrastructure

The purpose of this list is to discuss issues in the US National Spatial Data Infrastructure (NSDI). The National Research Council definition of NSDI is given as: The National Spatial Data Infrastructure is the means to assemble geographic information that describes the arrangement and attributes of features and phenomena on the Earth. The infrastructure includes the materials, technology, and people necessary to acquire, process, store, and distribute such information to meet a wide variety of needs.

Server: `listproc@grouse.umesve.maine.edu`
List: `NSDI-L@grouse.umesve.maine.edu`
Contact: `stevef@grouse.umesve.maine.edu` (Steven Frank)

2.6.26. QUAKE-L — General Earthquake Discussion

The focus of this mailing list is on the ways various national and international computer networks can help in the event of an earthquake. One of the basic problems discussed might be network reconfigurations which would be temporarily required; others might be in actually putting various groups in electronic contact with each other.

Public notebooks for the list will be available from the server (send the command "information database" to the server for details), and are available via anonymous FTP.

URL: `ftp://vm1.nodak.edu/LISTARCH/QUAKE-L.*`
IP: `134.129.111.1`
Server: `listserv@vm1.nodak.edu`
   `listserv@ndsuvm1.bitnet`
List: `QUAKE-L@vm1.nodak.edu`
   `QUAKE-L@ndsuvm1.bitnet`
Contact: `nu021172@vm1.nodak.edu`
Contact: `nu021172@ndsuvm1.bitnet` (Marty Hoag)

2.6.27. QUATERNARY List

This mailing list is for all interested in research in the Quaternary geological period, including geologists, geomorphologists, soil scientists, palaeoenvironmentalists, archaeologists, palaeontologists, geochronologists, palynologists, and others.

Server: `listserv@morgan.ucs.mun.ca`
List: `QUATERNARY@morgan.ucs.mun.ca`
Contact: `dgl@zeppo.geosurv.gov.nf.ca` (Dave Liverman)

2.6.28. RAILROAD List

To subscribe to the railroad list, send a message to `listserv@cunyvm.cuny.edu` with the line `subscribe railroad` in the body.

2.6.29. SEISML   Seismological Data Distribution

Seismological data for general distribution

Server: `listserv@bingvmb`
   `listserv@bingvmb.cc.binghamton.edu`
List: `SEISM-L@bingvmb`
   `SEISM-L@bingvmb.cc.binghamton.edu`
Contact: `fwu@bingvmb.bitnet` (Francis Wu)

2.6.30. SEISMD-L   Seismological Discussion

Seismological topics of general interest

Server: `listserv@bingvmb`
   `listserv@bingvmb.cc.binghamton.edu`
List: `SEISMD-L@bingvmb.bitnet`
   `SEISMD-L@bingvmb.cc.binghamton.edu`
Contact: `fwu@bingvmb.bitnet` (Francis Wu)

2.6.31. SOILS-L   Soil Science

A forum for the discussion of all subjects dealing with soil science. Soil physics, chemistry, genesis, classification, mineralogy, fertility, conservation, etc. may be discussed within this unmoderated group. The formation of this group has been sanctioned by The American Society of Agronomy and the Soil Science Society of America.

Server: `listserv@unl.edu`
List: `SOILS-L@unl.edu`
Contact: `jp@unl.edu` (Jerome Pier)

2.6.32. STAT-GEO   Quantitative Methods In Geosciences

Forum of quantitative methods in geosciences.

Server: `listserv@ufrj.bitnet`
   `listserv%ufrj.bitnet@vtbit.cc.vt.edu`

List: `STAT-GEO@ufrj.bitnet`
    `STAT-GEO@%ufrj.bitnet@cunyvm.cuny.edu`
Contact: `igg02001@ufrj.bitnet` (Hugo Richard)

2.6.33. **TGIS-L**   Temporal Topics in GIS Mailing List
TGIS-L is a listserver set up to facilitate discussion of all issues regarding temporal topics in GIS (Geographic Information Systems). TGIS-L has been established by joint effort of the ICA Interest Group on Temporal Topics in GIS and the US National Center for Geographic Information and Analysis. The ICA Interest group is chaired by Gail Langran (`langran@u.washington.edu`). The NCGIA's research initiative #10, on "Spatio-Temporal Reasoning and GIS", is co-led by Max Egenhofer (`max@mecan1.maine.edu`) and Reg Golledge (`golledge@ncgia.ucsb.edu`).

Postings to this list should focus on research, commentary, and business concerning spatiotemporal subjects. These include, but are not limited to: time in GIS; spatio-temporal reasoning; representing time on maps; dynamic cartography; temporal aspects of spatial cognition.

Server: `listserv@ubvm.cc.buffalo.edu`
    `listserv@ubvm.bitnet`
List: `TGIS-L@ubvm.cc.buffalo.edu`
    `TGIS-L@ubvm.bitnet`
Contact: `geodmm@ubvms.cc.buffalo.edu` (David Mark)

2.6.34. **TRANSIT** List
Send a message to `listserv@gitvm1.bitnet` with the message `subscribe transit` in the body to subscribe to the transit list.

2.6.35. **TRANSP-L**   Transportation Planning
Send a message to `listproc@gmu.edu` with the message `subscribe transp-l` in the body to subscribe to the transportation planning list.

2.6.36. **UIGIS-L**   GIS User Interface issues
The central theme of this discussion group is the issues about the user interface for GIS software.

Server: `listserv@ubvm.bitnet`
List: `UIGIS-L@ubvm.bitnet`

2.6.37. **URBAN-L**   Urban Planning
Send a message to `listserv@trearn.bitnet` with the message `subscribe urban-l` in the body, to subscribe to the urban planning list.

Server: `listserv@trearn.bitnet`
List: `URBAN-L@trearn.bitnet`

2.6.38. **VIGIS-L**   Virtual World Interfaces for GIS
VIGIS-L is a mailing list for those specifically interested in Virtual World Interfaces and their application to Geographic Information Systems.

Its purpose is to provide a forum for issues specifically surrounding the use of Virtual Worlds (Virtual Reality) Interfaces for Geographic Information Systems as well as any and all spatial information/decision support systems. The broad goal is to generate constructive discussions about how Virtual Worlds will be used in GIS, as well as approach the fundamental issue of why implement VR at all.

Server: `listserv@uwavm.bitnet`
List: `VIGIS-L@uwavm.bitnet`

2.6.39. **VOLCANO**   Volcano Discussion list
It carries some discussions about volcano-related issues, as well as the monthly Global Volcanism Network reports. The latter are published by a group of geologists at the Smithsonian; we receive the reports a few weeks before they come out in print. I also maintain a list of volcanologists called **VLIST**

FILE. VLIST contains names, e-mail addresses, research interests, job titles, and fax numbers for a hundred or so volcanologists and assorted fans.

If you would like to join volcano listserv, send a brief note to Jon Fink at `AIJHF@ASUACAD.BITNET`.

List: VOLCANO@asuacad.bitnet

Contact: `aijhf@asuacad.bitnet` (Jon Fink)

2.7. Bibliographies

2.7.1. NCGIA Publications

NCGIA publications, Initiatives, annual reports, and tech reports.

URL: `ftp://ncgia.ucsb.edu/pub/biblio`

IP: `128.111.254.105`

Contact: `postmaster@ncgia.ucsb.edu` or `raj@ncgia.ucsb.edu` (Richard A. Johnson)

The NCGIA Bibliographies can also be found at U Maine.

URL: `ftp://grouse.umesve.maine.edu/pub/NCGIA/Biblio`

Contact: `stevef@grouse.umesve.maine.edu`

2.7.2. Bibliography from the Tectonics and Topography Conference

This directory includes the bibliography from the Tectonics and Topography conference held on Aug 31 to Sept 4, 1992. The bibliography is in several formats: text, text for ProCite import, and macintosh EndNote. The macintosh version is compressed, and binhexed.

URL: `ftp://magic.ucsb.edu/pub/chapman`

Contact: `dwv@magic.ucsb.edu` (David Valentine)

2.7.3. EPA National Library

EPA National Library on-line database can be accessed for bibliographic searches.

URL: `telnet://epaibm.rtpnc.epa.gov`

IP: `134.67.180.1`

2.7.4. Multidiscipline Bibliographic Database

This contains a lot in geology but is not near as good as commercial databases like GeoRef.

URL: `telnet://database.carl.org`

3. Resources By Subject

3.1. Bulletin Board Systems (BBS)

BBS systems are often the best sources of good up-to-date and organized information. Because they are run by individuals who try to reach an audience every day with news and fresh perspectives, you get the benefit of an active site of information. Ask a question of the Sysop (the system operator of the BBS), and you'll get an answer within a day at least. They also tend to specialize in a particular field, so if you want to know something about that field, chances are the BBS is the place to check first, even before you go searching the Internet. Most BBS operators are often well aware of what's out there on the net already.

For example, GISnet BBS specializes in GIS resources, and even though it is not as big as the whole Internet, if you log in there you can usually find just the pointer you need to the multi-megabyte database you've been looking for. Even things that don't get saved on the Internet (like interesting message threads) are often archived here.

To reach BBSes, you need to use a modem and dial out over regular telephone lines.

3.1.1. The GeoInfo Network

GeoInfo Network is an association of BBS systems throughout North America that specialize in earth science or GIS interests.

CDMG Online	916-327.1208	Sacramento, CA
COGSnet	303-526.1617	Golden, CO
Computer Plumber	319-337.6723	Iowa City, IA
Computer Solutions	504-542.9600	Hammond, LA
Dark Matter	604-534-7667	Langley, BC
GeoFuel	416-829.0858	Oakville, ONT
GeoNet	316-265.6457	Witchita, KS
GISnet	303-447.0927	Boulder, CO
NASA MLP	206-871-3965	Port Orchard, WA
PreCambrian	602-881.5836	Tucson, AZ
PSN (Memphis)	901-360.0302	Memphis, TN
PSN (Pasadena)	818-797.0536	Pasadena, CA
PSN (San Jose)	408-226.0675	San Jose, CA
Snowshoe	304-572.2531	Snowshoe, WV
SurveyNet	207-549-3213	Whitefield, ME

3.2. Jobs in Earth Sciences

3.2.1. GIS Jobs Clearinghouse

Intended to be a simple listing of jobs related to GIS and other similar fields (image processing, GPS etc . . .). The archive will be accessible via gopher and WWW. This is NOT a new mailing list, rather an archive of submissions from those advertising positions. Please, only send announcements if your the originator of the announcement, this way I hope we can reduce the number of redundant posts. To post a send mail to: jobs@torpedo.forestry.umn.edu and please include the following on the subject line: job title, location (state, country, zip code) and a closing date.

Look under "Remote Sensing and GIS Information" on either server.

URL: `gopher://walleye.forestry.umn.edu:70/11/gopher`

URL: `http://walleye.forestry.umn.edu/0/www/main.html`

Contact: sdlime@soils.umn.edu (Steve Lime)

3.2.2. Federal Government Jobs

This site has a sub section of jobs listed by the Federal government. This includes many different offers, not just those related to earth sciences.

URL: `telnet://fedworld.gov`

3.2.3. The GeoInfo Network BBSes—Job conferences

The GeoInfo BBS network maintains a conference of jobs available in the earth sciences. Most of these are originally advertised over the Internet, but if you aren't following all the relevant Internet conferences, you can catch up here. See the listing of BBSes above to find the one nearest to you.

3.2.4. Jobs listed by keyword/geographic search

Current job announcements in many, many fields. The gopher index is searchable by geographic area, keyword (like gis), etc.

URL: `gopher://nero.aa.msen.com`

3.3. Programming—Algorithms Source Code and Data Formats

3.3.1. Computers & Geoscience Source Code

The IAMG will establish an ftp site effective June 1st, 1994. This service will provide Internet users access to programs and test data that have been published in the journals, Computers and Geosciences and Mathematical Geology. The service is intended to assist members in obtaining programs/data which have been previously difficult or time consuming to obtain.

Programs will be stored in both tar (UNIX) and zip (PKZIP-DOS) forms. Code access will be by Journal, Volume and Number. Thus, for Computers & Geosciences, the file `v20-5-10.zip` will contain programs published in Volume 20, Number 5, Paper/Note #10. The files are in the directory: `/pub/CG`.

For the Journal Mathematical Geology, program code from Volume 25, No. 5, Paper/Article #1 will be in file `v25-5-1` in directory `/pub/MG`.

URL: `ftp://imag.org`

Contact: `rsr@amthyst.dweomer.org` (Spencer Ramshaw)

3.3.2. Point In Polygon
Fastest Point in Polygon Test, Eric Haines, in *Ray Tracing News*, vol. 5, no. 3, September, 1992; `ftp://princeton.edu/pub/Graphics/RTNews/RTNv5n3.Z`

3.3.3. Voronoi Tessellation source code
Source code from the article *Spatial Data And The Voronoi Tessellation*, Dr. Dobbs Journal, Dec 1992

URL: `ftp://ftp.mv.com/pub/ddj/12.1992`

3.3.4. Viewshed Algorithms
`skatz@DSC.BLM.GOV` (Sol Katz 303-236-0101) writes:

"Look at yalemap (original and 2 prettified versions). It has a viewshed program written in f77. You can see how it works using cogsmap or skmap in the same directory. (skmap has better graphics)."

URL: `ftp://dsc.blm.gov/pub/gis/yalemap.zip`

Contact: `skatz@DSC.BLM.GOV` (Sol Katz 303-236-0101)

3.3.5. TIN "Linear Time Algorithm" Software
An article is published in IJGIS, 1993, Vol. 7, No. 6, pp. 501-524 describes a "linear-time algorithm". The associated DOS-executable program developed by the author is available.

URL: `ftp://shelf.ersc.wisc.edu/pub/CHIDTVD.ZIP`

3.3.6. Thiessen / Voronoi Polygons & Delauney Triangle Algorithms
C source code for calculating vectors for Thiessen Polygons:

URL: `ftp://netlib.att.com/netlib/voronoi/sweep2.Z`

The GRASS module, s.voroni.

URL: `ftp://pasture.ecn.purdue.edu/pub/mccauley/grass`

The NCSA 'MinMaxer' is a triangulation system that does, amongst others, Delaunay triangulation, which is the dual to Voronoi or Thiessen polygons.

URL: `ftp://ftp.ncsa.uiuc.edu/SGI/MinMaxer`

3.3.7. AML code for ARC/INFO 5.0, 6.11
URL: `ftp://dis2qvarsa.er.usgs.gov/amls`

3.3.8. AML code for GIRAS data
URL: `ftp://dis2qvarsa.er.usgs.gov/data/giras`

3.3.9. AML ftp site
There is a *very small* ftp site of AMLs at:

URL: `ftp://wigeo.wu-wien.ac.at/pub/acdgis-l/aml`

3.3.10. Coordinate Conversion Software
USGS General Cartographic Transformation package converted to C

URL: `ftp://edcftp.cr.usgs.gov/pub/software/gctpc`

3.3.11. Topographic Analysis source code (FORTRAN)
URL: `ftp://edcftp.cr.usgs.gov/pub/software/topo`

3.3.12. DCW to DXF conversion:
URL: `ftp://dsc.blm.gov/pub/gis/dcw2dxf.zip`

3.3.13. UNIX version of VPFView 1.1
(to view DCW data) is available from:

URL: `ftp://jupiter.drev.dnd.ca`
URL: `ftp://cc.drev.dnd.ca`
IP: 131.132.32.2
Contact: parento@cc.drev.dnd.ca (Marc Parenteau)

3.3.14. LAS (Land Analysis System) Documentation
URL: `ftp://edcftp.cr.usgs.gov/pub/software/las/doc`

3.4. Digital Data

3.4.1. ARC/INFO Coverages
380 ARC/INFO coverages online

URL: `ftp://gsb.igsb.uiowa.edu`

Contact: jgiglierano@gsbth-po.igsb.uiowa.edu (Jim Giglierano)

3.4.2. Counties

3.4.2.1. ARC/INFO Export Coverage of selected U.S. States.
URL: `ftp://csdokokl.cr.usgs.gov/pub/gis_data`
IP: 136.177.176.4
Contact: ahrea@csdokokl.cr.usgs.gov (Alan Rea, Hydrologist, USGS)

3.4.2.2. ARC/INFO export files of US statewide county coverages
The maps were derived from the Census TIGER files. As such, the data in metro areas may be the old, crude DIME data, but the rest of the boundaries are derived from USGS 1:100K DLGs.

URL: `ftp://dis2qvarsa.er.usgs.gov/state100`

3.4.2.3. County outlines as Versatec plot file
URL: `ftp://ftp.uu.net/graphics/maps/USmap.Z`
IP: 192.48.96.9

3.4.3. Micro World Databank II
URL: `ftp://ftp.uu.net/graphics/maps/wdb-ii.Z`
IP: 192.48.96.9

3.4.4. Census County Boundaries
Part 1 of the 1980 Census boundaries

URL: `ftp://ftp.uu.net/graphics/maps/Census.Part1.Z`
IP: 192.48.96.9

3.4.5. US Census Bureau Data
This is the main Bureau of the Census FTP site, and looks like it will be a rich source of population, business, health and other demographic data. It came on-line in March 1994.

URL: `ftp://ftp.census.gov`

3.4.6. US Hydrologic Units Data
This directory contains all the 1:100,000-scale and 1:250,000-scale data files of Hydrologic Units for the United States.

URL: `ftp://dis2qvarsa.er.usgs.gov/data/giras/hu`

3.4.7. GIRAS Land Use Data
This directory contains all the 1:100,000-scale and 1:250,000-scale data files of land use and land cover maps for the United States. These files were obtained from the National Mapping Division in GIRAS format and were compressed using the UNIX compress command.

URL: `ftp://dis2qvarsa.er.usgs.gov/data/giras/lu`

3.4.8. Digital Data on India
Digital data for India includes nationwide district-level data from the 1961, 1971, and 1981 censuses and from annual agricultural production statistics.

URL: `ftp://cwmills.umd.edu/pub/india`

3.4.9. Timezone Boundary Data
Arthur David Olson has created a public domain time zone database, but it does not include latitude/longitude boundaries.

URL: `ftp://elsie.nci.nih.gov/pub/tzcode94d.tar.gz:code`
URL: `ftp://elsie.nci.nih.gov/pub/tzdata94d.tar.gz:data`

3.4.10. EROS Data Center
This site has lots of useful things from software source code to vast amounts of data.

URL: `ftp://edcftp.cr.usgs.gov`

3.4.11. DLGs of US at 1:100,000 and 1:2,000,000 scale
Digital Line Graph data sets of USA.

URL: `ftp://edcftp.cr.usgs.gov/pub/data/DLG/`

3.4.12. US Land Use/Land Cover at 1:100,000 and 1:250,000 scale
URL: `ftp://edcftp.cr.usgs.gov/pub/data/LULC`

3.4.13. Digital Elevation Models (DEMs)

3.4.13.1. Software

3.4.13.1.1. MicroDEM—DEM Software
Microdem is a set of pascal programs with source code which do all kinds of things with DEM data, and includes one data set. The program is shareware and available from the author:
    Dr. Peter Guth PETMAR TRILOBITE BREEDING RANCH 252 Lower Magothy Beach Road Severna Park, MD 21146

URL: `ftp://ftp.blm.gov/pub/gis/microdem.zip`

3.4.13.1.2. GRIDPAK—3D Gridding Software
URL: `ftp://ahab.rutgers.edu/pub/gridpak`

3.4.13.1.3. SPLAT—Contouring Software
SPLAT is a contouring package.

The file to download is called `SPLATSFX.EXE` which is a self extracting (PK) archive of the program `SPLAT.EXE` and a short manual in windows write format.

URL: `ftp://cica.indiana.edu/pub/pc`

URL: `ftp://nic.funet.fi/pub/msdos`

3.4.13.2. Data

3.4.13.2.1. Mars DEMs
Mars DEM data (Valles Marineris region) sampled at a variety of spatial resolutions.

URL: `ftp://stardent.arc.nasa.gov/pub/`

IP: `128.102.21.44`

3.4.13.2.2. US 3-Arc-second DEMs
3 arc-second DEM data in 1 degree square segments for most of the U.S.

URL: `ftp://resdgs1.er.usgs.gov/dems`

IP: `130.11.52.55`

3.4.13.2.3. DEMs of USA 1:250,000 scale
URL: `ftp://edcftp.cr.usgs.gov/pub/data/DEM/250/`

3.4.13.2.4. ETOPO5 World Topographic Dataset
These files contain worldwide bathymetric and elevation data in meters with a 5 minute by 5 minute latitude/longitude data density.

URL: `ftp://walrus.wr.usgs.gov/pub/data/etopo5.northern.bat.Z (8.3 Mb)`

URL: `ftp://walrus.wr.usgs.gov/pub/data/etopo5.southern.bat.Z (7.9 Mb)`

IP: `130.118.7.254`

Contact: `norman@OCTOPUS.WR.USGS.GOV` (Norman Maher)

URL: `ftp://ahab.rutgers.edu/pub/gridpak/etopo5`

3.4.13.2.5. Map Datasets—DLG, DEM, TIGER USGS DLG
This is a gold mine of a site for mapping data. It is a DEM, DTM, TIGER Data exchange site for all kinds of public domain map data.

URL: `ftp://spectrum.xerox.com/pub/map/`

IP: `192.70.225.78`

Contact: `Moore.Wbst128@Xerox.Com` (Lee Moore)

3.4.13.2.6. DEMs of the San Francisco Area
The data have a horizontal resolution of 3.0 X 3.0 seconds of lat/long degrees and have a vertical resolution of 1.0 meters.

```
sf24.dem  38.0  37.0  -123.0  -122.0  SAN FRANCISCO, CA
sj13.dem  38.0  37.0  -122.0  -121.0  SAN JOSE, CA
sx24.dem  37.0  36.0  -123.0  -122.0  SANTA CRUZ, CA
zp13.dem  37.0  36.0  -122.0  -121.0  MONTEREY, CA
```

URL: `ftp://edcftp.cr.usgs.gov/pub/data/DEM`

IP: `130.118.7.254`

Contact: `norman@OCTOPUS.WR.USGS.GOV` (Norman Maher)

3.4.13.2.7. DEMs of Haiti and Madagascar
These are 30 arc-second DEMs created by EROS from the elevation contours from the Digital Chart of the World CD-ROM dataset.

URL: `ftp://edcftp.cr.usgs.gov/pub/data/30ASDCWDEM/`

3.4.14. CIA World Map database
The CIA World map database is a set of coastlines, rivers, political boundaries developed by the CIA years ago, and released via the Freedom of Information Act. The data was captured at a scale of 1:5,000,000 I believe. It's got a few errors as some counties have changed boundaries since its release, but it's not bad for world maps. The data are not topologically structured, so all you can get is lines, no polygons. Pity, that. This is all over the place too. A few sites that have it now are:

URL: `ftp://gis.queensu.ca/pub/gis/cia/`
URL: `ftp://ftp.cs.toronto.edu/doc/geography/`
URL: `ftp://ftp.uu.net/graphics/maps/WorldMap.tar.Z-split`

3.4.15. City Locations

3.4.15.1. World Cities
Coarse lat/long file for cities around the world.

URL: `ftp://gis.queensu.ca/pub/gis/city/`

3.4.15.2. World & US Cities
URL: `ftp://ftp.cs.toronto.edu/doc/geography/`

3.5. Environmental

3.5.1. GERMINAL project (GIS for Environmental Management and Planning)
Document follows developments on the GERMINAL project (GIS for Environmental Management and Planning). Subject headings are "Geographic Information Systems" and "Environment".

URL: `http://dgrwww.epfl.ch/GERMINAL/Germinal.html`

3.5.2. ANU—Australian National University—Bioinformatics
URL: `http://life.anu.edu.au:80/`

3.5.3. ANU—Landscape Ecology Services
URL: `http://life.anu.edu.au/landscape_ecology/landscape.html`

3.5.4. ERIN—Australian Environmental Resources Information Network
ERIN is experimenting with providing metadata through database queries, automatic generation of species distribution maps, biological modelling, many and varied documents, and actual geographic information bits and bytes. They also have links to all sorts of other interesting environmental and GIS servers and resources.

ERIN's purpose is to make environmental information available to the Commonwealth of Australia Department of Environment and associated agencies.

URL: `http://kaos.erin.gov.au/erin.html`
Contact: `davidc@ERIN.GOV.AU` (David Crossley)

3.5.5. HOLIT—Israel Ecological & Environmental Information System
URL: `http://www.huji.ac.il/www_teva/db000.html`

3.5.6. Environmental Science Gopher at UC Santa Cruz
URL: `gopher://scilibx.ucsc.edu:70/11/The Researcher/Science and Engineering/Environmental Science`

3.5.7. EnviroGopher at Carnegie Mellon University
URL: `gopher://envirolink.org/1/`

3.6. Forestry

3.6.1. Forest Management DSS software
HSG (Harvest Schedule Generator) is a spatially referenced forest inventory projection tool developed by Tom Moore and Cary Lockwood of the Petawawa National Forestry Institute. This tool is designed to assist forest managers and others in the design and evaluation of forest management strategies.

URL: `ftp://pi19.pnfi.forestry.ca/pub/hsglite`

3.6.2. Oregon State Univ, Forestry Sciences Laboratory
This gopher is maintained by the Forest Science Laboratory of Oregon State University, Corvallis, Oregon. The primary purpose is to allow users to find GIS (Geographic Information System) files among our rather extensive collection of geographic data.

The gopher operates solely as an index. This means that you will not be able to retrieve GIS files directly through the gopher system.

If you are interested in obtaining GIS data, we recommend that you first use the gopher to identify the particular files that you want. Once you have identified the files, please fill out the request form (if you do not have accounts on fsl machines) and email it to: `GIS-request@fsl.orst.edu`

When the available data are ready for transfer, you will receive a confirmation of the name of your file and the date it can be accessed in an anonymous ftp area for downloading. Data is made available within 1—2 working days of your request, although priority may be given to financial benefactors.

URL: `gopher://gopher.fsl.orst.edu:70/1`

3.7. Geography

3.7.1. Geographic Name Server
Zipcode, population, lat/long other stats from 1980 census for US cities. Enter name of city at the (non-existent) prompt and press Enter. Include state (as in Ipswich, MA) or you'll get that city's information in every state it is found. Type 'quit' to exit.

Tom Liebert (author of the GNS) reports: GNS covers only USA now, but I just received global city data from CIA RWDB2. I'll incorporate that fairly soon.

URL: `telnet://martini.eecs.umich.edu:3000`
IP: `141.212.99.9, 141.212.100.9`
Contact: `libert@eecs.umich.edu` (Tom Libert, GNS author)

3.7.2. Japan Geography
URL: `http://www.ntt.jp/japan/index.html`

3.7.3. Project GeoSim—Geography education software
URL: `http://geosim.cs.vt.edu/index.html`

3.7.4. Gazetter for the U.S.
URL: `http://wings.buffalo.edu/geogw`

3.7.5. Geography Datasets—US Census Data
The file Census.part1.Z contains part 1 of the 1980 US Census county boundaries. The other parts do not seem to be available. This site also contains a copy of the CIA World Databank II and a shell

archive file to create two C programs to compress and/or map the WDB data (`wdb-ii.z`) Note: This site is extremely fussy about the password you use. You must use your actual, full email address, or you won't be granted access.

URL: `ftp://ftp.uu.net/pub/Census`

IP: `192.48.96.9`

3.7.6. CIA World Fact Book

The CIA World Factbook contains summary information about the countries of the world including size and population,, commercial, military, and political data.

There are many places where this data set can be found on the Internet. The best way to find the latest versions is to use Veronica and search for "world factbook". Also note that this is updated each year.

URL: `ftp://ftp.cs.toronto.edu/doc/geography`

3.8. Geology & Geophysics

3.8.1. Mineralogy

3.8.1.1. Minerals Database

This is a database containing the names and chemical formulas of all currently accepted mineral species, 3507 or so of them. It is now available in a plain ASCII version which is easily importable in your favorite database program, and in a Microsoft RTF format.

URL: `ftp://c.scs.uiuc.edu`

Contact: `mcdonald@aries.scs.uiuc.edu` (Doug McDonald)

3.8.1.2. Mineral ID database

Mineral ID for the Macintosh computer is an interactive database of minerals, crystallographic systems, and mineralogy terms for both educational and reference purposes. For more information, e-mail me, and I will send you a full information sheet.

Contact: `liquori@lamar.ColoState.EDU` (Michael Liquori)

3.8.1.3. Rock forming mineral compositional database; PROBE software

URL: `ftp://perry.berkeley.edu/outgoing/donovan/`

3.8.1.4. Crystallography for the Macintosh

URL: `ftp://mac.archive.umich.edu/Crystal`

URL: `ftp://mac.archive.umich.edu/CrystalView`

Contact: `thomas.h.kosel.1@nd.edu` (Tom Kosel)

3.8.2. Earthquakes

3.8.2.1. NCEER Strong Motion Data Facility

URL: `telnet://strongmo:nceer@duke.ldgo.columbia.edu:23/8`

3.8.2.2. Center for Earthquake Research and Information (CERI Memphis St U)

URL: `gopher://gopher.ceri.memst.edu/1`

3.8.2.3. USGS Branch of Global Seismology and Geomagnetism

URL: `telnet://QED@neis.cr.usgs.gov`

3.8.2.4. Oklahoma Earthquake Catalog

URL: `gopher://wealaka.okgeosurvey1.gov:70/11/okeqcat`

3.8.2.5. Earthquake Information
The Usenet newsgroup ca.earthquakes is a good source of earthquake information and news.

Northern California

URL: `finger:quake@andreas.wr.usgs.gov`

Other sources

URL: `finger:quake@eqinfo.seis.utah.edu`
URL: `finger:quake@geophys.washington.edu`

Official office of emergency services bulletin site

URL: `telnet://oes1.oes.ca.gov:5501`

3.8.2.6. Geologic Faults Map Data
Digitized database of geologic faults (primarily for different parts of the U.S.) and California earthquake locations.

URL: `ftp://alum.wr.usgs.gov/pub/mapFaults data`
URL: `ftp://alum.wr.usgs.gov/pub/summaryEarthquake locations`

Contact: oppen@alum.wr.usgs.gov (David Oppenheimer)

3.8.2.7. Earthquake Maps & Charts of the Northridge earthquake
This site contains data, graphs, and maps relating to the Northridge Quake. They have been collected from sci.geo.geology and ca.earthquakes, and ftped from caltech. There are postscript (ps), GIF (gif), and text (txt) files.

URL: `ftp://ftp.stat.ucla.edu/pub/data/various/quake/`

3.8.2.8. World Earthquake Data via "Finger"
URL: `finger://quake@geophys.washington.edu`

3.8.3. USGS Digital Map Open-File Reports
The Geologic Division of the USGS (Central Region) has a server that functions as a repository for on-line publications. You can find the following digital map Open-file Reports:

```
ofr-92-0328: The digital geologic map of the Roswell Resource Area, New
Mexico, in ARC/INFO export format.
ofr-92-0507: The digital geologic map of Colorado in ARC/INFO export for-
mat.
ofr-90-0676: Interactive Macintosh display of petroleum exploration
through time across the continental United States.
```

URL: `ftp://greenwood.cr.usgs.gov/pub/open-file-reports/`
IP: `136.177.48.5`
Contact: gellis@ctr-dms1.cr.usgs.gov (Eugene Ellis)

3.8.4. Geologic finite-element software
Three finite-element programs for modeling plate deformation are now available by anonymous FTP. They can be used to model deformation of the lithosphere, formulate tectonic hypotheses, fit geodetic data, estimate long-term seismic hazard, study the rheology of the plates, or teach students.

Each program is accompanied by explanatory text files, sample input and output files, and accessory programs for help in preparing the input and plotting graphics from the output.

Source code (FORTRAN77) is available.

URL: `ftp://pong.igpp.ucla.edu/pub/pbird/read_me`

Contact: Peter Bird pbird@ess.ucla.edu

3.8.5. StereoNet for Windows
StereoNet for Windows is a program for plotting on stereonets and performing 3D analysis and recalculations. If you are working on any of the above named subjects a lot of time can be saved by letting your PC do this work. The plots are ready for publication when they come out of your printer.

Some features:
```
Schmidt or Wulff nets.
Plotting planar data, as great circles.
Plotting points, with a number of different symbols
Plotting density contours.
Plotting rose diagrams.
Plotting statistics (mean, girdle, pole to girdle)
Plotting slip linear plots
Color support, the user can define any color.
```
URL: `ftp://torsken.nfh.uit.no/stereo/`
IP: 129.242.211.254
Contact: `perivar@ibg.uit.no` (Per Ivar Steinsund)

3.8.6. USGS—United States Geological Survey
URL: `http://sun1.cr.usgs.gov`

3.8.7. Arizona Geologic Survey (AzGS)
URL: `gopher://dillon.geo.ep.utexas.edu:70/11/EarthScienceRes/Publications/AZ.GeolSurv`

3.8.8. El Paso Geological Society Publication list
URL: `gopher://dillon.geo.ep.utexas.edu:70/00/EarthScienceRes/Publications/ElPasoGS`

3.8.9. Computer Oriented Geological Society (COGS)
Archives Contains COGS diskettes and other software collected from COGSnet BBS including geologic, GIS, mapping, earth science software for the PC and Macintosh. Includes several mapping data sets of use to all, or pointers to where they can be found. GSMAP and MOSS can be found here.
URL: `ftp://ftp.csn.org/COGS/`
IP: 128.138.213.21
Contact: `bthoen@gisnet.com` (Bill Thoen)

3.8.10. Geological Symbol Font
Font in Adobe Type 1 and True Type formats (both for the PC) contains geological symbols. It has also been converted to a CorelDRAW "wfn" file so it may be installed as a symbol for FCorelDRAW 3.x and 4.x.
   Also CorelDRAW "pat" files containing geological patterns.
URL: `ftp://opal.geology.utoronto.ca/pub/geology/corel/symbols/:Fonts`
URL: `ftp://opal.geology.utoronto.ca/pub/geology/corel/patterns/:Patterns`
Contact: `charters@madhaus.uucp` (Jim Charters)

3.8.11. CIA World Databank-II Map Data
This is a data file of coastlines, countries, rivers, islands and lakes of the world compiled by the CIA and now de-classified into the public domain. It's a large database; over 12 megabytes, compressed! This file is broken up into 5 pieces, so you have to get them all separately and 'cat' them together. The file is tightly packed in a binary format, and to read it you will need to use the C program contained in the archive, `domap.c`. The national boundary data is out-of-date as there have been many changes in the world since the late 80's. However it seems to be the best source for free world map data.

URL: `ftp://sepftp.stanford.edu/`

3.8.12. Sunrise/Sunset Calculations
Calculate sunrise and sunset for anyplace not 'close' to the poles. The source includes both 'print to screen' and 'print to printer' versions. Executable versions are here too.

URL: `ftp://ftpnssl.nssl.uoknor.edu/pub/skaggs/sunrise.bas`

IP: `129.15.66.34`

3.8.13. World Paleomagnetic Database
Databases, programs and information related to paleomagnetism.

URL: `ftp://earth.eps.pitt.edu/pub`

IP: `130.49.3.1`

3.8.14. Magnetic Field Computing programs
URL: `ftp://ftp.ngdc.noaa.gov`

Contact: `npeddie@isdres.er.usgs.edu`

3.8.15. Geochemistry—NewPet Software
This is an ftp site for NewPet, a geochem/igneous petrology data handling program. Includes ternary plots. MS-DOS compatible shareware ($25 voluntary).

URL: `ftp://sparky2.esd.mun.ca/geoprogs`

IP: `134.153.11.101`

3.8.16. Geological Hypercard Stacks
Macintosh Hypercard stacks pertaining to geology: bedforms An application for geometric simulation of sedimentary structures produced by migrating bedforms over time. Companion to the book "Bedforms, Cross-Bedding, and Sedimentary Structures" by David M. Rubin, published by SEPM. QuickTime animations of selected figures from the book. Best viewed on a screen 640x480 pixels or larger, set to 256 *grays* (not colors). Each of these files is a HyperCard stack with instructions and a pattern for making a three-dimensional model of one or more interesting landforms:

```
earthquake_effects
effects_of_ice
island_coral_reefs
loma_prieta
seven_faults
volcano map projections:
```

Hypertext files on USGS map projections usa-exploration:

USA Exploration—USGS OFR 90-676. This application illustrates the history of oil and gas exploration in the United States from 1900 to 1986.

URL: `ftp://ftp.walrus.wr.usgs.gov/pub/mac`

IP: `130.118.7.254`
Contact: `dr@octopus.wr.usgs.gov`

3.8.17. University of Minnesota Soil Science Gopher
URL: `gopher://gopher.soils.umn.edu:70/11`

3.8.18. Time Dependent Topography Through the Glacial Cycle
This site contains data sets of topography and ice coverage during the last glacial maximum. The topography data set contains elevation at 1 Kyr intervals, with elevations in meters. The second data set contains ice-cover data at 1 Kyr intervals. Area of coverage is the entire globe in a 1 x 1 degree grid, with a temporal range of 21KBP to the present.

URL: `ftp://rainbow.physics.utoronto.ca/pub/iceA/README`

IP: `128.100.75.19` (unofficial)

3.8.19. Water Quality Data Directory
URL: `gopher://scilibx.ucsc.edu:70/7/waissrc:/.WAIS/water-quality.src`

3.8.20. IGWR—Institute for Ground Water Research
URL: `gopher://igwmc.mines.colorado.edu:3851`

3.9. Geographic Information Systems (GIS)

3.9.1. Tallahassee Freenet (Internet GIS BBS)
Select SCIENCE AND TECHNOLOGY CENTRE from their main menu.

URL: `telnet://freenet.fsu.edu`

3.9.2. USGS beginners tutorial on GIS
URL: `http://waisqvarsa.er.usgs.gov/wais/home.html`

3.9.3. GeoSim module (MigModel)
Project GeoSim is a multidisciplinary effort by members of Virginia Tech's Departments of Geography and Computer Science, and College of Education, to develop computer-aided education software for introductory geography at the college and high school levels. Supported by NSF and FIPSE (US Dept. of Education), GeoSim's goal is to produce major changes in undergraduate geography education by applying the immense capabilities of Geographic Information Systems (GIS) and simulation.

Project GeoSim's primary activity is the creation of a series of computerized laboratory modules applicable to virtually all introductory geography courses. The first module, Intlpop/Humpop is meant to teach the basics of demographics and population modeling.

Intlpop is an interactive simulation and Humpop is a multimedia tutorial on population issues. The version presently available runs under MS-DOS (Intlpop alone) or MS Windows (both Humpop and Intlpop together). Versions running under the X Window System and the Macintosh operating system should be available sometime during Spring 1994.

MigModel, a program for studying modeling of migration patterns between counties of the US, is now available in preliminary form. This program allows students to select several variables from a larger list that the student hypothesizes affect migration patterns. The patterns that would result if the hypothesis were true are compared against the actual migration patterns to determine the level of correlation.

URL: `http://geosim.cs.vt.edu/index.html`
URL: `ftp://geosim.cs.vt.edu`
IP: `128.173.40.85`
URL: `gopher://geosim.cs.vt.edu`
IP: `128.173.40.85`
Contact: `shaffer@vtopus.cs.vt.edu` (Cliff Shaffer)
Contact: `carstens@vtvm1.cc.vt.edu` (Bill Carstensen)

3.9.4. CERL/GRASS welcome file
URL: `http://baldrick.cecer.army.mil:80/welcome.html`

3.9.5. OzGIS Mapping System
OzGIS is a software system for displaying geographically referenced data, such as Census data or environment data, as maps and diagrams on screens, printers and plotters on an IBM PC compatible. The system can be used to analyze socio-economic data produced by censuses and surveys and to support management decisions associated with for example Government planning, marketing, sales, site and personnel location, advertising. Digitized map data (e.g.,Census boundaries, GIS) and attribute data (e.g., sales, environmental) are accepted as Ascii files and preprocessed (e.g., amalgamation, line thinning, polygon construction, subsetting) before display. Maps of polygons, lines and points can be displayed according to one or two attributes along with various overlays. About 130 menus provide extensive options for interactively designing the layout and appearance of the map, and for attribute

handling, classification, interrogation and saving maps. Maps can be output on plotters, printers and various file types. Applications such as territory definition and retail site catchment analysis are supported.

URL: `ftp://oak.oakland.edu`

IP: `141.210.10.117`

URL: `ftp://wuarchive.wustl.edu`

IP: `128.252.135.4`

URL: `ftp://archive.orst.edu`

IP: `128.193.2.13`

URL: `ftp://ftp.uu.net`

IP: `137.39.1.9`

URL: `ftp://nic.funet.fi`

IP: `128.214.6.100`

URL: `ftp://src.doc.ic.ac.uk`

IP: `146.169.3.7`

URL: `ftp://nic.switch.ch`

IP: `130.59.1.40`

URL: `ftp://archie.au`

IP: `139.130.4.6`

URL: `ftp://nctuccca.edu.tw`

IP: `140.111.3.21`

Contact: `lws@ITD0.DSTO.GOV.AU` (Lloyd Simons)

3.9.6. GRASS/Linux Support Group

The old address (`st00@siuemus`) is no longer valid. For information or technical support on GRASS/Linux, please send a message to the following new address.

Contact: `CCAO@SIUEMUS.BITNET`

Contact: `ahrensl@daisy.siue.edu`

> XIS Solutions
> Box 1459, SIUE
> Edwardsville, IL 62026
> Tel: 618-692-2090

3.9.7. GRASS GIS Source Code

In addition to the GRASS GIS source code, there is an extensive database for the Spearfish (South Dakota) area to be used with GRASS. Although intended for GRASS, some of the data could easily be used for other purposes. For example, Arc/Information can display GRASS raster data. The README in /grass says that it is open 24 hours a day, 7 days a week.)

URL: `ftp://moon.cecer.army.mil/grass`

IP: `129.229.1.16`

3.9.8. Idrisi Files FTP site

This is the ftp site for Idrisi support files.

URL: `ftp://midget.towson.edu`

The Idrisi FAQ file:

URL: `ftp://midget.towson.edu/IDRISI/OTHER`

3.9.9. Miscellaneous GIS source code

This site has been known to briefly contain some interesting-looking files on the subjects of GIS, MOSS, mapping and other code fragments and subroutines along the same lines.

URL: `ftp://ftp.blm.gov/pub/gis/`

IP: `158.68.32.62`

Contact: `skatz@dsc.blm.gov`

3.9.10. Hydrology

USGS Streamflow Data sets 1874-1988 This site contains data on USGS streamflow statistics from 1874 to 1988 (that's no typo... it's *1874*).

The USGS Open-File Report 92-129, "Hydro-Climatic Data Network (HCDN): A U.S. Geological Survey streamflow data set for the United States for the study of climate variations, 1874-1988", by J.R. Slack and Jurate Maciunas Landwehr is available here also, and serves as documentation for the data set. See the `1ST_READ.ME` file for details.

URL: `ftp://srv1rvares.er.usgs.gov/hcdn92`

IP: `130.11.51.209`

3.10. GPS & Geodesy

GPS satellite current constellation status.

URL: `finger://gps@geomac.se.unb.ca`

3.10.1. GPS & Loran Information Center, U.S. Coast Guard

This is a BBS accessed via the Fedworld Gateway.

URL: `telnet://fedworld.gov`

3.10.2. GPStech Mailing List

Mailing list for the discussion of GPS technical issues. The intended audience is earth scientists and geodesists interested in high-precision GPS geodesy.

The mailing list is accessible by sending a message to the server

Server: `gpstech-request@cotopaxi.stanford.edu`

Contact: Jeff Freymueller at Stanford

3.10.3. CANSPACE—Canadian Space Geodesy Forum

This site is one of the best for GPS and Geodesy information

URL: `gopher://unbmvs1.csd.unb.ca:1570/1EXEC%3aCANSPACE`

3.10.4. Earth Disc image

This is a 2500x2499 pixel full-disc 11.5um (infrared) image of the earth taken by the METEOSAT 4 satellite on 16 September 1993.

Rick Kohrs (`rickk@ssec.wisc.edu`) colored the image as follows. He used a threshold temperature to determine which pixels in the image corresponded to clouds. He then removed the cloud pixels from consideration. Since the temperatures over land and sea overlap, he used a base map to separate the remaining pixels into sea and land groups. At this point he had three partial images: (a) clouds, (b) unclouded sea, and (c) unclouded land. Based on temperatures he colored each of these separately using an appropriate fraction of the total number of cells available in an 8-bit color map. The combined image you see here uses the whole set of 256 colors.

URL: `ftp://ssec.wisc.edu/pub/dws/em930916.jpg` JPEG version

URL: `ftp://ssec.wisc.edu/pub/dws/em930916.gif` GIF version

IP: `144.92.108.61`

3.11. Mapping

3.11.1. GeoVu—Windows Mapping software

URL: `ftp://ftp.ngdc.noaa.gov/Acess_Tools`

Contact: `amh@ngdc.noaa.gov` (Allen Hittelman)

3.11.2. JHU/APL Digital relief maps of U.S.
URL: **http://ageninfo.tamu.edu/apl-us/**

3.11.3. WWW map for Japan
URL: **http://www.ntt.jp/japan/map**

3.11.4. VPFVIEW (DCW) program for UNIX (Sun workstations)
Program for UNIX systems to view maps from the DMA's Digital Chart of the World CDROM data set.
URL: **ftp://jupiter.drev.dnd.ca/pub/gis/vpfview**
IP: **131.132.32.2**

3.11.5. EPI-MAP GIS source and data
Thematic mapping system developed by the Center for Disease Control and Prevention in Atlanta, GA. (USA). Includes many data sets of various country political boundaries down to the state/province (2nd order) level. US counties are also included.
URL: **ftp://oak.oakland.edu/pub/msdos/mapping/emap***
IP: **141.210.10.117**

3.11.6. GMT—Generic Mapping Tools software source
URL: **ftp://kiawe.soest.hawaii.edu/pub/gmt**
IP: **128.171.151.16**

3.11.7. GRASS GIS source for LINUX
URL: **ftp://topquark.cecer.army.mil/pub/grass**
IP: **129.229.32.13**

3.11.8. KHOROS—Scientific Visualizaion Software
URL: **ftp://pprg.eece.unm.edu/pub/khoros/release**
IP: **129.24.24.10**

3.11.9. MapInfo & MapBasic Files
MapBasic applications, many with source code, data sets for MapInfo, and information files of tips and tricks for working with MapInfo. See also MAPINFO-L , the MapInfo mailing list.
URL: **ftp://ftp.csn.org/mapinfo/**
IP: **128.138.213.21**
Contact: bthoen@gisnet.com (Bill Thoen)

3.11.10. MOSS—PC GIS
PC MOSS executables and data.
URL: **ftp://ftp.csn.org/COGS/MOSS/**
IP: **128.138.213.21**
Contact: skatz@dsc.blm.gov (Sol Katz)

3.11.11. Sample ETOPO5 data set relief images
Texas A&M University
URL: **ftp://ageninfo.tamu.edu/11/apl-us**
IP: **128.194.173.6**

3.11.12. LINUX—UNIX on DOS platform
URL: **ftp://sc.tamu.edu**
IP: **128.194.167.3**

3.11.13. MAPGEN/PLOTGEN Mapping Software

This is the primary source of the MAPGEN/PLOTGEN public-domain software. Other source code of general interest, including the USGS General Cartographic Transformation Package (GCTP-II), is also available here. A newer projection package, proj4.2 is available here.

URL: **ftp://charon.er.usgs.gov/pub/**

IP: 128.128.40.24

Contact: gie@charon.er.usgs.gov (G.I. Evenden)

3.11.14. USGS General Cartographic Transformation Package

Source code for the USGS General Cartographic Transformation Package (GCTP-II). This software can be used to calculate lat/long conversions between various projections used on USGS maps.

URL: **ftp://isdres.er.usgs.gov/pub/usgs/gctp/**

IP: 130.11.48.2

3.11.15. Generic Mapping Tools (GMT) Software

Contains the Generic Mapping Tools (gmt) software by Paul Wessel for map projections, spatial interpolation, contouring, 3D perspective, raster processing (postscript). This is C code designed for UNIX workstations (Sun, DEC, SGI, and NeXT).

URL: **http://www.soest.hawaii.edu/soest/about.ftp.html**

URL: **ftp://kiawe.soest.hawaii.edu/pub/gmt/**

IP: 128.171.151.16

Contact: wessel@soest.hawaii.edu (Paul Wessel)

3.11.16. USGS Cartographic Software and Data Documentation

The National Mapping Division of the U. S. Geological Survey (NMD) provides a national series of base cartographic data. Computer software supporting these data is primarily in the FORTRAN language. The software programs are supported on a variety of mainframe, minicomputer, and workstation hardware platforms. This software was previously available to the general public only on 9-track magnetic tape or diskette through the Earth Sciences Information Center (ESIC) for a nominal reproduction and handling fee. Fifteen FORTRAN programs, sample data and job control language are now available on Internet using file transfer protocol (FTP). A limited amount of soft-copy computer program documentation is also available in both Word Perfect and ASCII.

URL: **ftp://nmdpow9.er.usgs.gov/**

IP: 130.11.52.92

Contact: mlinck@usgs.gov (Michael K. Linck, Jr.)

3.11.17. Oceanography Physical oceanography data

URL: **ftp://shrimp.jpl.nasa.gov**

3.11.18. Ocean Network Information Center

OCEANIC database—data about ocean currents for climatic change, subduction zones and deep sea dumping, among other things. A list of information and oceanographers involved in the WOCE project is also available. Also contains descriptions of the following data sets:

>   NODC data sets
>   NCAR data sets
>   Hawaii Sea Level Center data sets
>   JPL DAAC (formerly NODS)
>   ECMWF data sets
>   NSIDC data sets
>   University of Miami data sets
>   University of Rhode Island data sets
>   CDIAC data sets

URL: `telnet://oceanic@delocn.udel.edu`

URL: `gopher://diu.cms.udel.edu/`

URL: `http://diu.cms.udel.edu/`

IP: `128.175.24.1`

3.11.19. Marine and Aquatic Sciences Libraries (UC Santa Cruz)
URL: `gopher://gopher.ucsc.edu:70/11/The Library/Other Libraries/Marine and Aquatic Sciences Serials Lists`

3.11.20. National Oceanographic Data Center (NODC, NOAA)
URL: `gopher://gopher.nodc.noaa.gov:70/11/`

3.11.21. Virginia Coast Reserve Information System (VCRIS)
URL: `gopher://atlantic.evsc.virginia.edu:70/1`

3.11.22. Geological Survey Atlantic Marine Geology
This is a good gateway to other resources, Marine geology, Bathymetry, Great Lakes and more.

URL: `gopher://bramble.er.usgs.gov:70/1`

3.11.23. Bedford Institute of Oceanography (Canada) Gopher System
URL: `gopher://biome.bio.dfo.ca:70/1`

3.11.24. Ocean Network Information Center Software
Home of the World Ocean Circulation Experiment (WOCE) Data Information Unit (DIU). Files include programs to do various oceanographic computations.

URL: `ftp://delocn.udel.edu/FORTRAN`

IP: `128.175.24.1`

Contact: `walt@delocn.udel.edu`

3.11.25. East Coast Tidal Heights & Winds Database
From the file README at this site: "This account is intended to provide an easily accessible data base of tidal heights and winds along the U.S. east coast. This project of the FSU Sea Level Center is funded by C&GC, NOAA. The data set is at present still being accumulated: In the directory pub/Tidedata files labeled .hrly. are hourly data from standard NOAA tidal stations; monthly data are labeled .mon. etc Thus, fernand.mon.9791 is monthly data, Fernandina, Fla, 1897-1991; the data are in standard NOAA format: tides in hundredths of ** FEET** relative to the mean for 1960-1978 National Tidal Datum epoch. (missing data are 9999's) In the directory pub/Opcplot is a set of files from Dr Murray Brown; a flexible set of routines for plotting ocean data; see readme file. In the directory pub/Tides: a Shareware program "Tides" computes tidal heights and currents; in QuickBasic, for IBM PC-comps; In the directory pub/LiveAtlas is a set of files of the oceanographic atlas of Luyten & Stommel. Please see the readme file. In the directory pub the single file tsftdem.ftp is a set of files which constitute the "terribly slow Fourier transform" that recovers the low-frequency spectrum of a gappy data set (under Matlab)"

URL: `ftp://atlantic.ocean.fsu.edu/pub/Tidedata`

IP: `128.186.3.39`

Contact: `sturges@atlantic.ocean.fsu.edu`

3.11.26. Sea-surface temperature data (near real-time)
The data are AVHRR images within the radius of reception of the university's HRPT station, approximately 5S to 45N and 125W to 165E. Other tiles (windows) are available over California, Gulf of Mexico and West Atlantic as well.

URL: `ftp://satftp.soest.hawaii.edu/pub/avhrr/images`

IP: 128.171.154.29

Contact: sat_lab@soest.hawaii.edu

3.11.27. Digital relief images of USA
Topographic relief images created from the ETOPO5 data set by Ray Sterner.

URL: http://ageninfo.tamu.edu/apl-us/

URL: gopher://ageninfo.tamu.edu/11/apl-us

Contact: hmueller@amethyst.tamu.edu (Hal Mueller)

3.11.28. Color Shaded Relief Map of the U.S.
A color shaded relief map of the US is available as 60 GIF images.

Individual GIF images cover a 5 deg by 5 deg area. These images are being made available on a trial basis on our ftp site. Please do not copy more than 1 or 2 images during working hours (8:30 to 7:00 pm Eastern Standard Time) or they may have to be removed.

The elevation data is from ETOPO5 which has a horizontal resolution of 1/2 arc minute for both East/West and North/South, and a vertical resolution of 20 feet. The vector data (coastlines, rivers, boundaries) are from the world vector data base. There are some areas where the two data bases have minor differences in positioning, most noticeable for some rivers. The errors are not constant over the map and no attempt has been made to correct for them in this version of the map.

URL: ftp://fermi.jhuapl.edu/pub/gifmap

IP: 128.244.147.18

Contact: sterner@tesla.jhuapl.edu (Ray Sterner)

3.11.29. Diamondhead Oahu 3D GIF Image
Images of a honolulu dem file converted to several .gif files.

URL: ftp://ftp.cerf.net/pub/inbound/KV_TMP

3.11.30. 3D DEM images of San Francisco
Images of USGS San Francisco topography created with VisionForm's Vdm; JPEG compressed.

URL: ftp://ftp.cerf.net/pub/inbound/KV_TMP/README_SANF

Contact: jsquires@nic.cerf.net (James A. Squires)

3.11.31. Digital relief maps of U.S.
Created from the ETOPO5 data set (5 arc-minute resolution)

URL: http://www.doc.ic.ac.uk/public/geology/maps/gifmaps/

URL: ftp://src.doc.ic.ac.uk/geology/maps/gifmaps

IP: 146.169.2.10

3.11.32. Mid-East Maps from 1000 BCE to Gulf War
This service is primarily dedicated to information about Israel politics, and other government information, but the "graphics" option contains GIF maps of Israel and the nearby Arab states. Maps depict the limits of the Kingdom of David and Solomon of 1000 BCE to missile strikes during the Gulf War.

URL: gopher://israel-info.gov.il

3.11.33. US GeoData indexes
These indexes are the same as the graphic indexes showing the availability of the DEM 7.5' and 15' Units, DEM 1-Degree Units, DLG 7.5' and 15' Units, DLG 30' Units, LULC 30' Units, LULC 1-Degree Units, CD ROM Data, and also about 400 DOQ listings.

URL: ftp://greenwood.cr.usgs.gov/pub/open-file-reports/

IP: 136.177.48.5

Contact: gellis@ctr-dms1.cr.usgs.gov (Eugene Ellis)

3.11.34. Canadian Province Boundary Data
Coarse boundary file of Canada (self-extracting ZIP file). It is a DXF format file using lat/long coordinates.
URL: `ftp://gis.queensu.ca/pub/gis/canada-d.exe`

3.11.35. Color Shaded Relief Map Images
GIF images are made with ER Mapper.
URL: `ftp://earth.eps.pitt.edu/pub/ermapper/`
IP: `130.49.3.1`

3.12. Paleontology

3.12.1. University of California—Berkeley, Museum of Paleontology
URL: `gopher://ucmp1.berkeley.edu:70/1`

3.13. Remote Sensing

3.13.1. AVHRR Images—Western US
AVHRR (Advanced Very High Resolution Radiometer) images from 1989 through 7 Jan 1992 cover CO, WY, KS, NE, and NM, as well as parts of AZ, UT, OK, and TX. Since 7 Jan 1992, coverage includes these plus CA, OR, NV, WA, and MT, to 1000 km off Pacific coast. Total coverage of US for 1989-present will be available soon. West coast data from 1980-1985 will be available some time this year.

Images are 1024 lines x 1024 elements before 7 Jan 1992, 2560 lines x 1024 elements after. Images are 1 km resolution and 8-bit format.

Contact Tim Kelley by e-mail `kelley@sanddunes.scd.ucar.edu` or telephone 303/497-1221 for login, password, and manual. Service is free to Internet users and is funded by NASA.

URL: `telnet://sanddunes.scd.ucar.edu` (for login password, contact Tim Kelly)
Contact: `kelley@sanddunes.scd.ucar.edu` (Tim Kelly)

3.13.2. Satellite Images
URL: `http://web.nexor.co.uk/places/satelite.html`

3.13.3. SRSC—Space Remote Sensing Center satellite flood images (U.S./Europe)
URL: `http://ma.itd.com:8000/flood.html`

3.13.4. EROS Data Center, the USGS repository for Remote Sensing data
URL: `http://sun1.cr.usgs.gov/eros-home.html`

3.13.5. EROS—Remote Sensing Data Center
URL: `http://sun1.cr.usgs.gov/eros-home.html`

3.13.6. Institute for Photogrammetry—University of Stuttgart
URL: `http://hpux.bauingenieure.uni-stuttgart.de`

3.13.7. NASA—Images from the Voyager and Magellan missions
URL: `ftp://explorer.arc.nasa.gov/pub/SPACE/`
IP: `128.102.32.18`

3.13.8. Images of Planets
Planetary images from Magellean and Viking missions. News about other NASA missions.
URL: `ftp://explorer.arc.nasa.gov/pub/SPACE/GIF/`

Famous image of Earth taken by one of the Apollo missions to the moon:

URL: `ftp://explorer.arc.nasa.gov/pub/SPACE/GIF/earth.gif`

IP: `128.102.18.3`

3.13.9. Snow Cover Satellite Images

US Map of snow cover for the US, derived from 12km reduction of GOES data. Also 1km resolution snow cover maps of California and Nevada, Snow Water Equivalent and other images The National Operational Hydrologic Remote Sensing Center is now distributing satellite snow data derived from AVHRR and GOES for major portions of the U.S., southern Canada and Alaska. North America is split into 26 windows, each approx 1000x1000 pixels, at a resolution of 1.1 km/pixel. There are a number of types of GIF images in this directory: the Satellite Snow Cover Maps, weekly national and regional summaries and a special blow-up of the Upper Colorado basin.

URL: `ftp://snow.nohrsc.nws.gov/pub/`

IP: `192.46.108.1`

Contact: `tim@snow.nohrsc.nws.gov` (Tim Szeliga)

3.13.10. Space Shuttle Earth Observation Project Photography Database

Space Shuttle Earth Observation Project photography database of the Flight Science Support Office (FSSO). Contains references to over 120,000 photographs of Earth from space during the last 3 decades. Also some digitized images. These are in band-sequential format with a 512-byte header, and 512 x 512 bytes of red, green, and blue data layers. The images are stored in .DAT files and are binary. There are two types of photos available: 1024 x 1024 and 512 x 512. Some are 3 channel, Some are 1 channel. Note: Get the file 'pho.list' to see descriptions of selected images, and which are color and which are grey-scale. The 1024x1024 are 1 channel and the 512x512 are 3 channel. Adobe Photoshop (Macintosh) reads these just fine.

URL: `ftp://sseop.jsc.nasa.gov`

IP: `146.154.11.34`

Contact: `pitts@sn.jsc.nasa.gov` (Dr. David E. Pitts, Manager)

3.13.11. NOAA-11/12 Mosaic Images of North America

NOAA-11/12 mosaic GIF images of North America derived from HRPT (High Resolution Picture Transmission) data stream

URL: `ftp://rainbow.physics.utoronto.ca/pub/sat_images`

IP: `128.100.75.19` (unofficial)

Contact: `moore@rainbow.physics.utoronto.ca` (Professor G.W.K. Moore)

3.13.12. AVHRR sample images and viewers—U.S. Weather Service Hydrologic RS Center

URL: `ftp://snow.nohrsc.nws.gov/pub/avhrr_sample`

IP: `192.46.108.1`

3.13.13. Satellite images

URL: `http://web.nexor.co.uk/places/satelite.html`

3.14. Space & Planetary Science

3.14.1. CASS—Center for Advanced Space Studies

The Center for Advanced Space Studies (previously Lunar/Planetary Institute, or LPI) provides resources on geology, geophysics, astronomy and astrophysics. Support services are provided for other departments, such as publications, and computer. Materials on these topics are available. Menu driven—use VT100 emulation or equivalent.

URL: `telnet://cass:online@cass.jsc.nasa.gov`

URL: `http://cass.jsc.nasa.gov/CASS_home.html`

Contact: `bigwood@cass.jsc.nasa.gov` (David Bigwood)

3.14.2. SPAN—Space Physics Analysis Network

Space Physics Analysis Network (SPAN) Network Information Center (NIC), managed by the National Space Science Data Center (NSSDC), an online facility to provide a central source for information.

URL: `telnet://span_nic@nssdca.gsfc.nasa.gov`

3.14.3. NED—NASA/IPAC Extragalactic Database

NASA/IPAC Extragalactic Database

URL: `telnet://ned@ipac.caltech.edu`
IP: 131.215.139.35

3.14.4. Earth, space science data

URL: `ftp://huntress.jpl.nasa.gov`

3.14.5. JPL public information

URL: `ftp://pubinfo.jpl.nasa.gov/public/jplinfo`

3.14.6. The NASA Home Page

URL: `http://hypatia.gsfc.nasa.gov/NASA_homepage.html`

3.15. Standards

3.15.1. Spatial Data Standards documents

Documentation on the Distributed Spatial Data Library (DSDL), 1992 ASTM Spatial Data Standard, and policy statements.

URL: `ftp://dis2qvarsa.er.usgs.gov/docs`

(Mar 1993) Metadata Standard documents, FGDC definitions, minutes of ASTM, GIS/LIS and URISA meetings

URL: `ftp://dis2qvarsa.er.usgs.gov/metadata`

3.15.2. European Mapping Standards & Reference systems

MEGRIN (Multipurpose European Ground-Related Information Network) is an initiative of the Comité Européen des Responsables de la Cartographie Officielle—C.E.R.C.O.

The concept of MEGRIN is to be a service open to all of those who want to use in their own systems digital spatial data which are produced and administrated in other systems. There you can find information about national spatial information systems in Europe and the European Transfer Format (ETF)

(Note: this site may be closed after June 1, 1994)

URL: `telnet://megrin:megrin@v2.ifag.de`
IP: 141.74.240.1

3.15.3. Nova Scotia Land Information Standards Initiative

The Province of Nova Scotia, under the direction of the Department of Municipal Affairs, has formed the Nova Scotia Land Information Standards Committee. This committee has been established to address the issues surrounding the development of land-related information standards within Nova Scotia. The initiative is an open, consensus building one which has representation from a variety of organization including: federal, provincial, municipal and private sector. Efforts are now underway to develop a communication strategy to disseminate information regarding the activities of the committee and its associated task groups. If you or your organization are interested in the Nova Scotia standards initiative and would like additional information either on the process or how you might become involved, please contact Ed Light, Land Information Analyst, Department of Municipal Affairs, Land

Information Management Services Division [phone] (902) 424-3761; [fax] (902) 424-5872; or [e-mail] poirier@fox.nstn.ns.ca

Contact: **poirier@FOX.NSTN.NS.CA** (Mark Poirier)

3.15.4. FGDC metadata standard

The latest documents on the (US) Federal Geographic Data Committee's (FGDC) draft of the spatial metadata standard is available in WordPerfect (ver. 5.1), and postscript formats.

URL: **ftp://isdres.er.usgs.gov/GDC/**

IP: 130.11.48.2

URL: **ftp://waisqvarsa.er.usgs.gov/wais/docs/**

IP: 130.11.51.187

Contact: GDC@USGS.GOV

Contact: MDOMARAT@USGS.GOV (Michael A. Domaratz)

3.15.5. SDTS (FIPS 123) Function Library source code

Site contains the current Unix tar library of the FIPS 123 Function Library. load123.z is a compressed Unix tar archive of the library. install is a shell script to uncompress and unarchive it. The machine is slow or slower than ISDRES, but it's a UNIX machine and has the current library on it.

URL: **ftp://resdgs1.er.usgs.govl/public/sdts/fipslib/unixtar**

IP: 130.11.52.55

3.15.6. Spatial Data Transfer Standard

Contains all the text to the latest release of the Spatial Data Transfer Standard. The standard is quite extensive and covers every type of spatial data that you are ever likely to encounter. A must-read for GIS data developers! Includes postscript and ASCII text versions.

Articles about SDTS (ASCII, WordPerfect, or Postscript)

URL: **ftp://sdts.er.usgs.gov/pub/sdts/articles/**

Sample SDTS data sets including DLG-3, TIGER, and digital orthophoto quarterquadrangle (more to be added in future)

URL: **ftp://sdts.er.usgs.gov/pub/sdts/datasets/**

Public domain SDTS support software

URL: **ftp://sdts.er.usgs.gov/pub/sdts/software/**

SDTS standard ifself, the Topological Vector Profile, and the latest draft of the Raster Profile (ASCII, WortPerfect, or Postscript)

URL: **ftp://sdts.er.usgs.gov/pub/sdts/standard/**

IP: 130.11.52.170

Contact: sdts@usgs.gov

3.15.7. NMD Map Standards Documents (DLG, DOQ)

The National Mapping Division of the U.S. Geological Survey now offers certain of its computer software programs and associated documentation on Internet. The NMD provides a national series of base cartographic data. Computer software supporting these data is primarily in the FORTRAN language. The software programs are supported on a variety of mainframe, minicomputer, and workstation hardware platforms. This software was previously available to the general public only on 9-track magnetic tape or diskette through the Earth Sciences Information Center (ESIC) for a nominal reproduction and handling fee. Fifteen FORTRAN programs, sample data and job control language are now available on Internet using file transfer protocol (FTP). A limited amount of soft-copy computer program documentation is also available in both Word Perfect and ASCII. Additional documentation will be added. Any documentation not available via FTP can be obtained in hard copy from USGS's Earth

Sciences Information Center for a nominal charge. Ordering information and price quotes may be obtained by calling 1-800-USA-MAPS.

URL: `ftp://nmdpow9.er.usgs.gov/public`

IP: `130.11.52.92`

Contact: `mlinck@usgs.gov` (Michael K. Linck, Jr.)

3.15.8. Open Geodata Interoperability Specification (OGIS)
Draft specs (OGIS is sponsored by the Open GIS Foundation)

URL: `ftp://moon.cecer.army.mil/ogis/spec`

3.15.9. Metadata standards and minutes of GISLIS, ASTM, URISA meetings
URL: `ftp://dis2qvarsa.er.usgs.gov/metadata`

3.16. Transportation

3.16.1. Institute for Transportation Research and Education at the U. of North Carolina
URL: `http://itre.uncecs.edu`

3.17. Meteorology

Stern, Illana (1994), "Sources of Meteorological Data Frequently Asked Questions (FAQ)". Usenet news.answers (bi-monthly). digital text file, 68K

This is the best source for online meteorological resources. It is well-maintained, accurate, and pretty much the authoritative reference on the subject.

This document contains a good introduction to Internet use and resources, and specifically covers information on the following topics:

  1) Current weather (satellite images)
      a) North America
      b) Europe
      c) Pacific
      d) Other
  2) Current weather and forecasts (maps, radar, soundings)
  3) Current weather and forecasts (text)
  4) Special event information (may be transient)
  5) Other images
  6) Map data
  7) Research data and metadata
  8) Software
  9) Pointers to other resources

To receive this document via e-mail, send a message to `mail-server@rtfm.mit.edu` with the line:

  `send /pub/usenet/news.answers/weather/data/part1`

in the body. Other sources are listed below.

URL: `ftp://rtfm.mit.edu/pub/usenet-by-hierarchy/news/answers/weather/data/part1`

URL: `http://www.cis.ohio-state.edu/hypertext/faq/usenet/weather/top.html`

Contact: `ilana@ncar.ucar.edu` (Ilana Stern)

3.17.1. CDIAC—Climatic Data Sets Carbon Dioxide Information Analysis Center
Contains data sets of world-wide climatic data including Atmospheric CO_2 content, tree-core/precip. corrélations, historical air temp., pressure, precip. (some going back to the 1600's!) for world, global paleoclimate to 6000 B.P., historical weather station data back to 1800's, and more.

URL: `ftp://cdiac.esd.ornl.gov/pub`

URL: **ftp://suns01.esd.ornl.gov/pub**
IP: 128.219.24.36
Contact: OMNET: CDIAC
Contact: INTERNET: CDP@STC10.CTD.ORNL.GOV
Contact: BITNET: CDP@ORNLSTC

3.18. Wildlife

3.18.1. Fish and Wildlife Service (USFWS) WAIS Server

The following items can be found here:

1. A Catalog of Automated Information Systems (CAIS) of the FWS. This catalog of metadata (descriptive information) lists both active and proposed information systems. Contact points are included for each system.
2. The CAIS currently describes 87 information systems. A new version of the CAIS will be available by the end of June. This version will serve updated metadata on 120 systems.
3. A description of the various servers (WAIS, World Wide Web, Gopher, File Transfer Protocol, etc.) maintained by the FWS.
4. State codes, County codes, and USGS Hydrologic Units, as defined in FIPS publications 5-2, 6-4 and 103.
5. The latest copy of the "Content Standards for Digital Spatial Metadata" produced by the Federal Geographic Data Committee.
6. The President's Executive Order implementing the National Spatial Data Infrastructure.
7. A list of State fish and wildlife agency contacts for fish and wildlife information systems produced by the Fish and Wildlife Information Exchange.
8. The WinWAIS client software produced by the U.S. Geological Survey for accessing WAIS servers.
9. The MOSAIC client software for accessing World Wide Web servers.

The easiest way to establish communications with this WAIS server is to access the Directory of Servers, search for "wildlife" (without the quotes), and download the address information.

URL: **wais://USFWS_Region_9_Info_Res_Mgt_Data_Admin:1028/ /data/wais/spxwais/irmindex/irmserv**
IP: 164.159.126.3
Contact: fishera@mail.fws.gov (Dr. Alan R. Fisher)

3.18.2. USFWS Forensics Laboratory
URL: **ftp://ash.lab.r1.fws.gov/**
URL: **http://ash.lab.r1.fws.gov/**
Contact: mitchellStu@mail.fws.gov

3.18.3. USFWS National Wetlands Inventory
URL: **ftp://192.189.43.33**
Contact: herman@enterprise.nwi.fws.gov

3.18.4. USFWS Division of Information Resources Management Library Server

The library server is an automated mechanism for distributing information via Internet mail. The library server responds to requests for specific files. For more information, send an e-mail message to r9irmlib@mail.fws.gov with send help (without the quotes) as the subject.

URL: **mailto//:r9irmlib@mail.fws.gov**
Contact: fishera@mail.fws.gov

3.18.5. USFWS Division of Refuges WWW Server
URL: **http://bluegoose.arw.r9.fws.gov/**
Contact: furnisss@mail.fws.gov

A Guide to Environmental Resources on the Internet

15

Carol Briggs-Erickson

Toni Murphy

Version 1.2 Updated May 1994

Welcome to A Guide to Environmental Resources on the Internet by Carol BriggsErickson and Toni Murphy. This is a guide to resources of an environmental nature which can be found on the Internet and was written to be used by researchers, environmentalists, teachers and any person who is interested in knowing and doing something about the health of our planet.

The guide is arranged alphabetically by subject and then by the Internet tools used to locate those resources.

TABLE OF CONTENTS

1. Introduction
2. Major environmental organizations and networks
3. Subject resources
4. Regulations and Standards
5. Regional Concerns
6. Library Online Catalogs
7. Index (For those who prefer searching by tool)
8. Acknowledgements

1 Introduction

This guide is arranged primarily by subject, but since there are a number of resources that reside within databases that are available to the public covering the whole scope of environmental concerns, and a number of agencies that deal with environmental standards and regulations, we decided to give these agencies and databases their own sections. We also found some resources that deal with the ecology of one geographic area. These were also put into a separate section. Everything else that we found, we felt could be placed under one or two subject headings except for the resources found in the many online catalogs available by gopher and telnet. Time constraints kept us from listing the catalogs by subject, but each catalog included contains at least 50 resources pertaining to three or more of our subject topics. We searched for our resources using gopher, telnet, archie, veronica, ftp, world wide web and wais. We did not find much of relevance using www subject entry points; nor were there a great number of wais documents. What we did find using www and wais is listed under each subject.

Some of the files mentioned in this guide are in the GIF format. If you are not using Mosaic or other software that allows viewing of these image files, consult the following FAQ document on accessing software conversion programs.

URL: `file://bloom-picayune.mit.edu/pub/usenet-by-group/alt.answers/pictures-faq/part3`

2. Major environmental organizations and networks.

    2.1   Consortium for International Earth Science Information Network (CIESIN)

Contains environmental policies, conference information, full text of world treaties, WAIS searchable environmental sources.

Audience: Primarily earth scientists, but contains resources of interest to environmentalists, and researchers, ducators.

Rating: A good source for general issues; many of the documents are available from other Internet sources, e.g., EPA, UNCED.

URL: `gopher://gopher.ciesin.org`

The CIESIN Catalog Services at Polytechnic University is searchable by:

```
gopher gopher.isnet.is
Hytelnet
Other Resources
Miscellaneous Resources
GreenPages Pilot Project at Polytechnic University
GreenPages Pilot Project at Polytechnic University
```

URL: `gopher://solomon.technet.sg:70/11/Technet/hytelnet/sites2/oth000/oth065`

or

URL: `telnet://sirius.poly.edu` login: `gp`

    2.2   Environmental Protection Agency (EPA)

The EPA maintains searchable databases covering a wide range of environmental issues in its "Online Library System". In addition to a main, national catalog of citations, there are searchable databases on hazardous wastes, clean lakes, and environmental financing. The publication, Access EPA, is also available.

Audience: Researchers, consumers, environmentalists.

Rating: Very comprehensive coverage, large dataset.

URL: `telnet://epaibm.rtpnc.epa.gov` login: public menu: `1`

In addition, the EPA maintains a gopher site covering topics such as agriculture, air, water, land, and related environmental topics.

```
gopher North America
USA
Washington DC
USA Environmental Protection Agency
```

URL: `gopher://gopher.epa.gov`

Ongoing studies and reports are available through the Future Studies gopher and wais server.

URL: `gopher://futures.wic.epa.gov`

or

URL: `telnet://Server.wais.com/215/epafutures.src`

The EPA Office of Air Quality Planning and Standards also maintains a network of bulletin boards. (See 3.2)

    2.3   EcoNet

Large, fee-based network comprised of many environmental discussions, reports, articles, and documents. Resources include U. S. EPA press releases and weekly transcripts of "Living on Earth" documents. Resources include U. S. EPA press releases and weekly transcripts of "Living on Earth" (NPR's Environment news program.) Large, Worldwide coverage and membership. Some materials are archived and available via ftp.

Send a blank message to: `econet-info@igc.apc.org` for information.

URL: `file://bongo.cc.utexas.edu/pub/output/peacenet/Brochures/econet_brochure`

URL: `gopher://igc.apc.org`

URL: `http://www.econet.apc.org`

There are many discussion groups relating to environmental issues. Just a few include:

```
en.alerts
en.events
en.climate
en.energy
en.recycle
en.toxics
sc.natlnews (Sierra Club)
en.cleanair
```

2.4 Environmental Resources Information Network (ERIN)

Network linking the Australian Nature Conservation Agency, the Australian Heritage Commission, the Commonwealth Environment Protection Agency, and the Department of the Environment, Sport and Territories. Main focus is on endangered species, vegetation, and area studies. Resources include data sets, images (GIF), international agreements, legislation and conference information. Emphasis on the Australian environment; some world coverage.

URL: `http://kaos.erin.gov.au:80/erin.html`

URL: `gopher://kaos.erin.gov.au`

3. Subject resources

   3.1 Acid rain

   3.1.1 Telnet

   3.1.1.1 Classroom Earth

   Classroom Earth (An environmental education resource made possible by a grant from NASA) has an Acid Rain Online for teaching about the study of acid rain. Water sample data is entered by groups; the data can be downloaded and compared.

   URL: `telnet://classroom_earth.ciesin.org 2010 hit RETURN when connected`

   For additional resources on acid rain, consult section 3.6 Environment (general)).

   3.2 Air pollution

   3.2.1 LISTSERVS:

   SAFETY@UVMVM
   This is a group which discusses safety in all aspects. It is relevant here on topics of waste disposal (burning, etc.), and chemical hazards.

   3.2.2 EPA bulletin boards:

   URL: `telnet://ttnbbs.rtpnc.epa.gov`

   Some available bulletin boards

   CAAA—Clean Air Act Amendments
   EMTIC—Emission Measurement Technical Information Center emission test methods and testing information)
   AIRS—Air quality and emissions

BLIS—Compilation of air permits from air pollution control agencies.
NATICH—Information submitted by EPA, state and local agencies about air toxics programs
COMPLI—Stationary source and asbestos compliance policy
CHIEF—Latest information on air emission inventories and emission factors
ATPI—Current course offerings on air pollution

3.2.3 FTP sites:

3.2.3.1 ftp.cic.net
There are many good documents in the e directory at this site having to do with pollution and other environmental issues, useful to researchers.

URL: `file://ftp.cic.net/pub/e-serials/alphabetic/e/env-link/unocal.pollution.gz`
URL: `file://bongo.cc.utexas.edu/pub/output/peacenet/Brochures/econet_brochure`
URL: `file://ftp.cic.net/pub/e-serials/alphabetic/e/env-link/unocal.pollution.gz`
URL: `file://ftp.cic.net/pub/nircomm/gopher/e-serials/alphabetic/ex/env-link`

3.2.3.2 unix.hensa.ac.uk
The pollution datasets at this site are of value to researchers and environmental scientists and legislators.

URL: `file://unix.hensa.ac.uk/pub/statlib/datasets/pollution`

3.3 Alternative energy

3.3.1 LISTSERVS:

HYDROGENL@URIACC.URI.EDU
Discusses hydrogen as an alernative energy source. Some very lively discussions, but tends to be scientist oriented.

ENERGYL@TAUNIVM
Good discussion of alternative energy.

AE@SJSUVM1.SJSU.EDU
This alternative energy discussion group is "intended to provide a forum to discuss the current state of the art and future directions of alternative energy sources that are renewable or sustainable."

3.3.2 Newsletters:

3.3.2.1 Wind Energy Weekly, newsletter.
For free online subscription, e-mail Tom Gray (Internet/Bitnet: `tgray@igc.apc.org`) (EcoNet/PeaceNet: `tgray@igc`) (UUCP: `uunet!cdp!tgray`). Also available by gopher.

URL: `gopher://dale.ucdavis.edu:70/11/Committees and Organizations/Special Interest Groups/Instructional Technology Networking Consortium/Journals/Wind.Energy.Weekly`

3.3.3 FTP and gopher:

3.3.3.1 Center for Renewable Energy and Sustainable Technology (CREST)
This is an (emerging) educational resource center providing services and education focusing on renewable energy, energy efficiency, the environment, and sustainable development.

URL: `file://ftp.digex.net/pub/crest/ae-guide`
`gopher and www access: in development`

3.3.4 Telnet

3.3.4.1 Electric Ideas Clearinghouse BBS
This bbs is sponsored by the Washington State Energy Office, the U.S. Department of Energy. Though it provides document delivery to a limited number of western states, there are some citations which would be of interest to researchers, educators, and consumers in any location.

Discussion forums include ENVIRON, NEWS, WIND, SOLAR, and others. The searchable periodical database includes over 100 bulletins, newsletters, and trade journals.

URL: `telnet://eicbbs.wseo.wa.gov`

3.4 EcoSystems

3.4.1 LISTSERVS:

ECOSYSL@vm.gmd.de
Ecosystem theory in German

ECOLOGL@UMDD.UMD.EDU
Discussion group of the Ecological Society of America. Includes grant information, job postings, general news and discussion of ecological topics. Very active group.

ECOLOGY@EMUVM1
Politics and the environment. Discusses government policy, EPA rulings, etc.

3.4.2 FTP:
URL: `file://pencil.cs.missouri.edu/pub/student_envirolink/Ecosytem_Decay.txt`

(note the spelling of the word Ecosytem, type it exactly to get this document)

3.4.3 Gopher:
Coweeta Hydrologic Laboratory is a nice searchable bibliography on Ecosystems in the Coweeta LTER Site.

```
gopher sparc.ecology.uga.edu
Coweeta LTER Site
Bibliographic References
```

URL: `gopher://sparc.ecology.uga.edu/11/cwtsite/cwtbib`

3.5 Endangered species

3.5.1 FTP:

3.5.1.1 UN Treaty (1973) available via ftp and gopher.
Contains text on the international trade in endangered species of wild fauna and flora. Good for researchers and those interested in environmental law.

`ftp jade.tufts.edu`

`/pub/diplomacy/BH613.txt`

URL: `file://jade.tufts.edu/pub/diplomacy/BH613.txt`

3.5.1.2 Environmental Resources Information Network (ERIN)
The main focus is on endangered species, vegetation, and area studies. Resources include international agreements, legislation, and conference information. Emphasis on the Australian environment; some world coverage.

`gopher kaos.erin.gov.au`

URL: `http://kaos.erin.gov.au:80/erin.html`
URL: `gopher://kaos.erin.gov.au`

3.6   Environment (general)

3.6.1   LISTSERVS and newsgroups:

ENVSTL@BROWNVM.brown.edu
Environmental studies. Very busy list, good discussion.

ENVBEHL@POLYVM
Environment and human behavior. Moderately busy, some similar postings to ENVSTL

SFERL@UCF1VM
South Florida Environmental Reader (moderated) Pertains mainly to Southern Florida.

BIODIVL@BDT.FTPT.BR
Group interested in forming a biodiversity network. (Archives of this list available via gopher at gopherbdt.ftpt.br)

BIOSPHL@UBVM
Biosphere, ecology discussion list

`alt.earth.summit`

`sci.environment`

`sci.bio.ecology`

`clari.tw.environment`

3.6.2   Gopher:

3.6.2.1   EcoGopher at UVa
EcoGopher provides easy access to information from many environmental agencies and organizations all in one place. Using "katie"—keyword search of all text in EcoGopher. Researchers, environmentalists and teachers can find an abundance of resources. There are also several good resources available on the one page gopher menu.

```
gopher ecosys.drdr.Virginia.edu
    katie
```

URL: `gopher://ecosys.drdr.virginia.edu/1`
URL: `http://ecosys.drdr.virginia.edu/Environment.html`

3.6.2.2   World Health Organization (WHO)
Environmental health newsletter updated regularly.

URL: `gopher://gopher.who.ch/11/.ehe/.news`

3.6.2.3   CIESIN (See 2.1 above for description)
URL: `gopher://gopher.ciesin.org`

3.6.2.4   LTER (Long Term Ecological Research gopher)
Includes datasets, conferences, bibliographies, meeting abstracts, etc. Good for researchers, and environmental scientists.

URL: `gopher://lternet.edu`

3.6.2.5   CICNet gopher
Access to newsletters, keyword searching of databases, EcoNet documents, etc. Resource for researchers, environmental scientists, oceanographers and others.

URL: `gopher://gopher.cic.net`

3.6.2.6　World Bank gopher
The World Bank gopher has several resources pertaining to environmental issues.

URL: **gopher://ftp.worldbank.org:70/1**

3.6.3　Telnet:

3.6.31　PENPages
There are many good documents on the environment here that would be useful to teachers, researchers and environmentalists.

URL: **telnet://psupen.psu.edu**

login: your twoletter state code
keyword search: environment

3.6.3.2　Envirolink Network
There are some great bibliographies, statistical resources and other documents relevant for researchers and environmentalists at this site.

URL: **telnet://envirolink.org**

login: gopher

3.6.3.3　OLS database
The EPA mainframe is open 24hrs/day, except from 8:00 PM Sunday to 7:00 AM Monday (EST). The OLS database contains book citations, federal agency technical reports, indices, audiovisual materials, maps, journals and other documents. The National Catalog, Hazardous Waste, and Lakes databases can be searched by single keyword. They allow searchers to combine terms in a boolean type search.

URL: **telnet://epaibm.rtpnc.epa.gov**

```
select Public Access
select OLS
select 1
```

3.6.3.4　EnviroNet
This is a resource for space environment information. It contains handbook sections which are good resources for teachers and environmental researchers.

URL: **telnet://envnet.gsfc.nasa.gov**

login: envnet
passwd: henniker

3.6.3.5　SciLink
There are two discussion groups that are relevant here, "environment" and "earth." You can also send private messages to other SciLink users. This is a good resource for educators, environmentalists and students K-12.

URL: **telnet://scilink.org**

login: guest
passwd: guest

3.6.3.6　Compelling earth views
NASA photographs of the earth from space.

URL: **telnet://sseop.jsc.nasa.gov**

login: PHOTOS
password: PHOTOS

3.6.3.7 Fedworld

Though not a strictly environmental resource, Fedworld is rich in environmental papers and reports. All aspects of the environment can be found here in the form of research reports, documents, and files. Some of the NTIS reports include:

> Acid Precipitation
> Air Pollution
> Clean Coal Technologies
> Hazardous Material Data File
> Toxic Release Inventory on Tape
> Catalog of Environment Reports & Studies

In addition to NTIS information, PBSRCH files include research on environmental concerns (recycling, methane from solid wastes, acid mine drainage, etc.)

URL: `telnet://fedworld.gov`

3.6.4 Email:

3.6.4.1 Environmental Audit '90 Energy and Water Conservation (chart)

40 page discussion with charts to raise campus consciousnous towards the environment. Concise, interesting, good statistics, useful for those involved in college campus ecology and recyling programs.

email Julian Keniry (`julian@NWFDC.NWF.ORG`)

3.6.4.2 Good bibliography.

Relevant for researchers on environment and women's studies.

Title: Women and the Environmental Movement
Author: Jennifer L. Harder `jlharder@ucdavis.edu`

3.6.5 FTP:

3.6.5.1 EcoNet Energy & Climate Information Newsletter

Informative newsletter, useful to researchers and environmental scientists.

`ftp ftp.cic.net`

  `/pub/nircomm/gopher/e-serials/alphabetic/e/econet/ecix.gz`

URL: `file://ftp.cic.net/pub/e-serials/alphabetic/e/econet/ecixtc.gz`

3.6.5.2 GREENDISK

(introductory issue of environmental journal on computer diskette, subscription costs $35.00/year, disk envelopes and labels made of recycled materials)

Worth the cost, if you're buying environmental journals, without the guilt of killing trees. Relevant for researchers and general public.

`ftp igc.org`

  `/pub/GreenDisk`

URL: `file://igc.org/pub/GreenDisk`

Many other environmental newsletters and journals are available at the anonymous ftp site at `ftp.cic.net` in the directory `pub/nircomm/gopher/e-serials`. Included are:

> BEN (Botanical Electronic News)
> Biosphere (Newsgroup newsletter)
> Climate/Ecosystem Dynamics
> EnvLink
> ERIN (Newsletters of the Australian Environmental Resources Information Network) in PostScript format (maps and detailed drawings included)

LTER (Longterm Environmental Research) Data Management Bulletin and LTER Network News
South Florida Environmental Reader
University of Michigan Global Change Newsletter

3.6.5.3 Bibliography on the effects of fire on all aspects of the environment.
```
ftp life.anu.edu.au
   /pub/landscape_ecology/firenet/firebib/firebib.txt
```

URL: `file://life.anu.edu.au/pub/landscape_ecology/firenet/firebib/firebib.txt`

3.6.5.4 BASIC Software ftp:
Environmental programs, looked useful for educators and researchers. The program listed here compares ecological population relationships.
```
ftp netserv1.its.rpi.edu
   /pub/faculty/bungay/envir1/ecology.bas
```

URL: `file://netserv1.its.rpi.edu/pub/faculty/bungay/envir1/ecology.bas`

3.6.6 WWW:

3.6.6.1 The Environment (Community)
This WWW site provides links to several environmental resources.

URL: `http://www.einet.net/galaxy/Community/The-Environment.html`

3.6.6.2 Environment: HOLIT - a Hebrew language database.
We could not evaluate this database, because we do not speak Hebrew, but there seemed to be enough data here to check into it for those researchers able to read Hebrew.

URL: `http://galaxy.einet.net/hytelnet/WWW003.html`

3.6.7 General newsletters and serials: (which can be accessed via gopher and/or ftp)

3.6.7.1 Student Envirolink
env-link+forms@andrew.cmu.edu

3.6.7.2 Sense of Place
An electronic magazine produced by students at Dartmouth. Useful to students, educators and researchers.
e-mail to `SOP@dartmouth.edu` for notification of latest issue.

3.6.7.3 The Scientist
A biweekly newspaper dealing with the life sciences read by scientists and researchers. Some articles are relevant to educators and environmentalists.
```
gopher inforM.umd.edu
```
```
ftp ds.internic.net
   /pub/thescientist
```

URL: `file://ds.internic.net/pub/thescientist`

3.6.7.4 The Environmental Magazine
URL: `gopher://gopher.internet.com`

3.6.7.5 MEEMAN Archive (Environmental Journalism)
Database of environmental articles, citations and abstracts. Useful for researchers, environmentalists, and educators.

URL: `telnet://hermes.merit.edu`

login: `mirlyn`, choose `MEEM`

3.6.7.6 LTER (Longterm Environmental Research)
Data Management Bulletin)
Datasets, bibliography, bulletin boards. Data of interest to researchers, educators and environmental scientists.

URL: `gopher://lternet.edu`

3.7 Environment and Education

3.7.1 LISTSERVS:

`GRNSCHL@BROWNVM`
(Green School List)

`IAPWILD`
(World School for Adventure Learning) This listserv is limited to schools who wish to interact and exchange ideas with students, explorers and scholars around the world.

`ASEHL@TTUVM1`
American Society of Environmental Historians

`ENVSTL@BROWNVM`
Environmental studies discussion. This is a moderately active group discussing a variety of environmental issues often relating to education and teaching.

`SEACnet` (Student Environmental Action Coalition Network).
There are several mailing lists related to this group. To subscribe to any of them send a message to:

    listproc@ecosys.drdr.virginia.edu
    seac+discussion (General discussion list)
    seac+nafta (NAFTA discussion list)
    seac+highschool (High School Caucus list)
    subscribe seac+announce Jane Doe

3.7.2 Telnet:

3.7.2.1 Classroom Earth (See 3.1.1.1)
An environmental education resource possible by a grant from NASA. A good resource for educators and students k12.

URL: `telnet://classroom_earth.ciesin.org 2010`
hit RETURN when connected

3.7.3 Gopher:

3.7.3.1 EcoGopher (see also 4.3 Federal Register for Grant Funding)
URL: `gopher://ecosys.drdr.virginia.edu/1`

3.7.3.2 CTI Centre for Biology.
Educational software reviews relating to teaching. Includes pollution simulators and environmental programs. Relevant to educators, students and environmental scientists.

URL: `gopher://gopher.csc.liv.ac.uk/11/ctibiol`

3.7.3.3   EElink (Environmental Education)
　　　　　This site is rich in educational resources.

　　　　　URL: `gopher://nceet.snre.umich.edu`

3.7.3.4   ERIC lesson plans
　　　　　K12 lesson plans pertaining to science and the environment.

　　　　　URL: `gopher://ericir.syr.edu/11/Lesson/Science`

3.7.4   FTP:

3.7.4.1   Center for Renewable Energy and Sustainable Technology (CREST)
　　　　　This is an educational resource center which provides services and education focusing on renewable energy, energy efficiency, the environment, and sustainable development. The file "00index" contains a list of available files.

　　　　　URL: `file://ftp.digex.net/pub/crest`

3.7.4.2   Software reviews archives
　　　　　Reviews of programs in ecology. For students and educators.

```
gopher archives.math.utk.edu
Software
Life Sciences
Programs in Ecology
```

　　　　　URL: `file://archives.math.utk.edu/life.sciences/ecology/`

3.7.4.3   Solar energy factsheet for kids.
　　　　　Interesting solar energy facts for students and educators.

　　　　　URL: `file://sunsite.unc.edu/pub/academic/environment/alternative-energy/nc_solar_center/factsheets/slr4kids.fsh`

3.8   Forestry

　　3.8.1   LISTSERVS/newsgroups:

　　　　　FOREST@NIC.FUNET.FI
　　　　　send subscribe message to: `mailserver@nic.funet.fi`

　　　　　FMDSSL@PNFI.FORESTRY.CA
　　　　　Forest Management Decision Support System

　　　　　NATRESLIBL
　　　　　A discussion group for Natural Resources Librarians. Subscriptions and messages are sent to the list moderator, Anne Hedrich at: `annhed@cc.usu.edu`

　　　　　bionet.agroforestry

　　3.8.2   Gopher:

　　3.8.2.1   METLA
　　　　　Gopher system of Forestry, Environment and Natural Resource sponsored by the Finnish Forest Research Institute. Contains statistics on Finnish forestry.

　　　　　URL: `gopher://pihta.metla.fi/11`

3.8.2.2 University of British Columbia (UBC Press)
Mounts citations to its published books by subject; they publish books in environmental and resource studies and include a section on forestry.

```
gopher gopher.ubc.ca
Libraries and Information Sources
UBC Press
Books in Print
Forestry
```

URL: `gopher://gopher.ubc.ca:70/11/libraries/ubc-press/books-in-print/Forestry`

3.8.2.3 Publications and short articles are available through the Purdue Cooperative Extension.
gopher hermes.ecn.purdue.edu

```
PCE Gopher Information Server
Agriculture
Forestry and Natural Resources
```

URL: `gopher://hermes.ecn.purdue.edu`

3.8.2.4 The Ecological Data Exchange (EDEX)
URL: `gopher://yaleinfo.yale.edu:7000/11/Forestry/edex`

3.8.2.5 Forestry gopher at University of Minnesota
Contains reports on areas of forestry and conservation.

URL: `gopher://minerva.forestry.umn.edu`

3.8.3 Telnet:

3.8.3.1 PENPages (See 3.6.3.1 above for description)
Keyword search on forestry retrieved 112 documents.

URL: `telnet://psupen.psu.edu`

login: `your twoletter state code`

3.8.4 Bibliographies:
Title: Water Quality and Forestry
e-mail `wqic@nalusda.gov`

3.8.5 FTP:

3.8.5.1 1992 UNCED Forest Principles
UN Environmental Summit. Text of Agreement on Environment and Development.

URL: `file://life.anu.edu.au/pub/biodiversity/rio/unced.forest`

3.8.5.2 Usenet news discussion of agroforestry.
URL: `file://fly.bio.indiana.edu/usenet/bionet/agroforestry`

3.8.5.3 Canadian forestry
This document is a list of the people in charge of the Canadian Forestry Department.

URL: `file://relay.cs.toronto.edu/cadomain/registrationsflat/ca.forestry`

3.9 Greenhouse effect/Ozone depletion

3.9.1 Newsgroups:
sci.geo.meteorology
frequent discussions on ozone

3.9.2 Gopher:

3.9.2.1 British Columbia Atmosphere Caucus
A good source of information on the ozone.

```
gopher freenet.victoria.bc.ca
Atmospheric Ozone Information
```

URL: **gopher://freenet.victoria.bc.ca/11/atmosphere**

3.9.2.2 Ozone Depletion Gopher
Many reports on ozone are located at this site.

URL: **gopher://serra.unipi.it:2347/7?ozone+depletion**

3.9.3 FTP:

3.9.3.1 Introduction to the Ozone Layer.
Several documents explaining ozone depletion in layman's terms. Ozone depletion articles written by Robert Parson from U. of Colorado. Deals with physical properties of UV radiation xand ozone. He is admittedly not an expert in this field.

URL: **file://bloom-picayune.mit.edu/pub/usenet-by-group/sci.environment/ Ozone_Depletion***

3.9.3.2 Articles from ECO newsletter.
Useful to researchers.

URL: **file://pencil.cs.missouri.edu/pub/student_envirolink/ Greenhouse_Effects.txt**

3.9.3.3 Good article on solar collectors.
There are articles on solar homes, energysaving landscaping, and other alternative energy topics. Relevant for educators, environmentalists, students.

URL: **file://sunsite.unc.edu/pub/academic/environment/alternative-energy/ nc_solar_center/factsheets/aspvsite.fsh**

3.9.3.4 Tiempo is a bulletin on global warming and the Third World.
URL: **file://igc.apc.org./pub/ECIX/tiempo*** (there are several files: **tiempo1 - tiempo11**)

3.9.3.5 Ozone graphics.
Two GIF images of ozone levels and chlorine monoxide over the northern and southern hemisperes. Both maps were produced by the Microwave Limb Sounder aboard the Upper Atmosphere Research Satellite.

URL: **file://plaza.aarnet.edu.au/micros/pc/garbo/pc/gif-astro/ozone93a.gif**
URL: **file://plaza.aarnet.edu.au/micros/pc/garbo/pc/gif-astro/ozone93b.gif**

3.9.3.6 United Nations Treaties
Files containing the United Nations treaties on ozone: Vienna Convention for the Protection of the Ozone Layer (1985) and Montreal Amendment, London (1990).

URL: `file://wiretap.spies.com/Gov/Treaties/Treaties/ozone.85`
URL: `file://wiretap.spies.com/Gov/Treaties/Treaties/ozone.90`

3.9.4 Telnet:

3.9.4.1 PENPages (See 3.6.3.1 above for description)
URL: `telnet://psupen.psu.edu`
login: `your twoletter state code`
keyword search: `ozone layer`

3.10 Hazardous waste

3.10.1 LISTSERVS:

SAFETY@UVMVM
Discusses laboratory safety, hazardous waste disposal, etc) Very active and good discussion.

HAZMATL
A forum for facilitating a central resource of chemical information such as regulatory status, and toxicology information. Subscribe: `majordomo@csn.org`

3.10.2 Gopher:

3.10.2.1 Detailed factsheets of EPA's three hundred and fifty toxic substances.
URL: `gopher://ecosys.drdr.Virginia.edu:70/11/library/factsheets/toxics`

3.10.2.2 OSHA information
Occupational Safety and Health regulations.

`gopher ginfo.cs.fit.edu`
(see also 3.10.3.1 for additional gopher site)

URL: `gopher://ginfo.cs.fit.edu:70/1`

3.10.3 FTP:

3.10.3.1 SIRI
The Safety Information Resource on the Internet (SIRI). This is a gopher and ftp site which provides access to file libraries, a searchable index and gopher links to other safety related gopher sites. Though dedicated to a variety of safety issues, much information on issues regarding hazardous waste can be found here.

URL: `ftp://siri.uvm.edu/SIRI/SIRI_file_library/Text_files`

3.10.3.2 Hazardous Materials Reports
A database of the Hazardous Materials reports is available in three parts via ftp:

URL: `file://gandalf.umcs.maine.edu/pub/hazmat/hazmat_1`
URL: `file://gandalf.umcs.maine.edu/pub/hazmat/hazmat_2`
URL: `file://gandalf.umcs.maine.edu/pub/hazmat/hazmat_3`

3.11 Oceanic

3.11.1 LISTSERVS:

PACIFIC@BRUFPB
Discussion on all aspects of the Pacific Ocean. Not very active.

3.11.2   Gopher:

3.11.2.1   Woods Hole Oceanographic Institution
Bibliographies, oceanographic data and data from experiments reside on this gopher. Researchers and professional oceanographers will find this information relevant to their studies.

URL: `gopher://pearl.whoi.edu/11/WHOIdatabases`

3.11.3   Telnet/WWW

3.11.3.1   NOAA (National Oceanic and Atmospheric Administration)
This is an excellent source of oceanic data for researchers and educators.

URL: `telnet://esdim1.nodc.noaa.gov`

login: `noaadir`

or

URL: `telnet://gopher.esdim.noaa.gov`

login: `gopher`

Also available via WWW:

URL: `http://www.nodc.noaa.gov`

3.11.3.2   Oceanic Information Center
Oceanic has an easy to use interface. Kermit is compatible and OIC has directions for importing it from ftp sites and installing it.

URL: `gopher://diu.cms.udel.edu`

3.11.4   FTP:

3.11.4.1   Sea surface temperature data
URL: `file://aurelie.soest.hawaii.edu/pub/avhrr/images`

3.12   Recycling

3.12.1   LISTSERVS:

RECYCLE@UMAB
Recycling in practice. Good discussion.

NCIWL@YALEVM
Nutrient cycling issues. Not a lot going on here.

3.12.2   Telnet:
PENPages (See description 3.6.3.1 above)
Keyword search on `recycling`

URL: `telnet://psupen.psu.edu`

login: `your twoletter state code`

3.12.3   Gopher:

3.12.3.1   The Texas A&M University gopher
This gopher has a section on recycling. Contains nontechnical, consumer oriented information.

```
gopher gopher.tamu.edu
Browse information by subject
```

```
Recycling
Aggies for a Clean Tomorrow
```

URL: **gopher://gopher.tamu.edu/11/.dir/recycle.clean.dir**

3.13 Sustainable agriculture

3.13.1 LISTSERVS:

SUSTAGL@WSUVM1
Sustainable agriculture discussion group.

almanac@ces.ncsu.edu

Subscribe sanetmg (electronic conference of the Sustainable Agriculture Network) SAN is supported by a grant from the USDA's Sustainable Agriculture Research and Education (SARE) Program. There is a lot of information available through this network and a number of access points. For information, contact Gabriel Hegyes, SAN Coordinator: **ghegyes@nalusda.gov**

3.13.2 Telnet:
PENPages (See description 3.6.3.1 above)
Keyword search on sustainable agriculture retrieved over 50 documents.

URL: **telnet://psupen.psu.edu**

login: **your twoletter state code**

3.13.3 Bibliographies:
Title: Evaluation of Agricultural Best Management Practices
To order: e-mail **wqic@nalusda.gov**

3.13.4 FTP:

3.13.4.1 Very good sustainable agriculture bibliography
For researchers, farmers, and educators.

URL: **file://sunsite.unc.edu/pub/academic/agriculture/sustainable_agriculture/sanet/showcase.bibliography**

3.14 Water quality

3.14.1 LISTSERVS:

WATERL@SUVM1
This is a water quality discussion list. There is not a lot of activity on this one, but some interesting discussion.

AQUIFER@IBACSATA
Pollution and groundwater discharge. Not much discussion on this list.

A groundwater modeling discussion list is being developed. Interested participants may contact Sam Standring at **sstandring@fullerton.edu**

3.14.2 Email:

3.14.2.1 Environmental Audit '90 - Energy and Water Conservation (chart)
40 page discussion with charts to raise campus consciousnous regarding water usage. Concise, interesting, good statistics.

email Julian Keniry (**julian@NWFDC.NWF.ORG**)

3.14.2.2 Bibliographies:
Title: Water Quality and Forestry
To order: e-mail: **wqic@nalusda.gov**

3.14.3 FTP:

3.14.3.1 There are a number of relevant documents in the /gopher/ directory.
This document is relevant for environmentalists, and researchers, with emphasis on teaching.

URL: `file://ftp.cic.net/pub/great-lakes/natural-resources/Groundwater/GroundWaterStrategy.txt`

3.14.3.2 Grandwater Quality
There are an number of relevant documents on groundwater quality at this site, also, one of which is listed below.

URL: `file://sunsite.unc.edu/pub/academic/political-science/Community_Idea_Net/Cleaning-Up-Groundwater-Contamination`

3.14.3.3 Water Quality Database
Citations are available from each Extension Service in the Land Grant System. In addition, more than 350 complete documents are available for recovery online. That number is expected to reach 1,000 by the end of 1994.

```
gopher hermes.ecn.purdue.edu
Purdue Cooperative Extention Gopher
Environment
Water Quality
```

WAIS: info.cern.ch : waterquality.src

URL: `telnet://hermes.ecn.purdue.edu`
login: cerf
password: purdue

3.14.4.4 Universities Water Information Network (UWIN) (in development)
This network is sponsored by the Universities Council on Water Resources (UCOWR). Water resources publications and educational information. The citation databases are excellent for researchers and educators.

URL: `gopher://uwin.cwr.siu.edu`

This network also offers a Water Talk bbs where discussion groups include: Hydrology, International Issues, Water Quality, and Water Policy.

URL: `telnet://gopher.cwr.siu.edu`
or

URL: `telnet://bbsrelay.cwr.siu.edu`

(You will be greeted with login instructions.)

3.15 Wetlands

3.15.1 FTP:
Very good report on Great Lakes/St. Lawrence River Basin. Of interest to researchers and environmental legislators. There are several other environmental reports at this site under WaterAirLand.

URL: `ftp://ftp.cic.net/pub/great-lakes/natural-resources/wetlands.rep`

3.16 Wildlife

3.16.1 LISTSERVS:

CONSBIO@UWAVM.U.WASHINGTON.EDU
Discussion regarding conservation biology. Low volume.

CTURTLE@NERVM
Sea Turtle Biology and Conservation discussion group. Some active discussion on this list.

MARMAN@UVVM.UVIC.CA
Marine mammals research and conservation. Moderate activity.

WILDNET@TRIBUNE.USASK.CA
Send to: wildnetrequest@tribune.usask.ca

The moderator asks members to submit a brief biographical profile; this listing is available to members on request. It is valuable in identifying members of the group who may share common backgrounds and interests.

3.16.2 Telnet:
PENPages (see 3.6.3.1 above for description)
Keyword search on wildlife retrieved 50 very up-to-date documents.

URL: `telnet://psupen.psu.edu`
login: `your twoletter state code`

3.16.3 FTP:

3.16.3.1 sunsite.unc.edu
There are many good documents at this site about wild flora and fauna.

URL: `ftp://sunsite.unc.edu/pub/academic/agriculture/sustainable_agriculture/general`

URL: `ftp://sunsite.unc.edu/pub/academic/agriculture/sustainable_agriculture/discussion-groups/newsgroups/bionet.general`

Several Smithsonian wildlife pictures are available from this site as well.

URL: `ftp://sunsite.unc.edu/pub/multimedia/pictures/smithsonian/gif89a/science-nature`

files: eagle.gif, owls.gif, many others

3.16.3.2 Australian Wildlife Legislation
URL: `file://wiretap.spies.com/Gov/Aussie/wildlife.act`

4. Regulations and Standards

4.1 United Nations Environment Programme (ENEP)
UNCED, Agenda21, preconference documents

URL: `gopher://nywork1.undp.org`

URL: `ftp://info.umd.edu/inforM/Educational_Resources/AcademicResourcesByTopic/UnitedStatesAndWorld/International/UnitedNations`

WAIS info.cern.ch uncedagenda.src

4.2 Environmental Safety and Health Information Center (ESHIC)

ESHIC is a central repository for the Department of Energy. Tiger Team Assessment documents, plans, and assessments. It includes DOE documents concerning compliance, regulations, policy, training, and longterm planning.

URL: `gopher://dewey.tis.inel.gov:2019/1/`

4.3 Federal Register

Searchable by subject (Environ, Energy, Agriculture) and by agency.

URL: `gopher://gopher.counterpoint.com`

4.4 OSHA Document Citations

Searchable OSHA document citations.

URL: `gopher://ginfo.cs.fit.edu:70/1`

4.5 Federal Legislation via Library of Congress

The Library of Congress Information System contains federal legislation introduced in Congress since 1973. Information includes summaries and status of legislation. Searchable by subject (legislative), member's name, key words, bill number, public law number, committee name. Current file updated daily. This database has limited hours.

URL: `telnet://locis.loc.gov`

(no login required)

4.6 White House Press Releases on the Environment

Press releases, speeches and proclamations are available by subject at this location and many are included on the environment. An easy place to find relatively current information from the White House.

URL: `gopher://info.umd.edu:901/11/inforM/Educational_Resources/Government/United States/Executive/WhiteHouse/PressReleases/Environmen`

5. Regional Concerns

5.1 LISTSERVS:

COMPSYL@UIUCVMD
Midwest ecological issues

NATURAL@UCHCECVM
Ecology and environmental protection in Chile

MEH2OL@TAUNIVM.TAU.AC.IL
Devoted to water issues in the Middle East

SFERL@UCF1VM
South Florida environmental list

5.2 FTP:

5.2.1 Report of the Bi-national Program to Restore and Protect the Lake Superior Basin.
URL: `file://pencil.cs.missouri.edu/pub/student_envirolink/Lake_Superior_Basin_Project.txt`

5.2.2		GLIN Great Lakes Information Network
		URL: `gopher://gopher.great-lakes.net:2200/11`
		URL: `gopher://gopher.cic.net:2000/11/glin`
5.3		Gopher:

Texas Studies Gopher Armadillo, the Texas Studies Gopher, is designed to provide instructional resources and information about Texas natural and cultural history and the Texas environment. The site also includes several resources on environmental issues.

`gopher riceinfo.rice.edu`

URL: `gopher://riceinfo.rice.edu:1170/11/Texas/Environment`

5.4		Ejournals

`BEN@CUE.BC.CA`
Botanical/ecological information on Canada.
(subscribe: `ACESKA`)

5.5		Other regional information sites
5.5.1		Oregon environmental legislation

Text of Oregon environmental bills.

`gophergaia.ucs.orst.edu`

Oregon Legislative Information System Natural Resources

URL: `gopher://gaia.ucs.orst.edu:70/11/osu-i+s/OLIS/Natural Resources`

5.5.2		National Capital Freenet

Good Canadian source of environmental information.

URL: `telnet://guest@freenet.carleton.ca:23/`

at main menu, type: `go envir`

5.5.3		EcoNet (feebased)

Covers many areas: California, Hawaii, Florida, New York, Africa, Siberia, Scotland and others. Send blank message to: `econetinfo@igc.apc.org` for information.

5.5.4		Environmental News Network Briefings.

Environmental issues of Northwest U.S.

URL: `gopher://gopher.uidaho.edu/11s/e-pubs/enn`

6. Library catalogs

This is a selected listing of library catalogs with extensive environmental holdings. All can be reached through gopher and the following telnet addresses. If no login is specified, follow screen instructions when connected.

Acadia University
telnet: `auls.acadiau.ca`
login: `opac`
URL: `telnet://opac@auls.acadiau.ca`

Arizona State University
telnet: `carl.lib.asu.edu`
login: `carl`
URL: `telnet://carl@carl.lib.asu.edu`

Athabasca University
telnet: `aucat.athabascau.ca`
login: `aucat`
URL: **telnet://aucat@aucat.athabascau.ca**

Augusta College
telnet: `acvax.ac.edu`
login: `ACPAC`
URL: telnet://ACPAC@acvax.ac.edu

Bates College
telnet: `ladd.bates.edu`
URL: **telnet://ladd.bates.edu**

Boston University
telnet: `library.bu.edu`
login: `library`
URL: **telnet://library@library.bu.edu**

Brandeis University
telnet: `library.brandeis.edu`
login: `louis`
URL: **telnet://louis@library.brandeis.edu**

Brandon University
telnet: `library.brandonu.ca`
login: `libcat`
URL: **telnet://libcat@library.brandonu.ca**

Butler University
telnet: `ruth.butler.edu`
login: `iliad`
URL: **telnet://iliad@ruth.butler.edu**

California Institute of Technology
telnet: `libopac.caltech.edu`
login: `clas`
URL: **telnet://clas@libopac.caltech.edu**

California Polytechnic State U.
telnet: `library.calpoly.edu`
URL: **telnet://library.calpoly.edu**

California State University at Chico
telnet: `libcat.csuchico.edu`
URL: **telnet://libcat.csuchico.edu**

California State University at Fresno
telnet: `alis.csufresno.edu`
login: `remote`
URL: **telnet://remote@alis.csufresno.edu**

California State University at Hayward
telnet: `library.csuhayward.edu`
login: `library`
URL: **telnet://library@library.csuhayward.edu**

California State University at Long Beach
telnet: `coast.lib.csulb.edu`
login: `vt100, start`
URL: **telnet://vt100, start@coast.lib.csulb.edu**

California State University at Sacramento
telnet: `eureka.lib.csus.edu`
login: `library`
URL: **telnet://library@eureka.lib.csus.edu**

CARL Colorado Alliance of Research Libraries
search individual catalogs
telnet: `pac.carl.org`

(Two good opacs in this system for environmental resources are U. of Colorado at Boulder and Colorado School of Mines)

URL: **telnet://pac.carl.org**

Claremont Colleges
California
telnet: `blais.claremont.edu`
login: `library`
URL: **telnet://library@blais.claremont.edu**

Connecticut State University
telnet: `csulib.ctstateu.edu`
login: `csulib`
exit: h

URL: **telnet://library@blais.claremont.edu**

Dartmouth
telnet: `lib.dartmouth.edu`
exit: bye
URL: **telnet://lib.dartmout.edu**

Drake University
telnet: `lib.drake.edu`
login: `cowles`
URL: **telnet://cowles@lib.drake.edu**

Florida State University System
telnet: `luis.nerdc.ufl.edu`
login: `luis`
URL: **telnet://luis@luis.nerdc.ufl.edu**

Georgia State University
telnet: `library:gsu.edu`
exit: quit
URL: **telnet://library.gsu.edu**

Harvard University
telnet: `hollis.harvard.edu`
login: `hollis`
URL: **telnet://,hollis@hollis.harvard.edu**

Indiana University
telnet: `iuis.ucs.indiana.edu`
login: `guest`
choose: `IUCAT`
URL: **`telnet://guest@iuis.ucs.indiana.edu`**

Lawrence Livermore National Laboratory
telnet: `aish.llnl.gov`
login: `patron`
URL: **`telnet://patron@aish.llnl.gov`**

Loyola Marymount University
telnet: `linus.lmu.edu`
login: `library`
URL: **`telnet://library@linus.lmu.edu`**

Michigan State University
telnet: `hermes.merit.edu`
login: tab to command line, type `dial magic`
URL: **`telnet://magic@hermes.merit.edu`**

Northeastern University
telnet: `library.lib.northeastern.edu`
URL: **`telnet://library.lib.northeastern.edu`**

Pima College, Arizona
telnet: `libcat.pima.edu`
login: `lib`
URL: **`telnet://library@libcat.pima.edu`**

San Diego State University
telnet: `library.sdsu.edu 74`
URL: **`telnet://library@library.sdsu.edu`**

San Jose State University
telnet: `sjsulib.sjsu.edu`
login: `lib`
exit: `h`
URL: **`telnet://lib@sjsulib.sjsu.edu`**

Santa Clara University
telnet: `sculib.scu.edu`
login: `clara`
URL: **`telnet://clara@sculib.scu.edu`**

Sonoma State University
telnet: `vax.sonoma.edu`
login: `opac`
URL: **`telnet://opac@vax.sonoma.edu`**

Tufts University
telnet: `library.tufts.edu`
login: `tulips`
URL: **`telnet://tulip@library.tufts.edu`**

University of Alabama, Huntsville
Huntsville, Alabama

telnet: library.uah.edu
login: he
URL: **telnet://library@library.uah.edu**

University of Arizona
telnet: sabio.arizona.edu
login: sabio
URL: **telnet://sabio@sabio.arizona.edu**

University of Arkansas
Fayetteville, Ark.
telnet: library.uark.edu
login: library
URL: **telnet://library@library.uark.edu**

University of California
telnet: melvyl.ucop.edu
URL: **telnet://melvyl.ucop.edu**

University of Colorado at Colorado Springs
telnet: .arlo.colorado.edu
login: arlo
URL: **telnet://arlo@arlo.colorado.edu**

University of Hawaii at Manoa
telnet: starmaster.uhcc.hawaii.edu
login at enter class: lib
exit: //exit
URL: **telnet://lib@starmaster.uhcc.hawaii.edu**

University of Illinois at Urbana/Champaign
telnet: illinet.aiss.uiuc.edu
login: b
choose: luis
URL: **telnet://b@illinet.aiss.uiuc.edu**

University of Iowa
telnet: oasis.uiowa.edu
login: oasis
URL: **telnet://oasis@oasis.uiowa.edu**

University of Maine system
telnet: ursus.maine.edu
login: ursus
URL: **telnet://ursus@ursus.maine.edu**

University of Miami
telnet: stacks.library.miami.edu
login: library
exit: q
URL: **telnet://library@stacks.library.miami.edu**

University of Michigan
telnet: hermes.merit.edu
login: mirlyn
URL: **telnet://mirlyn@hermes.merit.edu**

University of Minnesota
telnet: `lumina.lib.umn.edu`
login: `PA`
URL: **`telnet://PA@lumina.lib.umn.edu`**

University of Northern Iowa
telnet: `starmaster.uni.edu`
login: `library, type 1 at service prompt`
URL: **`telnet://1,@starmaster.uni.ed`**

University of Notre Dame
telnet: `irishmvs.cc.nd.edu`
login: `library`
exit: `x`
URL: **`telnet://library@irishmvs.cc.nd.edu`**

University of the Pacific
telnet: `pacificat.lib.uop.edu`
login: `library`
URL: **`telnet://library@pacificat.lib.uop.edu`**

Wesleyan University, Connecticut College and Trinity College
telnet: `library.wesleyan.edu`
login: `luct`
exit: `stop`
URL: **`telnet://luct@library.wesleyan.edu`**

Williams College, Massachussetts
telnet: `library.williams.edu`
login: `library`
URL: **`telnet://library@library.williams.edu`**

Yale University
telnet: `umpg.cis.yale.edu port 6520`
URL: **`telnet://orbis@umpg.cis.yale.edu:6520`**

7. Index
   FTP sites

archives.math.utc.edu	*3.7.4.2*
aurelie.soest.hawaii.edu	*3.11.4.1*
bloompicayune.mit.edu	*3.9.3.1*
ds.internic.net	*3.6.7.3*
fly.bio.indiana.edu	*3.8.5.2*
ftp.cic.net	*3.2.3.1, 3.6.5.1, 3.6.5.2, 3.14.3.1, 3.15.1*
ftp.digex.net	*3.3.3.1, 3.7.4.1*
ftp.greatlakes.net	*5.2.2*
gandalf.umc.maine.edu	*3.10.3.2*
igc.apc.org	*2.3, 3.9.3.4*
igc.org	*3.6.5.2*
info.umd.edu	*4.1*
jade.tufts.edu	*3.5.1*
life.anu.edu.au	*3.6.5.3, 3.8.5.1*
netserv1.its.rpi.edu	*3.6.5.4,*
pencil.cs.missouri.edu	*3.4.2, 3.9.3.2, 5.2.1*
plaza.aarnet.edu.au	*3.9.3.5*
relay.cs.toronto.edu	*3.8.5.3*
siri.uvm.edu	*3.10.3.1*

sunsite.unc.edu	3.7.4.3, 3.9.3.3, 3.13.4.1, 3.14.3.2, 3.16.3.1
unix.hensa.ac.uk	3.2.3.2
wiretap.spies.com	3.9.3.6, 3.16.3.2

GOPHERS

dale.ucdavis.edu	3.3.2.1
dewey.tis.inel	4.2
diu.cms.udel.edu	3.11.3.2
ecosys.drdr.virginia.edu	3.6.2.1, 3.7.3.1,
ericir.syr.edu	3.8.2.4
freenet.carleton.ca	5.5.2
freenet.victoria.bc.ca	3.9.2.1
ftp.worldbank.org	3.6.2.6
futures.wic.epa.gov	2.2
gaia.ucs.orst.edu	5.5.1
ginfo.cs.fit.edu	3.10.2.2, 4.4
gopher.cic.net	3.6.2.5, 5.2.2
gopher.ciesin.org	2.1, 3.6.2.3
gopher.counterpoint.com	4.3
gopher.csc.liv.ac.uk	3.7.3.2
gopher.epa.gov	2.2
gopher.internet.com	3.6.7.4
gopher.isnet.is	2.1
gopher.tamu.edu	3.12.3.1
gopher.ubc.ca	3.8.2.2
gopher.uidaho.edu	5.5.4
gopher.who.ch	3.6.2.2
hermes.ecn.purdue.edu	3.8.2.3, 3.14.3.3
igc.apc.org	2.3
info.umd.edu	4.6
kaos.erin.gov.au	2.4, 3.5.1.2, 3.6
lternet.edu	3.6.2.4, 3.6.7.6
minerva.forestry.umn.edu	3.8.2.5
nceet.snre.umich.edu	3.7.3.3
nywork1.undp.org	4.1
pearl.whoi.edu	3.11.2.1
pihta.metla.fi	3.8.2.1, 3.11.2.1
riceinfo.rice.edu	5.3
serra.unipi.it	3.9.2.2
sparc.ecology.uga.edu	3.4.3
uwin.cwr.siu.edu	3.14.4.4

LISTSERVS

AE@SJSUVM1.SJSU.EDU	3.3.1
AQUIFER@IBACSATA	3.14.1
ASEHL@TTUVM1	3.7.1
BIODIVL@BDT.FTPT.BR	3.6.1
BIOSPHL@UBVM	3.6.1
COMPSYL@UIUCVMD	5.1
CONSBIO@UWAVM.U.WASHINGTON.EDU	3.16.1
CTURTLE@NERVM	3.16.1
ECOLOGL@UMDD.UMD.EDU	3.4.1
ECOLOGYL@EMUVM1	3.4.1
ECOSYSL@VM.GMD.DE	3.4.1
ENERGYL@TAUNIVM	3.3.1
ENVBEHL@POLYVM	3.6.1
ENVSTL@BROWNVM.BROWN.EDU	3.6.1, 3.7.1
FMDSSL@PNFI.FORESTRY.CA	3.8.1
FORESTL@NIC.FUNET.FI	3.8.1

GRNSCHL@BROWNVM	3.7.1
HAZMATL	3.10.1
HYDROGENL@URIACC.URI.EDU	3.3.1
IAPWILD@VM1.NODAK.EDU	3.7.1
MARMAN@UVVM.UVIC.CA	3.16.1
MEH20L@TAUNIVM.TAU.AC.IL	5.1
NATURAL@UCHCECVM	5.1
NATRESLIBL/annhed@cc.us.edu	3.8.1
NCIWL@YALEVM	3.12.1
PACIFIC@BRUFPB	3.12.1
RECYCLE@UMAB	3.12.1
SAFETYL@UVMVM	3.2.1, 3.10.1
SANETMG/almana@ces.ncsu.edu	3.13.1
SFERL@UCFIVM	3.6.1, 5.1
SUSTAGL@WSUVM1	3.13.1
WATERL@WSUVM1	3.14.1
WILDNET@TRIBUNE.USASK.CA	3.16.1

TELNET

classroom_earth.ciesin.org	2010 3.1.1.1, 3.7.2.1
eicbbs.wseo.wa.gov	3.3.4.1
envirolink.org	3.6.3.2
envnet.gsfc.nasa.gov	3.6.3.4
epaibm.rtpnc.epa.gov	2.2, 3.6.3.3
esdiml.nodc.noaa.gov	3.11.3.1
fedworld.gov	3.6.3.8
freenet.carleton.ca	5.5.2
gopher.cwr.siu.edu	3.14.4.4
gopher.esdim.noaa.gov	3.11.3.1
hermes.ecn.purdue.edu	3.14.3.7
hermes.merit.edu	3.6.7.5
locis.loc.gov	4.5
psupen.psu.edu	3.6.3.1, 3.8.3.1, 3.9.4.1, 3.12.2, 3.13.2, 3.15.2, 3.16.2
scilink.org	3.6.3.5
Server.wais.com	2.2
sirius.poly.edu	2.1
sseop.jsc.nasa.gov	3.6.3.6
ttnbbs.rtpnc.epa.gov	3.2.2

WWW

http://ecosys.drdr.virginia.edu	3.6.2.1
http://kaos.erin.gov.au	2.4, 3.5.1.2
http://vms.huji.ac.il	3.6.6.2
http://www.econet.apc.org	2.3
http://www.einet.net	3.6.6.1
http://www.nodc.noaa.gov	3.11.3.1

8. **Acknowledgments**

Our many thanks to Dr. Kenneth Linton and James Kane of Muskegon Community College, clients who were instrumental in helping us identify relevant resources for this guide. We would also like to thank Joe Janes and Lou Rosenfeld, our families who were so patient, various and sundry furry critters, whoever invented the fax machine and Alexander Graham Bell.

We received a tremendous response from the environmental community. The following people were instrumental in the compilation of this guide by contributing their suggestions, reports, and expertise. Our heartfelt thanks to:

>Barber, Rob (State University New York)
>Berbara, Ricardo (United Kingdom)
>Beverstock, Dave (Environmental Research Institute of Michigan)

Bouwmans, Ivo (Delft University Clean Technology Institute, The Netherlands)
Brien, Marilyn (Texas)
Budde, Bernard (The Netherlands)
Chenery, Mary Faeth (LaTrobe University)
Cushman, John (New York Times)
Diekmann, Jens
Dombrowski, Janet (National Geographic Society Library)
Endacott, Phil
Feild, Junior (Auburn University)
Finlay, Jeff (St. Peter's College)
Fredericks, Eldon (U. S. Department of Agriculture)
Gray, Tom (EcoNet; editor 'Wind Energy Weekly')
Gronbeck, Christopher (Center for Renewable Energy and Sustainable Technology [CREST])
Gross, Louis (University of Tennessee)
Harder, Jennifer L. (UC Davis)
Hegyes, Gabriel A. (Sustainable Agriculture Network)
Hinchman, Ray (Argonne National Laboratory)
Hunt, Ronn (U. S. Department of Energy)
Ip, David (Canadian Forest Service)
Jaroch, Ed
Jascourt, Stephen
Keniry, Julian.
Klein, Matt (Ball State University)
Koch, ErnstChristian (KaiserslauternUniversity, Germany)
Kool, Richard (British Columbia Ministry of Environment, Lands and Parks)
Krug, Gretchen (SILS University of Michigan)
Lang, Anthony (University of Toronto, Canada)
Lawrence, Kevin
Lerner, Joshua (San Joaquin Valley Endangered Species Recovery Planning)
Line, Mark (Open Pathways)
Link, Terry (Michigan State University)
Lynch, Maureen (Environmental Protection Agency)
Makuch, Joseph. (Water Quality Information Center)
Mclaren, Doug (University of Kentucky)
Morris, Joyce
Nickerson, Gord (Library Software Archives)
Pellinen, Matti (Finnish Association for Nature Conservation, Finland)
Phillips, Dave (New York)
Rose, Michael
Rowe, Stewart
Sackman, Gleason (Moderator of InterNic nethappenings)
Sagady, Alex (American Lung Association)
Sandmeyer, Robert
Spiegel, Erica
Srinivas, Ravi (Syracuse University)
Stein, Michael (EcoNet)
Stewart, Tom
Taylor, Leon (Tulane University)
Teeter, Robert
Truong, Tri (University of Texas)
Visser, Clyde R.
WandesfordeSmith, Geoffrey.
Weaver, Mike (Environmental Protection Agency)
Webster, Barry (Ann Arbor)
Whittington, Jim

Woods, Eric
Yeakley, Alan
Yurman, Dan

Standard Disclaimer:

We do not guarantee that the information found in this guide will be available to everyone, or that it will not have moved or been removed by its owner by the time that this guide is published. We make no claim that this guide is totally comprehensive on any of the subjects that we have included here. We found an abundance of information on environmental topics; due to time constraints not all of this information could be included. Additionally, there may well be resources that we were unable to find, or that were added after this guide was published. At this time, we intend to update the guide every six months or so. And to this end we ask that users of this guide would inform us of omissions and/or new resources as they are found.

    Carol BriggsErickson (cbriggs@sils.umich.edu) and Toni Murphy (murphyt@sils.umich.edu)

Internet/Bitnet Health Sciences Resources

16

Lee Hancock
Educational Technologist
Educational Techology
A Division of Dykes Library
University of Kansas Medical Center

Copyright © Lee Hancock 1993. This document is copyrighted for non-commerical distribution only. Please retain complete credits with any distribution copies or partial copies. Thank you.

Please send any comments, suggestions, corrections, additions, deletions to Le07144@Ukanvm or Le07144@Ukanvm.cc.ukans.edu Thank you.

I also owe a special debt of gratitude to Vivian (Jenny) Jacobson for her assistance in putting together this edition. At her suggestion we put the this list into a database format of her design. She also was also of a tremendous assistance in getting this information into the database. The ascii output is still a little rough, but by the next update I should have the report bugs out. So please try to ignore any format errors this time. Around midnight I start missing details.

LISTSERV DISCUSSION GROUPS

AAVLD-L
Description: Forum for discussion between veterinary diagnostic laboratories and members of the AAVLD.
Access: Electronic Mail
Bitnet Address: `listserv@UCDCVDLS`

ABUSE-L
Description: The ABUSE-L list was formed to serve as a forum for professionals for discussion of topics related to child abuse.
Electronic Mail
Contact: Ann S. Botash, MD botasha@vax.cc.hscsyr.edu
   Director, Child Abuse Referral and
   Evaluation Program
   SUNY Health Science Center at Syracuse
   750 East Adams Street
   Syracuse, NY 13210
Bitnet Address: `listserv@UBVM`
Internet Address: `listserv@UBVM.CC.BUFFALO.EDU`

ACT-UP
Description: ACT-UP was set up for the discussion of the work being done by the various act-up chapters worldwide, to announce events, to exchange ideas related to aids activism, and, more broadly, to discuss the politics of AIDS and health care.
Access: Electronic Mail
Contact: Lenard Diggins (owner)
Bitnet Address: `act-up-request@world.std.com`

ADA-LAW
Description: This list is a discussion about any aspect of the disability-related laws.
Access: Electronic Mail
Contact: wtm@sheldev.shel.isc-br.com
Bitnet Address: `listserv@NDSUVM1`
Internet Address: `listserv@VM1.NODAK.EDU`

ADDICT-L
Description: ADDICT-L exists for the mature discussion of the various addictions experienced by a large portion of society. The focus of this list is to provide an information exchange network for individuals interested in researching, educating or recovering from a variety of addictions. It is not the intent of this list to focus on one area of addiction, but rather to discuss the phenomena of addiction as it relates to areas of various types of addictions.
Access: Electronic Mail
Contact: Owner: David Delmonico: ddelmoni@kentvm.kent.edu
Bitnet Address: `listserv@kentvm`
Internet Address: `listserv@VM1.NODAK.EDU`

ADMIN-L
Description: NYS Department of Health.
Access: Electronic Mail
Bitnet Address: `listserv@ALBNYDH2`

ADMIN-L
Description: Adirondack Medical Records Association discussion list. This list is private. Contact the owner to request subscription.
Access: Electronic Mail
Contact: Owner: bdk01@albnydh2
Bitnet Address: `listserv@ALBNYDH2`

AGEING
Description: BIOSCI Aging electronic conference.
Access: Electronic Mail
Internet Address: `listserv@DARESBURY.AC.UK`

AGRIS-L
Description: The Food and Agriculture Organization Library.
Access: Electronic Mail
Bitnet Address: `listserv@IRMFAO01`

AHL
Description: American Health Line News Service.
Access: Electronic Mail
Bitnet Address: `listserv@GWUVM`

AI-MEDICINE-REQUEST
Description: A discussion list for the areas of medical informatics that deal with AI, like CAI or decision support. Computer scientists and engineers with interest in biomedical and clinical research, and of physicians with interest in medical informatics. AI in Medicine is a broad subject area which encompasses almost all research areas in artificial intelligence. For the purposes of this e-conference, AI in Medicine may

be defined as "computed-based medical decision support" or "computer-assisted medical decision making". All requests to be added to or deleted from this e-conference, problems, questions, etc., should be sent to: AI-MEDICINE-REQUEST@VUSE.VANDERBILT.EDU

Access: Electronic Mail
Contact: Owner: Serdar Uckun, MD serdar@vuse.vanderbilt.edu
Internet Address: listserv@VUSE.VANDERBILT.EDU

AIDS

Description: This is a redistribution list for the Usenet newsgroup Sci.Med.AIDS. Mail to the list is automatically forwarded to the moderator team for the newsgroup

Access: Electronic Mail
Contact: Owner: aids@cs.ucla.edu—Moderator Team
Bitnet Address: listserv@RUTVM1
Internet Address: listserv@RUTGERS.EDU

AIDS-STAT

Description: This discussion list is for the distribution of AIDS statistics from various agencies. The prime information being distributed will be the Center for Disease Control's monthly AIDS Surveillance Report.

All requests to be added to or deleted from this distribution list, problems, questions, etc., should be sent to: AIDS-STAT-REQUEST@WUBIOS.WUSTL.EDU

Access: Electronic Mail
Contact: Owner: David Dodell ddodell@stjhmc.fidonet.org
Internet Address: listserv@WUBIOS.WUSTL.EDU

AIDS-STAT-REQUEST

Description: AIDs statistics.
Access: Electronic Mail
Internet Address: listserv@WUBIOS.WUSTL.EDU

AIDS_INTL

Description: This is a discussion list for the International Committee for Electronic Communication on AIDS (ICECA). The purpose of ICECA is to foster international coordination of electronic activities on AIDS. It also tries assist individuals and organizations who are interested to participate electronically and to identify and arrange activities.

Access: Electronic Mail
Contact: Owner: Michael Smith mnsmith@umaecs
Bitnet Address: listserv@RUTVM1
Internet Address: listserv@RUTGERS.EDU

AIDSNEWS

Description: The AIDSNews Forum is used for the discussion of any issue relating to AIDS/ARC. AIDS Treatment News reports on experimental and alternative treatments, especially those available now. It collects information from medical journals, and from interviews with scientists, physicians and other health practitioners, and persons with AIDS or ARC; it does not recommend particular therapies, but seeks to increase the options available. The ethical and public-policy issues around AIDS treatment research will also be examined. AIDS Treatment News, Northern Lights Alternatives, and many other publications are also distributed to this e-conference.

To protect privacy the subscriber e-conference is kept confidential. If you have any problems subscribing to the e-conference send mail to the Coordinator.

Access: Electronic Mail
Contact: Owner: Michael Smith mnsmith@umaecs

Bitnet Address: **listserv@RUTVM1**

Internet Address: **listserv@RUTGERS.EDU**

ALCOHOL

Description: This is an alcohol and drug studies discussion group. ALCOHOL is a unique e-conference offering the BITNET Community a chance to voice their opinions about the abuse of alcohol, illegal and other commonly abused drugs. The e-conference is open to anyone, but contributions from the psychological and medical professions are encouraged. Students are especially encouraged, as they may provide some fresh insight.

Access: Electronic Mail

Contact: Owner: Phillip Charles Oliff fxx1@lmuacad

Bitnet Address: **listserv@LMUACAD**

ALS

Description: This is a discussion list for those interested in ALS Amyotrophic Lateral Sclerosis, or Lou Gehrig's Disease). This list has been set up to serve the world-wide ALS community. That is, ALS patients, ALS support/discussion groups, ALS clinics, ALS researchers, etc.. Others are welcome (and invited) to join. THIS IS NOT A LISTSERV SETUP. For more information, please send email to: BRO@HUEY.MET.FSU.EDU (Bob Broedel).

Access: Electronic Mail

Contact: bro@huey.met.fsu.edu (Bob Broedel)

Internet Address: **BRO@HUEY.MET.FSU.EDU**

AMALGAM

Description: The AMALGAM list distributes information about chronic mercury poisoning from dental "silver" tooth fillings.

Access: Electronic Mail

Contact: Herausgeber:
Siegfried Schmitt
Klosterweg 28
D-76131 Karlsruhe
uj21@dkauni2.bitnet
uj21@ibm3090.rz.uni-karlsruhe.de

Bitnet Address: **listserv@DEARN**

Internet Address: **listserv@VM.GMD.DE**

AMALGAM

Description: Dental AMALGAM and MERCURY Poisoning distribution list. Only book reviews and article abstracts will be published. Send your contributions to AMALGAM@IBMVM.RUS.UNI-STUTTGART.DE or to AMALGAM@DS0RUS11 via email. (in English, French or German).

Access: Electronic Mail

Bitnet Address: **AMALGAM@DS0RUS11**

Internet Address: **IBMVM.RUS.UNI-STUTTGART.DE**

AMIA-37

Description: American Medical Informatics Association discussion list. This list coordinates email for the members of the American Medical Informatics Association's Professional Specialty Group on Emergency Medicine Anesthesiology, and Critical Care (PSG-37). This group focuses on issues pertinent to the application of medical informatics within the patient care continuum represented by these medical specialties.

Access: Electronic Mail

Contact: Owner: Ron Benoit rbenoit@count.ab.umd.edu

AMIED-L
Description: American Medical Informatics Association Education PSG
Access: Electronic Mail
Internet Address: `listserv@VM1.MCGILL.CA`

ANHODD
Description: A mail list for the exchange of information between drug scientists, to share skills and resources and identify potential research partners.
Access: Electronic Mail
Internet Address: `listserv@CC.UTAS.EDU.AU`

ANEST-L
Description: This list is a vehicle for the discussion of topics related to anesthesiology and collection of any information related to anesthesiology.
Access: Electronic Mail
Contact: Owner: Andrew M. Sopchak `sopchaka@snysyrv1`
Bitnet Address: `listserv@UBVM`
Internet Address: `listserv@UBVM.CC.BUFFALO.EDU`

AOBULL-L
Description: New York state Department of Health area office.
Access: Electronic Mail
Bitnet Address: `listserv@ALBNYDH2`

APASD-L
Description: APA Research Psychology Network. The APA Science Directorate Funding Bulletin is designed to alert subscribers to research and training funding sources for psychology.
Access: Electronic Mail
Contact: Owners: Deborah Segal `apasddes@gwuvm`
Cheri Fullerton `apasdcf@gwuvm`
Bitnet Address: `listserv@VTVM2`

APASPAN
Description: APA Scientific Grassroots Network discussion list.
Access: Electronic Mail
Contact: Owner: Cheri Fullerton `apasdcf@gwuvm`
Bitnet Address: `listserv@GWUVM`

APSSCNET
Description: A discussion list for the American Psychological Society Student Caucus.
Access: Electronic Mail
Internet Address: `listserv@VM1.MCGILL.CA`

ASLING-L
Description: American Sign Language List.
Access: Electronic Mail
Bitnet Address: `listserv@YALEVM`

AUDITORY
Description: Research in auditory perception discussion list. As of this date, the list is closed to new members.
Access: Electronic Mail
Contact: Owner: Dan Ellis `dpwe@media.mit.edu`
Bitnet Address: `listserv@MCGILL1`

AUTISM
Description: This is a discussion list devoted to the xDevelopmentally Disabled. Autism's purpose is to provide a forum for those who are Developmentally Disabled, their teachers, and those interested in this area. The list provides a forum for the understanding and treatment of all types of Developmental Disability and to further Networking among those so handicapped to increase their interaction with the rest of society.
Access: Electronic Mail
Contact: Owner: Bob Zenhausern `drz@sjuvm.bitnet`
Bitnet Address: `listserv@SJUVM`

AVHIMA-L
Description: AVHIMA-L (American Veterinary Health Information Management).
Access: Electronic Mail
Internet Address: `listserv@VMD.CSO.UIUC.EDU`

BACKS-L
Description: A discussion list concerning research on low back pain, and resulting disabilities.
Access: Electronic Mail
Contact: Owner: Elizabeth H. Dow `edow@moose.uvm.edu`
Internet Address: `listserv@MOOSE.UVM.EDU`

BEHAVIOR
Description: Behavioral and Emotional Disorders in Children discussion list.
Access: Electronic Mail
Contact: Owners: Samuel A. DiGangi `atsad@asuacad`
Robert B. Rutherford Jr. `atrbr@asuacad`
Bitnet Address: `listserv@ASUACAD`

BHRD-L
Description: New York state Bureau of Health Resource Development.
Access: Electronic Mail
Bitnet Address: `listserv@ALBNYDH2`

BIOCIS-L
Description: Biology Curriculum Innovation Study.
Access: Electronic Mail
Bitnet Address: `listserv@SIVM`

BIOESR-L
Description: Biological applications of Electron Spin Resonance.
Access: Electronic Mail
Bitnet Address: `listserv@UMCVMB`

BIOMCH-L

Description: Biomechanics and Movement Science listserver. This list is intended for members of the International, European, American, Canadian and other Societies of Biomechanics, ISEK (International Society of Electrophysiological Kinesiology), and for all others with an interest in the general field of biomechanics and human or animal movement. For the scope of this list, see, e.g., the Journal of Biomechanics (Pergamon Press), the Journal of Biomechanical Engineering (ASME), or Human Movement Science (North-Holland). BIOMCH-L is operated under the Patronage of the International Society of Biomechanics.

Access: Electronic Mail

Contact: Technical help can be obtained by sending the command send biomch-l guide to LISTSERV@HEARN or LISTSERV@NIC.SURFNET.NL

Bitnet Address: **listserv@HEARN**

Internet Address: **listserv@NIC.SURFNET.NL**

BIOMED-L

Description: Association of Biomedical Communication Directors. BIOMED-L is a international discussion list for Directors of Biomedical Communications Centers in Medical Schools, Veterinary Schools and Schools of Allied Health Sciences. Topics of discussion may include Center Administration, Instructional Development, Medical Informatics, Medical Illustration, Biomedical Photography, Computer Graphic Imaging, Television Production, and other relevant issues. BIOMED-L is a private forum.

Access: Electronic Mail

Contact: Bill Hillgartner (owner)

Bitnet Address: **BIOMED-L@VM1.MCGILL.CA** (list)

AD38@@MUSICA.MCGILL.CA (listserv)

BIOMED-L

Description: This is a discussion list concerning the topic of Biomedical Ethics. Since the field of medicine and medical technology are rapidly changing and the field is so broad, it is difficult to have clearly delineated rules as to what should and should not be discussed. Possible topics for this list might include: paternalism, fetal cell transplant, the right to die, AIDS, suicide, patient autonomy, abortion, drug legalization, euthanasia, respirator withdrawal, transplants, allocation of scarce resources and many others too numerous to list here. The discussions may be ethical, philosophical, religious, political, social or even, in some cases, personal. Open discussion, disagreement, and dissent is encouraged. Open flames are most certainly NOT.

Access: Electronic Mail

Contact: Owner: Bill Sklar 86730%lawrence.Bitnet@vm1.nodak.edu

Bitnet Address: **listserv@NDSUVM**

Internet Address: **listserv@VM1.NODAK.EDU**

BIOMET-L

Description: Bureau of biometrics at albnydh2.

Access: Electronic Mail

Bitnet Address: **listserv@ALBNYDH2**

BISEXU-D

Description: BISEXU-L Digest.

Access: Electronic Mail

Bitnet Address: **listserv@BROWNVM**

BISEXU-L
Description: This is a mailing list for discussion of issues of bisexuality. Cordial and civilized exchange of relevant ideas, opinions & experiences between members of all orientations is encouraged—we do not discriminate on the basis of orientation, religion, gender, race, etc.. Not intended in the spirit of separatism from other lists devoted to lesbian, gay issues.

Access: Electronic Mail
Contact: Owner: Elaine Brennan e1406010@brownvm
Bitnet Address: `listserv@BROWNVM`

BLIND-L
Description: Computer use by and for the sight impaired discussion list. This list is intended to provide a forum for discussion of computer use by the blind and visually impaired. Topics relating to use of VM/CMS and PCs are of particular interest, but discussion of other systems is also welcome.

Access: Electronic Mail
Contact: Owner: Daniel P. Martin dmartin@uafsysb
Bitnet Address: `listserv@UAFSYSB`

BOSTON-RSI
Description: Repetetive stress injuries.
Access: Electronic Mail
Internet Address: `listserv@world.std.com`

BRAIN-L
Description: Mind-Brain discussion group.
Access: Electronic Mail
Contact: Owner: Chris Westbury chris@ego.psych.mcgill.ca
Bitnet Address: `listserv@MCGILL1`

BRAINTMR
Description: A forum to discuss topics related to all types of brain tumors whether benign or malignant. Information and experiences are shared among patients, their supporters, all kinds of medical professionals, and researchers who study brain tumor growth/treatment.

Here are just a few examples of how BRAINTMR could be used:

    For patients and families dealing with the same tumor type to "meet."
    To find out WHO is doing WHAT brain tumor research.
    To address emotional aspects of patients' brain tumor treatment.
    To discuss the impact of brain tumors on individuals, society and the practice of medicine
    To discuss other intracranial malformations (such as the AVM).

Access: Electronic Mail
Contact: Owner: Samantha Scolamiero samajane@athena.mit.edu
    Listowner & Brain Tumor Survivor (cpa/brainstem epidermoid)
    182 Redington Street
    Swampscott, MA 01907-2135 USA
    Home Phone: 617/593-5095.
Internet Address: `listserv@MITVMA.MIT.EDU`

BRCTR
Description: Braille Research Center forum.
Access: Electronic Mail
Bitnet Address: `listserv@ULKYVM`

BRIT-L

Description: Behavioral research in transplantation.

Access: Electronic Mail

    Mike Renfro

        `frog@ksuvm`

Bitnet Address: `listserv@KSUVM`

BRTHPRNT

Description: A list provided to aid communication among and between the primary audience of birthparents of adopted children. Others are welcome to join the discussion but are advised that the primary mission of the list is to provide a forum for birthparents to discuss issues that pertain to them. The list will remain officially unmoderated but subscribers should remember that it is a listowner's duty to keep lists focused.

Access: Electronic Mail

Contact: Owner: Nathan Brindle `nbrindle@indycms.bitnet`

    `nbrindle@indycms.iupui.edu`

Bitnet Address: `listserv@INDYCMS`

Internet Address: `listserv@INDYCMS.IUPUI.EDU`

C+HEALTH

Description: The C+Health discussion group is intended to promote sharing of information, experiences, concerns, and advice about computers and health. This list is intended to promote sharing of information, experiences, concerns, and advice about computers and health. Anecdotal evidence, media reports, and some formal studies suggest that computer users are at risk from misuse and overuse of computers. Eyestrain, headache, carpal tunnel syndrome, and other apparently computer-related maladies are increasing. And it would appear that many institutions have been slow to respond with education, training, office and lab design, etc.

Access: Electronic Mail

Contact: Owner: Kimberly Updegrove `kimu@dairp.Upenn.Edu`

Bitnet Address: `listserv@IUBVM`

Internet Address: `listserv@IUBVM.UCS.IND.IANA.EDU`

CADUCEUS

Description: This is a History of Medicine Collections Forum. CADUCEUS is a moderated discussion group organized for members of the Archivists and Librarians in the History of Health Sciences, and other individuals interested in medical history collections. CADUCEUS is a moderated discussion group organized for the members of the Association of Librarians in the History of the Health Sciences, and other individuals interested in medical history collections. To subscribe, send a request to: `CADUCEUS@UTMBEACH.BITNET`

Access: Electronic Mail

Contact: Owner: Inci Bowman

Bitnet Address: `listserv@UTMBEACH`

Internet Address: `listserv@BEACH.UTMB.EDU`

CANCER-L

Description: This list is a public list for the discussion of CANCER related topics.

Access: Electronic Mail

Contact: Owner: Susan Rodman `u0ac3@wvnvm.bitnet`

Bitnet Address: `listserv@WVNVM`

CANCHID

Description: The Canadian University Consortium on Health in International Development (CUCHID) is a multi-campus consortium including medical schools and others devoted to research and projects in the area of health and developing countries. Its actual work deals with health and vulnerable groups, be they in poor or rich countries. High on the current agenda is work on the role of tobacco, as a health hazard to all and, in particular, as the source of "life style" illness for the young in developing countries.

Access: Electronic Mail

Internet Address: `listserv@VM1.YORKU.CA`

CDMAJOR

Description: Communication Disorder discussion List.

Access: Electronic Mail

Bitnet Address: `listserv@KENTVM`

CEMS-L

Description: Collegiate Emergency Medical Services.

Access: Electronic Mail

Bitnet Address: `listserv@MARIST`

CERTAN-L

Description: NIH/DCRT—CERTAN Acquistion Project. This Listserv is to be used to communicate information regarding NIH's/DCRT reprocurement. The list will handle potential vendor questions.

Access: Electronic Mail

Contact: Owner: Eddie Suiter `esi@nihcu`

Bitnet Address: `listserv@NIHCU`

CFS-L

Description: This list concerns Chronic Fatigue Syndrome. The discussions seek to serve the needs of persons with chronic fatigue syndrome by enabling a broad range of CFS-related topics. Subscription is open and the list is unmoderated. Please note that any advice which may be given on this list regarding diagnoses or treatments, etc., reflects only the opinion of the individual posting the message; people with CFS ought to consult with a licensed health care practitioner who is familiar with the syndrome.

CFS is an illness characterized by debilitating fatigue and a variety of flu-like symptoms. The condition is also known as chronic fatigue immune deficiency syndrome (CFIDS), myalgic encephalomyelitis (ME) and by other names, and in the past has been known as chronic Epstein-Barr virus (CEBV).

Access: Electronic Mail

Contact: Owner: Roger Burns Bitnet: `Bfu@nihcu.bitnet`
Internet: `rburns@cap.gwu.edu`
Compuserv: `73260.1014@compuserve.com`
Genie: `r.burns34@genie.geis.com`

Bitnet Address: `listserv@NIHLIST`

Internet Address: `listserv@LIST.NIH.GOV`

CFS-MED

Description: Chronic Fatigue Syndrome/CFIDS medical list.

Access: Electronic Mail

Bitnet Address: `listserv@NIHLIST`

Internet Address:

CHMINF-L
Description: Chemical Information Sources.
Access: Electronic Mail
Bitnet Address: `listserv@IUBVM`

CLAN
Description: Cancer Liaison and Action Network.
Access: Electronic Mail
Contact: Owner: Jean-Claude Salomon `salomon@frmop11`
Bitnet Address: `listserv@FRMOP11`

CLGSG-L
Description: Coalition of Lesbian and Gay Student Groups.
Access: Electronic Mail
Bitnet Address: `listserv@RICEVM1`

CMEDSSOC
Description: Canadian Medical Student Societies.
Access: Electronic Mail
Bitnet Address: `listserv@UTORONTO`

CMTS-L
Description: CMTS-L, Chemical Management and Tracking Systems, is a discussion group focused on the formation of a chemical management and tracking system at Cornell University. CMTS-L will also act as a forum at the international level for the exchange of ideas concerning the efforts at various educational and commercial organizations engaged in the establishment of chemical management and tracking systems.

There are many of us attempting to design, fund and implement chemical inventory and tracking systems, waste management systems, chemical recycling/exchange lists and other applications of computers to chemical management. The idea for this new list arose during the 11th Annual College Hazardous Waste Conference held at Stanford last month. It was apparent that many individuals at numerous institutions were working on various aspects of this problem, along with the regulatory problems associated with research scale use of chemicals and the resulting chemical waste at educational and research institutions.

Hopefully, this list will allow us to work together to solve some common problems associated with the large scale introduction of computerized chemical management systems. Any information or threads of conversations related to the topics described above are acceptable for posting to CMTS-L.

Access: Electronic Mail
Contact: Tom Shelley `tjs1@cornell.edu`
Environmental Health and Safety
Cornell University
118 Maple Ave., Ithaca, NY 14850.
(607) 255-4862
Internet Address: `listserv@cornell.edu`

CNRG
Description: Canadian Nurses Research Group.
- networking for nurse researchers.
- has discussion groups for particular topics, e.g., "caring."

Access: Electronic Mail

Contact: Apply to: Judy Wuest, University of New Brunswick, Canada;
   wuest@unb.ca
   Sue Holmes: sholmes@cariboo.bc.ca
Internet Address: See Contact

COCAMED
Description: Computers in Canadian Medical Education discussion group.
Access: Electronic Mail
Contact: Owner: Grace Paterson grace.paterson@dal.ca
Bitnet Address: **listserv@UTORONTO**

COGSCI-L
Description: The Cognitive Science Discussion Group consists of faculty and students in a variety of disciplines, including Psychology, Philosophy, Linguistics, Computer Science, Music and others interested in the study of cognition, broadly defined. The group has biweekly meetings in the Behavioral Science Building at York, with presentations or discussions.
Access: Electronic Mail
Contact: Owner: Michael Friendly friendly@yorkvm1.bitnet
Bitnet Address: **listserv@MCGILL1**

Name: COMMDIS
Description: This lists subscrption request must be sent to COMSERVE@RPIECS. Send the following command to that address to begin your subscription: Join Commdis Your name
Access: Electronic Mail
Contact: Owner: support@rpitsvm (Comserve Support Staff)
Bitnet: **listserv@COMSERVE.RPIECS**

COMPMED
Description: COMPMED is an unmoderated, open forum for the discussion of comparative medicine, laboratory animals (all species) and related subjects. This list is open to any email user with an interest in laboratory animals and biomedical research. Subject matter may range from, but is not limited to:

- News items
- Meeting announcements
- Research issues
- Information requests
- Veterinary/husbandry topics
- Job notices
- Animal exchange information
- Book reviews

Access: Electronic Mail
Contact: Owner: Ken Boschert ken@wudcm.wustl.edu
Bitnet Address: **listserv@WUVMD**
Internet Address: **listserv@WUVMD.WUSTL.EDU**

COMPUMED
Description: Computers in Medicine. Software and Hardware Developments in Medicine. List members include Medical administrators in hospitals and universities, software developers, government officials in the sciences and social services, students in medical facilities, and software and hardware suppliers to government, hosital centres and universities.

Access: Electronic Mail
Bitnet Address: `listserv@SJUVM`
Internet Address: `listserv@SJUVM.STJOHNS.EDU`

COMSERV
Description: Communication in health care.
Subgroup: COMMDIS. Speech disorders discussion list.
Access: Electronic Mail
Contact: Subscriptions to the COMMDIS list must be sent to `COMSERVE@RPIECS`. Send the following command to that address to begin your subscription: `Join Commdis your name`
Bitnet Address: `listserv@RPIECS`
Internet Address: `Comserve@vm.its.rpi.edu`

CONFLIST
Description: University of California at San Francisco School of Medicine Conference List.
Access: Electronic Mail
Bitnet Address: `listserv@UCSFVM`

CONFOCAL
Description: Confocal Microscopy List.
Access: Electronic Mail
Contact: Owner: Robert Summers `summers@ubmed.buffalo.edu`
Bitnet Address: `listserv@UBVM`

CONSLIN
Description: Discussion on Biological Conservation.
Access: Electronic Mail
Bitnet Address: `listserv@SIVM`

COSTAR
Description: Members of the AMIA Comp Med Rec Work Group list may be interested in subscribing to a complementary list which will focus on propagating news, questions, answers and debate relating to the COSTAR (Computer STored Ambulatory Record), which was first developed at the Massachusetts General Hospital for the Harvard Community Health Plan. It is now in the public domain and has been implemented in 500 sites world wide including a network of 23 Canadian and US Multiple Sclerosis research clinics.
Access: To subscribe to this list send a request to: `costar-cmrs-request@unixg.ubc.ca`
Contact: Donald Studney MD `studney@unixg.ubc.ca`
Department of Medicine
University Hospital
2211 Wesbrook Mall, Vancouver BC
CANADA V6T 2B5
voice: 604 822-7142
fax: 604 822-7141
Internet Address: See Access

COSTAR-CMRS
Description: COSTAR focuses on propagating news, questions, answers and debate relating to COSTAR (the Computer STored Ambulatory Record), which was first developed at the Massachusetts General Hospital for the Harvard Community Health Plan. It is now in the public domain and available from:

COSTAR Users' Group
23715 W. Malibu Road
Suite 248
Malibu, CA 90265
Phone: 800 869-6301, or (310) 465-9322

COSTAR has been implemented in 500 sites world-wide including a network of 23 Canadian and US Multiple Sclerosis research clinics. Several of these sites use the HL-7 protocol for data exchange.

Access: To subscribe to this list send a request to: **costar-cmrs-request@unixg.ubc.ca**

Contact: Listowner:
Donald Studney **MDstudney@unixg.ubc.ca**
Department of Medicine
University Hospital
2211 Wesbrook Mall, Vancouver BC
CANADA V6T 2B5
voice: 604 822-7142
fax: 604 822-7141

Internet Address: **listserv@UNIXG.UBC.CA**

CPAE

Description: The Center for Professional and Applied Ethics (CPAE) is an academic for discussing issues related to professional and applied ethics. Topic areas include: Health Care, Business, Media, Law, Public Policy, Public Administration, Sport, Environment, Computing, Education.

Access: Electronic Mail

Contact: Ron Barnette (owner)

Internet Address: **listserv@CATFISH.VALDOSTA.PEACHNET.EDU**

CPRI-L

Description: Computerized Patient Records Institute discussion list.

Access: Electronic Mail

Contact: Owner: Lee Hancock **Le07144@ukanvm**

Editor: Deanie French **dv02@swtexas**

Internet Address: **listserv@UKANAIX.CC.UKANS.EDU**

CROMED-L

Description: Croatian Medical discussion list. The intention of this e-conference is to inform an international community on current events in Croatia, particularly in the sphere of medicine. The intention is also to establish Email as a tool for easier organization of gathering medical and humanitarian help.

Access: Electronic Mail

Contact: Ministry of Health
Republic of Croatia
Office for Cooperation between World Health
Organization and the Republic of Croatia
8. maja 42,
41000 YU-Zagreb
Phone: +38 41 430 621
Fax: +38 41 431 067
(Internet) **whocro@uni-zg.ac.mail.yu**

Bitnet Address: **listserv@AEARN**

CRYONICS

Description: Cryonic Life Support. Cryonic suspension is an experimental procedure whereby patients who can no longer be kept alive with today's medical abilities are preserved at low temperatures for treatment in the future. This list is a forum for topics related to cryonics, which include biochemistry of memory, low temperature biology, legal status of cryonics and cryonically suspended people, nanotechnology and cell repair machines, philosophy of identity, mass media coverage of cryonics, new research and publications, conferences, and local coverage.

Access: Email Addresses `cryonics@whscad1.att.com` (list)
`kqb@whscad1.att.com` (listserv)

Contact: Kevin Q. Brown (owner)

Internet Address: `cryonics@whscad1.att.com` (list)
`kqb@whscad1.att.com` (listserv)

CUSSNET

Description: Computer Users in the Social Sciences (CUSS) is a discussion group devoted to issues of interest to social workers, counselors, and human service workers of all disciplines, including clinical health care settings.

Access: Electronic Mail

Internet Address: `listserv@STAT.COM`

CYAN-TOX

Description: The Cyanobacterial Toxins discussion list. This list is a forum for exchange of information about cyanobacterial toxins, toxic cyanobacteria (blue-green algae) and related topics. It can also be used as a notice board. People interested in the field are welcome and encouraged to join Cyan-ox.

Access: Electronic Mail

Contact: Owners: Tom Lanaras `cdaz02@grtheun1`
Jussi Meriluoto `jmeriluoto@finabo`

Bitnet Address: `listserv@GREARN`

CYSTIC-L

Description: The CYSTIC-L discussion group will focus on the holistic impact of cystic fibrosis. While much of the list will be devoted to discussions of new medical advances as well as possible therapeutic and nutritional treatments, the list should also have a less rigorous side to it.

It will also be a forum for CF patients to vent about frustrating encounters with the medical-industrial complex, to discuss ways of countering bias that might exist in job or school-related activities, and just to talk in general about the myriad of factors that make our lives quite different from those with functional chloride

If you forward this on to a list that might like to know about it, please contact the owner, below, to avoid over-reproduction. Of course, passing this along to anyone who might be interested is the entire purpose this message is being posted ...

Access: Electronic Mail

Contact: Owner: Antony Dugdale `antdug1@minerva.cis.yale.edu`

Bitnet Address: `listserv@YALEVM`

Internet Address: `listserv@YALEVM.CIS.YALE.EDU`

D-ORAL-L

Description: An international forum for discussions of problems facing scientists and clinicians that deal with human and mammalian oral microbiota. Microbiology discussions include the prevalence of, and diseases caused by oral microbiota, physiology and genetics of virulence factors, host response to and virulence factors, autoimmune oral diseases, and the effects of aging on immune response.

Access: Electronic Mail

Contact: Owner: `spitznagel@utmem1.utmem.edu`
`caz@cu.nih.gov`
Dr. John Spitznagel
`jks@giskard.Uthscsa.Edu`

Bitnet Address: `listserv@NIHLIST`

D-PERIO

Description: Informational conversation of NIDR grantees or potential grantees on the general topic of periodontal disease.

Access: Electronic Mail

Contact: Co-owners: Dennis Mangan `ufd@nihcu`
Thomas Murphy `tgl@nihcu`

Bitnet Address: `listserv@NIHLIST`

DBLIST

Description: Databases for Dentistry discussion list.

Access: Electronic Mail

Contact: Owner: John Zimmerman `johnz@umab`

Bitnet Address: `listserv@UMAB`

DCVDLS

Description: American Assoc of Vet Lab Diagnosticians.

Access: Electronic Mail

Bitnet Address: `listserv@UCDCVDLS`

DDFIND-L

Description: Forum for Information Networking on Disability.

Access: Electronic Mail

Bitnet Address: `listserv@GITVM1`

DEAF-L

Description: Discussion list for issues concerning the hearing impaired.

Access: Electronic Mail

Owner: Roy Miller `ge0013@siucvmb`

Bitnet Address: `listserv@SIUCVMB`

DEAFBLND

Description: Dual sensory impairment (deaf-blindness) is the topic of this forum. The mission of DEAFBLND is to share information, inquiries, ideas, and opinions The list is open to professionals in the field, to individuals with DSI, and to their families and friends.

Access: Electronic Mail

Contact: Owner: Bob Moore `str002@ukcc`

Bitnet Address: `listserv@UKCC`

DENTAL

Description: Dental Test List.

Access: Electronic Mail

Bitnet Address: `listserv@UMAB`

DENTAL-L

Description: Cosine Project—Dental Research unit.

Access: Electronic Mail

Bitnet Address: `listserv@IRLEARN`

DENTALMA

Description: Dentistry related articles reports and techniques. There is also a FILELIST available in conjunction with this discussion list. To obtain the FILELIST, send either a `GET DENTALMA FILELIST` or `IND DENTALMA` to `LISTSERV@UCF1VM`

Access: Electronic Mail
Contact: Owner: Karl-Johan Soderholm soderhol@uffsc
Bitnet Address: `listserv@UCF1VM`

DEVIANTS

Description: Social Deviants. The workings of the Great Wok and all things deviant from accepted social norm are discussed here. Occasionally disgusting, but not always, it is the home of ranting, experimental reports, news clippings and other related items. Medical curiosities, cults, murders and other phenomena are well in place here.

Access: Electronic Mail deviants@csv.warwick.ac.uk (list)
   deviants-request@csv.warwick.ac.uk (listserv)
Internet Address: See Access
   `deviants@csv.warwick.ac.uk`
   `deviants-request@csv.warwick.ac.uk`

DIABETES

Description: International Research Project on Diabetes.
Access: Electronic Mail
Contact: Owner: Martin Wehlou wehlou@fgen.rug.ac.be
Bitnet Address: `listserv@IRLEARN`

DIABETIC

Description: Open Discussion forum for DIABETIC patient concerns. This forum is open to all users on this and any other node to aid diabetic persons in the exchange of views, problems, anxieties, and other aspects of their condition. As this is a public forum, all messages are subject to review by any one who might request a copy. This list was started in response to comments from some of the users of `DIABETES@IRLEARN` that perhaps a separate forum for diabetic patient questions and comments could be made available.

Access: Electronic Mail
Contact: Owner: R N Hathhorn sysmaint@pccvm
Bitnet Address: `listserv@PCCVM`

DIARIA

Description: El Centro Nacional de Informacion de Ciencias Medicas le ofrece el servicio de Informacion Diaria elaborado por el Grupo de Informacion Especial.
Access: Electronic Mail
Internet Address: `listserv@INFOMED.CU`

DIARRHOE

Description: DIARRHOE is a mailing list for information exchange and discussions on all aspects related to diseases, disorders, and chemicals which cause diarrhoea in humans and animals.
Access: Electronic Mail
Bitnet Address: `listserv@SEARN`
Internet Address: `listserv@SEARN.SUNET.SE`

DIET

Description: Support and Discussion of Weight Loss.
Access: Electronic Mail
Contact: Owner: Roger Campbell campbell@ubvm
Bitnet Address: `listserv@NDYCMSI`

DISRES-L
Description: This is the disability research list covering any kind of disability-related research.
Access: Electronic Mail
Contact: Owners: Gary Woodill `fcty7310@ryerson`
Grant Davis `gdavis@utoroise`
Bitnet Address: `listserv@RYERSON`
Internet Address: `listserv@RYEVM.RYERSON.CA`

DOHMEM-L
Description: New York state Deparment of Health memorandam.
Access: Electronic Mail
Bitnet Address: `listserv@ALBNYDH2`

DOWN-SYN
Description: A listserv mailing list for discussion of Down Syndrome. This mailing list will be gatewayed with the correpsonding Usenet newsgroup called `bit.listserv.down-syn`. I am also starting a Fidonet conference called "Down-Syn" which will also be gatewayed with this mailing list.
Access: Electronic Mail
Contact: Bill McGarry (203) 926-6187
Bitnet Address: `listserv@NDSUVM1`
Internet Address: `listserv@VM1.NODAK.EDU`

DRUGABUS
Description: Drug Abuse Education Information and Research. A forum for issues related to community drug abuse education and the epidemiology and study of drug abuse. It is run by the Office of Substance Abuse Studies at the University of Maryland at Baltimore.
Access: Electronic Mail
Contact: Owner: Trent Tschirgi `ttschirg@umab`
Bitnet Address: `listserv@UMAB`

DRUGHIED
Description: Drug Abatement Research Discussion. This list is for individuals interested in prevention issues, programs and news related to alcohol and other substance abuse in higher education.
Access: Electronic Mail
Contact: Owner: Deanie French `dv02@swtexas`
Bitnet Address: `listserv@TAMVM1`

DSSHE-L
Description: The Discussion group on Disabled Student Services in Higher Education DSSHE-L is a LISTSERV discussion group formed to serve as a communication vehicle for those interested in the provision of services to students with disabilities in Higher Education.
Access: Electronic Mail
Bitnet Address: `listserv@UBVM`

DTEP-L
Description: Drug Abuse Education Information and Research.
Access: Electronic Mail
Bitnet Address: `listserv@UAMB`

EASI

Description: Disability Access to Libraries. EASI (Equal Access to Software and Information) is starting the list to:
1. provide a forum to share questions and answers about how to make libraries more accessible.
2. provide a platform from which to reach libraries which are not yet considering seriously the question of access for users with disabilities.
3. provide a platform from which to lobby vendors of electronic library services to create tools that are already highly acessible.
4. encourage electronic networks and network information services to make their facilities as accessible as possible to users with disabilities.
5. create and provide services to assist libraries and information providers with resources to assist them in becoming more disability accessible.

Access: Electronic Mail

Contact: Dick Banks rbanks@uwstout.edu (or rbanks@uwstout.Bitnet).

Bitnet Address: `listserv@SJUVM`

Internet Address: `listserv@SJUVM.STJOHN.EDU`

EBCBCAT

Description: Catalogue of biological software.

Access: Electronic Mail

Bitnet Address: `listserv@HDETUD1`

ECGRP-L

Description: Technology and Social Behavior Group.

Access: Electronic Mail

Bitnet Address: `listserv@PSUVM`

EGRET-L

Description: EGRET-L is a moderated listserver for the discussion of topics relating to the epidemiological software package EGRET. It is hoped that this forum will be used to enhance the use of EGRET by the exchange of tips, shortcuts, news and information about problems among the users of this package. It is especially desirable that EGRET-L be used as a resource for new and experienced users to turn to for help when problems are encountered or when they come up with novel applications of the software.

Access: Electronic Mail

Contact: Owners: Stephen P. Baker sbaker@umassmed.ummed.edu
David Avery david@dartcms1

Bitnet Address: `listserv@DARTCMS1`

Internet Address: `listserv@DARTCMS1.DARTMOUTH.EDU`

EHS-L

Description: Environmental Health System.

Access: Electronic Mail

Contact: jjm03@albnydh2
dls13@albnydh2

Bitnet Address: `listserv@ALBNYDH2`

ELDERS

Description: An Elders list has been set up at St Johns University in New York developed for the creation of projects, for discussion of social and political issues, finding new friends and for elders to act as electronic grandparents and elder mentors.

Our membership consists of elders—those over 55 years of age—from a wide range of backgrounds, but with a common purpose—a place where knowledgable people can reach others and where anyone with questions can write for relevant information.

Elder Centre

A Resource Centre for elders is being developed on a gopher where information on organisations, agencies, etc. will be stored and retrieved. St. Johns University is the home of a series of lists devoted to education for everyone. An ever increasing library has been built on many topics on St Johns' gopher.

Access: Electronic Mail

Contact: Owner: Pat Davidson, Co-listowner, Isle of Wight.
xuegxaa@csv.warwick.ac.uk
Elaine Dabbs, Co-listowner, Sydney, Australia.
edabbs@extro.ucc.su.oz.au

Bitnet Address: `listserv@SJUVM`

Internet Address: `listserv@SJUVM.STJOHNS.EDU`

EMBINFO

Description: EMBNet (European Molecular Biology Network) EBCBBUL.

Access: Electronic Mail

Bitnet Address: `listserv@IBACSATA`

EMED-L

Description: A list for health care professionals in Emergency Medicine. This list functions as an automatic mail/distribution system for the exchange of information and issues relating to a particular subject—in this case—emergency medicine. As a member of the list you will be able to pose questions or opinions that will automatically be distributed to all other members of the list. As the list grows, you will be able to seamlessly communicate with members throughout the country—if not the world. This list is sponsored by the Emergency Medicine group at UCSF.

Access: To subscribe to the list send an email message to
`majordomo@itsa.ucsf.edu`

Leave the subject area blank (it will be ignored anyway). In the body of the message just type the following:
`subscribe emed-l@itsa.ucsf.edu your_email_address`

Contact: moderator: Chris Barton cbarton@itsa.ucsf.edu

Internet Address: See Access

EMERG-L

Description: This is an informational network for the exchange of educational topics concerning all branches of emergency services worldwide.

Access: Electronic Mail

Contact: Owners: Marist EMS hzal@marist
Joey J. Stanford grjs@marist

Bitnet Address: `listserv@MARIST`

EMFLDS-L

Description: Electromagnetics in Medicine, Science & Communication This is a list of those interested in electromagnetic fields as they pertain to our new "Electromagnetic Society." Vast scientific literature has been published in recent years on the biological interactions of EM Fields with biological systems. This includes data on 60 Hz to microwave radiation.

Access: Electronic Mail

Contact: Owner: David Rodman oopdavid@ubvms

Bitnet Address: `listserv@UBVM`

EMSA-L

Description: European Medical Students Area-List. EMSA-L is free of charge and open to all medical students. We will try to distribute news about the health care system in Europe and try to discuss political, ethical and clinical aspects of medicine. After the approval of the GA we can also distribute information about EMSA over this list and try to give EMSA publicity.

Access: To subscribe EMSA-L you send an Email message to:
> emsa-l-request@orion.informatik.uni-freiburg.de

Internet Address: `listserv@ORION.INFORMATIK.UNI-FREIBURG.DE`

EMSNY-L

Description: Emergency Medical Services. EMSNY-L is a list devoted to discussion of emergency medical services issues of concern to providers in New York State and elsewhere. Queries will be answered by knowledgeable field providers. Where appropriate, State EMS staff will respond. Files available include the State BLS protocols, the rules and regulations, DNR (do not resuscitate) regulations and policy statement, and hospital emergency department regulation.

Access: Electronic Mail

Contact: Owner: Mike Gilbertson `meg04@albnydh2`

Bitnet Address: `listserv@ALBNYDH2`

ENVBEH-L

Description: This a forum on Environment and Human Behavior. It is meant to encourage discussion on a variety of topics concerning the relations of people and their physical environments, including architectural and interior design and human behavior, environmental stress (pollution, catastrophe) and behavior, human response to built and natural settings, etc.. It is open to anyone and any relevant topic.

Access: Electronic Mail

Contact: Owner: Richard Wener `rwener@polyvm`

Bitnet Address: `listserv@POLYVM`

EXPER-L

Description: Experiences on Viral Attacks.

Access: Electronic Mail

Bitnet Address: `listserv@TREARN`

EYEMOV-L

Description: Eye Movement Network. Subscribers are investigators representing a range of research interests in eye movements.

Access: Electronic Mail

Contact: Owner: Dennis Carmody `CARMODY_D@SPCVXA.SPC.EDU`
Saint Peter's College

Bitnet Address: `listserv@SPCVXA`

Internet Address: `listserv@SPCVXA.SPC.EDU`

FACSER-L

Description: Facilities and Services Discussion List. This list is for the discussion of topics related to facilities and services, including: Physical plant operations, Security and public safety, Transportation and parking, Telephone, Mail service, Environmental health and safety, Capital planning, Facilities utilization.

Access: Electronic Mail

Contact: Roman Olynyk (owner)

Internet Address: `listserv@WVNVM.WVNET.EDU`

FAM-MED
Description: Use of computer technology in the teaching and practice of Family Medicine.
Access: Electronic Mail
Contact: Owner: Paul Kleeburg, M.D. paul@gacvax1
Bitnet Address: listserv@GACVAX1
Internet Address: listserv@GAC.EDU

FAMCOMM
Description: Marital/family & relational communication discussion list. Subscriptions to this list must be sent to COMSERVE@RPIECS (Bitnet) Send the following command to that address to initiate your subscription: Join FamComm Your name
Access: Electronic Mail
Contact: owner: support@rpitsvm (Comserve Support Staff)
Bitnet Address: listserv@RPIECS

FAMILY-L
Description: Academic family medicine discussion.
Access: Electronic Mail
Contact: Owner: Joe Stanford fcmjoe@mizzou1
Bitnet Address: listserv@MIZZOU1

FAMLYSCI
Description: For researchers and scholars focusing on family science, marriage and family therapy, family sociology, and the behavioral science aspects of family medicine. To join the mailing list, send a request to the Coordinator: Greg Brock: gwbrock@ukcc.Uky.Edu
Access: Electronic Mail
Contact: Coordinator: Greg Brock gwbrock@ukcc.uky.edu
Bitnet Address: listserv@UKCC
Internet Address: listserv@UKCC.UKY.EDU

FAO-BULL
Description: Food and Agriculture Organization, AFCO Tech.
Access: Electronic Mail
Bitnet Address: listserv@IRFMA001

FAO-DOC
Description: Food and Agriculture Organization
Access: Electronic Mail
Bitnet Address: listserv@IRFMA001

FAO-INFO
Description: The Food and Agriculture Organization INFO List.
Access: Electronic Mail
Bitnet Address: listserv@IRFMA001

FAOLIST
Description: Food and Agriculture Organization Open Discussion.
Access: Electronic Mail
Bitnet Address: listserv@IRFMA001

FEMISA

Description: FEMISA is conceived as a list where those who work on or think about feminism, gender, women and international relations, world politics, international political economy, or global politics, can communicate.

Access: Electronic Mail

Internet Address: `listserv@MACH1.WLU.CA`

FET-NET

Description: A discussion list concerning research in fetal and perinatal care. Target Group: Those investigators concerned with basic and/or clinical research in fetal and neonatal physiology. Aims of this distribution list:

- Fast circulation of new research information.
- Better international contacts and cooperation.
- Announcement of scientific meetings in this field.
- Distribution of abstracts and programs for scientific meetings.
- Questions/discussions about theoretical and practical matters in our field of research.
- Questions and announcements about fetal-research funding
- All other information related to fetal physiology: the latest news, gossip, etc...

Access: Electronic Mail

Contact: Owners: Bouke Woudstra/Jan Aarnoudse `fetalnet@rug.nl`
Bouke Woudstra `xpvkbouke@rug.nl`

Bitnet Address: `listserv@HEARN`

FIBROM-L

Description: FIBROM-L is a discussion forum for the disease/syndrome known as fibromyalgia/fibrositis. It is an opportunity for researchers, physicians, patients, family and friends of patients and other interested persons to discuss this condition. FIBROM-L is an unmoderated list open to all interested subscribers. It is supported by the Computing and Communications Services Office (CCSO) of the University of Illinois at Urbana-Champaign (UIUC).

Access: Electronic Mail

Contact: Owners: Sandra Bott `sbott@vmd.cso.uiuc.edu`
Molly Mack `mollym@vmd.cso.uiuc.edu`

Internet Address: `listserv@VMD.CSO.UIUC.EDU`

FINAN-HC

Description: Health Care Financial Matters Discussion List. This "list" is designed to enhance the exchange of information and ideas among members interested in teaching and research in health care finance. "Finance" is broadly interpreted to include accounting, economics, and insurance. While most discussions will focus on United States issues, international concerns are encouraged. Membership applicants should "introduce" themselves by speaking about their relevant interests and/or experiences.

Access: Electronic Mail

Contact: Owner: Robert Woodward `rsw@wubios.wustl.edu`

Bitnet Address: `listserv@WUVMD`

FIT-L

Description: FIT-L is a discussion list for exchanging ideas, tips, any type of information about wellness, exercise, and diet.

Access: Electronic Mail

Contact: Owner: Chris Jones `jones@etsuadmn`

Bitnet Address: `listserv@ETSUADMN`

FITNESS
Description: Fitness and the IUPUI campus.
Access: Electronic Mail
Bitnet Address: `listserv@NDYCM`

FO-GCG
Description: INFO-GCG: GCG Genetics Software Discussion.
Access: Electronic Mail
Bitnet Address: `listserv@UTORONTO`

FORENS-L
Description: Forens-L is an unmoderated discussion list dealing with forensic aspects of anthropology, biology, chemistry, odontology, pathology, psychology, serology, toxicology, criminalistic, and expert witnessing and presentation of evidence in court.
Access: Electronic Mail
Contact: Owner: M. Yasar Iscan `iscan@fauvax`
Bitnet Address: `listserv@FAUVAX`
Internet Address: `listserv@ACC.FAU.EDU`

FORENSIC
Description: Forensic medicine, anthropology, death investigation, mortality statistics, accident and safety research discussion list.
Access: Electronic Mail
Contact: Owner: David Broudy `dbroudy@unmb`
Bitnet Address: `listserv@UNMVMA`

FORUMBIO
Description: Forum on molecular biology.
Access: Electronic Mail
Bitnet Address: `listserv@BNANDP11`

FREE-L
Description: A conference for free exchange of information regarding the issues of fathers' rights. These issues arise in the context of divorce, custody disputes, and visitation and child-support arrangements.
Access: Electronic Mail
Contact: Owners: Anne P. Mitchell `shedevil@vix.Com`
    Dale Marmaduke `idqm400@indycms`
Bitnet Address: `listserv@INDYCMS`
Internet Address: `listserv@INDYCMS.IUPUI.EDU`

FSDNURSE
Description: Federal Service Doctoral Nurses List. FSDNURSE is a network discussion group for Federal Service Nurses with Doctoral Degrees. It serves doctoral prepared active duty and reserve nurses in the Army, Navy, Air Force, as well as doctoral prepared nurses in the Red Cross, Veterans Administration, and US Public Health Service.

FSDNURSE has been established to enable network-based discussions that can enhance and enrich consultations among Federal Service Nurses. Send subscription requests to and forward questions regarding FSNURSE To:

P. Allen Gray, Jr., RN, PhD
gray@vxc.Uncwil (Bitnet)
GRAY@VXC.UNCWIL.EDU (Internet)
307 Church Street
Wilmington, NC 28401
Phone: (919) 251-8518
Fax: (919) 395-3863

Access: Electronic Mail

Contact: Owner: P. Allen Gray gray@vxc.uncwil.edu
Doug Cutler uncdwc@uncvm1

Bitnet Address: `listserv@UNCVM1`

GEGSTAFF

Description: This list is open to the discussion of all topics relating to sexuality and gender in Geography. Discussions of theoretical and empirical work/issues are welcome as are book reviews, calls for papers, and information on conferences.

Access: Electronic Mail

Bitnet Address: `listserv@UKCC`

Internet Address: `listserv@UKCC.UKY.EDU`

GENDER

Description: Study of communication and gender discussion list. Subscriptions to this list must be sent to COMSERVE@RPIECS. Send the following message to COMSERVE@RPIECS to begin your subscription: `Join Gender Your name`.

Access: Electronic Mail

Contact: Owner: `support@rpitsvm (Comserve Support Staff)`

Editor: Karla Tonella kdtonell@vaxa.weeg.uiowa.edu

Bitnet Address: `listserv@RPIECS`

GENETICS

Description: Genetics is dedicated to the discussion of clinical human genetics. Its focus is on the diagnosis, management and counseling of conditions of known or possible genetic origin, and the clinical application of genetic technologies in obstetrics, pediatrics and medicine. Genetics is open to all persons interested in clinical human genetics, including health care providers (clinicians, nurses, and other health professionals) and consumers (interested laypeople). Genetics is owned and coordinated by a Board-certified Clinical Geneticist (Luis Fernando Escobar, MD) and an interested layperson (John B Harlan)

Access: Electronic Mail

Contact: Owners: Editorial: Luis Fernando Escobar M.D.
ized100@indyvax
ized100@indyvax.iupui.edu
Administrative: John B Harlan
ijbh200@indyvax
ijbh200@indyvax.iupui.edu

Bitnet Address: `listserv@INDYCMS`

Internet Address: `listserv@INDYCMS.IUPUI.EDU.INDYCMS`

GEOGFEM

Description: This list is open to the discussion of all topics relating to gender issues in Geography. Discussions of theoretical and empirical work/issues are welcome as are book reviews, calls for papers, and information on conferences.

Access: Electronic Mail

Bitnet Address: `listserv@UKCC`

Internet Address: **listserv@UKCC.UKY.EDU**

GERINET

Description: Geriatric Health Care Discussion Group. This is a mailing list of those interested in geriatric health care. It is intended to have multidisciplinary representation (e.g., physicians, nurses, social workers, physical therapists, occupational therapists, psychologists, speech the rapists, lawyers, nursing home administrators, etc.) of individuals concerned about the well-being of elders.

Access: Electronic Mail

Contact: Owner: Robert S. Stall, M.D. drstall@ubvms.cc.buffalo.edu

Bitnet Address: **listserv@UBVM**

Internet Address: **listserv@UBVM.CC.BUFFALO.EDU**

GFULMED

Description: This is for discussion of the Grateful Med software package issued by NIH.

Access: Electronic Mail

Bitnet Address: **listserv@NDSUVM1**

Internet Address:

GLB-MEDICAL

Description: Homosexuality and the Medical Profession. GLB-MEDICAL is a new electronic discussion group devoted to issues related to homosexuality and the medical profession. Personal anecdotes, opinions, original research, news and requests for information about the topic are all welcomed. Discussion may include (but isn't limited to):

- being OUT (or not) in medical school, to colleagues, or to patients
- discrimination experienced by gay, lesbian, or bisexual physicians
- examples, effects, and causes of discrimination experienced by glb patients
- glb suicide, addiction, abuse, gaybashing, STD's, and the medical profession's responses
- glb education in medical school
- the medical profession's role in public education on glb issues

Confidentiality will be respected regarding the usernames on the mailing list. Queries concerning the list or requests for items to be posted anonymously may be addressed to the moderator.

Access: Electronic Mail glb-medical@ac.dal.ca (list)
  mailserv@ac.dal.ca (listserv)

Contact: Moderator: Kevin Speight
  kevinsp8@ac.dal.ca

Internet Address: **glb-medical@ac.dal.ca (list)**
  mailserv@ac.dal.ca (listserv)

GMRLIST

Description: Greater Midwest Region Health Science Libraries.

Access: Electronic Mail

Bitnet Address: **listserv@UICVM**

Internet Address: **listserv@UICVM.UIC.EDU**

GNOME-PR

Description: Human Genome Program Bulletin Board.

Access: Electronic Mail

Internet Address: **listserv@DARESBURY.AC.UK**

GNOME-PR

Description: BIOSCI Human Genome Program E-conference. The National Institute of Health's Human Genome Program is also planning to start a newsgroup for the discussion of genome-related issues.

Access: Electronic Mail

Contact: Owner: Jane Peterson `jp2@nihcu`

Bitnet Address: `listserv@IRLEARN`

Internet Address: `listserv@IRLEARN.UCD.IE`

GOMED-L

Description: Ontario Medical Education Group.

Access: Electronic Mail

Bitnet Address: `listserv@QUCDN`

Internet Address: `listserv@QUCDN.QUEENSU.CA`

GRADNRSE

Description: The GradNrse is a discussion for practicing nurses. It is moderated and originates at Kent State University, Kent, Ohio, USA. It is intended to provide practicing nurses worldwide a place to give and get information about practice situations from their colleagues.

Access: Electronic Mail

Contact: Owner: Linda Q. Thede, RN, MSN, `lthede@kentvm`

Bitnet Address: `listserv@KENTVM`

Internet Address: `listserv@KENTVM.KENT.EDU`

GRANOLA

Description: The GRANOLA list is a forum for discussion of vegetarian-relevant issues. Topics include but are not limited to the following: exchange of really cool recipes, discussion of the various types of vegetarianism, nutrition information, a supportive atmosphere, animal rights issues, cookbook recommendations, tips on surviving as a vegetarian on meal plan.

Access: Electronic Mail

Contact: Owner: Derrell Early `bestuur@vtvm2`

Bitnet Address: `listserv@BROWNVM`

GRANTS-L

Description: NSF Grants & Contracts Bulletin Board.

Access: Electronic Mail

Bitnet Address: `listserv@JHUVM`

H-PROMO

Description: Health Promotion Research List.

Access: Electronic Mail

Bitnet Address: `listserv@RYERSON`

HALRC-L

Description: Health Affairs LRC

Access: Electronic Mail

Contact: Owners: Sally Binkowski `sbinkowski@uncsphvx`
Doug Cutler `uncdwc@uncvm1`

Bitnet Address: `listserv@UNCVM1`

HC-L
Description: HC-L HEALTHCOM/VM Discussion.
Access: Electronic Mail
Bitnet Address: `listserv@ALBNYDH2`

Name: HEALTH-ED-REQUEST
Description: A conference area dealing with Health Education. Any topic dealing with ideas, problems, or solutions is acceptable.
Access: Electronic Mail
Internet Address: `listserv@STJHMC.FIDONET.ORG`

HEALTH-L
Description: HC-L HEALTHCOM/VM Discussion International Discussion on Health Research,
Access: Electronic Mail
Contact: Owner: Jill Foster `jill.foster@newcastle.ac.uk`
Internet Address: `listserv@IRLEARN.UCD.IE`

HEALTHCO
Description: Communication in health/medical context discussion list.
Access: Electronic Mail
> `HEALTHCO@RPICICGE.BITNET` (list)
> `COMSERVE@VM.ECS.RPI.EDU` (listserv)

Subscriptions to this list must be sent to `COMSERVE@RPITSVM` (bitnet) or `COM SERVE@VM.ITS.RPI.EDU` (internet). Send the following command to that address to initiate your subscription: `Join HealthCo Your name`

Contact: Owner: `support@rpitsvm` (Comserve Support Staff).
Bitnet Address: `HEALTHCO@RPICIGE`
Internet Address: `COMSERVE@VM.ECS.RPI.EDU`

HEALTHMGMT
Description: HEALTHMGMT is an unmoderated Internet discussion forum for those interested in the practice, research, and education of management in health care and health service organizations. Discussions on issues pertaining to the management and administration of all health-related organizations, including hospitals, health systems, HMOs, nursing homes, health care networks, etc., and debates about current issues and events in health care and their impact on health care organizations and research are all welcomed. Management practitioners, researchers, and educators interested in health care issues are all encouraged to participate. Enrollment is open to anyone interested in these issues. HEALTHMGMT is also the electronic discussion list for the Health Care Administration Division of the Academy of Management.

Potential uses of HEALTHMGMT include (but are not limited to):

- Requests for information, literature references, or help on any management-related health care issue (such as TQM, hospital organization design, nursing home administration, HMO pricing structures, etc).
- Discussions or debates on topics of interest to the members of the list (e.g., the impact of managed competition on health care organization, the tax-exempt status of hospitals, assessment of new technology in hospitals)
- Notices for professional meetings for management practitioners or academics. If you come across a notice for an interesting professional meeting, please post some information about it.
- Postings for jobs. Anyone aware of job openings (practitioner or academic) in the health care management area is encouraged to post this information.
- Calls for papers. Any calls for papers are especially encouraged.

HEALTH SCIENCES 315

- Book reviews: Read a good health care book lately? Share your opinions.
- Course design and syllabi: share your educational ideas with your colleagues.
- Archives: Every submission to HEALTHMGMT is automatically archived and made available for retrieval from the HEALTHMGMT listserver or the Management Archive gopher server.

Access: Electronic Mail

Internet Address: **listserv@CHIMERA.SPH.UMN.EDU**

HEALTHNET

Description: An Internet discussion list for applications of high speed communication networks in Canadian Health Care.

HEALTHNET is an internet forum for discussion of issues surrounding high speed networking inititives focussing on (but not specific to) Canadian health care. Anyone who is working on or with an interest in these initatives is invited to join and contribute (for example: health care personnel and adminstrators, physicians, technologists, government officials etc).

Potential uses of HEALTHNET include (but are not limited to):

- Discussion of the use of networks (such as the Internet) for health care applications. Applications may include items such as Medical Electronic Data Interchange(EDI) for billing over The use of community health information networks and the use of network technology in the study of health outcomes.
- Discussion of issues such as privacy and security over networks, the application of remote diagnosis, radiographic transmissions etc.
- Announcement of programs involving computer networks and Healthcare facilities, health ministries etc in Canada.
- Requests for information regarding network initatives, service providers, government programs and so on.
- Job postings and RFP's—anyone aware of job openings or who wish to post an RFP for a healthcare network initiative are encouraged to do so.

Access: Electronic Mail

Contact: Michael Pluscauskas (x-man@mgcheo.med.uottawa.ca)
Internet Health Care Applications Consultant
Industry Canada, Ottawa
Telephone: (613) 998-6639.

Internet Address: **listserv@CALVIN.DGBT.DOC.CA**

HEALTHPLAN

Description: White House Health Plan. This Internet mailing list is a conduit through which the White House sends health-reform announcements directly to health professionals and others with electronic mailing addresses.

Access: Electronic Mail Addresses:
HEALTHPLAN@IGC.APC.ORG (list)
SFREEDKIN@IGC.APC.ORG (listserv)
Steve Freedkin (owner)

Contact: Steve Freedken, sfreedkin@igc.apc.org

Internet Address: **SFREEDKIN@IGC.APC.ORG**

HEALTHRE

Description: Health Care Reform. The purpose of Health Reform (HealthRe) is to share information and opinions, ideas and inquiries that relate to the topic of health care reform. While this is high in the political life of the United States at the present, observations, comments, or opinions on health care reform in other countries are welcome.

Access: Electronic Mail

Contact: Co-Listowners: Eleftheria Maratos-Flier
        `emarat@ha rvarda.harvard.edu`
        Rick Narad
        `rnarad@oavax.csuchico.edu`
        Bob Moore
        `str002@ukcc`

Bitnet Address: `listserv@UKCC`

Internet Address: `listserv@UKCC.UKY.EDU`

HELPNET

Description: Network Emergency Response Planning.

Access: Electronic Mail

Bitnet Address: `listserv@NDSUVM1`

HERB

Description: Medicinal and Aromatic Plants discussion list. This list is semi-officially supported by the ANADOLU UNIVERSITY MEDICINAL PLANTS RESEARCH CENTRE (TBAM)
    26470 ESKISEHIR / TURKEY
    Tlf-Net:+90 (22) 150580 ext.3661
    Fax-Net:+90 (22) 150127

Bitnet: `TBAM@TRANAVM2`
    `D54@TRANAVM1`

Contact:Owners: Suleyman Aydin `d54@tranavm1`
    Huryasa Aslan `huryasa@tranavm1`

Bitnet Address: `listserv@TRANAVM2`

HGML-L

Description: Human Gene Mapping Library.

Access: Electronic Mail

Bitnet Address: `listserv@YALEVM`

HHSCOM-L

Description: Although open to subscription, the list is primarily for staff within the U.S. Department of Health and use of the resources available on the Internet, improving HHS use of communication technology, and improving HHS access to information available within and outside of the Department.

Access: Electronic Mail

Contact: Listowner: Bob Raymond, `OSASPE.SSW.DHHS.GOV`
    Office of the Assistant Secretary for Planning and Evaluation.
    Telephone: (202) 690-7316

Bitnet Address: `listserv@NIHLIST`

HHSCTL-L

Description: US Dept of HHS: Reducing Internal Regulation. The list includes those staff persons within the U.S. Department of Health and Human (HHS) who are participating in a Department-wide effort to reduce internal regulations. Internal regulations or controls are rules imposed on HHS organizations, their managers, or staff that require approval of plans or activities, or provide detailed guidance on how to do something, or require detailed reporting on their activities.

    This control reduction effort is part of the Department's Continuous Improvement Process established in mid-1993 National Performance Review and to identify other ways to improve all Departmental activities. The National Performance Review and President Clinton's Executive Order on internal regulation requires that Federal agencies reduce these regulations by 50 percent by September 1996.

The purpose of the list is to provide a means for communicating proposals and developments related to the effort to regulation reduction effort. This is one of a number of activities within the Department whose purpose it is to implement and build upon the recommendations of the National Perfornamce Review recommendations. Other activities may also have established lists.

Access: Electronic Mail

Contact: Listowner: Bob Raymond, Bobr@osaspe.ssw.dhhs.gov
Office of the Assistant Secretary for Planning and Evaluation
Phone: (202) 690-7316.

Bitnet Address: **listserv@NIHLIST**

HIM-L

Description: The purpose of HIM-L is to:
- A. facilitate the transition of "medical record" practitioners to "health information managers."
- B. discuss current legislative, accreditation, and regulatory issues affecting the HIM field.
- C. provide a forum for health information management educators to share educational strategies.
- D. develop joint student projects within and between HIM programs.
- E. provide interaction for HIM students with educators and students from other HIM programs
- F. provide an opportunity for HIM students to practice using a listserv.

Access: Electronic Mail

Internet Address: **listserv@FIONA.UMSMED.EDU**

HL-7

Description: HL-7 is an electronic conference designed to foster communication concerning technical, operational, and business issues involved in the use of the HL-7 interface protocol. It is also intended as a forum for the HL-7 Working Group members who are participating in the specification of the interface protocol. Health Level Seven is an application protocol for electronic data exchange in health care environments.

This HL-7 (Health Level Seven) Conference is *not* an official part of the HL-7 Working Group and Executive Committee. Official inquiries concerning HL-7 (Health Level Seven) should be sent directly to: Health Level Seven, P.O. Box 66111, Chicago, IL 60666-9998, fax: (708) 616-9099. In accordance with current CREN regulations, commercial activity (such as the selling of software) will be prohibited. Subscription to this conference is open to *anyone* interested.

Access: Electronic Mail

HL-7@VIRGINIA.EDU (list)

HL-7-REQUEST@VIRGINIA.EDU (listserv)

HL-7-REQ@VIRGINIA (Bitnet)

David John Marotta (owner)

All requests to be added to or deleted from this e-conference, problems, questions, etc., should be sent to: HL-7-REQUEST@VIRGINIA.EDU (Internet)

Contact: Owner: David John Marotta,
Medical Center Computing,
Stacey Hall
Univ of Virginia
Box 512 Med Cntr
Charlottesville VA 22908
(804) 982-3718 wrk
(804) 924-5261 msg
(804) 296-7209 fax
djm5g@virginia.edu
djm5g@virginia

Internet Address: **HL-7-REQUEST@VIRGINIA.EDU**

HMATRIX-L

Description: A discussion of online health science resources. Of primary interest, but not limited to, are resources available on the Internet. Discussions included where to find information, sounds, images and software of interest to the health professional and interested layperson. We're interested in not only what's available where, but also the quality of resource.

Access: Electronic Mail

Contact: Listowner: Lee Hancock le07144@ukanvm
le07144@ukanvm.cc.ukans.edu

Internet Address: **listserv@UKANAIX.CC.UKANS.EDU**

HOLISTIC

Description: Discussion list dedicated to providing information and discussion on holistic concepts and methods of living which provide a natural way of dealing with the challenges of life.

Access: Electronic Mail

Contact: Curt Wilson (owner)

Bitnet Address: **listserv@SIUCVMB**

Internet Address: **listserv@SIUCVMB.SIU.EDU**

HQ-L

Description: HealthQuest Products Discussion List HQ-L (HealthQuest Products Discussion List) is a list to discuss software created and supported by HealthQuest. Examples include, but are not limited to: Clinical Data Editor (CDE), Clinipac, Medical Records Enhancement/Abstract, Patient Accounting (Medipac and/or Medipac III), Patient Appointments, Patient Management (PM), and Trendstar.

Access: Electronic Mail

Contact: Owner: Jeff Schlader jschlade@psuhmc

Bitnet Address: **listserv@PSUHMC**

HSNETM-L

Access: Electronic Mail

Internet Address: **listserv@MIZZOU1.MISSOURI.EDU**

HSPBED-L

Description: Hospital Bed Availability in NY State.

Access: Electronic Mail

Bitnet Address: **listserv@ALBNYDH2**

HSPNET-D

Description: Hospital Computer Network Discussion Group.

Access: Electronic Mail

Bitnet Address: **listserv@ALBNYDH2**

HSPNET-L

Description: Hospital computer network discussion group HSPNET-L provides consultation, a monthly digest, and a database of hospital networks. It emphasizes restoration and extension of consulting for rural hospitals by connection to major medical centers. All aspects (hardware, software, staff training, confidentiality of patient data, etc) will be covered. Particular attention will be paid to existing networks both in the USA and abroad.

HSPNET-D is the Digest of HSPNET-L

All requests to be added to or deleted from this e-conference, problems, questions, etc., should be sent to the owner.

Access: Electronic Mail
Contact: Owner: Donald F. Parsons M.D. `dfp10@albnyvm1`
Bitnet Address: `listserv@ALBNYDH2`

HUMAGE-L

Description: Humanistic Effects of Aging.
Access: Electronic Mail
Bitnet Address: `listserv2ASUACAD`

HUMBIO-L

Description: Humbio-L is an unmoderated discussion list dealing with biological anthropology, adaptation, environmental stress, biological race, growth, genetics, paleoanthropology, skeletal biology, forensic anthropology, paleodemography, paleopathology, primate biology & behavior.
Access: Electronic Mail
Contact: Owner: M.Y. Iscan `iscan@fauvax`
Bitnet Address: `listserv@FAUVAX`
Internet Address: `listserv@ACC.FAU.EDU`

HUMEVO

Description: Human Evolutionary Research, moderated by the International Institute for Human Evolutionary Research at George Washington University in Washington, DC, examines human biological evolution, adaptation, variation, and evolutionary medicine. Sub-areas include interactive newsletter, hotline, bulletin board, cooperation column, research, and education.
Access: Electronic Mail
Contact: Owner: Noel T. Boaz `boaz@gwuvm`
Bitnet Address: `listserv@GWUVM`

HYPBAR-L

Description: HYPBAR-L is an e-conference to provide an unmoderated environment where issues, questions, comments, ideas, and procedures can be discussed. In a broad sense, this includes virtually anything dealing with medicine in relation to diving and HyperBaric Medicine. The explicit purpose of HYPBAR-L is to provide timely interchange between subscribers, to provide a forum where interesting questions can be addressed within the context of interactive exchange between many individuals, to discuss the evolution and application of HyperBaric and Diving Medicine, to announce professional meetings, calls for papers, and any additional information that would be of interest.
Access: Electronic Mail
Contact: Owner: Derrell Early `bestuur@vtvm2`
`csm1al@technion`
Bitnet Address: `listserv@TECHNION`
Internet Address: `listserv@TECHNION.TECH NION.AC.IL`

HYPERMED

Description: Biomedical Hypermedia Instructional Design discussion list.
Access: Electronic Mail
Contact: Owner: Kent Hisley `khisley@umab`
Bitnet Address: `listserv@UMAB`

IAPSY-L

Description: Interamerican Psychologists List (SIPNET). IAPSY is intended to facilitate and encourage communication and collaboration among psychologists throughout the Americas and the Caribbean, and to aid the Interamerican Society for Psychology/Sociedad Interamericana de Psicologia in its activities. The languages of the list are English, French, Portuguese and Spanish (the languages of the ISP).

Access: Electronic Mail

Contact:Owner: Bob Pfeiffer `grape@albnyvm1`

Bitnet Address: `listserv@ALBNYVM1`

IBDlist

Description: IBDlist is a moderated mailing lists which discusses all aspects of Inflammatory Bowel Diseases, with particular emphasis on Crohn's disease and Ulcerative Colitis. Anyone with an interest in these diseases, whether direct or indirect is welcome. This list will also act as a clearinghouse for information and discussion of current treatments, research, and other information related to IBDs. This list is not restricted to those suffering from one of the diseases or directly linked to IBD patients.

Access: Electronic Mail

Contact: Owner: Thomas Lapp

Internet Address: `IBDLIST-REQUEST%MVAC23@UDEL.EDU`

ICECA

Description: International Committee for Electronic Communication on AIDS (ICECA). The purpose of ICECA:

- to foster international coordination of electronic activities on AIDS.
- to assist individuals and organizations who are interested to participate electronically.
- to identify and arrange activities.

Subscription to this list is limited to committee members. Mail may be sent to the committee by anyone. Further information about ICECA may be obtained from the list owner.

Access: Electronic Mail

Contact: Owner: Michael Smith `mnsmith@umaecs`

Bitnet Address: `listserv@RUTVM1`

IMIA-L

Description: International Medical Informatics Assn. Board.

Access: Electronic Mail

Bitnet Address: `listserv@UMAB`

IMMNET-L

Description: Medical Immunization Tracking systems. IMMNET-L is an electronic bulletin board service designed to facilitate a national discussion about immunization tracking systems. State and local health agencies are specifically invited to participate. The purpose of agencies to share experiences in system design and implementation and is intended to encourage the development of standards for coding and data exchange. Other possible discussion topics could include algorithms for evaluation of compliance and reviews of commercial software.

Access: Electronic Mail

Contact: James E. Levin, MD, PhD `jlevin@umnhcs`
`jlevin@simvax.labmed.umn.edu`

Bitnet Address: `listserv@DARTCMS1`

Internet Address: `listserv@DARTCMS1.DARTMOUTH.EDU`

IMMUNE

Description: This list is a support group for people with immune-system breakdowns (and their symptoms) such as Chronic Fatigue Syndrome, Lupus, Candida, Hypoglycemia, multiple allergies, learning disabilities, etc. and their significant others, medical caretakers, etc.. The group is unmoderated and open to anyone anywhere in the world (no arguments about whether or not these disabilities exist).

All requests to be added to or deleted from this e-conference, problems, questions, etc., should be sent to: `IMMUNE-REQUEST@WEBER.UCSD.EDU`

Access: The address for posting is `immune@weber.ucsd.edu`, whereas to join, send a request to `immune-request@weber.ucsd.edu` (a human address).

Contact: Owner: Cyndi Norman `cnorman@ucsd.edu`

Internet Address: **`immune-request@WEBER.UCSD.EDU`**

INCLEN-L

Description: The purpose of this e-conference is to provide units of the International Clinical Epidemiology Network presently connected by electronic mail, with a vehicle for questions and comments to an "expert" in different aspects of clinical epidemiology.

Access: Electronic Mail

Contact: Owner: `cliftonj@mcmaster`

Bitnet Address: **`listserv@MCMVM1`**

INFO-AIDS

Description: Acts as a clearinghouse for information, and discussion on AIDS, including alternative treatments, political implications, etc. Exchanges files with `AIDNEWS@RUTVM1`.

Access: Electronic Mail

Internet Address: **`listserv@RAINBOW.UUCO`**

INGEST

Description: Ingestive Disorders Mailing list.

Access: Electronic Mail

Contact: Owners: henry kissileff `hrkom@cuvmb`
Jerry B. Altzman `jauus@cuvmb`

Bitnet Address: **`listserv@CUVMA`**

INHEALTH

Description: International Health Communication discussion list. InHealth is a Comserve hotline.

Access: Electronic Mail Addresses
`INHEALTH@VM.ECS.RPI.EDU` (list)
`LISTSERV@VM.ECS.RPI.EDU` (listserv)

For more information send this message to `COMSERVE@RPIECS` (bitnet) or `COM SERVE@VM.ECS.RPI.EDU` (Internet): Help Topics Hotlines

Contact: `support@rpitsvm` (Comserve Editorial Staff)

Bitnet Address: **`listserv@RPIECS`**

Internet Address: **`listserv@VM.ECS.RPI.EDU`**

INHIB

Description: Growth inhibitory molecule theme research group.

Access: Electronic Mail

Contact: Owner: Dr. Lisa McKerracher `cyla@musica.mcgill.ca`

Internet Address: **`listserv@VM1.MCGILL.CA`**

INJURY-L

Description: The Center for Rural Emergency Medicine and the Injury Control Center of West Virginia University have established a discussion list on the Internet for injury research, epidemiology, intervention, prevention and other related issues. The list is open to all persons who share these interests.

Access: Electronic Mail

Contact: Paul M. (Mike) Furbee
Research Coordinator
Center for Rural Emergency Medicine
P.O. Box 9151
Robert C. Byrd Health Sciences Center
Morgantown, WV 26506
(304) 293-6682
furbee@wvnvm.wvnet.edu

Bitnet Address: `listserv@WVNVM`

Internet Address: `listserv@WVNVM.WVNET.EDU`

IOOB-L

Description: Discussion list dedicated to industrial/organizational psychology and organization behavior (IOOB).

Access: Electronic Mail

Contact: Owners: John L. Cofer cofer@utkvx
Harold Pritchett harold@uga

Bitnet Address: `listserv@UGA`

IRAMED

Description: This group is for general medical discussions/questions.

Access: Electronic Mail

Internet Address: `listserv@JERUSALEM1.DATASRV.CO.Il`

JMEDCLUB

Description: Medical Journal Discussion Club.

Access: Electronic Mail

Bitnet Address: `listserv@BROWNVM`

Internet Address: `listserv@BROWNVM.BROWN.EDU`

KINST-L

Access: Electronic Mail

Bitnet Address: `listserv@ULKYVM`

L-HCAP

Description: Technology for the handicapped.

Access: Electronic Mail

Bitnet Address: `listserv@NDSUVM1`

LACTACID

Description: This is a mailing list for discussion and information exchange on ALL aspects related to the biology and uses of lactic acid bacteria; e.g., in human beings and animals (e.g., in new-borns, oral cavity, vaginal tract, etc) in fermented foods (cheese, pickles, sauerkraut, etc.) in animal feeds (ensilage) in the production of polysaccharides and others (e.g., dextran).

Access: Electronic Mail

Contact: Owner: Eng-leong Foo
eng-leong_foo_mircen-ki%micforum@mica.mic.ki.se

Bitnet Address: `listserv@SEARN`

Internet Address: `listserv@SEARN.SUNET.SE`

LAIDOFF

Description: So, you've been laid off? Stress related issues.

Access: Electronic Mail
Bitnet Address: `listserv@ARIZVM1`

LASMED-L

Description: The purpose of this forum is to gather all relevant information on the subject of lasers in medicine in Israel and to distribute it quickly through the computer network.

Access: Electronic Mail

Contact: Owner: Joseph van Zwaren de Zwarenstein
    jo%ilncrd.bitnet@cunyvm.Cuny.Edu
    jo@ilncrd

Bitnet Address: `listserv@TAUNIVM`

Internet Address: `listserv@TAUNIVM.TAU.AC.IL`

LD-L

Description: Veterinary Laboratories. This list has been created to provide a forum for discussion between veterinary diagnostic laboratories and members of the AAVLD. Topics such as test standardization, fees, diagnostic information assistance, animal health surveillance, reports on conferences and symposia are especially welcomed. Discussions related to specific cases should be approached within the limits of diagnostic medicine and restrict discussions of therapy or treatments.

Access: Electronic Mail

Contact: Jim Case DVM,Ph.D (owner)

Bitnet Address: `listserv@UCDCVDLS`

LD-LIST

Description: Learning Disability Information Exchange List. LD-List is an open, unmoderated, international forum that provides an information exchange network for individuals interested in Learning Disabilities. Subscribers include persons with Learning disabilities, family members and friends, educators and administrators, researchers, and others wishing to know more about this disease. Any topic related to Learning Disabilities is appropriate for discussion.

Access: To subscribe, send an email message to
    LD-List-Request@East.Pima.edu. In the BODY of the note say ONLY: SUBSCRIBE.

Contact: LD-List-Owner@East.Pima.edu

Note: Ray Harwood is acting as list owner temporarily; the LD-List-Owner address will always point to the "current" list owner.

Internet Address: `listserv@EAST.PIMA.EDU`

LHU-L LIST

Description: The NYS Dept of Health's mission to safeguard the health of the citizens of NY has necessitated the collection a wide variety of data from the Local Health Units. Efforts are underway to find ways to make the process simpler and more efficient. Some of the ways that have supply PC applications having uniform user interfaces, and improve delivery of information electronically. It is the goal of this list to open up a convenient channel for members to openly discuss the problem even though we are spread out across the entire state and have very busy schedules.

Some of the subscribers to the list are from Local Health Units, members of various divisions in the Health Department who collect the data and members of Information Systems and Health Statistics who manage the Healthcom computer network. The LHU-L list's success depends on the free exchange of ideas, questions, answers, problems and solutions. Please feel free to join and contribute.

Access: Electronic Mail

Contact: Listowner: Barry Krawchuk, bdk01@albnydh2

Bitnet Address: `listserv@ALBNYDH2`

LIS-MEDICAL

Description: Of interest to UK health sciences librarians on LIS-MEDICAL. We have an agreement with Nancy Start about a similar arrangement for MEDLIB-L. It means that UK people don't all have to subscribe to the US list, and they only get messages of international interest forwarded to LIS-MEDICAL. LIS-MEDICAL has around 250 members, mostly from the UK but with an increasing number of overseas subscribers.

Access: Electronic Mail

Contact: Martin Lewis
University of Sheffield Health Sciences Library
Sheffield S10 2JF
JANET: m.j.lewis@sheffield.ac.uk
tel: (0742)766222x3025
fax: (0742)780923

Internet Address: listserv@SHEFFIELD.AC.UK

LIST-HEALTHPLAN

The LIST.HEALTHPLAN Internet Electronic Mailing List

Description: LIST.HEALTHPLAN is an Internet electronic mailing list for receiving, via electronic mail, announcements from the White House regarding health-care reform. It is a *one-way* channel. Subscribers receive, as electronic mail, announcements from the White House regarding health-care reform. The welcome letter sent to new subscribers tells how to subscribe to discussion list, receive back postings from LIST.HEALTHPLAN, and edit/remove your subscription. SAVE IT FOR REFERENCE.

Access: To subscribe, send a message with the Subject: SUBSCRIBE LIST.HEALTHPLAN to sfreedkin@igc.apc.org (Steve Freedkin). For information *only* send a message with the Subject: SEND WELCOME LETTER ONLY. If you don't know how to set the Subject: line in the message header ask your local system administrator/support person.

Contact: Steve Friedkin sfreedkin@igc.apc.org

Internet Address: See Access

LIVE-EYE

Description: Color and Vision Discussion Forum, LIVE-EYE is to be used as a discussion forum. It will not be closely monitored. This is an excellent place to conduct discussions on any topic relevant to color science and/or vision research. LIVE-EYE is an adjunct to the Color and Vision Network (CVNet).

Access: Electronic Mail

Contact: Owner: cvnet@vm1.yorku.ca

Bitnet Address: listserv@YORKVM1

Internet Address: listserv@VM1.YORKU.CA

LPN-L

Description: Laboratory Primate Newsletter List.

Access: Electronic Mail

Bitnet Address: listserv@BROWNVM

LTCARE-L

Description: This interest group seeks to identify, share, and discuss research findings relevant to public policy on disability (both physical and cognitive), aging and long-term care. The group is interested in the characteristics of long term care systems, including eligibility for services, participation rates, socio-economic status of participants, organizational and financial arrangements, service use, and costs. An area of major emphasis is how changes in public policy would affect programs (e.g., Medicare, Medicaid, Older Americans Act) benefitting frail elderly and other experience of States in the USA and other nations in providing long-term care are welcomed. This list is maintained in the office of the Assistant

Secretary for Planning and Evaluation (ASPE) located in the U.S. Department of Health and Human Services (DHHS).

Access: Electronic Mail

Contact: Listowner: Robert Clark bobc@osaspe.ssw.dhhs.gov

Bitnet Address: **listserv@NIHLIST**

MAXLIFE-L

Description: MaxLife-L is a list for those working toward a positive, healthy life style while at the same time choosing to avoid heavy consumerism. It is for people who choose their activities with careful consideration to the pleasure they bring as well as all their costs. Please note that this is a MAILSERV and not a listserv server.

Access: Address posts for the list to: maxlife@email.unc.edu or maxlife@gibbs.oit.unc.edu

Contact: Penny Ward crunchy@email.unc.edu
Sharon Gordon gordonse@iris.uncg.edu

Bitnet Address: **mailserv@UNCG**

Internet Address: **listserv@GIBBS.OIT.UNC.EDU**

MED-TECH

Description: Forum for discussions, postings, etc., for the Clinical Laboratory Sciences.

Access: Electronic Mail

Contact: Owner: Robert Lathrop G563@Music.Ferris.Edu
Ferris State University
Big Rapids, Michigan 49307

Bitnet Address: **listserv@FERRIS**

Internet Address: **listserv@VM1.FERRIS.EDU**

MEDFORUM

Description: Medical Student Organization/Policy Forum.

Access: Electronic Mail

Bitnet Address: **listserv@ARIZVM1**

MEDINF-L

Description: Biomedical Informatics Discussion Group. E-conference for people working in medical data processing/medical informatics. All other requests to be added to or deleted from this e-conference, problems, questions, etc., should be sent to: PL_REI%DHVMHH1.BITNET@CUNYVM.CUNY.EDU

Access: Electronic Mail

Contact: Owner: Prof. Dr. Claus O. Koehler dok205@dhddkfz1

Bitnet Address: **listserv@DEARN**

MEDLIB-L

Description: MEDLIB-L is a forum for librarians in the health sciences. Discussion includes practical and theoretical issues in both the public and technical service areas. This list may be used to exchange ideas, questions, concerns and announcements of particular interest to health sciences librarians.

Access: Electronic Mail

Contact: Owner: Nancy Start hslstart@ubvm

Bitnet Address: **listserv@UBVM**

MEDMAC-fL

Description: Discussion list of the 3d Medical Faculty of the Charles University, Prague. 3d is public health, epidemiology, immunology, basic sciences. Most of the communications are in Czech. The list is closed.

Access: Electronic Mail

Contact: Dr. Milan Jira
Internet Address: `listserv@EARN.CVUT.CS`

MEDNETS

Description: Medical Telecommunications Networks. A forum to discuss medical telecommunication networks in the areas of clinical practice, medical research, and administration. The e-conference is intended to be used for ongoing discussions, information searches, contact searches, surveys, and so on.

Archives: `LISTSERV@NDSUVM1` or `LISTSERV@VM2.NODAK.EDU` also available via anonymous ftp to `VM1.NODAK.EDU` (134.129.111.1) with any password. After you are connected enter CD MEDNETS to access the archives (our file system is NOT hierarchical so to go back to the "root" you would enter CD ANONYMOUS)

Access: Electronic Mail

Contact: Owner: Marty Hoag nu021172@ndsuvm1

Bitnet Address: `listserv@NDSUVM1`

Internet Address: `listserv@VM1.NODAK.EDU`

MEDPHS-REQUEST

Description: A list to foster electronic communication between medical physicists, open to interested others.

Access: Electronic Mail

Internet Address: `listserv@RADONC.DUKE.EDU`

MEDPHY-L

Description: EFOMP Medical Physics Information Services.

Access: Electronic Mail

Bitnet Address: `listserv@AWIIMC12`

Internet Address: `listserv@VM.AKH-WIEN.AC.AT`

MEDPHYS

Description: Medical Physics. An attempt to foster electronic communication between medical physicists, open to interested others. Medical physics is a somewhat opaque but widely used synonym for radiological physics—the physics of the diagnostic and therapeutic use of radiation in medicine. At present most of the subscribers are involved in radiotherapy.

Access: Email Addresses

    medphys@radonc.duke.edu (list)

    medphys-request@radonc.duke.edu (listserv)

Internet Address: `medphys-request@radonc.duke.edu`

MEDSTU-L

Description: Medical student discussion list. This is an open list, but the two listowners respectfully request that the e-conference be limited to students in medical schools.

Access: Electronic Mail

Contact: Owners: Art St. George stgeorge@bootes.unm.edu
    stgeorge@unmb

David Goldstein dgoldst@bootes.unm.edu
    dgoldst@unmb

Bitnet Address: `listserv@UNMVMA`

Internet Address: `listserv@UNMVM.EDU`

MEDSUP-L

Description: Medical Support List.

Access: Electronic Mail

Bitnet Address: **listserv@YALEVM**

Internet Address: **listserv@YALEVM.CIS.YALE.EDU**

MENOPAUS

Description: Menopause Discussion List. MENOPAUS is an open list is for the discussion of menopause, and the sharing of remedies and personal experiences related to menopause. It's open to women of all ages and other interested parties. While the list is meant to be a casual discussion list, people from the medical community are also welcome.

Access: Electronic Mail

Contact: Judy Bayliss (owner)

Bitnet Address: **listserv@PSUHMC**

Internet Address: **listserv@PSUHMC.MARICOPA.EDU**

MHCARE-L

Description: Discussion of topics pertaining to Managed Health Care and Continuous Quality Improvement.

Access: Electronic Mail

Contact: Owner: Andrew Balas medinfab@mizzou1

Bitnet Address: **listserv@MIZZOU1**

Internet Address: **listserv@MIZZOU1.MISSOURI.EDU**

MI-EDUC

Description: Education in Medical Informatics.

Access: Electronic Mail

Bitnet Address: **listserv@UMAB**

MI-STDNT

Description: Students in Medical Informatics.

Access: Electronic Mail

Bitnet Address: **listserv@UMAB**

Internet Address:

MICEE-L

Description: Medical Informatics in Central & Eastern Europe (English language).

Access: Electronic Mail

Contact: Jan Vejvalka jan.vejvalka@lfmotol.cuni.cz
   Head of Informatics, Charles University Hospital Motol

Internet Address: **listserv@LFMOTOL.CUNI.CZ**

MICZ-L

Description: Medical Informatics in Czech Republic (and language).

Access: Electronic Mail

Contact: Jan Vejvalka jan.vejvalka@lfmotol.cuni.cz
   Head of Informatics, Charles University Hospital Motol

Internet Address: **listserv@LFMOTOL.CUNI.CZ**

MINHLTH

Description: Minority Health Issues in the US. The purpose of this list is fourfold:
   1. For researchers who either directly or correctly look at issues of minority health, from a variety of perspectives and fields to network.
   2. For announcements of meetings fellowships, graduate school opportunities, workshops, etc.

3. To discuss and answer specific questions and issues in minority health research
4. To discuss and share perspectives on research in this area in general and in health care of minorities.

Access: Electronic Mail
Contact: Michelle Murrain (owner)
Internet Address: `listserv@DAWN.HAMPSHIRE.EDU`

MIS-L

Description: NYS Department of Health Management Information.
Access: Electronic Mail
Internet Address: `listserv@ALBNYDH2`

MOBILITY

Description: MOBILITY is a list to help disabled persons gain access and mobility. Topics for discussion include the following:
1. Mobility doe not include just access to Public transportation. It is also our ability to get around using wheelchairs, and our own cars or vans.
2. Mobility also means communications. What about cell phones? I am presently trying to get NYNEX to start a special Emergency Life Line Mobile Service for those Cell Subscribers who have special parking permits or handicapped mass transit ID cards. Or whose doctor say a cell phone might be needed for the disabled person's health and safety. This will give these disabled persons the safety and ability to use a cell phone at a vastly reduced rate, giving them quick and efficient mergency communications if their motorized wheelchair or car or van breaks down.
3. Mobility will also be discussed as it relates to socializing and dating.
4. And we will also be discussing education and employment and how it relates to mobility.
5. Finally, you will help us with your views and news on mobility.

Access: Electronic Mail
Contact: Robert Mauro `rmauro@delphi.com`
Bitnet Address: `listserv@SJUVM`

MOL-EVOL

Description: Molecular-Evolution Bulletin Board.
Access: Electronic Mail
Internet Address: `listserv@DARESBURY.AC.UK`

MORPHMET

Description: Biological Morphometrics Mailing List.
Access: Electronic Mail
Contact: Owners: Leslie F. Marcus `lamqc@cunyvm`
     `bigcu@cunyvm`
Bitnet Address: `listserv@CUNYVM`

MOTOL-L

Description: Discussion list of the Motol Medical Faculty, in Czech language.
Access: Electronic Mail
Contact: Jan Vejvalka `jan.vejvalka@lfmotol.cuni.cz`
     Head of Informatics, Charles University Hospital Motol
Internet Address: `listserv@FMOTOL.CUNI.CZ`

MOTORDEV

Description: Human Motor Skill Development.

Access: Electronic Mail
Bitnet Address: `listserv@UMDD`
Internet Address:

MPSYCH-L
Description: Society for Mathematical Psychology.
Access: Electronic Mail
Bitnet Address: `listserv@BROWNVM`

Name: MSLIST-L
Description: Multiple Sclerosis Discussion/Support.
Access: Electronic Mail
Bitnet Address: `listserv@NCSUVM`

MUCO-FR
Description: Cystic Fibrosis discussion list—France (Mucoviscidoses).
Access: Electronic Mail
Contact: Owner: Michel Jorda `jorda@frcism51`
 `jorda@frsun12`
Bitnet Address: `listserv@FRMOP11`

MxDIAG-L
Description: Dedicated to molecular diagnostic applications in pathology. If your work involves molecular techniques as applied to human diseases, especially to diagnostics, this list should provide a useful place for discussion of topics of interest to you. xHere is the mission statement of this service:

> This list will provide a forum to exchange information for those physicians and scientists interested in the application of modern molecular techniques to the field of pathology, especially in the area of diagnostics. The list will not be moderated in order to encourage participation. All information relevant to molecular pathology/diagnostics including technical discussions, regulatory information, meeting announcements, managerial issues, etc. are appropriate for this list.

Access: Electronic Mail
Bitnet Address: `listserv@ALBNYDH2`

NARA-L
Description: A list created to improve internal communication among NARA staff on issues of technology and electronic interchange. Topics include use of the NIH e-mail accounts, Internet resources of interest to NARA staff, and other NARA news.
Access: Electronic Mail
Contact: Owner: `ozh@nihcu`
Bitnet Address: `listserv@NIHLIST`

NAT-HLTH
Description: NAT-HLTH Health Issues of Native Peoples.
Access: Electronic Mail
Internet Address: `listserv@TAMVM1.TAMU.EDU`

NCE-RESP
Description: Network of Centers of Excellence in Respiratory Health discussion list.
Access: Electronic Mail
Contact: Owner: Whitney Devries `whitney@christie.meakins.mcgill.ca`

Bitnet Address: **listserv@MCGILL1**

NCIW-L
Description: Nutrient Cycling Issues.
Access: Electronic Mail
Bitnet Address: **listserv@YALEVM**

NEUCHILE
Description: Chilean Neuroscience Discussion List (Lista de discusion sobre Neurociencias) (at Yale).
Access: Electronic Mail
Contact: Owner: Adrian Palacios palacios-adrian@yale.edu
Bitnet Address: **listserv@CUNYVM**

NEUR-SCI
Description: Neuroscience Bulletin Board.
Access: Electronic Mail
Internet Address: **listserv@DARESBURY.AC.UK**

NEURL
Description: Neuroscience Strategic Planning.
Access: Electronic Mail
Bitnet Address: **listserv@UICVM**
Internet Address: **listserv@vievm.vic.edu**

NEURO1-L
Description: Neuroscience Information Forum.
Access: Electronic Mail
Contact: Owner: #m01ejn@luccpua
Bitnet Address: **listserv@UICVM**
Internet Address: **listserv@UICVM.UIC.EDU**

NEURON
Description: A list in digest form dealing with all aspects of neural networks especially natural systems, neurobiology, neuroscience...etc.
Access: Electronic Mail
Internet Address: **listserv@CATTELL.PSYCH.UPENN.EDU**

NEUS582
Description: Methods in Modern Neuroscience discussion list.
Access: Electronic Mail
Contact: Owner: u59950@uicvm
Bitnet Address: **listserv@UICVM**
Internet Address: **listserv@vicvm.vic.edu**

NEWS-L
Description: NYS Department of health news.
Access: Electronic Mail
Bitnet Address: **listserv@ALBNYDH**

NEXT-MED

Description: NeXT Medical Applications. NeXT-Med is open to end users and developers interested in medical solutions using NeXT computers and/or 486 systems running NEXTSTEP. Discussions on any topic related to NeXT use in the medical industry or relating to health care is encouraged.

Access: Email Addresses

    `NeXT-Med@ms.uky.edu` (list)

    `next-med-request@ms.uky.edu` (listserv)

Internet Address: **`NeXT-Med@ms.uky.edu`** (list)

    `next-med-request@ms.uky.edu` (listserv)

NIATRN-L

Description: National Institute of Aging Population Researchers and Trainees List. Involves people performing research on aging and the aged.

Access: Electronic Mail

Contact: Owners: James McNally `st403145@brownvm`

Bitnet Address: **`listserv@BROWNVM`**

NIH-GUIDE

Description: NIH Grants and Contracts Distribution List.

Access: Electronic Mail

Bitnet Address: **`listserv@UBVM`**

NIH-GUIDE

Description: NIH Guide List (TCSVM).

Access: Electronic Mail

Bitnet Address: **`listserv@TCSVM`**

NIH-L

Description: NIH Redistribution List.

Access: Electronic Mail

Bitnet Address: **`listserv@WSUVM1`**

NIHDIS-L

Description: NIH Guide Discussion List. This is a discussion list for institutional hubs who are participating in the E-Guide program and others who are interested in sharing information about how E-Guide material is used at the institutional level to disseminate and make available NIH policy information.

Access: Electronic Mail

Contact: Owner: Jim Jones `jimj@jhuvm`

Bitnet Address: **`listserv@JHUVM`**

NIHDOC-L

Description: NIH Guide List (LSUVM).

Access: Electronic Mail

Bitnet Address: **`listserv@LSUVM`**

NIHGDE-L

Description: NIH Guide Primary Distribution—NIH Guide University of Washington distribution list. This List controls the PRIMARY DISTRIBUTION of the electronic form of the "NIH Guide for Grants & Contracts" from the NIH to institutions participating in this program. As the program is currently defined, each institution on this list will receive one copy of each publication sent and is in turn responsible for "redistributing" or "making available" the publication for others at that institution by whatever means the institution deems appropriate.

The Bitnet address of this list is NIHGDE-L@JHUVM. The Internet address of this list is NIHGDE-L@JHUVM.HCF.JHU.EDU. This list has no formal peers, however some "institutional representatives" on this list are LOCAL List Server lists. These lists may have different list header options than this list and are not managed by the NIH.

If you have questions about this NIH program, would like further information on how to participate in this program, or if you need to reports problems, suggestions, or concerns, please Contact:

> Ms. Becky Duvall (301) 496- 5366
> Institutional Liason Office (q2c@nihcu)
> National Institutes of Health
> Building 31, Room 5B31
> 9000 Rockville Pike
> Bethesda, Maryland 20892

Access: Electronic Mail
Contact: Owners: John Paul Elrod jpe@jhuvm
Kevin Callahan kcd@nihcu
Bitnet Address: **listserv@JHUVM**

NIHGUIDE

Description: NIH Listing of Available Grants and Contracts.
Access: Electronic Mail
Bitnet Address: **listserv@UMAB**
Internet Address: **listserv@UMAB.UMD.EDU**

NNLM-SEA

Description: National Network Library of Medicine SEA.
Access: Electronic Mail
Bitnet Address: **listserv@UMAB**
Internet Address: **listserv@UMAB.UMD.EDU**

NRSING-L

Description: Nursing Informatics discussion list.
Access: Electronic Mail
Contact: Owners: Gordon Larrivee larrivee@umassmed
John Schiwitz john@umssmdvm
Internet Address: **NIC.UMASS.EDU**

NUCMED-REQUEST

Description: Discussion of Nuclear Medicine and related issues. Of particular concern is the format of digital images.
Access: Electronic Mail
Internet Address: **listserv@UWOVAX.UWO.CA**

NURCENS

Description: NURCENS is a network discussion group for nurses associated with or interested in nursing centers (nurse run clinics affiliated with schools of nursing). NURCENS has been established to enable computer network based discussions that can enhance and enrich consultations among nurses about nursing centers.

Forward questions regarding NURCENS to:
P. Allen Gray, Jr., RN, PhD
gray@vxc.uncwil (Bitnet)
gray@vxc.uncwil.edu (Internet)
307 Church Street
Wilmington, NC 28401
Phone: (919) 251-8518
Fax: (919) 395-3863

Access: Electronic Mail
Contact: Owners: P. Allen Gray gray@vxc.ucwil.edu
Doug Cutler uncdwc@uncvm1
Bitnet Address: **listserv@UNCVM1**

NURSE-L

Description: Nursing School project.
Access: Electronic Mail
Bitnet Address: **listserv@EMUVM1**

NURSENET

Description: A Global Forum form for Nursing Issues. NURSENET is an open, unmoderated, global electronic conference for discourse about diverse nursing issues in the areas of nursing administration, nursing education, nursing practice, and nursing research. While unmoderated, we hope that subscribers will volunteer to introduce and host topics in areas of their interest and expertise.

We can use this space to make announcements, share ideas, papers, bibliographies, resources, to take polls, review books, ask for opinions, and to create community.

When you subscribe, you will receive The NURSENET Guide which contains useful commands and information.

Access: Electronic Mail
Contact: List Manager: Judy Norris jnorris@oise.on.ca
Bitnet Address: **listserv@UTORONTO**
Internet Address: **listserv@VM.UTCC.UTORONTO.CA**

NUTEPI

Description: Nutritional epidemiology discussion list.
Access: Electronic Mail
Contact: Owner: Gert Mensink mensink@db0tui11
Bitnet Address: **listserv@DBOTUI1**

OCC-ENV-MED-L

Description: OCCUP-ENV-MED provides a forum for announcements, dissemination of text files and academic discussion. The forum is designed to allow presentation of clinical vignettes, synopses of new regulatory issues and reports of interesting items from publications elsewhere (both the medical and the nonmedical journals).

The Association of Occupational & Environmental Clinics represents the first nucleus of members for the list, and will use the list for announcements. AOEC members are either:

A. interested clinics with approved credentials documenting expertise in Occupational & Environmental Medicine
B. individuals interested in sharing this topic, but who have no requirement to show advanced training or expertise.

Professional affiliations of the Mail-list subscribers will include:
- Occupational Physicians and Nurses
- Industrial Hygienists
- Government Public Health officials
- University investigators and regulators in
- Occupational & Environmental Medicine diseases.

Topics may include:
- Case Presentations, ending with "what do I do next?"
- Ethical concerns
- Requests for technical expertise, usually free and off-the-cuff.
- Requests for collaborators, either research or business.
- Announcements of hot topics, including regulatory issues, case reports with effect on usual practice, news events.
- Job postings and requests for offers.

Access: To place your name on the mail list, send a special message to the following internet address: `mailserv@mc.duke.edu`. Include just a single line message that says:

`SUBSCRIBE FirstName LastName`

Please put in your full name in quotes.

Contact: Gary Greenberg, MD Occ-Env-Med Sysop `green011@acpub.duke.edu`
Bitnet Address:
Internet Address: `MAILSERV@MC.DUKE.EDU`

OMERACT

Description: The OMERACT list is focused on Outcome Measures in Rheumatoid Arthritis Clinical Trials. Target group: rheumatologists, methodologists, physicians involved in drug regulation, physicians in industry. Purpose: to stimulate discussions around themes related to Outcome Measures in Rheumatoid Arthritis Clinical Trials. These discussions have been the focus of several conferences: The name OMERACT was coined for such a conference in Maastricht, The Netherlands in 1992.

Topics discussed include:
- Validation of outcome measures in the WHO/ILAR core set;
- Use of indices (aggregate measures) in trials;
- Discussion of new measures such as utilities and psychosocial measures; (economic and toxicity).

Although the main focus is on Rheumatoid Arthritis, discussions on other disease (groups) are also welcome, e.g., Osteoarthritis.

Access: Electronic Mail
Contact: Maarten Boers, M.D., PhD, MSc
`boers@intmed.Rulimburg.Nl`
Dept Int Med/Rheumatology,
University Hospital
PO Box 5800
6202 AZ Maastricht
The Netherlands
voice phone: +3143 877004; fax: +3143 875006.

Bitnet Address: `listserv@HEARN.BIT`
Internet Address: `listserv@NIC.SURFNET.NL`

ORADLIST

Description: Oral Radiology discussion list.

Access: Electronic Mail
Contact: Owners: `iadescw@mvs.oac.ucla.edu`
`iadescw@uclamvs.bitnet`
`csmiddw@mvs.oac.ucla.edu`
`csmiddw@uclamvs.bitnet`
Bitnet Address: `listserv@UCLACN1`

OXYGEN-L

Description: Oxygen Free Radical Biology and Medicine Discussion.
Access: Electronic Mail
Contact: Owners: Lillian Novela `c467414@mizzou1`
Olen R. Brown `vetorb@mizzou1`
Bitnet Address: `listserv@UMCVMB`

PANET-L

Description: Medical Education and Health Information discussion list. This discussion list is intended to provide a forum for the sharing of those seeking "Health for All in the Year 2000." The Dominant language is English, although some information appears in Spanish. Membership is open to all nationalities and health care disciplines, although emphasis is on Latin America and the field of medicine. The e-conference is a collaborative effort between the Health Manpower Development Office (HSM) of the Pan American Health Organization and the Panamerican Federation of Associations of Medical Schools (PAFAMS).
Access: Electronic Mail
Contact: Owners: Wendy Steele `steele@mcs.nlm.nih.gov`
`pafams@yalevm`
Bitnet Address: `listserv@YALEVM`
Internet Address: `listserv@YALEVM.CIS.YALE.EDU`

PARKINSN

Description: Parkinson's Disease Information Exchange Network. PARKINSN is an open, unmoderated, international forum that provides an information exchange network for individuals interested in Parkinson's Disease. Subscribers include persons with Parkinson's disease, family members and friends, health care workers, researchers, and others wishing to know more about this disease. Any topic related to Parkinson's disease is appropriate for discussion.
Access: Electronic Mail
Contact: Barbara Patterson `patterso@fhs.csu.mcmaster.ca`
Internet Address: `listserv@VM.UTCC.UTORONTO.CA`

PARKINSON

Description: PARKINSON is an open, unmoderated, international forum that provides an information exchange network for individuals interested in Parkinson's Disease. Subscribers include persons with Parkinson's disease, family members and friends, health care workers, researchers, and others wishing to know more about this disease. Any topic related to Parkinson's disease is appropriate for discussion.
Access: Electronic Mail
Contact: Manager: Barbara Patterson `patterso@fhs.csu.mcmaster.ca`
Internet Address: `listserv@VM.UTCC.UTORONTO.CA`

PBLIST

Description: The PBLIST list exists to promote discussion of problem-based learning (PBL) in health sciences education. Topics may include case-writing; tutoring and training of tutors; collaboration between departments and institutions; student perspectives on PBL; research and experiences with PBL in various courses and institutional settings; evaluation methods; and the fostering of collegial relationships in support of the goal of this list. The owners hope that interpersonal computing will enhance the use of PBL in health sciences education and bring together those educators and students who wish to share their thoughts on this subject.

Access: Send email command to MAILSERV@UTHSCSA.EDU or MAILSERV@UTHSCSA.BITNET

Contact: Owners/Moderators: Tom Deahl deahl@thorin.uthscsa.edu
Bill Hendricson hendricson@uthscsa.edu

Bitnet Address: listserv@UTHSCSA

Internet Address: listserv@UTHSCSA.EDU

PEDIATRIC-PAIN

Description: This is an international forum for discussion of any topic related to pain in children. Appropriate subjects might include: clinical problems or questions, research problems or proposals, announcements of meetings, book reviews, and political or administrative aspects of children's pain management and prevention.

Access: Electronic Mail. To subscribe, send an e-mail message to: MAILSERV@ac.dal.ca with the first line of the body of the message: subscribe

Internet Address: listserv@AC.DAL.CA

PHARM

Description: Pharmacy Mail Exchange is a general discussion list for pharmacists and workers in related fields. Subscribers receive details of access to a BBS which includes a directory of email users, and software directory.

Access: Electronic Mail

Contact: Owner: Paul Hodgkinson
Dept of Pharmacy
Leicester Polytechnic
(Janet) phh@leicp.ac.uk

Internet Address: listserv@DMU.AC.UK

PHYSIO

Description: Physiotherapy discussion.

Access: Electronic Mail

Internet Address: MAILBASE@MAILBASE.AC.UK

PHYSL-TR

Description: Physiology Discussion List.

Access: Electronic Mail

Bitnet Address: listserv@TRITU

Internet Address: listserv@CC.ITU.EDU.TR

PLAY-L

Description: PLAY-L focuses on the multidisciplinary study of play, games, and sport in diverse sociocultural contexts. Topics may include (but are not limited to) the nature of the ludic, children's play, animal play, adult games, amateur or professional and celebrations, joking and humor, mass-mediated images and representations of play, narratives of play, play in fiction, the global, national, regional, or local organization.

Access: Electronic Mail

Contact: Owner: Alan Aycock aycock@hg.uleth.ca

Internet Address: listserv@HG.ULETH.CA

POP-BIO

Description: Population Biology is a synthesis of population ecology and population genetics, pursuing a unified theory to explain the structure, functioning and evolution of populations of living beings. Such populations are very complex systems, exhibiting a variety of phenomena that we still do not master. Just to quote a famous example, multiannual density cycles (e.g., in lemmings) have not received a satisfactory explanation, despite decades of debated studies and speculations. Population Biology is a very active field, encompassing such diverse approaches as tenacious, harsh field work to track long term demographic and genetic fluctuations, or sophisticated conversations with a computer about strange attractors possibly causing chaos in the density fluctuations.

Topics that can be discussed include: ecology, population genetics, systematics, evolution, morphometry, interspecific competition, sociobiology, mathematical modelling, population regulation, pest control, chromosomal evolution, social behavior, statistical methodology in population study, population management of endangered species, applications of molecular biology techniques, etc., and, last but not least, your own topic. There is no restriction on the species: viruses, protokaryotes, plants, animals (including man), mythic or extinct species, computer-simulated species. Technical problems, book reviews, meeting announcements and so on are also welcome.

The names of the new groups are:

Internet: POPULATION-BIOLOGY

Bitnet: POP-BIO

Usenet: bionet.population-bio

If you wish to participate in the group, please send your subscription request to the appropriate BIOSCI node below. More information on BIOSCI can also be requested at the addresses below:

BIOSCI%NET.BIO.NET@VM1.NODAK.EDU (Internet, USA)

BIOSCI@NET.BIO.NET (BitNet, USA)

BIOSCI@IRLEARN.UCD.IE (Internet, Ireland)

BIOSCI@UK.AC.DARESBURY (Janet, U.K.)

BIOSCI@BMC.UU.SE (EARN/Internet, Sweden)

Access: Electronic Mail

Contact: Moderator: Vincent Bauchau
(Internet) VINCENT%BUCLLN11.BITNET@VM1.NODAK.EDU
(Bitnet) VINCENT@BUCLLN11

Internet Address: **listserv@DARESBURY.AC.UK**

PRENAT-L

Description: Perinatal outcomes discussion list. The primary purpose of this listserv is to share information on perinatal health data and information resources for NYS, including birth and death data, hospitalization data, health status measures, program participation, congenital malformations registry data, and data on maternal risk factors. National and other-level data may also be pertinent. This listserv is one of the products resulting from a RWJ Foundation-funded project to improve health data for policy making. It was developed as one way to make health data resources more accessible to the health policy and research community. Many of the have been involved in this project and advised on ways to improve maternal and infant data. Contributors will make some summary tables available, will notify members of new reports or studies that they feel will be of interest, and will report on other data initiatives in which they are involved or know about.

Access: Electronic Mail

Contact: Owner: Michael Zdeb msz03@albnydh2

Bitnet Address: **listserv@ALBNYDH2**

PSI-L

Description: PSI-L is a forum for discussing experiences, questions, ideas, or research having to do with psi (e.g., ESP, out-of-body experiences, dream experiments, and altered states of consciousness). This list is mainly about the nature of psi; if you're interested in debating whether psi exists, this isn't the place to do it. We're interested in hearing about personal experiences, and considering why and how these different phenomena happen, the connections between them, how to bring them about and what psychological or philosophical implications they have.

Access: Electronic Mail

Contact: Owner: Lusi N. Altman `lnaqc@cunyvm`
`lnaqc@cunyvm.cuny.edu`

Bitnet Address: `listserv@RPITSVM`

PSYART

Description: Institute for Psychological Study of the Arts.

Access: Electronic Mail

Bitnet Address: `listserv@NERVM`

PSYC

Description: Psychology, neuroscience, behavioral psychology.

Access: Electronic Mail

Bitnet Address: `listserv@PUCC`

PSYCGRAD

Description: Psychology Graduate Student discussion forum. Now among each other efficiently and free of charge. The primary purpose is to provide a medium through which graduate students in the field of psychology can communicate.

Access: Electronic Mail

Contact: Owner: Matthew Simpson `054340@uottawa`

Bitnet Address: `listserv@UOTTAWA`

PSYCHE-D

Description: Discussion for those interested in the subject of consciousness. It is hoped that it will allow members to share ideas, do common research and so on. PSYCHE-D, the discussion list, will also be used to discuss articles that appear in the journal PSYCHE, but in addition members are invited to speak on other related themes.

Access: Electronic Mail

Contact: Owner: David Casacuberta `ilff3@cc.uab.es`

Bitnet Address: `listserv@NKI`

PSYCHIATRY

Description: Unmoderated discussion forum dealing with issues in psychiatry and abnormal psychology. This mailbase list has been set up with the aim of utilizing the vast resources of the Internet on behalf of everyone interested in issues in psychiatry and abnormal psychology. As with any discussion forum its value will be proportional to the effort that those contributing to it are prepared to make in provoking stimulating and thoughtful debate.

The forum was judged to be necessary because many of the findings and viewpoints in the fields of psychiatry and abnormal psychology are both controversial and easily misinterpreted, resulting in a lack of empathy and understanding between those pursuing radically different approaches to the aetiology and pathophysiology of mental illness. It is hoped that the forum will act as a bridge between those taking a biomedical viewpoint of the study and treatment of psychopathology, and those taking a more existential or psychodynamic viewpoint.

It is hoped in particular that amicable discussion will encourage and support an attitude of mutual respect, producing a more collaborative approach to these difficult issues, so narrowing the unacceptably wide gulf that now separates the opposing camps.

All of those wishing to share personal insights, research findings, philosophical outlooks, clinical case notes, or simple anecdotes on any of the following, are cordially invited to contribute:

- Methodology: clinical case histories, scientific experimentation, laboratory models, statistical and analytical methods, meta-analysis.
- Current and past research papers, unpublished findings.
- Epidemiology of mental illness.
- Concepts of abnormality: The underlying philosophy of psychiatry and abnormal psychology.
- The history of perceived causes of abnormal behaviour: possession and witchcraft, physical causes, psychogenic causes.
- The real life experience of mental illness.
- Conflicting Approaches? The Biomedical approach, the psychodynamic approach, the environmental model: behavioural and cognitive approaches.
- Psychiatric Nomenclature
- Psychometric Testing—Psychological classification and assessment.
- Specific Disorders: Personality disorders, neuroses, paranoid states, affective disorders, schizophrenia, organic disorders, eating disorders, sexual dysfunction and abnormality, psychoactive substance abuse, psychosomatic illness, behavioural disorders in children.
- Diagnosis, classification, sympptomatology, and prognosis of mental illness.
- Psychoneuroimmunology, psychoneuroendocrinology.
- Disorders of the nervous system and psychopathology.
- Psychiatric emergencies.
- Psycotherapeutic techniques.
- Alternative approaches: meditation, relaxation, etc.
- Physical treatments: psychopharmacology, electro-convulsive therapy, aversion therapy, psychoneurosurgery, etc.
- Mental illness and the legal system: uses and abuses of psychiatry.
- Mental illness and society: community care, the history of mental health care, the public perception of the mentally ill.
- Psychopathology and creativity.
- Aetiology: genetics, neuroanatomy, neurophysiology.
- Reviews of new publications, journal articles, conferences. Have you read a stimulating reappraisal, or cogent exposition of your speciality? If so, let us know.
- Assessment of contributors to the development of psychology and psychiatry: Charcot, Freud, Jung, Adler, Bleuler, Kraepelin, Meyer Erikson, Fromm, Rogers, Perls, Frankl, Skinner, Ellis, Laing et al.

The basic underlying philosophy of this forum is: "There is someone wiser than any of us, and that is all of us." This would also be an appropriate motto for the Internet, and I would be very happy to hear from anyone who would like to assist in compilation of a resource guide, register of research interests, or any other such extension to the services offered by this list that would be productive in making it a more useful tool to the subscribers.

Access: Send subscription request to MAILBASE@MAILBASE.AC.UK
Contact: Ian Pitchford I.Pitchford@Sheffield.ac.uk
Internet Address: **mailbase@mailbase.ac.uk**

PSYLAW-L

Description: Psychology and Law, international discussion.
Access: Electronic Mail
Bitnet Address: **listserv@UTEPA**

QADATA-L
Description: New York State Department of Health: Data.
Access: Electronic Mail
Bitnet Address: `listserv@ALBNYDH2`

QML
Description: Quantitative Morphology List. This is an open, unmoderated mailing list to support researchers and clinicians in the field of quantitative morphology. This can include (but is not limited to): queries for help with technical or professional problems; pointers to interesting recent publications; summaries and abstracts of your own recent work; news of upcoming meetings; news about job openings or other professional opportunities; and news about granting agencies or programs.
Access: Electronic Mail
Contact: Owner: Dean Pentcheff `dean2@tbone.biol.scarolina.edu`
Internet Address: `listserv@TBONE.BIOL.SCAROLINA.EDU`

QUALRS-L
Description: Qualitative Research for the Human Sciences.
Access: Electronic Mail
Contact: Owners: David Quarterman `dlq@uga`
Harold Pritchett `harold@uga`
Bitnet Address: `listserv@UGA`

RADSIG
Description: Radiology Special Interest Group.
Access: Electronic Mail
Contact: Owner: `rowberg@locke.hs.washington.edu`
Bitnet Address: `listserv@UWAVM`

RBMI
Description: Groupe de Recherche en Biologie Moleculaire.
Access: Electronic Mail
Bitnet Address: `listserv@FRORS13`

RBMI
Description: Groupe de Recherche en Biologie Moleculaire.
Access: Electronic Mail
Bitnet Address: `listserv@FRULM11`

RECOVERY
Description: Recovery is intended as a forum and support group for survivors of childhood sexual abuse, incest and/or their SO's. Postings are published in digest format and contributors may post anonymously. The emphasis is on healing and recovery through the use of the Twelve Steps of Alcoholics Anonymous as adapted for our purposes.
Access: Electronic Mail
Internet Address: `listserv@WVNVM.WVNET.EDU`

RESADM-L
Description: A forum for individuals involved in research administration for discussion of a wide variety of research administration issues including changes in federal regulations, interpretation and implementation of private and federal sponsor regulations, indirect costs, budget caps, new grant programs and anything

else that would generally be of interest to research administrators. The forum is intended to give research administrators a way to "compare notes" and to share policies, procedures and information that help to get the job done in this increasingly complex field.

Typical members would include members of the Society of Research Administration and NCURA, but participation in the list would by no means be limited to members of these groups.

Access: Electronic Mail
Contact: Owner: Elizabeth Mazzella `eam01@albnydh2`
Bitnet Address: `listserv@NIHLIST`

RESEARCH

Description: Extramural Funding. Research news from Temple University. The RESEARCH list is for those people (primarily at educational institutions) who are interested in applying for outside funding support. That is, support from government agencies, corporations, foundations etc. This list attempts to assist faculty in locating sources of support and also to forward information regarding the latest news from potential sponsors. As an example, National Science Foundation, National Institutes of Health.

Access: Electronic Mail
Contact: Owner: Eleanor Cicinsky
Bitnet Address: `listserv@TEMPLEVM`

REVES

Description: Network on Health Expectancy.
Access: Electronic Mail
Bitnet Address: `listserv@FRMPO11`

RHCFRP-L

Description: Residential Health Care Facilities discussion list.
Access: Electronic Mail
Bitnet Address: `listserv@ALBNYDH2`

RISK

Description: Provided as a means of electronically distributing communications related to issues concerning the general topic of risk management and insurance. Originally created as a discussion group of the American Risk and Insurance Association, but non-members may subscribe. Of interest to hospital risk managers.

Access: Electronic Mail
Internet Address: `listserv@UTXVM.CC.UTEXAS.EDU`

SAFETY

Description: SAFETY is for people interested in the various environmental, health and safety issues and problems on college and university campuses. These can include life safety issues (fire protection, trip and fall and other general safety issues), chemical safety issues (waste disposal, laboratory safety, meeting regulations), biological hazards and radiation safety.

Access: Electronic Mail
Internet Address: `listserv@UVMVM.UVM.EDU`

SAIS-L

Description: Science Awareness and Promotion. The SAIS List was formed in hopes of creating a forum for exchanging innovative ideas about making science more appealing to students. Science has brought to humankind better health, improved communication, better transportation and other advancements that raise the standard of living. It is imperative that students see the potentialities of science, whether harmful or beneficial, in order to judge how best to use science in their own lives and in the best interests of society.

Access: Electronic Mail
Internet Address: `listserv@UNB.CA`

SCHIZ-L: CLINICAL AND BASIC SCIENCE RESEARCH IN SCHIZOPHRENIA

Description: SCHIZ-L is an unmoderated discussion list devoted to schizophrenia research. The objective of the list is to provide a forum for communications among researchers and others interested in this mental illness. It is hoped that this forum will facilitate discussion of both published and unpublished findings and ideas, foster potential collaborations between investigators, and develop into an information resource for those in this field.

Access: Electronic mail
Contact: Owner: Steve Daviss sdaviss@cosy.ab.umd.edu
Bitnet Address: `listserv@UMAB`
Internet Address: `listserv@UMAB.UMD.EDU`

SCHIZOPH (Schizophrenia Information Exchange Network)

Description: SCHIZOPH is an open, unmoderated, global electronic conference that provides an information exchange network on issues related to schizophrenia. Subscribers include people and organizations interested in, or working on, issues related to schizophrenia. These include family and friends, researchers, healthcare providers, support and advocacy groups. Any topic related to schizophrenia is appropriate for discussion. We can use this space to make announcements, share ideas, papers, bibliographies, resources, experiences, etc.

Access: Electronic Mail
Contact: Owner: Chris Glover cglover@oise.on.ca
Internet Address: `listserv@VM.UTCC.UTORONTO.CA`

SCODAE

Description: Communications Network for Pharmacy-School-Based Programs of Substance Abuse Education.
Access: Electronic Mail
Contact: Owners: Trent Tschirgi ttschirg@umab
Anthony Tommasello ttommase@umab
Bitnet Address: `listserv@UMAB`

SCR-L

Description: Study of Cognitive Rehabilitation.
Access: Electronic Mail
Contact: Owner: Joe Silsby birpjoe@mizzou1
Bitnet Address: `listserv@MIZZOU1`

SENIOR

Description: Senior health & living discussion group. Senior is dedicated to the discussion of all issues relating to the health and lives of senior citizens. It is intended to serve in part as a networking tool to facilitate enhancement of senior health and life by matching senior citizen needs with existing services. Senior is open to all persons interested in the health and lives of senior citizens, including health care providers, social service providers, gerontologists, and others.

Access: Electronic Mail
Contact: Owner: John B Harlan ijbh200@indyvax.iupui.edu
ijbh200@indyvax
Bitnet Address: `listserv@INDYCMS`

SHS

Description: Student Health Services discussion list. The purpose is to promote the widespread and rapid exchange of information among the medical and administrative staffs of student health services of institutions of higher education.

Access: Electronic Mail
Contact: Owners: Dr. Jo G. Sweet `sweet@utkvx`
Bruce Delaney `pa6460@utkvm1`
Bitnet Address: **`listserv@UTKVM1`**
Internet Address: **`listserv@UTKVM1.UTK.EDU`**

SKEPTIC

Description: Analysis of the Paranormal. This list is a discussion group designed for philosophers, psychologists, natural and biological scientists, writers, etc. to take a 'skeptical' and scientifically informed look at claims of the paranormal, etc. i.e., Creationism, Health Fraud, witchcraft, crypto-zoology. Anything that might appear in *The Skeptical Inquirer* is fair game. There are no paranormal topics that cannot be discussed here, but it would be extremely nice if the discussions could be kept *rigorous* ...

Access: Electronic Mail
Contact: Taner Edis (owner)
Internet Address: **`listserv@JHUVM.HCF.JHU.EDU`**

SLEEP-L

Description: For discussion of sleep disorders. Membership is restricted to health care providers involved in academic or clinical pursuits related to sleep or discussion of sleep disorders. Membership is restricted to health care providers involved in academic or clinical pursuits related to sleep.

Access: Electronic Mail
Bitnet Address: **`listserv@QUCDN`**

SLFHLP-L

Description: Self-Help research discussion group. SLFHLP-L was created to provide a forum for those who are interested in researching self-help / mutual-aid. People from many different fields and backgrounds participate in the list: social workers, community psychologists, socologists, community health workers, self-help clearinghouses, graduate students, and others. The list is used to ask questions or share information on research ideas, designs and methodologies, to report interim or published results, to make announcements.

Access: Electronic Mail
Contact: `owner-slfhlp-l@vmd.cso.uiuc.edu` (owner)
Internet Address: **`listserv@VMD.CSO.UIUC.EDU`**

SMDM-L

Description: SMDM-L is the electronic bulletin board service for members of The Society for Medical Decision Making and others interested in the theory and practice of decision making. The online community draws from a diversified group including physicians and other heath care professionals, students, hospital and health administrators, policy analysts, health economists, educators, computer analysts, psychologists and medical ethicists. Discussion topics include the analysis of decision making as it applies to clinical practice, to the establishment of health care policies, and to the administration of health care programs. In addition, the service will post announcements of general interest to the decision making community. SMDM-L is a moderated list with subscription open to all.

Access: Electronic Mail
Contact: Owner: James E. Levin, MD, PhD `jlevin@simvax.labmed.umn.edu`
Bitnet Address: **`listserv@DARTCMS1`**
Internet Address: **`listserv@DARTCMS1.DARTMOUTH.EDU`**

SMOKE-FREE

Description: SMOKE-FREE is a support discussion list for people recovering from addiction to cigarettes. Anybody with an interest in quitting smoking or in helping others quit is encouraged to join the discussion.

Access: Electronic Mail

Contact: Owner: Natalie Maynor maynor@ra.msstate.edu

Internet Address: **listserv@RA.MSSTATE.EDU**

SMS-SNUG

Description: Shared Medical Systems (SMS) National User Group (SNUG) Conference SMS-SNUG is an electronic conference designed to foster communication concerning technical, operational, and business issues involved in the use of the SMS Inc. products. The e-conference is sponsored by the University of North Carolina Hospitals Information Systems Division. The e-conference is also supported by the University of North Carolina Office of Information Technology. Our thanks to their management and staff for permission to use their VM system for the e-conference and for assistance in setting it up. While intended as a forum for SMS users, Shared Medical staff participation is welcomed and solicited. Subscription is open to anyone interested.

Access: Electronic Mail

Contact: Owners: Lyman A. Ripperton III
Technical Services Manager
Information Services Division
The University of North Carolina Hospitals
Chapel Hill, NC 27514
Phone: 919/966-3969

Bitnet Address: **listserv@UNVCM1**

Internet Address: **listserv@GIBBS.OIT.UNC.EDU**

SNURSE-L

Description: The student nurses conference list. This list has been established as an effort to initiate undergraduate nursing students to a world of electronic health data. SNURSE-L has a number of different goals lined up:
1. The collection and processing of health data.
2. Discussion of trends and issues in nursing.
3. Enhanced communication between undergraduate student nurses.
4. An area for communication among nursing student leaders.

Access: Electronic Mail

Contact: Owner: Dan Fisher fisherd@scsud.ctstateu.edu

Bitnet Address: **listserv@UBVM**

Internet Address: **listserv@UBVM.CC.BUFFALO.EDU**

SOCWORK

Description: Social Work Discussion List.

Access: Electronic Mail

Contact: Owner: Harry Chaiklin inmate@umab

Bitnet Address: **listserv@UMAB**

SOREHAND

Description: Discussion of Carpal Tunnel Syndrome and Tendonitis

Access: Electronic Mail

Contact: Owner: Richard Karpinski owner@ccnext.ucsf.edu

Bitnet Address: **listserv@UCSFVM**

SOS-DATA

Description: Social Science Data List.

Access: Electronic Mail

Contact: Owners: Dave Sheaves uirdss@uncvm1.oit.unc.edu
  Doug. Cutler uncdwc@uncvm1.oit.unc.edu
  Jim Cassell cassell@uncvm1.oit.unc.edu
Bitnet Address: **listserv@UNCVM1**

SPHALB-L
Description: SUNYA/DOH/AMC School of Public Health.
Access: Electronic Mail
Bitnet Address: **listserv@ ALBNYDH2**

SPORTPSY
Description: Exercise and Sports Psychology.
Access: Electronic Mail
Contact: Owner: Michael Sachs v5289e@templevm
Bitnet Address: **listserv@TEMPLEVM**

SSSSTALK
Description: This list provides a network through which professional researchers, clinicians, educators and students in the field of sexuality can communicate freely, professionally, and efficiently.
Access: Electronic Mail
Contact: Owner: Betty Harris bah6017@tamvenus
Bitnet Address: **listserv@TAMVM1**
Internet Address: **listserv@TAMVM1.TAMU.EDU**

STOPRAPE
Description: Sexual Assault Activist List. STOPRAPE is a list created for the purpose of connecting anti-rape campus activists from all over the country. The goal of the list is to have a fast and effective way to share information about assault on our various campuses and to open a dialogue on possible solutions to the endemic violence against women on campus.
Access: Electronic Mail
Contact: Owner: M. Moore Robinson st102199@brownvm
  Jenny Fallesen st801517@brownvm
Bitnet Address: **listserv@BROWNVM**

STROKE-L
Description: CerebroVascular Accident. The purpose of the Stroke Lists is to share information and opinions, ideas and inquiries that relate to the topic of stroke.
Access: Electronic Mail
Contact: Owner: Bob Moore str002@ukcc.uky.edu
Bitnet Address: **listserv@UKCC**
Internet Address: **listserv@UKCC.UKY.EDU**

STUT-HLP
Description: STUT-HLP is intended to be a support list for people who stutter and their families. It is *not* intended to be an academic discussion list, since other lists (stutt-l stutt-x) currently exist to serve that purpose. The idea for STUT-HLP grew from my observation that the current lists that are available for stuttering seem to serve the needs of academics rather than people who stutter.
Access: Electronic Mail
Contact: Owner: Robert W. Quesal mfrwq@uxa.ecn.bgu.edu
Bitnet Address: **listserv@ECNUXA**
Internet Address: **listserv@BGU.EDU**

STUTT-L

Description: Stuttering: Research and Clinical Practice Stuttering: Research and Clinical Practice Mailing list to facilitate the exchange of information among researchers and clinicians working on the problem of stuttering. Researchers are encouraged to submit descriptions of current projects (purpose, procedures, results if any, current status) and to raise questions that may be of interest to other researchers. Clinicians are encouraged to describe unusual cases.

Access: Electronic Mail

Contact: Owner: Woody Starkweather v5002e@templevm

Bitnet Address: `listserv@TEMPLEVM`

STUTT-X

Description: For those who study stuttering.

Access: Electronic Mail

Bitnet Address: `listserv@ASUACAD`

SUNYHC-L

Description: SUNY Health Council Discussion.

Access: Electronic Mail

Bitnet Address: `listserv@BINGVMB`

Internet Address: `listserv@BINGVMB.CC.BINGHAMTON.EDU`

SUNYSPHL

Description: State University of New York School of Public Health.

Access: Electronic Mail

Bitnet Address: `listserv@ALBNYDH2`

TBI-SPRT

Description: Traumatic Brain Injury list exists for the exchange of information by survivors, supporters, and professionals concerned with traumatic brain injury and other neurological impairments which currently lack a forum. We know from our own experience that one of the main difficulties people dealing with tbi face is that their time is mostly dominated by the survivor's recovery process. Accessing support groups or networking of any kind can seem like one more thing to add to a packed schedule.

Access: Electronic Mail

Contact: Owner: Len Burns lburns@cats.ucsc.edu
   labyris@gorn.echo.com

Bitnet Address: `listserv@SJUVM`

Internet Address: `listserv@JUVM.STJOHNS.EDU`

TDR-SCIENTISTS

Description: TDR stands for "UNDP/WorldBank/WHO Special Programme for Research and Training in Tropical Diseases".

The List is a cost-free media for TDR Communications Unit to propagate important public information texts to any e-mail users connected to the Internet, with interest in TDR. The List may also serve as an informal Forum among TDR scientists to exchange ideas/information which may be helpful to each other. Messages should be short (Remember in some countries users are paying for e-mail per every word they receive!). In mid-1993 when WHO became a full Internet node, a number of WHO Divisions, including TDR, started to experiment with the new facilities. One of which is Mail-Reflector. It enables an e-mail based distribution list or discussion list. TDR-SCIENTISTS List was announced in October 1993 issue of TDR News.

This is an experimental List `<TDR-SCIENTISTS@who.ch>`. It is planned that sometime in 1994 WHO would acquire an Internet software which simulates functions of Listserv (of Bitnet type). Until then, a human host or two are looking after the traffic.

FAQ: some of the Frequently Asked Questions are:

Q. Give me the list of all subscribers.

A. Please wait until the List is put on a Listserv type. There are subscribers who wish to remain anonymous. Listserv will take care of this requirement nicely by giving a "conceal option" to subscribers.

Q. If I have a question to TDR officials, can I send them e-mail directly?

A. E-mail is considered by the TDR secretariat as "an experimental communication mode, somewhere between Voice- mail and Fax". All TDR professionals have an account `<lastname@who.ch>`. E-mail communications from developing countries are taken as a substitute of Fax, so you can send even OFFICIAL notes (except of course where a signature is legally required).

Access: Send your request to join TDR-SCIENTISTS to `tdr-scientists-REQUEST@who.ch`. N.B.: Note the word request.

Contact: (For more information on TDR itself, write to TDR Communications, WHO, 1211 Geneva 27, Switzerland or send e-mail to `TDRNEWS@who.ch`.) An auto-response address was created. Send any message to `tdr-scientists-INFO@who.ch`. The machine will respond by ending this text.
Bob Hata `hata@who.ch`
K. Hata, Ph.D. `hata@who.ch`
Management Officer (Networking)
UNDP/WorldBank/WHO Special Programme
Tropical Diseases Research (TDR)
WHO, 1211 Geneva 27, Switzerland

Internet Address: `tdr-scientisits-REQUEST@who.ch`

TELEMED

Description: Discussion group for providing brief news on Telemedicine and discussing related issues.

Access: Electronic Mail

Internet Address: `listserv@LEON.NRCPS.ARIADNET.GR`

THICVA-REQUEST

Description: Provides for the discussion of Traumatic Head Injuries, Cerebrovascular Accidents, and other related Intracranial Malformations.

Access: Electronic Mail

Internet Address: `listserv@STJHMC.FIDONET.ORG`

THPHYSIO

Description: Thermal Physiology. Mailing list for accelerating exchanges of information between scientists working in the field of thermal physiology, such as relevant advices, queries, and ideas. The list is also a good place to ask questions of general interest; stimulating discussion on recent results or publications; and to provide an easy and cheap way to forward general announcements.

Access: Electronic Mail

Contact: Owner: Michel Jorda `jorda@frsun12`

Internet Address: `listserv@FRMOP11.CNUSC.FR`

TIPS

Description: Teaching In the Psychological Sciences. A forum for the open discussion of all aspects of teaching in psychology.

Access: Electronic Mail

Internet Address: `listserv@FRE.FSU.UMD.EDU`

TRDEV-L

Description: Provides a forum for the exchange of information on training and the development of human resources. Training is designed to improve human work performance on the job, and development. Could be of interest to hospital human resource managers.

Access: Electronic Mail

Contact: Owner: Jeffery Allen `jma110@psuvm`

Bitnet Address: `listserv@PSUVM`

TRNSPLNT

Description: Organ Transplant TRNSPLNT is a discussion list for organ transplant recipients and anyone else interested in the issues, experiences and realities of living with an organ transplant. Over the last 30 years, the number of transplants performed each year has grown steadily in both absolute numbers and type of organs transplanted. Though there are hospital, clinical and pharmaceutical industry-sponsored newsletters, there are few, if any, completely independent discussion forums for those who have experienced this.

Access: Electronic Mail

Contact: Dan Flasar
Systems Manager
General Clinical Research Center (GCRC)
St. Louis, MO
Washington University School of Medicine
Recipient of 3 kidney transplants.
`danf_cm@wugcrc.wustl.edu`
`sysflasar@wugcrc.wustl.edu`

Bitnet Address: `listserv@WUVMD`

Internet Address: `listserv@WUVMD.WUSTL.EDU`

TWINS

Description: Even though the term 'twins' issued, it is meant to represent twins, triplets, etc. The purpose is to provide an open forum for the discussion of issues related twins.

Access: Electronic Mail

Contact: Owner: Jeffery Allen `jma110@psuvm`

Internet Address: `listserv@ATHENA.MIT.EDU`

ULDENT-L

Description: U of L Dental School Faculty/Staff Discussion.

Access: Electronic Mail

Bitnet Address: `listserv@ULKYVM`

URBANITES

Description: Urban self sufficiency. The purpose of this mailing list is to discuss and promote self-sufficiency in everyday life in many forms. This includes but is not limited to basic needs such as food, shelter, health, and safety. A unique aspect of this list, however, unlike many others, is that we will concentrate on the city and urban/semi-burbs applications of traditional self-sufficiency technology.

Access: Email Addresses
`URBANITES@PSYCHE.MIT.EDU` (list)
`strata@FENCHURCH.MIT.EDU` (listserv)

Contact: Owner: Stephen G. Wadlow `sgw@silver.lcs.mit.edu`

Internet Address: See access `URBANITES@PSYCHE.MIT.EDU` (list)
`strata@FENCHURCH.MIT.EDU` (listserv)

UVHINF-L

Description: UVic Health Info Science Bulletins.

Access: Electronic Mail

Contact: Owners: Leslie Wood `his@uvvm`
Deborah Needley `his2@uvvm`

Bitnet Address: `listserv@UVVM`

Internet Address: `listserv@UVVM.UVIC.CA`

VALIDATA

Description: VALIDATA is an electronic conference on topics related to psychological measure development, testing, and validation. It is established to provide a forum for the exchange of ideas on the creation and improvement of multi-item individual difference measures of unobservable psychological constructs. The discussion is essentially unmoderated and the following topics are especially encouraged:

- Uses of confirmatory factor analysis tools in measure purification.
- Face validity opinions.
- Constructs in need of measurement improvement.
- Psychometric problems in existing scales.
- Techniques for improving MTMM studies.

Goals include advancing this area, improving methodology, encouraging new scale development, and improving overall value of psychological measurement scales.

Validata announced by the Marketing Department at the College of Business of Florida State University through a cooperative effort with the Department of Management and Marketing at the University of Alabama.

Access: Electronic Mail

Contact: Owner: Leisa Reinecke Flynn, `lflynn@postoffice.cob.fsu.edu`
Department of Marketing
College of Business
Florida State University
Tallahassee, FL 32306-1042
Phone: (904) 644-4294

Bitnet Address: `listserv@UA1VM.BITNET`

Internet Address: `listserv@UA1VM.UA.EDU`

VEGGIE

Description: Vegetarianism. If you are interested in vegetarianism, veganism, fruitarianism, macrobiotics, whole/natural foods, health/fitness, cooking, etc., this new mailing list may be for you! (We are a "dissident" spin-off of Granola, another vegetarian mailing list.) Our list is called "VEGGIE" to be inclusive of vegans, fruitarians, lacto-, ovo-, ovo-lacto-vegetarians, vegetable-lovers, those simply interested in vegetarianism or veggie recipes, etc! You do not have to be a vegetarian to join!

Access: Electronic Mail

Contact: Owner: Penny Ward

Internet Address: `listserv@GIBBS.OIT.UNC.EDU`

VETADM-L

Description: Veterinary Hospital Administration issues.

Access: Electronic Mail

Bitnet Address: `listserv@TAMVM1`

VETCAI-L
Description: Veterinary Medicine Computer Assisted Instruction.
Access: Electronic Mail
Bitnet Address: `listserv@KSUVM`

VETHIS-L
Description: Veterinary Hospital Information Systems.
Access: Electronic Mail
Bitnet Address: `listserv@UIUCVMD`

VETINFO
Description: Discussion of Informatics in Veterinary Medicine.
Access: Electronic Mail
Bitnet Address: `listserv@UCDCVDLS`

VETLIB-L
Description: Veterinary Medicine Library issues.
Access: Electronic Mail
Bitnet Address: `listserv@VTVM2`

VETMED-L
Description: Veterinary Medicine.
Access: Electronic Mail
Bitnet Address: `listserv@UGA`

VETMICRO
Description: Veterinary Microbiology discussion Group.
Access: Electronic Mail
Bitnet Address: `listserv@UCDCVDLS`

VETMYCOP
Description: Veterinary Mycoplasma Discussion Group.
Access: Electronic Mail
Bitnet Address: `listserv@UCDCVDLS`

VISION-L
Description: Eye movement research discussion list.
Access: Electronic Mail
Internet Address: `listserv@ADS.COM`

VISION-LIST
Description: Expert Systems and Vision. Discussion group for artificial intelligence vision researchers. The list is intended to embrace discussion on a wide range of vision topics, including: physiological theory, computer vision, artificial intelligence technology applied to vision research, machine algorithms, industrial applications, robotic eyes, implemented systems, ideas, profound thoughts.
Access: Send subscription message to the
`Vision-List-Request@ADS.COM` listserv.
Contact: Tod Levitt (owner)
Internet Address: `Vision-List-Request@ADS.COM`

VSTAT-L

Description: Vital Statistics kept at the NY State Dept of Health.

Access: Electronic Mail

Contact: Co-listowners: EBC Maillog `ebc@albnydh2`
Pam Akison `pja01@albnydh2`

Bitnet Address: `listserv@ALBNYDH2`

WHONCD-L

Description: WHO COLLABORATING CENTERS ON NON-COMMUNICABLE DISEASES DISCUSSION GROUP

The Division of Health and Development of the Pan American Health Organization (PAHO) is pleased to announce to all participants at WHO Collaborating Centers on Non Communicable Diseases that the discussion group list WHONCD-L has been deployed at `db2.nlm.nih.gov` server as a part of the recommendation of the meeting.

Access: Electronic Mail

Contact: Dr. Carlos A. Gamboa `gamboa@nlm.nih.gov`

Internet Address: `listserv@DB2.NLM.NIH.GOV`

WHSCL-L

Description: Health Sciences Library Discussion.

Access: Electronic Mail

Contact: Owners: `osakb@emuvm1 libsf@emuvm1`

Bitnet Address: `listserv@EMUVM1`

WITSENDO

Description: Endometriosis. WITSENDO is a moderated mailing list which discusses all aspects of Endometriosis with particular emphasis on coping with the disease and its treatment. Anyone with an interest in this disease is welcome to participate whether or not they actually suffer from the disease. The list will act as a clearinghouse for information exchange and promote discussion of current treatments, research and educational literature. Professional (medical) comments are of course, most welcome.

Access: Electronic Mail

Contact: Owner: `david@dartcms1`

Bitnet Address: `listserv@DARTCMS1`

Internet Address: `listserv@DARTCMS1.DARTMOUTH.EDU`

WMN-HLTH

Description: The Center for Women's Health Research is starting an electronic newsletter and discussion group for people who are interested in women's health and can access email on internet or bitnet.

Access: Electronic Mail

Contact: Owner: Shirlee Cooper `shirlee@carson.u.washington.edu`

Bitnet Address: `listserv@UWAVM`

Internet Address: `listserv@UWAVM.U.WASHNGTON.EDU`

WU-AIDS

Description: `Sci.Med.AIDS` Newsgroup.

Access: Electronic Mail

Contact: Owner: Michael Smith `mnsmith@umaecs`

Bitnet Address: `listserv@WUVMD`

WUNIHG-L

Description: Washington University NIH Guide Distribution.

Access: Electronic Mail

Contact: Owner: Ken Robin `p84103kr@wuvmc`

Bitnet Address: `listserv@WUVMD`

Y-RIGHTS

Description: Children's/Adolescent's Rights List. Also distributed in a weekly format.

Access: Electronic Mail

Contact: Owner: `drz@sjuvm`

Bitnet Address: `listserv@SJUVM`

USENET NEWS GROUPS

These are news groups subscribed to by universities. They can also be accessed via telnet and Gopher at various sites around the world.

ALT NEWSGROUPS

Description: `alt.support.arthritis`

A discussion of issues concerning arthritis sufferers

`alt.education.disabled`

A discussion of issues concerning the disabled.

`alt.recovery`

12 step groups (such as AA, ACA, GA, etc.)

BIONET NEWS GROUPS

Description: Unlike most Usenet newsgroups, the bionet newsgroups all have gateways into non-listserver mailing lists. The cross-posting of articles to more than one newsgroup is discouraged, since at this time the e-mail subscribers will get multiple copies of any cross-posted articles. These mailing lists are administrated by David Kristofferson's BIOSCI service, which is funded by the US National Science Foundation for the express purpose of supporting computer networking among biologists. By supporting personal e-mail subscriptions to the bionet newsgroups, BIOSCI has effectively formed a bridge between biologists with e-mail and those with Usenet (once familiar with Usenet, few people have the patience for e-mail subscriptions). David Kristofferson is responsible for proposing the creation of the bionet domain of Usenet and starting many of the bionet newsgroups. Requests for e-mail subscriptions to bionet newsgroups are handled by `biosci@net.bio.net` (for requests from he Americas) and `biosci@daresbury.ac.uk` (for all others).

BioSci

Three important items follow: BIOSCI archive searching by e-mail, the BIOSCI FAQ, and the BIOSCI User Address Directory form. If you have not yet listed yourself in our e-mail address directory, please take a few minutes to complete and return the form below. If your address information has changed since you listed yourself, please send us an updated form.

Sincerely,

Dave Kristofferson

BIOSCI/bionet Manager

`kristoff@net.bio.net`

Searching BIOSCI Archives with Waismail

E-mail users can search the BIOSCI archives by using our waismail e-mail server. For instructions send the message help to `waismail@net.bio.net`. Leave the Subject: line blank. Other methods of searching the archives via WAIS and gopher are described in the BIOSCI FAQ.

BIOSCI FREQUENTLY ASKED QUESTIONS (FAQ) SHEET

New users of BIOSCI/bionet may want to read the "Frequently Asked Questions" or "FAQ" sheet for BIOSCI. The FAQ provides details on how to participate in these forums and is available for anonymous FTP from

URL: `ftp://net.bio.net/BIOSCI/biosci.FAQ`

for retrieval by gopher

URL: `gopher://net.bio.net:70/`

It may also be requested by sending e-mail to: `biosci@net.bio.net` (use plain English for your request).

The FAQ is also posted on the first of each month to the newsgroup BIONEWS/`bionet.announce` immediately following the posting of the BIOSCI information sheet. A FAQ describing administrative details of the bionet newsgroups is available from

`biosci@net.bio.net` or

`biosci@daresbury.ac.uk`

and appears regularly in the bionet.announce newsgroup. Note: rules for forming new bionet newsgroups differ somewhat from those used elsewhere in Usenet. Various other FAQs dealing with the interests of specific newsgroups are posted in those newsgroups. Tom Schneider's FAQ for bionet.info-theory is available by anonymous ftp from

URL: `file://ncifcrf.gov/pub/delila/bionet.info-theory.faq`

`bionet.general`

General BIOSCI discussion

`bionet.genome.chrom22`

Discussion of Chromosome 22

`bionet.journals.contents`

Biology Journals Contents

`bionet.immunology`

Discussion concerning immunology research

`bionet.molbio.ageing`

Cellular and organismal ageing

`bionet.molbio.bio-materix`

Computer applications to biological databases

`bionet.molbio.embldatabank`

EMBL Nucleic acid database discussion

`bionet.molbio.genbank`

Information concerning the GenBank Nucleic acid

`bionet.molbio.genbank.updates`

Moderated. GenBank updates

`bionet.molbio.gene-linkage`

Discussions about genetic linkage analysis

`bionet.molbio.evolution`

How genes and proteins have evolved

`bionet.molbio.genome-program`

Discussion of Human Genome Project issues

`bionet.molbio.hiv`

Discussion concerning the molec. biology of HIV

`bionet.molbio.methds-reagnts`

Requests for information and lab reagents

`bionet.neuroscience`

Research issues in the neurosciences

`bionet.molbio.proteins`

Research on proteins and protien databases

`bionet.sci-resources`

Information about funding agencies

BITNET LISTSERV ECHOS

Description: As with all of the bit.listserv news groups, these are echos of the corresponding Bitnet mailing lists.

> `bit.listserv.aidsnews`
> `bit.listserv.autism`
> `bit.listserv.deaf-l`
> `bit.listserv.l-hcap`
> `bit.listserv.mednews`
> `bit.listserv.psycgrad.`

MISC NEWSGROUPS
Description:

> `misc.emerg-services`
>> Emergency services discussion group
>
> `misc.handicap`
>> This newsgroup covers all areas of disabilities, technical, medical, educational, legal, etc.

SCI NEWSGROUPS
Description:

> `sci.bio`
>> Biology and related sciences discussion
>
> `sci.bio.technology`
>> Discussion of technology in biology
>
> `sci.med`
>> Medicine and its related products and regs.
>
> `sci.med.aids`
>> AIDS: treatment, path./biol., HIV prevention
>
> `sci.med.nurs`
>> Nursing discussion
>
> `sci.med.physics`
>> Physics in medicine discussion
>
> `sci.med.radiol`
>> Radiology discussion
>
> `sci.med.telemedicine`
>> Medical Networking—Hospital Networks
>
> `sci.psychology`
>> Psychology issues
>
> `sci.psychology.digest`
>> Psychology issues in digest form
>
> `sci.med.occupational`
>> Occupational Injuries discussion.

TALK NEWSGROUPS
Description: `talk.abortion`
>> Abortion issues discussion

```
talk.politics.drugs
```
The politics of drug issues

DOCUMENTS

These are pointers to significant documents (files) concerning health related subjects.

California Initiative
Description: The version proposed in California—returns huge amounts of authority and responsibility to the consumers and providers (meaning doc and other direct deliverers of services, NOT health plans, insurance companies, any third-party managers)
Access: e-mail Ask for the full text of the California Initiative.
Internet Address: **`DAEMON@IGC.APC.ORG`**

CLINTON HEALTH PLAN AND RELATED DOCUMENTS
Description: HEALTH PLAN

This is the book which President Clinton displayed while giving his talk. It consists of: `A letter, The Table of Contents, The forward, and chapter1 chapter2 chapter3 chapter4 chapter5 chapter6 chapter7 chapter8 chapter9 conclusion appendix1 and appendix2.`

Legislation is also available, but it is very large. Even broken down into sub-files these would probably break your mailers:

```
legis.00   7348(8)
legis.01   353502(8)
legis.02   164323(8)
legis.03   175588(8)
legis.04   180416(8)
legis.05   159408(8)
legis.06   114074(8)
legis.07   111585(8)
legis.08   75373(8)
legis.09   36520(8)
legis.10   23391(8)
legis.11   30496(8)
legis.12   6083(8)
```

The President's "Health Security Act" and "The President's Report to the American People" are now available electronically and in print and will soon be available on CD-ROM. Please note that document may not be available at every site immediately. Some sites may require up to 24 hours to make the report available. If you are unsuccessful with one site, don't hesitate to try another.

Table of Contents
    I. Retrieving an electronic version—at no charge
        A. Retrieval via electronic bulletin board
        B. Retrieval via electronic mail
        C. Retrieval via gopher or telnet
        D. Retrieval via anonymous file transfer protocol (ftp)
        E. Retrieval via state-of-the-art access methods
    II. Retrieving electronic versions—for a fee.
        CDROM
        Commercial Services
    III. Retrieving a paper copy—for a fee.

I. RETRIEVING AN ELECTRONIC VERSION—NO CHARGE

A—VIA ELECTRONIC BULLETIN BOARDS
1. Bulletin Board at Fedworld (National Technical Info. Service)
   Set software parameters for: N-8-1
   Dial: (9600 baud) 703-321-8020

B—VIA ELECTRONIC MAIL
The Health Security Act and "The President's Report to the American People" is divided into sections. This allows you to select sections of interest.

1. **almanac@ace.esusda.gov** (Extension Service, USDA)
   To retrieve all or part of the Legislation or Report via email, send one or more of the lower-case commands listed below on the right to: almanac@ace.esusda.gov

To Retrieve:	Type:
The Health Report	send health-book catalog
Health Legislation	send health-legis catalog
(This is being made more email able, Currently LARGE documents)	
The Need for Reform:	send hsa need4
The Health Security Plan Executive Summary:	send hsa 10pgr
The Preliminary Health Plan Summary:	send hsa summary
President's Address before Joint Session of Congresson "Health Security for All Americans".	send hsa speech
This document:	send hsa help

C—VIA Gopher or telnet

1. Americans Communicating Electronically
   URL: `gopher://cyfer.esusda.gov:70/11/ace/policy/health-book`

   Gopher Path: `Americans Communicating Electronically/National Policy Issues/Health Care ReformAgenda/The President's Report to the American People`

   For more information about ACE send E-mail to: info@ace.esusda.gov

2. University of North Carolina's SunSITE Archive
   URL: `gopher://calypso-2.oit.unc.edu:70/11/sunsite.d/politics.d/health.d`

   Gopher Path: `Worlds of SunSITE/US and World Politics/National Health-Security Act`

3. FedWorld.gov—National Technical Information Service
   URL: `telnet://fedworld.gov`

   After registering, select from the menu:
   ```
   S-Select a Library
   w-house Library
   ```

   The Health Care Security Plan Summary documents are named as follows in the FedWorld System:

Title:	Filename:
The Need for Reform	need4ref.txt
Preliminary Health Plan Summary	ummary.txt

   All of the above files, compressed
in ASCII text	hplan.zip
in WordPerfect format	hplanwp.zip
in MS Word format	hplandoc.zip

   For further information about FedWorld, call: 703-487-4650.

4. U.S. Department of Commerce
   URL: `telnet://ebb.stat-usa.gov`

   Login: `trial`

Select the following menu options: Presidential Health Security Plan

Files are named: `HSA01.txt`
`HSA02.txt`
`HSA03.txt`
`HSA04.txt`

This Economic Bulletin Board is available via telnet, temporarily at no charge.

For information, call: 202-482-1986

D—VIA ANONYMOUS-FTP
1. University of North Carolina's SunSITE Archive
   URL: `ftp://sunsite.unc.edu/pub/academic/political-science/Health-Security-Act`

E—VIA WORLD WIDE WEB
1. University of North Carolina's SunSITE Archive
   URL: `http://sunsite.unc.edu/nhs/NHS-T-o-C`

HSA ANALYSIS/CLINTON HEALTHPLAN

Description: A long and detailed analysis of the Clinton Health Care Security Act, prepared by Allan Bergman and Bob Griss of United Cerebral Palsy Association.

This document reflects proposals in the September 7th plan, but does not include all the changes contained in the October 27th legislation. They will be revising and updating the analysis in the next few weeks; however, the enclosed document is 90-95% accurate.

This analysis is based on a preliminary draft of the President's health reform proposal dated September 7, 1993 unless otherwise specified. The Consortium for Citizens with Disabilities (CCD) adopted five principles as the basis for a disability perspective on health care reform (see Appendix #1). These are: (1) non-discrimination; (2) comprehensiveness; (3) appropriateness; (4) equity; and (5) efficiency.

Access: Gopher

Contact: Allan Bergman or Bob Griss,
United Cerebral Palsy,
1522 K Street, Suite 1112,
Washington, D.C. 20005,
202-842-1266/800-USA-5UCP.

If you have problems connecting with the MCHNET gopher or would like an electronic copy of this document sent to you via InterNet, contact `John_Reiss@qm.server.ufl.edu`

URL: `gopher://QM-Server.ichp.ufl.edu:70/I:ICHP`
    `Gopher`
Server: `Health Security Act:Analysis:UCPA Analysis 11/93`

LIST.HEALTHPLAN

Description: Users of the Alliance for Progressive Computing (APC) networks, including PeaceNet, EcoNet, HomeoNet, and LaborNeton the Institute for Global Communications (IGC) system, may read any of the past postings in the conference LIST.HEALTHPLAN.

The directories listed below are both broken down into 1993 and 1994 subdirectories.

Access: FTP & Gopher

URL: `gopher://calypso.-2.oit.unc.edu:70/11/sunsite.d/politics.d/health.d`

URL: `ftp://sunsite.unc.edu/pub/academic/political-science/whitehouse-healthcare.archive`

NEUROSCIENCE INTERNET RESOURCE GUIDE, v 1.0

Description: This document aims to be a guide to existing, free, Internet-accessible resources helpful to neuroscientists.

Access: FTP, Gopher and WWW
Gopher Path: University of Michigan/Clearinghouse for Subject Oriented Research Guides/All Guides/Neurosciences
Contact: Please forward your comments, congratulations, info about missed resources, corrections, etc. to
nirg@umich.edu
Compiled by:
Sheryl Cormicle & Steve Bonario
School of Information and Library Studies, University of Michigan
URL: `ftp://una.hh.lib.umich.edu/inetdirsstacks/neurosci:cormbonario`
`gopher://una.hh.lib.umich.edu/inetdirstacks/neurosci:cormbonario`
`http://http2.sils.umich.edu/Public/nirg/nirg1.html`

WHITE HOUSE HEALTH PLAN

Description: The White House health plan
Access: FTP—Gopher
Gopher Path: Educational Resources/Academic Resources by Topic/United States and World Politics, Culture and History/United States/Executive/White House/Press Releases/Health Care
URL: `gopher://gopher inform.umd.edu:901/11/inforM/Educational_Resources/AcademicResources ByTopic/UnitedStatesAndWorld/United_States/Executive/WhiteHouse/PressReleases/HealthCare`

Electronic Publications

Journals and Newsletters available online. Some are table of contents, others full text.

AIDS ALERT FOR HEALTH CARE WORKERS

Description: AIDS Alert for Health Care Workers is an index to journal articles and occasional papers that address the occupational health and safety concerns of health care workers who are providing care for patients with AIDS. The Alert is annotated and compiled by Charlotte Broome of the Ryerson Polytechnical Institute's education and Life Sciences Library. Issues of the Alert will appear three to four times per year.
Access: The ALERT is distributed electronically by the Institute for AIDS Information.
`libr8508@ryerson`
Contact: Bob Jackson,
Librarian for Education & Life Sciences:
`libr8508@ryerson`
Correspondence: Ryerson Polytechncial Institute
Library, Education & Life Sciences
350 Victoria Street, Toronto,
Ontario, Canada M5B 2K3
Bitnet Address: `libr8508@RYERSON`

ALS DIGEST

Description: This publication covers all aspects of Amyotrophic Lateral Sclerosis (ALS), "Lou Gehrig's Disease". This includes ALS patients, patient supporters, physicians, support groups, research centers, etc.
Access: To subscribe, unsubscribe, or to contribute notes, send email to bro@huey.met.fsu.edu (Bob Broedel).
Contact: bro@huey.met.fsu.edu (Bob Broedel).
Internet Address: `bro@huey.met.fsu.edu`

BIOLINE PUBLICATION

Description: BIOLINE PUBLICATIONS is collaborating with the Tropical Data Base in Campinas, Brazil, and working closely with publishers of Journals and Newsletters, and authors of papers and reports worldwide who wish to cooperate in this venture.

Using the Internet, readers may browse and search without cost through large quantities of abstracts, summaries and contents lists, using simple menus, or keywords and phrases to search across the whole system. Bioline Publications uses state of the art, easy to use gopher software of growing application

Full text and associated graphics of material of interest can be ordered online and e-mailed to the reader's computer. Links are made direct from Bioline Publications' main menu to other bibliographic information on the Internet. Selecting a menu item connects users directly to the site of choice. Public domain and shareware software that may be of help in using Bioline Publications is available for retrieval direct from the main menu. Usage and searching instructions are available online.

Access to Journal abstracts, report summaries and contents lists is available free to all; readers must subscribe to Bioline Publications in order to receive the full text/graphics of documents of interest. Additional registration with the publishers of commercial journals is necessary if full text and graphics of scientific papers are required. Information on registration is available from the main menu of Bioline Publications. The cost of commercial journals is considerably less than the printed version.

The system starts up with a group of Journals (Biotechnology Letters, Biotechnology Techniques, Binary, Biopolicy International, Biotechnology and Development Monitor), a number of Newsletters, reports (including conference reports, Biodiversity Convention, EEC Directives, US Guidelines, culture collection information, shipping regulations). A futher four Journals (Biocontrol Science and Technology, Food and Agriculture Immunology, Nanobiology, The Genetic Engineer and Biotechnologist), additional Reports and Newsletters will be available within a few weeks; more will be added as the system grows, adding value for the user.

Bioline Publications welcomes requests from publishers, editors, authors and conference organisers interested in using the system for wider distribution of material of interest to the bioscientist. It also welcomes comments from the Internet community and suggestions for improvement.

Access: Gopher
Gopher Path: Publications/Bioline Publications
Contact: `bio@biostrat.demon.co.uk` or Bioline Publications
Stainfield House
Stainfield, Bourne, Lincs
PE10 0RS, UK.
Tel:+44 778 570618
Fax:+44 778 570175
URL: `gopher://gopher.bdt.ftpt.br:70/11/.bioline`

BIOMEDICAL LIBRARY ACQUISITIONS BULLETIN (AFFECTIONATELY KNOWN AS BLAB)

Description: This publication is directed to the acquisition of material for biomedical libraries.
Access: Send email to David Morse—`dmorse@hsc.usc.edu` and request to be added to their mailing list.
Contact: dmorse@hsc.usc.edu
Internet Address: **DMORSE@HSC.USC.EDU**

CATHARSIS

Description: Catharsis is a monthly newsmagazine that focuses on the personal health, intellect and creativity of those within the CFS/CFIDS/M.E. community. The contributors to Catharsis range from people with CFIDS or other challenges and disABILITIES, spouses and family members, and those who share an interest about CFIDS and related problems.

Catharsis is edited by Molly Holzschlag who has been a patient and worked in the support, education and advocacy realms of CFIDS for nearly a decade.

Access: Back issues of Catharsis can be obtained by sending the command GET CFS-CATH ### (where ### is a particular edition number, e.g., to get edition no. 1, use GET CFS-CATH 001) as the text of a message to the Internet address of the Listserv, i.e., LISTSERV@SJUVM.STJOHNS.EDU or to LISTSERV@SJUVM

Contact: Catharsis is always seeking contributions and subscribers who have material are particularly encouraged to send it in. Please email all contributions to Cathar-M@sjuvm.stjohns.edu or see Catharsis for other details regarding submissions.

Internet Address: listserv@sjuvm.stjohsjuvm.edu

CFS-NEWS

Description: The CFS-NEWS electronic newsletter focuses on medical news about CFS/CFIDS/ME and is issued at least once each month. It is based at the NIHLIST Listserv.

Access: e-mail subscribe your_name

Bitnet Address: listserv@NIHLIST

Internet Address: listserv@LIST.NIH.GOV

CFS-NEWS (CHRONIC FATIGUE SYNDROME NEWSLETTER CFIDS/ME)

Description: This independent newsletter seeks to serve the CFS community by quickly disseminating information about current medical research on CFS. It will be issued about once each month to give updates on these developments. Other CFS topics of interest to the readership will also be covered. Advice and contributions of news items are welcome. Chronic fatigue syndrome is an illness characterized by debilitating fatigue and a variety of flu-like symptoms. The condition is also known as chronic fatigue immune deficiency syndrome (CFIDS), myalgic encephalomyelitis (ME) and by other names, and in the past has been known as chronic Epstein-Barr virus (CEBV).

Archives of CFS-NEWS back issues can be listed by sending the command INDEX CFS-NEWS to LISTSERV@NIHLIST or to LISTSERV@LIST.NIH.GOV

Access: To Subscribe send the following command to LISTSERV@NIHLIST or to LISTSERV@LIST.NIH.GOV (in the BODY of email): SUB CFS-NEWS your full name

Bitnet Address: Listserv@nihlist

Internet Address: Listserv@list.nih.gov

CFS-WIRE

Description: The CFS-WIRE list is where support groups exchange newsletter articles and other news. Subscription is open to all, although support group representatives need to register to be able to post messages. Registration information is sent with the general subscription.

Access: To subscribe, use the usual Listserv procedure.

Bitnet Address: listserv@SJUVM

Internet Address: listserv@SJUVM.STJOHNS.EDU

DEAF MAGAZINE LIST

Description: Weekly Deaf Magazine.

Access: To sign up mail to deaf-request@clark.net leaving the subject blank and including the following command in the body: SUB DEAF firstname lastname

Contact: Nathan Prugh deaf-admin@clark.net

Internet Address: listserv@REQUEST@CLARK.NET

DISASTER RESEARCH

Description: This is an electronic newsletter dealing with hazards and disasters. Includes articles on recent events and policy developments, ongoing research, upcoming meetings—as well as queries, responses, and ongoing discussion among readers.

Access: Send email to HAZARDS@VAXF.COLORADO.EDU requesting subscription.

Internet Address: listserv@HAZARDS@VAXF.COLORADO.EDU

EUITnews

Description: EASI is dedicated to assisting higher education in developing computer support services for people with disabilities. This is an experiment in providing short, frequent updates directly to you (by email or fax). Let us know if you missed previous messages and want copies. Let us know if you have colleagues who also want to receive EUITNEWS. Please allow us two weeks for updating our lists.

PUBLICATIONS—(all available in ASCII): EASI currently has four publications available.

1. COMPUTERS AND STUDENTS WITH DISAABILITIES: NEW CHALLENGES FOR HIGHER EDUCATION is a detailed overview of how individuals with disabilities can use computers in post-secondary education.
2. COMPUTER ACCESS FACTS gives basic information on disability legislation, demographics and adaptive computer technology.
3. EASI FIXES covers computer access considerations in software development.
4. EASI OUTREACH brochure talks about EASI activities and how to become involved. EASI is currently developing a legal issues brochure and a publication on how to convert electronic text to Braille documents.

EUITNEWS also has an email list, hosted by the University of Michigan, which allows people to send questions or information to the entire EASI email list. This is often used by people who are looking for specific answers to questions on what type of hardware or software is available to help individuals with disabilities. Join the EMAIL list by contacting `jim_knox@um.cc.umich.edu`

Electronic Document Service: EASI has established an electronic document service that offers several documents about disabilities and computer use by individuals with disabilities. Among the documents available are an introduction to the EASI library, a sign-up flyer for people who want to become more involved, various EASI brochures, facts about the Americans with Disabilities Act, information on electronic access to library systems, and a document on how computers can be designed to be more accessible.

Access: Send email to `euitedit@bitnic.educom.edu` or `euitedit@bitnic.easi` and request a subscription.

Contact: `easi@educom`

Internet Address: **EUITEDIT@BITNIC.EASI**
EUITEDIT@BITNIC.EDUCOM.EDU

GOVERNMENT ELECTRONIC PUBLICATIONS

Description: NEWSLETTERS:

- AIDS BBS (run by Ben Gardiner)
  URL: `gopher://itsa.ucsf.edu:70/11/.i/.q/.d`
  Gopher Path: `Bio and Medical gophers and Information Sites/HIV/AIDS Gophers and Databases`

- CDC Daily Summaries
  URL: `gopher://odie.niaid.nih.gov:70/11/aids/cdcds`
  Gopher Path: `AIDS Related Information/CDC Daily Summaries`

- CDCStatistics
  URL: `gopher://vector.intercon.com:70/11/gaystuff/QRD/aids`

- Morbidity and Mortality Weekly Report (MMWR)
  URL: `gopher://cwis.usc.edu/11/The_Health_Sciences_Campus/Periodicals/mmwr`

- National AIDS Clearinghouse
  URL: `gopher://odie.niaid.nih.gov:70/11/aids/cdcnac`
  Gopher Path: `AIDS Related Information/CDC National AIDS Clearinghouse`

- National Commission on AIDS
  URL: `gopher://odie.niaid.nih.gov:70/11/aids/nca`

- NIAID Press Releases
  URL: `gopher://odie.niaid.nih.gov:70/11/aids/npr`

- Study Recruitment Information
  URL: **gopher://odie.niaid.nih.gov:70/11/aids/sri**
- Veterans Administration AIDS Information Newsletter
  URL: **gopher://odie.niaid.nih.gov:70/11/aids/vaain**

PEER-REVIEWED ELECTRONIC JOURNALS:
- Complexity International (Complex Systems Research)
  URL: **http://life.anu.edu.au/ci/ci.html**

ARCHIVES & EXTRACTS OF PEER-REVIEWED PRINT JOURNALS:
- Protein Science
  URL: **ftp://ftp.uci.edu/protein**

NEWSPAPERS, NEWSLETTERS, AND DISCUSSION GROUPS BIOSCI
- Biocomputing News
  URL: **http://beta.embnet.unibas.ch/basel/bcnews/default.html**
- EMBNet
  URL: **http://beta.embnet.unibas.ch/embnet/info.html**
- Discover: The World of Science
  URL: **gopher://gopher.enews.com:2100/11/category/sciences/General/discover**

  Gopher Path: gopher.internet.com/Electronic Newsstand (tm)/Titles arranged by Subject/Science—Ecology, Gardening, general/General/Discover
- Drosophila Information Newsletter
  URL: **http://ftp.bio.indiana.edu:70/11/Flybase/news**

  Gopher Path: gopher.cic.net/Electronic Serials/Alphabetic List/D/Drosophila
- GenTools
  URL: **gopher://gopher.gdb.org:70/77/.INDEX/gentools**
- Human Genome Newsletter (U.S. DOE)
  URL: **http://merlot.gdb.org/11/Genome/hgnews**

MORE INFORMATION ON ELECTRONIC JOURNALS, JOURNAL INDEXES AND DATABASES
- National Animal Genome Research Program Newsletter
  URL: **http://probe.nalusda.gov:8000/animal/NAGRPnews/index.html**
- Bionet News Archives
  URL: **gopher://ftp.bio.indiana.edu/11/Network-News**
- The Scientist
  URL: **http://ds.internic.net/11/pub/the-scientist**
- Swiss Node of the EMBnet
  URL: **http://beta.embnet.unibas.ch**
- World Health Organization Library Digest for Africa
  URL: **http://gopher.who.ch:70/11/.hlt/.digest**
- SeqAnalRef
  URL: **gopher://gopher.gdb.org:70/77/.INDEX/seqanalref**

BIOLOGICAL JOURNALS TABLES OF CONTENTS:
- AIDS ALERT, AIDS NEWS, and AIDS NEWS SERVICE
  URL: **gopher://gopher.cic.net/11/e-serials/general/science/medical/aids**

  Gopher Path: Electroic Serials/General Subject Headings/Science/medical/aids

- Browse several International Journals
  URL: `gopher://gopher.genethon.fr:70/11/Biblio/Journaux`

  Gopher Path: `Bibliography/Journaux`

- CICNet Electronic Journal Indices
  URL: `gopher://gopher.cic.net/11/e-serials/general`

- Harvard Biological Laboratories
  URL: `http://golgi.harvard.edu/homepage.genome`

- Medicine Journals
  URL: `gopher://gopher.cic.net/11/e-serials/general/science/biology`

- Science
  URL: `gopher://gopher.internet.com:2100/1GOPHER://1/category/science`

- WWW Servers for Biosciences
  URL: `http://golgi.harvard.edu/biopages.html`

HISTORY AND ANALYSIS OF DISABILITIES NEWSLETTER

Description: Covers news, conferences, seminars, books, articles, theses, research, organizations, analysis, etc. on history of disabilities and disabled persons, conceptual analysis of disability issues. Produced 2 to 3 times per year. Sponsored by History of Disabilities Network, Centre for Independent Living, Toronto (CILT), and ALTER -International Society for the History of Disabilities (Paris). Available in paper copy for $10 (US or Canadian funds) for four issues.

Access: Send email to `FCTY7310@RYERSON` to request subscription.

HSP DIGEST

Description: This is a monthly edited digest of the listserv unmoderated group `HSPNET-L@ALBNYDH2`.

Access: Send email to `LISTSERV@ALBNYDH2` with the following the message: `afd add hsp digest`

INFORMATION TECHNOLOGY AND DISABILITIES

Description: *Information Technology and Disabilities* (ISSN 1073-5127) is a new, quarterly electronic journal devoted to all aspects of computer use by persons with disabilities. It is intended to fill a void in the professional literature by bringing together articles by educators (K through College), librarians, human resources and rehabilitation professionals, as well as campus computing and other professionals concerned with the effective use of technology by people with all kinds of disabilities.

The premier issue of *Information Technology and Disabilities* reflects the breadth of coverage that the journal's editorial board plans to maintain in future issues. Feature articles include a case study of an accessible CD-ROM workstation at the Seattle Library for the Blind, a profile of the St. John's University UNIBASE system, including the many rehabilitation resources housed there, and an article on the Royal Society for the Blind (Australia), which provides excellent screen design principles for enhanced accessibility. Feature articles are supplemented by news of interest to computer users with disabilities as well as educators, librarians, rehabilitation and other professionals interested in the uses of new and emerging technologies by people with disabilities.

Access: The first issue of *Information Technology and Disabilities* will appear on January 15, 1994. Individual subscriptions are free of charge, and two subscription options are available:

1. Receive ENTIRE ISSUE AUTOMATICALLY. Please note: individual issues will range from 75 to 150 pages.

   address e-mail message to: `listserv@sjuvm.stjohns.edu`

   leave subject line blank, send the following one line message: sub itd-jnl John Smith

2. The journal will be made available at the St. John's University gopher. To receive each issue's TABLE OF CONTENTS ONLY:

   address e-mail message to: `listserv@sjuvm.stjohns.edu`

   leave subject line blank, send the following one line message: sub itd-toc Jane Doe

The Table of Contents will provide abstracts of articles as well as explicit instructions for using the gopher-based version of Information Technology and Disabilities.

Contact: SUBMISSION OF ARTICLES *Information Technology and Disabilities* is a peer-reviewed journal. Requests for authors' guidelines should be submitted to:
Tom McNulty
Editor-in-Chief
Bobst Library, New York University
70 Washington Square South
New York, N.Y. 10012
voice: 212/998-2519
TDD (leave message): 212/998-4980
e-mail to: `mcnulty@acfcluster.nyu.edu`
`mcnulty@nyuacf (bitnet)`

JOURNAL OF NIH RESEARCH

Description: Life Sciences Research and News about the National Institutes of Health. The Journal of NIH Research is edited for doctoral level scientists engaged in life sciences research that is funded by the National Institutes of Health.

Each issue contains the following sections:

Life sciences news.

Research: including original research reviews, summaries of significant initiatives, (such as AIDS and the human genome project);

Notes for the bench scientist (legal issues, ethical questions, NIH resources and funding news, and technological advances in instrumentation and other lab equipment, procedures and techniques.)

Access: Gopher

Gopher Path: `Electronic Newsstand (tm)/Titles Arranged by Subject/Health/Journal of NIH Research`

URL: `gopher://gopher.internet.com:2100/11/collected/nih`

LYMENET-L

Description: The Lyme Disease Electronic Mail Network. Subscribers to LymeNet-L receive The LymeNet Newsletter approximately twice a month. This publication provides readers with the latest research, treatment and political news about the Lyme disease epidemic. Lyme Disease is now the fastest growing infectious disease in the United States. In 10 short years, this little known bacterial infection has claimed half a million victims and the number of new patients continues to spiral upward with no relief in sight. It is estimated that in 1991, 100,000 Americans contracted this dangerous disease. If left untreated, LD can cause permanent nerve, musculoskeletal and cardiac damage.

Access: Electronic Mail

Back issues can be obtained via 2 methods:

Internet users may use anonymous FTP at: `ftp.Lehigh.EDU:/pub/listserv/lymenet-l/Newsletters/x-yy` where `x` is the volume number and `yy` is the issue number

URL: `http://www.ii.vib.no/~magnus/lists/LymeNet-L.html`

Internet and Bitnet users may use the listserver by sending it this command:

`get LymeNet-L/Newsletters x-yy` where x is the volume number and yy is the issue number

The LymeNet Newsletter is automatically crossposted to the `sci.med` UseNet group.

The Newsletter is suitable for both scientific and patient communities, as it contains sections for each. We will complete volume 1 by releasing issue #27 soon.

The Newsletter has been in publication since January '93. Volume 2 will begin in late January '94.

Contact: Marc Gabriel
Editor-in-Chief, The LymeNet Newsletter
`mcg2@lehigh.edu`

MEDNEWS—Health Infocom Newsletter

Description: This newsletter contains health oriented news articles from around the globe. The HEALTH INFOCOM NEWSLETTER is published once a week. The newsletter is usually quite large, so to facilitate network movement, it is broken up into multiple sections. These are always clearly marked.

Access: Send an email to `LISTSERV@ASUACAD.BITNET` with the line

Sub MEDNEWS FirstName LastName

MIDWIFERY

Description: MIDWIVES ARRIVE ON THE ELECTRONIC FRONTIER

Midwifery Today, a small press magazine located at 390 High Street, Eugene, Oregon, combines one of humanity's oldest professions, midwifery, with some of today's newest methods of communication and networking. In January, the magazine staked its claim on the electronic frontier with an account on America Online and an e-mail address of `Midwifery@aol.com`

Today, for this gives the staff another way to communicate with midwives and other birth practitioners around the world. Although the magazine is small, it has subscribers in 20 different countries and has covered midwifery in areas as diverse as Bali, Russia and Japan. In addition, plans are in full swing for an international Pacific Rim Conference, "Weaving a Global Future," to be held in Hawaii in February 1995.

The international reach of internet mail is important to Midwifery. Midwifery Today's electronic outreach extends beyond simply having an E-mail address. The magazine itself actively encourages midwives to use computers and to go online, with articles like "Midwifery in the Information Age," by Linda R. Barnes, MS, CNM, and "PC, IBM, Mac, DOS--Making Sense of the Alphabet Soup," by Daphne Singingtree, CM, both in the Winter 1993 issue. An article about midwives online, also by Singingtree, is slated for the Spring 1994 issue, now in production.

Founded in 1986, Midwifery Today, Inc. publishes a quarterly magazine filled with up-to-date information on the many issues surrounding birth and midwifery care. Midwifery Today magazine promotes the exchange of ideas and knowledge between many different kinds of birth practitioners, from medical doctors to lay midwives to childbirth educators. A strong editorial emphasis is teaching women about alternatives in pregnancy and childbirth: including a woman's right to have her children where and how she chooses.

Access: Anyone with full internet access can read Midwifery Today's subscription, submission and conference information on the Nightingale Nursing Gopher at the University of Tennessee and the University of Warwick Nursing Gopher, in England. (See Gophers section). The Nightingale Gopher also has the bibliography and references for "Guidelines for Serving Disabled Women," a two-part series which appeared in the Autumn and Winter 1993 issues.

Contact: MIDWIFERY TODAY
Midwifery information:
Jan Tritten
P.O. Box 2672, Eugene OR 97402
Editorial information: Jan Tritten
1-503-344-7438 1-800-743-0974
Kimberley Mangun, `midwifery@aol.com`

NATIONAL LIBRARY OF MEDICINE PUBLICATIONS

Description: National Library of Medicine publications.
Access: Gopher—World Wide Web
URL: `gopher://gopher.nlm.nih.gov:70/11/`

NIBnews

Description: This is a biomedical informatics monthly newsletter. Covers Brazilian (and eventually South American) activities, people, information, events, publications, software, and computer applications in health care, medicine and biology. Each issue contains about 100 lines in English. There is a longer printed version, available through postal mail to anyone wishing to receive it.

Access: Send email to either `sabbatini@bruc.Bitnet` or
`sabbatini@ccvax.unicamp.br` and request a subscription.

ONLINE JOURNAL OF CURRENT CLINICAL TRIALS

Description: Searchable database of current clinical trials

Access: Gopher

Gopher Path: `Research Facilities/D. Samuel Gottesman Library/Online Journal of Current Clinical Trials`

URL: `gopher://gopher.aecom.yu.edu/00/facilities/gottesman/Online Journal of Current Clinical Trials`

ONLINE JOURNAL OF KNOWLEDGE SYNTHESIS FOR NURSING

Description: Published by Sigma Theta Tau, premiered at the Biennial Convention in November 1993.

Access: Demo disks are available. A subscription (1 year) costs $60.00.

Contact: Sigma at 317-634-8171 or e-mail the editor, Jane Barnsteiner at `barnstnr@son.nursing.upenn.edu`

PHNFLASH

Description: PHNFLASH is an electronic newsletter on key population, health, and nutrition issues, produced by the Population, Health and Nutrition Department in the World Bank. This department is solely responsible for its content.

Access: Send an email message to the `listserver@tome.worldbank.org` to request a subscription.

PSYCHE

Description: This is an interdisciplinary journal of research on consciousness This journal relates to the PSYCHE-L discussion group on `LISTSERV@NKI.BITNET`

PSYCHE is a refereed electronic journal dedicated to supporting the interdisciplinary exploration of the nature of consciousness and its relation to the brain.

PSYCHE publishes material relevant to that exploration from the perspectives afforded by the disciplines of cognitive science, philosophy, psychology, neuroscience, artificial intelligence and anthropology. Interdisciplinary discussions are particularly encouraged.

PSYCHE publishes a large variety of articles and reports for a diverse academic audience four times per year. As an electronic journal, the usual space limitations of print journals do not apply; however, the editors request that potential authors do not attempt to abuse the medium. Psyche also publishes a hardcopy version simultaneously with the electronic version. Long articles published in the electronic version may be abbreviated, synopsized or eliminated from the hardcopy version.

Access: Send email `LISTSERV@NKI.BITNET` with `SUBSCRIBE PSYCHE-L YOUR NAME` as the message.

Contact: Patrick Wilken, Executive Editor of PSYCHE:
Email: `x91007@phillip.edu.au`

PSYCOLOQUY

Description: This publication covers all aspects of psychology, neuroscience, behavioral biology, etc. PSYCOLOQUY is a refereed electronic journal which is intended to implement peer review on the networks in psychology and its related fields (cognitive science, neuroscience, behavioral biology, linguistics, philosophy).

PSYCOLOQUY is not only implementing peer review (i.e., refereeing)for submissions, but also "scholarly skywriting," i.e., interactive peer feedback, likewise refereed, on accepted contributions (max length: 500 lines).

Access: Send email to `LISTSERV@PUCC.BITNET` with the following one-line message `SUB PSYC YOUR NAME` PSYCOLOQUY is also available on Usenet as the moderated newsgroup `sci.psychology.digest`

PSYGRD-J (THE PSYCHOLOGY GRADUATE STUDENT JOURNAL: THE PSYCGRAD JOURNAL)

Description: The purpose of the journal is to publish, from the graduate student perspective, professional-level articles in the field of psychology. The PSYCGRAD Journal is primarily published and written by graduate students in psychology. It is targeted for anyone interested in the field of psychology.

Volumes of the journal are each compiled by a member of an editing team. Each member is responsible for a specific topic area. All submissions are subject to the editing process. Subscriptions are open to the public. After you have subscribed, postings to the project can be sent to **PSYCGRAD@UOTTAWA.BITNET** or **PSYCGRAD@ACADVM1.UOTTAWA.CA**

Access: Send email to `LISTSERV@UOTTAWA.BITNET` or `LISTSERV@ACADVM1.UOTTAWA.CA` with the following:
   `SUB PSYGRD-J YOUR NAME`

Contact: Matthew Simpson `054340@uottawa.Bitnet`
   `054340@acadvm1.uottawa.ca`

REPETITIVE STRAIN INJURY (RSI) NETWORK NEWSLETTER

Description: RSINET—The Repetitive Strain Injury Network The RSI Network is a bimonthly newsletter of information for people concerned about carpal tunnel syndrome, tendinitis, and other repetitive strain injuries. It covers software, hardware, publications, ergonomic resources, worker's compensation, legislation, employment services, practitioners, personal stories of RSI sufferers, and more.

Access: FTP

URL: `ftp://sunsite.unc.edu/pub/docs/typing-injury/rsi-network`

SBIS NEWSLETTER

Description: This is the official bimonthly news publication of the Brazilian Society for Health Informatics. The language is Portuguese.

Access: Contact by email to request subscription.

Contact: Monica P. Ramos, SBIS' Executive Secretary,
   `epm@brfapesp.Bitnet` or Fax (+55 11 572-6601)

THE AMERICAN POLITICAL NETWORK

Description: The publication produces a daily summary of health care news and miscellaneous health care items. It's available via modem dial-in (request the number at the time of subscription) or through internet distribution.

Access: Call (703) 237-5130 and request to be put on their mailing list.

THE BLIND NEWS DIGEST

Description: The BLIND NEWS DIGEST is an electronic-mail only digest of articles dealing with blindnews or any type of vision impairment. The articles are from the Usenet newsgroup and misc.handicap. It is also gatewayed with the Fidonet conference, BlinkTalk. Other non-vision related articles from the `misc.handicap` newsgroup are carried in the Handicap Digest mailing list (L-HCAP)

Access: Send email to **WTM@BUNKER.SHEL.ISC-BR.COM** and request to be added to their mailing list. Relates to listserv list **BLINDNWS@NDSUVM1**

Contact: `WTM@BUNKER.SHEL.ISC-BR.COM`

THE HANDICAP DIGEST

Description: The HANDICAP DIGEST is an electronic-mail only digest of articles relating to all types of issues affecting the handicapped. The articles are taken from the Usenet newsgroup, the Handicap News. (misc.handicap) and various Fidonet conferences such as ABED, BlinkTalk SilentTalk, Chronic Pain, Spinal Injury, Rare Conditions, and several others. Relates to listserv list **L-HCAP@NDSUVM1**

Access: Send email to **WTM@BUNKER.SHEL.ISC-BR.COM** to request subscription.

Databases

Data archives

ALCOHOLISM RESEARCH DATABASE
Description: Project CORK collection on alcoholism and substance abuse on the Dartmouth College Library Online System.

Access: telnet

URL: `telnet://LIB.DARTMOUTH.EDU` SELECT FILE `CORK` once connected to the system

ASTRA
Description: An Access System for Databases Distributed on EARN/BITNET. The ASTRA service maintains multiple databases called META databases. Each one has an abstract containing information about the contents, i.e., title, name of the authors, a brief description of the database, the main arguments dealt with in the database and the language. Of interest to those in the health sciences is the ONCO database.

ONCO database

This bibliographic list keeps track of the work concerning ongoing research related to the Oncology field in Italy. The list includes work from different research groups at various institutions. The language is English.

NETWORK ACCESS AND USAGE

The ASTRA database is accessible by EARN/BITNET and non- EARN/BITNET users. For EARN/BITNET users, user interfaces for IBM VM/CMS and DEC VAX/VMS are developed. Also a batch language format has been developed for non-EARN/BITNET users and users of different operation systems.

To access the ASTRA system the EARN/BITNET users must have the user interface on their disk. The user interface can be obtained from `ASTRADB@ICNUCEVM` with the following commands:

For IBM VM/CMS   `GET ASTRA EXEC`
For DEC VAX/VMS   `GET ASTRA PAS`

After the files are received and stored on the disk, the server is accessed by entering:

For IBM VM/CMS   `ASTRA`
For DEC VAX/VMS   `RUN ASTRA`

Detailed information on the system can be retrieved by getting the file `ASTRA INFO` from `ASTRADB@ICNUCEVM`

Access: See Description

Contact: `astra@icnucevm`

Bitnet Address: `ASTRA@ICNUCEVM`

BIOCOMPUTING, BIOZENTRUM, UNIVERSITY OF BASEL. ARCHIVE OF BIOLOGICAL DATABASES
Description: First time users should access the directory biology/database and read the file DATABASES.TXT for a listing and description of the databases available.

Access: telnet

URL: `telnet://MODL.UNIBAS.CH`

BIOETHICS ONLINE SERVICE
Description: This section provides information on the following topics:
1. Description of the Service
2. Instructions

3. Questions or Problems?
4. Legal Notice
5. Credits
6. Routes of Access to the Service

1. DESCRIPTION OF THE SERVICE:

The Bioethics Online Service is an information resource of the Center for the Study of Bioethics and the Health Information Technology Center (HITC) of the Medical College of Wisconsin (MCW).

The Bioethics Online Service consists of:
a. The Bioethics Database
b. The Bioethics Center and Wisconsin Ethics Committee Network (WECN) News and Announcements section
c. The Bioethics Online E-mail Service

The features of the service are available for use through the Internet or by accessing the Medical Information Network (MIN) of the Health Information Technology Center at the Medical College of Wisconsin. The Bioethics Database is an update service providing information on current bioethics topics, including news reports, abstracts of pertinent journal articles, legislative actions and court decisions, with intermittent commentary. The information is searchable by key words.

The Bioethics Center and Wisconsin Ethics Committee Network (WECN) News and Announcements section posts news from the Bioethics Center, including speakers, conferences, journal clubs, and other presentations. It also posts news of the Wisconsin Ethics Committee Network, and information about its Speakers Bureau. A second feature of this section is a case discussion area.

The Bioethics Online E-mail Service allows users to send messages worldwide to those users of the Bioethics

Online Service who have E-mail addresses through the Medical College of Wisconsin or have Internet addresses. You must have an Outreach Account or a Post Account through the Medical College of Wisconsin, or have an Internet address to be able to utilize the Bioethics Online E-mail Service.

2. BIOETHICS ONLINE SERVICE DATABASE INSTRUCTIONS:

Using the Bioethics Database gopher:

The Bioethics Database menu has several numbered options. Select an option with the up/down arrow keys and <return>. Note that each menu entry ends with a special symbol. These symbols identify each menu entry as follows:

/	Item is a directory
.	Item is a text file
<?>	Item is a search index
<CSO>	Item is a CSO phone book
<TEL>	Item is a telnet session
<))	Item is a sound (looks like a speaker)

By noting the symbols at the end of each entry you will know what to expect when selecting a given menu choice. For example, if the menu entry you select ends with a "/", you will see another directory of choices; if it is a ".", a text file is presented; etc. (Note: The Bioethics Database does not support <CSO> or <) entries.)

After viewing a text file, you have the option of saving it to a file, printing it, or sending it to someone's mailbox (Note: MIN users without accounts are only provided the mail option). All printing occurs remotely at the ITS (Information Technology Systems) computer room. Please do not print files unless you are a local MCW user. All output is retrieved at the MCW ITS office.

The Bioethics Database is menu driven and very user friendly. A help screen is always available by typing "?". Traverse up menu levels with "u" (for up). Quit at any time with "q".

The Search Index

When you select a search index you are prompted for the word(s) to search on. The Bioethics Database supports natural language queries. All matches are ranked based on the number of matches found. For example, to search for articles on ethics or AIDS you could type: Index word(s) to search for: ethics aids. Search specifications are not case sensitive

Additional information on this service is available by typing "?" at any menu.

3. QUESTIONS OR PROBLEMS?

If you have technical questions or problems, please contact the MCW Information Technolgy Systems office.

Bioethics Online Service users with E-mail (MCWConnect or MCW Post Accounts) or Internet users may send comments or questions to: biohelp@its.mcw.edu

Otherwise you may send comments or questions to:

> Bioethics Online Service c/o Information Technology
> Systems Medical College of Wisconsin
> 8701 Watertown Plank Road
> Milwaukee, WI 53226
> (414) 257-8700.

You may also send comments or questions about the content of the service to:

> Arthur R. Derse, M.D., J.D.
> Bioethics Online Service Director
> Center for the Study of Bioethics
> Medical College of Wisconsin
> 8701 Watertown Plank Road
> Milwaukee, WI 53226
> (414) 257-8498
> aderse@its.mcw.edu

4. LEGAL NOTICE:

The Bioethics Online Service provides information of a general nature regarding current ethical, legal and legislative information. None of the information contained in the Bioethics Online Service is intended as ethical or legal advice or opinion relative to specific matters, facts, situations or issues and additional facts and information or future developments may affect the subjects addressed. The Bioethics Online Service is a copyright of the Center for the Study of Bioethics at The Medical College of Wisconsin. The Internet gopher is an information retrieval program distributed by the University of Minnesota.

5. CREDITS:

The Bioethics Online Service is made possible with the help of:
- Perry Brunelli, Technical Director and Acting Director, ITS
- Rob Gatter, J.D., Abstracter
- Mary Olson, Abstracts Editor
- Sean Castro, Technical Assistant
- Larry Roscoe, Technical Assistant
- Jay A. Gold, M.D., J.D., M.P.H. Abstracter Emeritus

6. ROUTES OF ACCESS to the MCW Bioethics Online Service:

a. Access by modem and telephone line to MCW:

i. For those with an MCWConnect Account at MCW: dial 1-800-699-3282 or 414-266-5777 at any baud rate. At the prompt (HITC>) type c outreach and press enter. At the menu select

Internet and press enter. At the next menu, select `Gopher` and enter. Finally, select `Bioethics Online Service` and press enter.

ii. For those with a Post Account at MCW: dial 414-266-5777 at any baud rate. At the prompt (`HITC>`) type `c post` (without the quotes) and press enter, then at the prompt (`post>`) type `bioethics` and press enter.

iii. For those who have neither a Post Account or an MCWConnect Account at MCW:

Obtain an MCWConnect Account from MCW. An MCWConnect Account provides access to the Bioethics Online Service, including a Bioethics Online E-mail account, and access to Internet which includes access to a cornucopia of medical databases, library resources, discussion groups, and electronic mail.

Best of all, this MCWConnect Account can be reached toll- free at 1-800-699-3282. It may also be reached by dialing 414-266-5777.

An MCWConnect Account subscription is $18/year (which includes password, login insructions, user support, and first 2 hours of connect time. Online connect time is $9/hour.

To get further information about MCWConnect or to apply for an account contact the Library Systems Office at MCW at 414-778-4290.

Wisconsin Ethics Committee Network members may also reach the Bioethics Online Service Database and Bulletin Board (minus the all the other capabilities including e-mail and Internet access) by dialing: 414-266-5777 At the prompt (`HITC>`) type `c min` and press enter, then select the `Bioethics Online Service` option on the menu.

All Wisconsin Ethics Committee Network members are encouraged to take best advantage of the service by obtaining an MCWConnect Account.

b. Access using the Internet:

i. Using a UNIX-based system with a gopher client: If you are accessing the Internet through a UNIX based system and have a gopher client, you may access the Bioethics Online Service by typing: gopher post.its.mcw.edu 72

ii. Using UNIX-based system utilizing telnet (without a gopher client) : If you are accessing the Internet through a UNIX based system but do not have a gopher client, you may access the Bioethics Online Service by typing: telnet min.lib.mcw.edu. Then select the "Bioethics Online Service" on the menu URL:

Any questions? Send e-mail to `biohelp@post.its.mcw.edu`

Access: telnet, gopher, and dial-up modem
Gopher Path: `Health and Clinical Information (+Bioethics Online Service)/MCW Bioethics Online Service`
Contact: Arthur R. Derse, M.D., J.D. Associate Director for Medical and Legal Affairs, Center for the Study of Bioethics, MCW, and Director
URL: `gopher://post.its.mcw.edu:72/1`

BIOSIS

Description: BIOSIS contains citations from a number of biological publications providing worldwide coverage of research in the biological and biomedical sciences. The database is comprised of over 500,000 citations covering over 9,000 primary and monograph titles.

Access: A password is needed to access this database, for help call the OCLC User Contact Desk at 1-800-848-5800.

CANCERNET

Description: CancerNet is a quick and easy way to obtain, through electronic mail, cancer information from the National Cancer Institute (NCI). CancerNet lets you request information statements from the NCI's Physician Data Query (PDQ) database, fact sheets on various cancer topics from the NCI's Office of Cancer Communications, and citations and abstracts on selected topics from the CANCERLIT database. Selected information is also available in Spanish. You can access CancerNet through a number of different networks including BITNET and Internet. There is no charge for the service unless your local computer center charges for use of e-mail. The CancerNet Contents List changes at the beginning of each month as new statements and other information is included.

Access: see instructions below

If you have any problems accessing CancerNet, you may call 1-301-496-7403 or send a message to `cheryl@icicb.nci.nih.gov` on the Internet.

Instructions

1. Address your mail message to:

    `cancernet@icicb.nci.nih.gov`

If you are not on Internet, you may have to change the format of the address. Consult your systems manager for the correct address format.

2. In the body of the message:

    a. If you need the CancerNet contents list, enter `help` to receive the most current list (substitute the word `spanish` if you want the contents list in Spanish).

    b. If you have the CancerNet contents list and would like to request a particular statement or piece of information, enter the code from the Contents List for the desired information. If you want more than one piece of information, enter the code for each piece of information desired on a separate line within the message.

Note: Individual statements may exceed 100K and some mail systems are limited in the size of the mail messages a user can receive. Please check your mail and storage capacity prior to submitting requests.

The information in CancerNet is also available on several Gopher servers as well as a number of secondary distributor sites. To access a gopher server if you have Gopher client software on your host computer or PC, point to `gopher.nih.gov`. CancerNet can also be accessed via telnet to `gopher.ncc.go.jp` (160.190.10.1), using `gopher` as the logon and password (additional gopher public access sites can also be accessed via telnet). You may have to go through several menus and submenus to access CancerNet on a gopher server. For a complete listing of all gopher and secondary sites, request item cn- 400030 from CancerNet.

If you have any further questions, send an e-mail message to:

    Cheryl Burg
    Building 82, Room 103A
    CancerNet Project Manager
    National Cancer Institute
    9000 Rockville Pike BLDG 82 Room 103A
    Bethesda, Maryland 20892
    Internet: `cheryl@icicb.nci.nih.gov`
    Phone: (301) 496-8880
    Fax: (301) 480-8105
    Internet Address: See description
    URL: `telnet://gopher.ncc.go.jp`

CDC WONDER

Description: What is CDC WONDER?

CDC WONDER is software for DOS based microcomputers that creates a fast and efficient electronic link between CDC and public health practitioners.

It is distributed free and uses a toll free number to connect to the CDC in Atlanta. It was originally created to connect local, county, and state public health officials to national databases. It is now available to all public health practitioners. The data available through CDC WONDER come from the National Center for Health Statistics of the Centers for Disease Control and Prevention, the National Cancer Institute, the National Institute for Occupational Safety and Health, the Census Bureau, etc.

Currently, CDC WONDER only runs on DOS based machines. They plan to port CDC WONDER to otherplatforms shortly. There will also be Internet access sometime later this year.

According to the CDC documentation, user specified tables can be created from the following data sets:

- AIDS Microfiche Data Summary
- AIDS Public Use
- Mortality Data:
- US Mortality by county, age, ICD code, year
- Associated Morbidity
- Comorbidity Multiple Cause of death data
- ENGLAND AND WALES MORTALITY
- CBA CEA Bibliography
- NHIS PAP Smear Data
- National Hospital Discharge Survey (Data elements available not specified in the documentation)
- NHIS Tobacco Use Data SEER (Cancer surveillance data set for 10 sites, combined to estimate national rates for age-race-gender-year stratum) Sexually Transmitted Disease Morbidity US Census

One limit of the WONDER system for those outside CDC is that it has to be accessed by modem, as access over the net is not yet available.

Access: email: **WRH2@opsirm8.em.cdc.gov**
This is not an automated email server, so just ask for a user registration form for Wonder. Please be sure to include a US Mail address.
Phone: 404-332-4569
You will be answered by Wonder User Support.
Request registration material.
fax: 404-488-7593
Send a note asking for registration material. Please be sure to include a US Mail address. The reason you cannot register automatically is the requirement for a physical signature to access some of the databases they provide.

Contact: Dan Rosen
Public Health Information Systems Branch
Information Resources Management Office
Centers for Disease Control and Prevention
4770 Buford Highway
MS F-51
Atlanta, GA 30341-3724
`dhr0@opsirm8.em.cdc.gov`
phone:404-488-7521
fax:404-488-7593

Internet Address: `wrh2@opsirm8.em.cdc`

CHAT

Description: CHAT (Conversational Hypertext Access Technology) is a natural language information system. This information retrieval technology developed by Industry Canada. Please note that your interactions with CHAT are being recorded. You will have a chance to leave comments at the end of your session.

There are information files available on the following topics:

- AIDS (Acquired Immune Deficiency Syndrome)
- Epilepsy
- Alice (A simulated conversation)
- Maur (A simulated conversation with a dragon)

- Spectrum Management Program of Industry Canada
- Caenorhabditis Genetics Center (CGC)

Access: telnet

Contact: For information about CHAT, download the file /pub/chat/info.page from debra.dgbt.doc.ca using anonymous ftp, or contact: Thom Whalen: (613) 990-4683 thom@debra.dgbt.doc.ca, Andrew Patrick: (613) 990-4675, andrew@debra.dgbt.doc.ca

URL: `telnet://debra.dgbt.doc.ca`

Login: CHAT

EUROPEAN MOLECULAR BIOLOGY LABORATORY, Heidelberg, Germany

Description: The EMBL Network File Server enables network access to the following:

- EMBL Nucleotide Sequence Database—The newest nucleotide sequence data created at EMBL and GenBank since the latest full release of the EMBL database
- DNA sequence alignments and consensus sequences
- Free software for molecular biologists
- Reference lists of relevance to molecular biology General documents with importance to molecular biology
- Documents describing the services of the EMBL Data Library.

Access: EMAIL—HELP

Bitnet Address: `netserv@embl-heidel`

FEDERAL FOOD AND DRUG ADMINISTRATION

Description: This is the FEDERAL FOOD AND DRUG ADMINISTRATION's Internet link to its databases. The user will find reports and press releases on everything the FDA is responsible for. There is an online users manual.

Access: telnet

URL: `telnet://150.148.8.48`

Login: BBS

FEDWORLD: NATIONAL TECHNICAL INFORMATION SERVICE

Description:

FedWorld (TM)
National Technical Information Service
A database of government databases.
Of interest are the following:

The Health Security Plan

ALF (USDA)	National Agricultural Library
CIC-BBS (GSA)	Consumer Information
CRS-BBS (Dept of Justice)	Amer. With Disabilities Act Info
NADAP (US Navy)	Navy Drug and Alcohol Abuse prevention
NDB-BBS (Dept of Agricul)	Human Nutrition Information Service
WTIE-BBS (EPA)	Wastewater Treatment Info Exchange
OASH-BBS (HHS)	Health & AIDS Information & Reports
NIDR Online (NIH)	Nat. Institute of Dental Research
NIHGL (NIH)	Nat. Inst. of Health Grant Line BBS
DRIPSS (EPA)	Drinking Water Info Processing Support
PIM BBS (EPA)	Pesticide Information Network
HSETC MD (U.S. Navy)	Naval Health Sci Edu & Training Command
ACF-BBS (HHS)	Admin. for Children and Families

HEALTH SCIENCES 375

BHPr-BBS (HHS)	Medical & Health Services Information
ABLE INFORM (Dof Ed)	Disability & Rehab Data & Info
Quick Facts! (NIAAA/HHS)	Alcohol Abuse & Alcoholism Information
RSA-BBS (RSA)	Rehabilitation Services Administration
NBCI-BBS (USDA)	Natl Biological Control Institute

Access: telnet
URL: `telnet://FEDWORLD.GOV`

GAO DAILY AND MONTHLY LISTING OF REPORTS

Description: The U.S. General Accounting Office, Congress' Watchdog agency, now has available a daily electronic posting of released reports. The "GAO Daybook" is the daily listing of released GAO reports and the "Reports and Testimonies Issued in Month/Year", includes abstracts of the items issued that month, arranged by subject.

Access: Telnet

Contact: Ordering information is included in the GAO menu. Any questions or comments can be sent to gao@cap.gwu.edu Please do not use this address for ordering reports.

URL: `telnet://CAP.GWU.EDU`

login: guest

password: visitor at main menu, type go gao

GENBANK

Description: These two addresses provide access to nucleotide and protein sequence databases. The sequences are from the literature and direct submissions. RETRIEVE allows you to retrieve a sequence using a gene name, GENBANK accession number (from Medline or another database) or other descriptive information. BLAST is a program that matches a sequence to sequences already in the database. Messages to either must be formatted in a very specific way. To receive directions for each send an email message with the word HELP in the body of the message.

Access: EMAIL

Internet Address: `RETRIEVE@NCBI.NLM.HLH.GOV`
`BLAST@NCBI.NLM.HLH.GOV`

HRO DISSEMINATION NOTES (HUMAN RESOURCES DEVELOPMENT AND OPERATIONS POLICY)

Description: The following issues of HRO DISSEMINATION NOTES are available through the PHNFLASH Listserv.

File Name		Title
HR0	a)	Tobacco Death Toll
HR1	b)	The Benefits of Education for Women
HR2	c)	Poverty & Income Distribution in Latin America
HR3	d)	Acute Respiratory Infections
HR5	e)	From Manpower Planning to Labor Market Analysis
HR6	f)	Enhancing Investments in Education through Better Nutrition and Health
HR7	g)	Indigenous People in Latin America
HR8	h)	Developing Effective Employment Services
HR9	I)	Social Security: Promise and Pitfalls in Privatization Experience in Latin America
HR10	j)	Making Motherhood Safe
HR11	k)	Indigenous People & Socio Economic Development in Latin America: The Case of Bolivia
HR12	l)	World Population Surpasses 5.5 Billion in 1993
HR14	m)	Alcohol-Related Problems: An Obstacle to Human Capital Development?

HR15	n)	Hidden Hunger I
HR16	o)	Hidden Hunger II--Micronutrient Malnutrition
HR17	p)	Barriers and Solutions to Closing the Gender Gap
HR18	q)	Higher Education, Innovation and Market Response: The Singapore Experience

Access: You must subscribe to the PHNFLASH newsletter in order to retrieve these files (see the newsletter section of this document.) Send a message to `Listserv@tome.worldbank.org` (World Bank staff can simply type `@listserv`) and in the text body, type: `get PHNFLASH filename`. Unfortunately the Listserv cannot handle multiple requests, so you have to send separate request for each issue.

Contact: PHNLINK Team `PHNLINK@worldbank.org`

Internet Address: `LISTSERV@TOME.WORLD`

INFOMED—ELECTRONIC INFORMATION STATISTICAL YEARBOOK OF HEALTH 1991—CUBA

Description: Infomed has distributed the table of the Statistical Yearbook of the Ministry of Public Health 1991. These tables contain the principle indicators of Health in Cuba. The tables are in ASCII files. All of these files are in Spanish.

Yearbook tables:

To obtain a table from the yearbook, send an electronic message to `LISTSERV@INFOMED.CU` without a subject and with the following content in the body of the message:

`GET ANUARIO <name of table>`

A list of the tables follows with the name of the file that contains them. You can only request up to 10 tables in the same message. If you have any difficulty, request the help file. Example:

You will receive the table by email.

Table of Contents of the Yearbook Mortality.

CMT-11	Death rates by age group
CMT-13	Mortality by age group and province
CMT-12	Principal causes of death for all ages
CMT-34	Years of potential life lost per 1000 inhabitants 1-64 years, rates of mortality according to selected causes of death
CMT-53	Rates of mortality according to selected causes of death by province
CMT-5	Principal causes of death by sex
CMT-1	Perinatal mortality
CMT-2	Perinatal mortality by province
CMT-52	Selected indicators of mortality under 5 years of age, also under 5 years of age by province
CMT-15	Infant mortality by province
CMT-16	Principal causes of death under 1 year of age
CMT-17	Principal causes of death from 1-4 years of age
CMT-18	Principal causes of death from 5-14 years of age
CMT-19	Principal causes of death from 15-49 years of age
CMT-20	Principal causes of death from 50-64 years of age
CMT-21	Principal causes of death from 65 years of age or more
CMT-22	Mortality due to heart disease
CMT-22A	Mortality due to heart disease by sex
CMT-23	Mortality due to malignant tumors
CMT-33	Mortality due to malignant tumors by sex
CMT-24	Accidental deaths by selected causes
CMT-24A	Accidental deaths by selected causes by sex
CMT-25	Mortality by infectious and parasitic diseases

CMT-26	Mortality by infectious and parasitic diseases by province
CMT-27	Mortality by acute diarrhetic diseases
CMT-28	Mortality by acute diarrhetic diseases by province
CMT-29	Maternal mortality by apparent cause
CMT-30	Maternal mortality by apparent cause by province
CMT-32	Mortality by reportable diseases

Access: See instructions above.

Internet Address: `LISTSERV@INFOMED.CU`

JOHNS HOPKINS GENETIC DATABASES

Description: 1. Genome Data Base (GDB) (Human chromosome mapping)

2. OMIM Data Base. Online Mendelian Inheritance in Man. (Inherited disorders and traits)

Network access is supported. However, users must first contact the Welch Medical Library at Johns Hopkins University to obtain a user id and password. Telephone (301) 955-9637 to obtain a user id and password, or contact `HELP@WELCH.JHU.EDU`

Access: Users must first contact GDB/OMIM User Support at Johns Hopkins University to obtain a user id and password.

Telephone (410) 955-7058 to obtain an account, or contact `help@gdb.org`

Access: telnet, ftp, gopher, wais
WAIS databases:
`gdb-citation.src`
`gdb-contact.src`
`gdb-locus.src`
`gdb-map.src`
`gdb-mutation.src`
`gdb-polym.src`
`gdb-probe.src`
`gdb.src`
WWW server: coming soon!

Contact: Ken Fasman, Ph.D.
Informatics Director
Genome Data Base
Johns Hopkins University School of Medicine
2024 E. Monument St.
Baltimore MD 21205
`ken@gdb.org`

URL: `telnet://gdb.gdb.org`
`ftp://ftp.gdb.org`
`gopher://gppher.gdb.org`

MEDLARS

Description: This is the NATIONAL LIBRARY OF MEDICINE DATABASES. You will be issued a user i.d. and password in order to access MEDLINE as well as the other 24 databases maintained by the National Library of Medicine. For online access informaiton, e-mail to the MEDLARS Management Section: `mms@nlm.nih.gov`

Access: See description

Internet Address: `mms@nlm.nih.gov`

MEDLINE

Description: MEDLINE is one of over 20 databases available from the National Library of Medicine.

Access: MEDLINE is accessible via the Internet. An account is required for billing purposes. The user is issued a user i. d. and password. For more information, email to `REF@NLM.NIH.GOV`. There is an algorithm for pricing. Since it is paid for by taxes, the prices are modest and have just DECREASED to about $17.00/hr. You can also get information about a software package available for $30 called GRATEFUL MED which allows untrained database searchers and health professionals a menu-driven means of performing searches on many of their databases. In addition, an enhancement to the original program called LOANSOME DOC allows you to order copies of articles that you wish to read from participating medical libraries. It is available for both IBM, compatibles and Mac computers. For information about GRATEFUL MED/LOANSOME DOC, email to: GMHELP@GMEDSERV.NLM.NIH.GOV

Once you get your user i.d./password (which is free) you can search databases directly at the telnet site listed below. Those institutions which make MEDLINE or other databases available for their students/faculty/clientele pay royalty fees and contractually can only allow members of that institution to search FREE.

URL: `telnet://medlars.nlm.nih.gov`

MISSING CHILDREN'S FORUM

Description: Contains known information about, and pictures of, children who are missing. The database is maintained by the National Center for Missing and Exploited Children (NCMEC). This mirror of the files contained in the CompuServe Forum is maintained as a public service by Maxwell Labs in order to provide access to this information for Internet users. The database contains pictures of the children in GIF format and text files containing information about their disappearance.

Access: World Wide Web (In the near future Gopher and anonymous ftp access will be added.)

It appears as if the site is still under construction. Missing Children's Hotline: 1-800-THE-LOST (1-800-843-5678) (24 hours, 7 days).

URL: `http://inept.scubed.com:8001/public_service/missing.html`

NATIONAL ARCHIVES AND RECORDS ADMINISTRATION—THE CENTER FOR ELECTRONIC RECORDS

Description: Health and Social Services Data. Provides datasets on magnetic media. Health-related data deposited in the Center incorporate both biomedical and sociological information.

Access: email

    Reference Staff
    Center for Electronic Records (NNX)
    National Archives and Records Administration
    Washington D.C. 20408
    Phone: (202) 501-5579

Bitnet Address: `TIF@NIHCU`

Internet Address: `TIF@CU.NIHCU.GOV`

NICOLAS DATABASE—NETWORK INFORMATION CENTER ON-LINE AID SYSTEM

Description: E-mail addresses for Health Agencies (Revised Oct 17, 1991)

Organization: Federal/State, Private: International, National (Agencies, Institutions), State/Province/City.

Access: For further info about nodes send a message to listserv at BITNIC (USA) or HEARN (Europe) `GET NODENTRY Node_name` Address enquiries: `Info-nets@Think.COM` (to subscribe on Bitnet `SUB INFONETS full_name` to any LISTSERV or on Internet mail request to `info-nets-request@think.com`) and `Help-net@templevm.bitnet`. For a full general account obtain `HOSTINFO NOTES` (send command to listserv at `JHUVM GET HOSTINFO NOTES`) this covers WHOIS, database searches for regions, topics or individuals, etc. It is especially useful to search the NIC database.

Contact: (800) 235-3155)

URL: `telnet://NIC.DDN.MIL`

PENNINFO

Description: This is a massive collection of information on the university, libraries, networks, computing resources, electronic texts, and MEDINFO database.

Access: telnet

URL: `telnet://PENNINFO.UPENN.EDU`
    `ftp://penninfo.srv.upenn.edu`

RESTRICTION ENZYME DATABASE (REBASE)
Description: Directory: repository or REBASE (Restriction Enzyme Database). The database contains both data and literature citations.
Access: FTP
Contact: Dr. Richard Roberts, Cold Spring Harbor Laboratory (ROBERTS@CSHL.ORG).
URL: **ftp://ncbi.nlm.nih.gov/repository/REBASE**

SOUTH EAST FLORIDA AIDS INFORMATION NETWORK
Description: Users may search for AIDS Information by any of the following:

```
P > PERSON/ORG/RESEARCH
O > Organization TYPE
M > MEDICAL Specialty
R > Research SITE
T > Research TYPE
A > Res ELIGIBILITY
H > HEALTH&SOCIAL Serv
B > Mental HEALTH Serv
E > EDUC & Info Serv
Q > QUIT
```

This project is sponsored in part by the National Library of Medicine.

Access: telnet
URL: **telnet://CALLCAT.MED.MIAMI.EDU**
login: LIBRARY
    Select L on main menu
    Select 1 on next menu
    SEFAIN Database

FTP SITES

These sites hold retrieveable files.

1990 CENSUS
Description: 1990 Census information, arranged state by state. Commands and file names are case-sensitive; be sure to capitalize as above. At the next asterisk, type `ls` or `dir` to get a list of the contents. To get the file you want, type `get filename`, where `filename` is the name of the file. Type quit to quit. The contents of INFO are also available for reading on line if you telnet to `info.umd.edu` and follow the directions.
Access: FTP
URL: **ftp://info.umd.edu/info/Government/US/Census-90**

AMALGAME
Description: Macintosh demos and XFCN PrintZ files. Files in English and French versions
Access: FTP

Contact: BENOIT@MEDENT.UMONTREAL.CA
(514) 343-6111 ext 3418
Universite de Montreal

URL: `ftp://amalgame.medent.umontreal.ca/pub/multimed_mac_demo`
`ftp://amalgame.medent.umontreal.ca/pub/multimed_mac_xfcn`

ANESTHESIOLOGY ARCHIVES

Description: The archive site for Anesthesiology contains files and programs of interest to anesthesiologists. Files include the complete bibliography of the Society for Neurosurgical Anesthesiology and Critical Care and a neuroanesthesia manual.

Access: FTP

Contact: Keith J Ruskin, MD
Department of Anesthesiology
NYU Medical Center
keith@mcan00.med.nyu.edu
ruskin@acf1.nyu.edu
(212)263-5072

URL: `ftp://gasnet.med.nyu.edu`

ARCHIVE OF BIOLOGY SOFTWARE AND DATA: INDIANA UNIVERSITY

Description: The main area of concentration of this archive is molecular biology. The archive contains software for the Macintosh, VAX- VMS, Unix, MS-DOS and other important operating systems. It is recommended that you transfer and read the file Archive.doc first. This file gives considerable information about, and instructions for using the archive.

Access: FTP

URL: `ftp://ftp.bio.indiana.edu`

BIOCOMPUTING SURVIVAL GUIDE

Description: Biocomputing Survival Guide is designed for the rare user of molecular biology computer programs. Basic operations of login procedures, file handling and transfer, and the GCG key programs are explained for both UNIX and VMS operating systems.

Access: Gopher

The Guide is available as a MS-WORD document from the EMBnet file server, and as printed version you can most conveniently obtain the Guide from the "Materialausgabe" at the Biozentrum ground floor, by sending a request to EMBnet Switzerland, or, internationally, to Paula Maki-Valkkila, CSC, Tietotie 6, P.O.Box 405, 02101 Espoo, Finland. The Biocomputing Survival Guide is a DIN A 5 booklet . The Biocomputing Tutorial (the black book) is no longer available but a new book will be available in the bookstores early 1994 (Humana Press).

GOPHER provides you with an easy way to access the GCG program documentation: Type the name of the program (gopher) on the command line, and select item 5 (GCG Software Documentation) by moving the cursor with the arrow keys to this item. Then, hit <RETURN> and select the first item by hitting <RETURN> again. You may search any keyword (e.g., sequence search) after typing it in and hitting <RETURN> again. You will obtain a list of all sections in the manual which contain the desired keyword. GOPHER will be featured in a future release of Biocomputing NEWS. From within the WWW program, a link to the top level of the bioftp gopher is available. Note that we must restrict the access to this part of the gopher to Basel University due to copyright reasons.

URL: `gopher://bioftp.unibas.ch`

BIOMEDICAL COMPUTER LABORATORY

Description: The Biomedical Computer Laboratory (BCL) is designated as a "Resource for Biomedical Computing" by the National Institutes of Health's National Center for Research Resources (NCRR). A significant portion of the activities at the BCL are supported by NCRR's Biomedical Research Technology Program (BRTP) which promotes the application of advances in computer science and technology, engineering, mathematics, and the physical sciences to research problems in biology and medicine by supporting the development of advanced research technologies. In addition to supporting the development of new or improved technologies, the BRTP resource program encourages the use of those developments in collaborative research with biomedical research investigators nationally through both collaborative interactions and service-oriented relationships.

BCL program emphasis is on quantitative imaging including positron-emission tomography (PET) image reconstruction utilizing estimation-maximization (EM) methods, computational optical-sectioning microscopy, shape modeling and segmentation, electron- microscopic autoradiography (EMA), image acquisition and quantitative analysis of DNA electrophoretic gels and autoradiogram, and parallel processing. The resource invites program participation by research investigators with relevant scientific interests. The participation can be either as a research collaborator or as a user of resource capabilities. A collaboration involves two-way interaction of mutual benefit, whereas user service provides a primary benefit to the user. Investigators wishing to explore the possibility of interactions with the resource at Washington University should contact us by mail, telephone, FAX, or email (preferred). Information may also be obtained via an anonymous FTP server on the Internet on which the Resource maintains public information including a list of publications available, selected publications, and software.

Access: FTP

Contact: Kenneth W. Clark
Telephone: (314) 362-2135
Coordinator of Resource Extramural Activities
FAX: (314) 362-0234 Biomedical Computer Laboratory
Email: INFO@WUBCL.WUSTL.EDU
Washington University School of Medicine
700 S. Euclid Avenue
St. Louis, MO 63110 USA

URL: ftp://wubcl.wustl.edu/pub

DATA FILES IN THE NATIONAL ARCHIVES AND RECORDS ADMINISTRATION

Description: The Center for Electronic Records of the U.S. National Archives has updated the FTP-able file containing the Center's "Title List: A Preliminary and Partial Listing of the Data Files in the National Archives and Records Administration" TITLE.LIST.DEC1793

Since last updated in September, entries for the following major series have been included: the 1980 Census of Population and Housing, STFs 1D, 3C, 3D, and 3F (Bureau of the Census); and the [Southeast Asia] Combat Area Casualties Current File, as of November 1993 (Office of the Secretary of Defense).

September's update included the following major series: the Institutional Investor Study, 1969-1971 (Securities and Exchange Commission), Bureau of Justice Statistics data files, National Medical Care Expenditure Surveys (Agency for Health Care Policy Research), and the Defense Wage Fixing data files, 1974-1991 (Office of the Secretary of Defense).

Access: FTP

Contact: THEODORE J. HULL
Archives Specialist, Archival Services Branch Center for Electronic Records, National Archives & Records Admin.
Washington, DC 20408
202-501-5579
Internet: tif@cu.nih.gov
bitnet: tif@nihcu
Please send research mail to:
Reference Services,
Center for Electronic Records (NSXA),
The National Archives at College Park,
8601 Adelphi Road,
College Park, MD 20740-6001.
The Center's general telephone number is 301-713-6630.

URL: ftp://ftp.cu.nih.gov/nara-electronic

FALL PREVENTION SUPPORT

Description: Tactilitics, Inc. the makers of the RN+ OnCall Bed Monitoring system, has established a Fall Prevention data site on the Internet. This data site is used to support the Fall Prevention Network and to support RN+ OnCall users. The information available includes research abstracts, RN+ product announcements, and Fall Prevention Network support services for practicing nurses and quality assurance persons. This data site is provided as a public service to fall prevention professionals.

Access: FTP

URL: `ftp://ftp.csn.org/RH+`

GOVERNMENT ACCOUNTING OFFICE (GAO)

Description: This site contains the Transition Reports released by the GAO on January 8, 1993, in the Anonymous FTP directory GAO-REPORTS at NIH (cu.nih.gov). They are intended to give the incoming congress and administration an overview of problems facing the nation.

ABSTRACT.FIL is a file with abstracts for each of the 28 reports. A-REPORT.LST is a file with the information below.

TRANSITION REPORTS OF HEALTH RELATED ISSUES

Health Care Reform. OCG-93-8TR. December 1992. 34 pp.(The file is CG08T93.TXT 34841 Bytes)

Health and Human Services Issues. OCG-93-20TR. December 1992. 33 pp. (The file is CG20T93.TXT 36319 Bytes)

So that they can keep a count of report recipients, and user reaction, please send an email message to KH3@CU.NIH.GOV and include, along with your email address, the following information:

1. Your organization.
2. Your position/title and name (optional).
3. The title/report number of the above reports you have retrieved electronically or ordered by mail or phone.
4. Whether you have ever obtained a GAO report before.
5. If you copy a report onto another bulletin board--if so, which report and bulletin board.
6. Other GAO report subjects you would be interested in. GAO's reports cover a broad range of subjects such as major weapons systems, energy, financial institutions, and pollution control.
7. Any additional comments or suggestions.

Access: FTP

URL: `ftp://ftp.cu.nih.gov/gao-reports`

HANDICAP

Description: This is an anonymous FTP site that contains only disability-related files and/or programs. There are about 40 directories with over 500 files/programs covering all types of disabilities. The "Handicap BBS List", a list of 800 BBS's carrying disability-related information, originates here.

Access: FTP

URL: `ftp://handicap.shel.isc-br.com`

HL7 CODE (CPMC)

Description: The HL7 Import/Export (hl7imex) provides a collection of functions that can be reused in programs to support HL7 Standard version 2.1. Functions support building, encoding and retrieval operation with HL7 messages.

HL7 is written in C and has been implemented at Columbia Presbyterian Medical Center (CPMC) for AIX (RS/6000). It has also been compiled and run on other systems/platforms (DOS, VMS, Sun OS, etc.)

Access: FTP

If you are unable to access the Internet you can obtain a copy of the software on a DOS formatted diskette by contacting:

Mark D. McDougall
Executive Director
Health Level Seven
900 Victors Way, Suite 122
Ann Arbor, MI 48108 USA
Phone (313) 665-0007
FAX: (313) 665-0300

Contact: Robert Sidelir `sidelir@cprvs.cpmc.columbia.edu`

URL: `ftp://cucis.cis.columbia.edu/pub/hl7`

IMMUNIZATION TRACKING

Description: Anonymous ftp directory for immunization tracking
Access: FTP
URL: `ftp://dorothy.cis.unf.edu/pub/immunization`

IUBIO ARCHIVE FOR BIOLOGY

Description: Molecular biology is the area of concentration, and it is also a home for Drosophila research data. It will include software for Macintosh, VAX-VMS, Unix, MS-DOS and any other important computer operating systems. Access to the archive is via anonymous FTP programs that connect to computers on the Internet.

Access: FTP
URL: `ftp://ftp.bio.indiana.edu`

LIMB—Listing of Molecular Biology databases

Description: A collection of information about the content and maintenance of a large number of databases of interest to the molecular biology community.

1) `metabolism`—A collection of notes and datasets relating to intermediate metabolism. Maintained by Peter Karp, NCBI. This collection includes the Enzyme Data Bank, maintained by Amos Bairoch, Centre Medical Universitaire, Geneva, Switzerland.

2) `mol-model`—A central data repository where workers in the field of macromolecular modelling can deposit and retrieve parameter sets, potential energy functions, and associated data relevant to molecular modelling applications. Maintained by Jay Ponder, Washington University, and David States, NCBI.

Access: `FTP FTP.BIO.INDIANA.EDU`
   Directory /molbnio/data
File: `list-of-molbio.text`
Also available via email—`LIMB@LANF.GOV` with a request
Contact: Gifford Keen, Los Alamos National Laboratory.
URL: `ftp://ftp.bio.indiana.edu/molbio/data/list-of-molbio.txt`

M-MEDIA

Description: This archive contains a library of medical applications created in Authorware for both the Mac and the PC. It came online Sept. 30, 1992 and invites public domain uploads. Several README files provide more information.

Access: FTP
URL: `ftp://m-media.muohio.edu/m-media`

MAC ARCHIVES SECTION AT THE UNIVERSITY OF MICHIGAN

Description: Directory /mac/etc/medical

The Mac Archives at University of Michigan collection area for medicine and the health sciences. As of this writing, the collection is small. The contents are gradually growing in the AMSA public domain software library, but these files are a few years old. They are seeking any Macintosh programs, utilities, demonstrations, or computer aided instruction related to the health sciences. Anyone developing any type of Macintosh medical software, and would like to make it available to the rest of the world, can send it to them.

SUBMITTING FILES TO THE MEDICAL SECTION OF THE ARCHIVES

The best way to get files to the archive is to FTP. Put them into the incoming directory, then email ERICM@UMICH.EDU and let him know that the file is there. This way he'll know there are health science files waiting within the directory, and also who to contact if the files don't work "as advertised."

Access: FTP

Contact: As of this writing the medical section of the archives is being maintained by Eric Meininger (ERICM@UMICH.EDU) Questions, problems and comments regarding the medicalarchive specifically should be sent to ERICM@UMICH.EDU. General mac.archive questions should be sent to COMMENTS@MAC.ARCHIVE.UMICH.EDU

URL: ftp://archive.umich.edu/mac

MEDTBOOK

Description: ASYMETRIX has set up the following directories on their FTP site. If anyone feels that they can allow others to SEE/USE/COMPARE what they have done, then use the UPLOAD directory to PUT the files. What is required is a text file description of the book and any other claims, disclaimers that are warrented. Perhaps a quick note to the list stating that you have uploaded some work, OR if you prefer a note to me and I will forward to the medical toolbook list—in which case make the subject line include MTBOOK LIST so that I can filter these out from the other messages.

Room for 250Mb of files is not a problem. All uploads should be uploaded to the /pub/medtbook/medicine/uploads directory. Include a text file with application to aid placement in correct subdirectory.

Access: FTP

Contact: John D. Hendriks
Faculty of Medicine
jdh@medicine.newcastle.edu.au
University of Newcastle
NSW 2308 Australia

URL: ftp://asymetrix.com/pub/medtbook/medicine
/pub/medtbook/medicine/uploads
/pub/medtbook/medicine/anatomy
/pub/medtbook/medicine/pharmacology
/pub/medtbook/medicine/community
/pub/medtbook/medicine/biochemistry
/pub/medtbook/medicine/physiology
/pub/medtbook/medicine/medicine
/pub/medtbook/medicine/paediatrics
/pub/medtbook/medicine/pathology
/pub/medtbook/medicine/psychiatry
/pub/medtbook/medicine/reproductive
/pub/medtbook/medicine/oncology
/pub/medtbook/dentistry
/pub/medtbook/veterinary

MIRROR FTP SITE FOR PUBLIC DOMAIN MEDICAL SOFTWARE

Description: This mirror site is maintained by the University of North Carolina. The directory structure and files contained in Campinas are exactly duplicated. The FTP resource for public domain medical software, documents and conferences established by the Center for Biomedical Informatics of the State University of Campinas, Brazil, now has a full mirror site which can be accessed more easily by users located in North America and Europe.

The original anonymous-access FTP node is CCSUN.UNICAMP.BR or 143.106.1.5 under the directory pub/medicine. It contains the following subdirectories:

1. pub/medicine: Contains 50+ public domain software for IBM-PCs
2. pub/medicine/conferences: Contains original announcements and programs for medical informatics conferences for the next 3 years
3. pub/medicine/documents: Papers, user guides, bibliography, reports, etc. on MI
4. pub/medicine/neuralnets: Documents and public domain software for neural network applications in medicine and biology

Access: FTP

URL: `ftp://sunsite.unc.edu/pub/academic/medicine/brazil-mirror`

NATIONAL CENTER FOR BIOTECHNOLOGY INFORMATION

Description: Compiled by The National Institutes of Health. The respository's directory is a collection of databases and software which has been deposited with the NCBI and made available for distribution "as is". The databases and software are not officially supported or maintained by the NCBI and the NCBI does not assume responsibility for the accuracy, validity, or reliability of the software. Each collection of software will typically be stored in individual directories containing README files for file descriptions and contact names. The following is a partial list of directories which are presently available in the NCBI repository:

TFD—Transcription Factor Database. A relational database of transcription factors maintained by David Ghosh, NCBI.

NGDD—Normalized Gene Designation Database. Normalized gene maps for E.coli, Salmonella, Bacillus Subtilus, Pseudomonas aeruginosa, and Caulobacter crescentus from Yvon Abel and Robert Cedergen.

EPD—Eukaryotic Promoter Database. NA POL II promoters active in higher excoriates. Maintained by Philipp Bucher, Stanford University.

Prosite: a dictionary of sites and patterns of proteins. Both the Handbook and a User Manual are available.

Access: `FTP GENBANK.BIO.NET`

Login: `anonymous`

Password: `guest`

Directory: `pub/db/prosite`

Files: `prosite.txt` (User Manual) `prosite.doc` (Handbook)

URL: `ftp://genbank.bio.net`

NIH SERVER

Description: Several directories with files from the National Institutes of Health.

Access: FTP

Contact: phone 1-301-496-5525 from 9am-3pm (Eastern Time USA) for help.

URL: `ftp://ftp.cu.nih.gov`

Password: `guest or anonymous`

NLM PUBLICATIONS SERVER

Description: Currently contains: NLM Current Bibliographies in Medicine, AIDS Bibliographies, UMLS documentation, chapters of the Online Services Reference Manual and NLM fact sheets.

Access: FTP

Contact: Suggestions, comments, or questions may be submitted by email to `FTPADMIN@NLMPUBS.NLM.NIH.GOV`

URL: `ftp://nlmpubs.nlm.nih.gov`

login: `nlmpubs`

SCIENTIST ON NSFNET

Description: The Scientist files are updated every two weeks. File numbers correspond to date of publication.

>Example: `the-scientist-921207`
>is: The Scientist of Dec. 7,. 1992

>Typing `get*` retrieves a listing of all files in The Scientist directory of NSFnet. TS files are about 3000 lines long. Once they are downloaded, it's easy to scroll to the next article by searching for the demarcator.

Access: The Scientist via NNSC Info-Server, which is an automatic program that delivers information by electronic mail. To request The Scientist from the Info-Server, send a message to:

>`INFO-SERVER@NNSC.NSF.NET`

>No subject field is needed The text of the request must be in the following special format:

Request: The-Scientist
Topic: `the-scientist-921207` (if you want the December 7 issue)
>or

Topic: `the-scientist-index` (if you wish to see the list of Scientist files)
Request: END
>You can request up to 20 topics in one request, each topic on a separate line. The NNSC Info-Server is now configured to split documents into a maximum size of 40,000 bytes (40K). The reason is that some important mail gateways reject messages longer than an arbitrary limit, and others have difficulty with long messages from time to time. This is why a Line or Byte Limit on the second line of your request is needed.

Access: FTP
URL: `ftp://NNSC.NSF.NET`

THE UCI MEDICAL EDUCATION SOFTWARE REPOSITORY

Description: This is a FTP site at the University of California for the collection of shareware public domain software and other information relating to medical education.

>The Repository currently offers both MSDOS and Macintosh software, and hopes to support other operating systems (UNIX, MUMPS, AMIGA). Uploads are welcome. They actively solicit information and software found useful in local medical education whether developed by an instructor or student.

>After uploading software, please send email to Steve Clancy (`SLCLANCY@UCI.EDU`) (for MSDOS) or Albert Saisho (`SAISHO@UCI.EDU`) (for MAC) describing the files) the uploaded files and any other information they might need.

>Note that they can only accept software or information that has been designated as shareware, public-domain or that may otherwise be distributed freely. Please do not upload commercial software! Doing so may jeopardize the existence of this FTP site.

Access: FTP
Contact: Steve Clancy, M.L.S. `SLCLANCY@UCI.EDU`
>Albert Saisho, M.D. `SAISHO@UCI.EDU`

URL: `ftp://ftp.uci.edu/med-ed`

VOXEL-MAN 3D

Description: Interactive atlas of skull and brain. Those who would like to have an impression of its functionality may get interactively generated sample images via FTP.

Access: Images are available via anonymous ftp at `FOKUS.UKE.UNI-HAMBURG.DE (134.100.96.5)` in the directory `[anonymous.voxelman.images]`. BINARY transfer mode! The server is a VAX/VMSsystem, so some aspects are somewhat special:

>commands
>common UNIX FTP server   this FTP server

```
cd voxelman          cd [.voxelman]
cd voxelman/images   cd [.voxelman.images]
cd ..                cd [-]
```
file size are in "blocks" of 512 bytes.

URL: `ftp://fokus.uke.uni-hamburg.ed/voxelman`

Gopher

I've tried to make this as comprehensive as possible by giving an index of all health related gopher sites, followed by descriptions of the more significant ones.

- medical gophers (an index of medical gophers)

Description: CWRU Medical School- Department of Biochemistry

URL: `gopher://biochemistry.bioc.cwru.edu`

- Cornell Medical College gopher

URL: `gopher://med.cornell.edu`

- Cancernet PDQ information

URL: `gopher://gopher.nih.gov`

- Icgebnet, International Center for Genetic Engineering and Biotechnology

URL: `gopher://genes.icgeb.trieste.it`

- Idaho State University College of Pharmacy

URL: `gopher://pharmacy.isu.edu`

- Ruralnet gopher, Marshall University School of Medicine Gopher Server for Rural Health Care Resources & Information

URL: `gopher://ruralnet.mu.wvnet.edu`

- Stanford University Medical Center

URL: `gopher://med-gopher.stanford.edu`

- University of Michigan Medical Center

URL: `gopher://gopher.med.umich.edu`

- University of North Dakota School of Medicine

URL: `gopher://gopher.med.und.nodak.edu`

- University of Texas Health Science Center at Houston

URL: `gopher://gopher.uth.tmc.edu/11/nsc_info`

OTHER BIO-GOPHERS RELEVANT TO MEDICAL RESEARCH:

- American Physiological Society

URL: `gopher://gopher.uth.tmc.edu`

- Arabidopsis AAtDB Gopher Server

URL: `gopher://weeds.mgh.harvard.edu`

- Australian Natl Botanic Gardens

URL: `gopher://155.187.10.12`

- Base de Dados Tropical (Tropical DB) Campinas, Brasil

URL: `gopher://bdt.ftpt.br`

- BioInformatics at the Australian National University
URL: `gopher://life.anu.edu.au`

- Bedford Institute of Oceanography in Darthmouth, Nova Scotia
URL: `gopher://biome.bio.ns.ca`

- Biodiversity and Biological Collections
URL: `gopher://huh.harvard.edu`

- Biology Gopher at OSU (Microbial Germplasm Database)
URL: `gopher://gopher.bcc.orst.edu`

- Brookhaven Protein Data Bank
URL: `gopher://pdb.pdb.bnl.gov`

- Caenorhabditis elegans Genetics Center (CGC)
URL: `gopher://elegans.cbs.umn.edu`

- CIC Electronic Serials for Science
URL: `gopher://gopher.cic.net/11/e-serials`

- CIESIN Global Change Gopher
URL: `gopher://gopher.ciesin.org`

- CGEBnet Int.Center
URL: `gopher://genes.icgeb.trieste.it`

- DNA DataBank of Japan (DDBJ) NIG, Mishima
URL: `gopher://gopher.nig.ac.jp`

- EMBnet BioBox Finland
URL: `gopher://finsun.csc.fi`

- EMBnet BioInformation Resource
URL: `gopher://bioftp.unibas.ch`

- EMBnet BioInformation Resource (EMBL)
URL: `gopher://felix.embl-heidelberg.de`

- EMBnet BioInformation Resource (France)
URL: `gopher://coli.polytechnique.fr`

- EMBnet BioInformation Resource (The Netherlands)
URL: `gopher://camms1.caos.kun.nl`

- EMBnet BioInformation Resource (UK)
URL: `gopher://s-crim1.dl.ac.uk`

- EcoGopher at U of Virginia
URL: `gopher://ecosys.drdr.virginia.edu`

- Genethon (CEPHB Human Polymorphism)
URL: `gopher://gopher.genethon.fr`

- Human Genome Mapping Project Gopher
URL: `gopher://hgmp.mrc.ac.uk`

- Institut Pasteur's Mycobacterium Database (MycDB) (France)
URL: `gopher://arabidopsis.pasteur.fr`

- National Cancer Center, Tokyo JAPAN

- National Science Foundation Gopher
URL: `gopher://stis.nsf.gov`

- National University of Singapore
URL: `gopher://nuscc.nus.sg/11/`

- IUBio Biology Archive, Indiana University
URL: `gopher://ftp.bio.indiana.edu`

- UH PIR server (Houston, experimental)
URL: `gopher://evolution.bchs.uh.edu`

- USDA Extension Service's Gopher Server
URL: `gopher://ra.esusda.gov`

- University of Western Australia Virology Gopher
URL: `gopher://virus.microbiol.uwa.edu.au`

- University of Wisconsin Biotechnology Center
URL: `gopher://calvin.biotech.wisc.edu`

- University of Wisconsin-Madison, Medical School
URL: `gopher://msd.medsch.wisc.edu`

- World Data Center on Microorganisms
URL: `gopher://fragrans.riken.go.jp`

AIDS RELATED INFORMATION

- Description: Aids Information on the NIAID gopher
    - FOCUS: A Guide to Research and Counseling
    - AIDSNews
    - CDC National AIDS Clearinghouse
    - National Commission on AIDS
    - CDC Daily Summaries
    - NIAID Press Releases
    - Morbidity and Mortality Weekly Report (MMWR)
    - AIDS Tx News
    - Study Recruitment Information
    - Veterans Administration AIDS Information Newsletter
    - AIDS Alert
    - Ben Gardiner's AIDS BBS
    - CDC Statistics

URL: `gopher://odie.niaid.nih.gov/11/aids`

Health And Medicine Releated Gophers With Descriptions

AMERICAN PHYSIOLOGICAL SOCIETY

Description: Overview of the American Physiological Society

Introduction

The American Physiological Society is devoted to fostering scientific research--with special emphasis on studying the ways the body functions--to education, and to the dissemination of scientific information. Through its activities, it plays an important role in the progress of science andthe advancement of knowledge. At the time of its founding in 1887 the Society had 28 members. It now has Approximately 7,500 members and is continuing to grow. The membership of the Society includes Nobel laureates and members of the National Academy of Sciences.

Most members have doctoral degrees in physiology, medicine (or other health professions), or both. They work in medical schools, either in physiology departments, in other basic science departments, or in clinical units. The remainder of the regular members are employed in hospitals, undergraduate schools, industrial organizations, private foundations, and government. The APS is governed by an elected Council consisting of the President, the President-Elect, the immediate Past President, and six elected Councillors. The Society maintains a staff and offices in Bethesda, Maryland. Management of the affairs of the Society is the responsibility of a full-time Executive Director appointed and compensated by and responsible to the Council. As a nonprofit scientific organization, the Society is tax exempt.

Access: Gopher
URL: `gopher://gopher.uth.tmc.edu:3300/11/`

ANESTHESIOLOGY INTERNET GOPHER

Description: Contains information of interest to those interested in the fields of anesthesiology and critical care. Includes bibliographic information, position announcements, lecture notes, case studies, and research abstracts. This Gopher also houses the archives of ANEST-L listserv list.

Top Level Directory:

```
About this Gopher
Anest-L Archive
Boards Keywords
Book Reviews
Case Archive
Faculty Positions
Internet Medical Resources
Lecture Notes
Research Abstracts
Tidbits
```

Access: Gopher. Messages and updates to the Gopher are announced on the ANEST-L mailing list.
Contact: Andrew M. Sopchak, M.D.
State University of New York
Health Science Center at Syracuse
Department of Anesthesiology
750 East Adams Street
Syracuse, NY 13210
Email: `GOPHER@EJA.ANES.HSCSYR.EDU`
URL: `gopher://eja.anes.hscsyr.edu/1`

ARABIDOPSIS RESEARCH COMPANION

Description: This is a Gopher Server provided by the AAtDB Project at Department of Molecular Biology, Massachusetts General Hospital and USDA/NAL Digital Equipment Corporation. AAtDB, An Arabidopsis Thaliana Database, is a collection of information on the model plant system Arabidopsis. The Arabidopsis-BioSci is a database of all the messages transmitted over the BioSci usenet group and associated mailing list.

The Arabidopsis thaliana (AAtDB), Caenorhabditis elegans (ACEDB) and Arabidopsis-BioSci WAIS indices provide fast access to every word in these databases. This Gopher server is also connected to several other Internet Gophers around the world as well as providing access to their WAIS and FTP servers of interest to biologist. Further searching instructions are available on the Gopher.

This server includes all messages since March of 1991 from the `BIONET.GENOME.ARABIDOPSIS` usenet newsgroup and the `ARAB-GEN@GENBANK.BIO.NET` mailing list.

Top level Gopher menu:
```
About the AAtDB Research Companion
Commonly Asked Questions about Gopher
Help Searching the WAIS databases indicated with "<?>"
Arabidopsis Information (thale cress)
Caenorhabditis Information (nematode)
Massachusetts General Hospital—Molecular Biology
FTP Archives for Molecular Biology
Global Biological Information Servers
Global Biological Information Servers by Topic
Global Information Services
North American Weather Forecasts
Search menu titles of the MolBiol/MGH Gopher Server
Veronica, Keyword Searches of Gopher Menus Worldwide
```
Access: Gopher
URL: **gopher://weeds.mgh.harvard.edu**

AUSTIN HOSPITAL, MELBOURNE, AUSTRALIA

Description: This Gopher is run by the PET Centre to make information available to the Austin Hospital and Medical Community. It will include access to images produced by the PET Scanner, as well as telephone directories and other information.

Gopher Directory:
```
About the Austin Hospital Gopher
Questions About Gopher
Guides to using gopher, FTP, etc
Research Related Information
Medicine/Medical Science Information and Resources
Library Catalogues
Digital Image Library
General Information and Resources
Other Gopher Information Servers
Program and File Archive Sites For Biology
Program and File Archives
Subject Oriented Gopher Information
Telephone and E-mail Directories
Local Time and Date in Melbourne, Australia
```
Access: Gopher
Contact: If you have any problems using the Austin Hospital Gopher, send e-mail to gopher@austin.unimelb.edu.au, or paper mail to Daniel O'Callaghan, PET Centre, Austin Hospital, Heidelberg, Vic, 3084.
URL: **gopher://gopher.austin.unimelb.edu.au**

BAYLOR COLLEGE OF MEDICINE GENOME CENTER

Description: This Gopher is run by the Systems Support Center at Baylor College of Medicine.
Contact: gopher@bcm.tmc.edu
URL: **gopher://kiwi.imgen.bcm.tmc.edu**

BIOFTP EMBnet SWITZERLAND

Description: The biology software used here is the GCG program package, and William Pearson's FASTA program suite. The main usage of GCG is currently still VMS bound, therefore, remote submission of jobs from VAX/VMS is possible in a transparent fashion.

The Hierarchical Access System for Sequence Libraries in Europe (HASSLE) is developed on this sytem as far as the UNIX flavour goes.

The gopher software on this computer was originally taken from Don Gilbert's distribution and has been modified in order to allow the use on all databases needed within this server, such as EMBL, SWISSPROT, etc. This server is not financed for use as international or national resource. If you like it, send me a mail, and I could use it as justification that I need more funding.

Access: Gopher
Contact: Reinhard Doelz doelz@urz.unibas.ch

```
GOPHER MENU
    About Gopher, and this bioftp site
    Biology subject tree in Gopher
    DIBUG [Discover Insight Biosym User Group] Mailing list
    EMBNet BioInformation Resource Switzerland
    GCG Software Manual
    Infoservers in European Countries
    If you have suggestions or problems....[7Jan94, 1kb]
    development site of GOPHER (U Minnesota)
    selected USENET News
```

URL: **gopher://bioftp.unibas.ch**

BIOINFORMATICS RESOURCE GOPHER

Description: The file `GeneID.info.txt` gives instructions on how to access and use the GeneID server. This file also contains references to the GeneID paper. If you don't have access to that paper, the file `GeneID.paper.sit.hqx` contains an early MSWord version of the paper.

Contact: Steen Knudsen
Email: `STEEN@BIR.CEDB.UWF.EDU`
URL: **gopher://dna.cedb.uwf.edu**

BIOSCI ARCHIVES GOPHER

Description: GOPHER MENU (Partial directory listing)

```
        ACEDB
        ADDRESSES
        AGEING
        AGROFORESTRY
        RABIDOPSIS
        IO-INFO
        BIO-JOURNALS
        BIO-MATRIX
        BIO-SOFTWARE
```

URL: **gopher://net.bio.net/11/BioSci/Bionet Biology Newsgroups Server**

BROOKHAVEN NATIONAL LABORATORY PROTEIN DATA BANK

Description: This is an experimental gopher server at the Protein Data Bank. They are trying to provide convenient and useful search methods, graphics, and some analysis information.

Access: Gopher
URL: **gopher://pdb.pdb.bnl.gov**

CAMIS (Center for Advanced Medical Informatics at Stanford)

Description: This document describes the CAMIS Gopher and the files available through this information source. There is an experimental and dynamic nature to this Gopher, and we regret any inconvenience caused by this. There are also files that may only be accessed by members of the local community that this Gopher serves.

WHAT IS CAMIS

CAMIS is an acronym for the Center for Advanced Medical Informatics at Stanford. CAMIS is a shared computing resource supporting research activities in biomedical informatics at the Stanford University School of Medicine.

WHAT'S IN THE CAMIS GOPHER

1. Local (CAMIS) Title Search

    This is an index search of the directory and document names in the CAMIS Gopher. This is a great tool for locating files and directories that are relevant to your needs. It is especially useful if you know something is available in this Gopher, but you forgot where it is. NOTE You may use partial words, Boolean variables and quotation marks in this search (see The Test Searching Capabilities directory in this directory for more information).

2. INTERNET-WIDE TITLE SEARCH

    This is an index search similar to the Local (CAMIS) Title Search, but for the entire Internet. There is currenty no Boolean capability nor partial word or phrase searching.

3. ABOUT THE CAMIS GOPHER

    Contains information about the CAMIS Gopher, Gopher in general, and several Gopher clients in particular, as well as a directory for testing the searching capabilities of this Gopher server.

4. BIO-MEDICAL AND RELATED GOPHERS

    This directory contains pointers to other Gopher sources that include "Medical Schools", "Medical Publications, Genetic Engineering, Computational Biology, etc."

5. CAMIS (CENTER FOR ADVANCED MEDICAL INFORMATICS AT STANFORD)

    This directory contains information such as "Technical Report Abstracts", the "SMI Publication List", a schedule of colloquia, journal club, seminars and other documents and resources useful to student and staff of the Section on Medical Informatics (SMI).

6. COMPUTING INFO

    This directory contains computing information for the Section on Medical Informatics (SMI) community as well as that of the Knowledge Systems Laboratory (KSL). Additionally, pointers to information outside SMI and KSL are included. These include various index searches of various Frequently Asked Question (FAQ) archives.

    The UNIX man pages are currently not indexed, but we hope to do this in the future.

7. FIND PEOPLE, PLACES, PROGRAMS, PHONE NUMBERS

    This directory contains location services which can be helpful in finding e-mail addresses, programs at ftp sites, area codes, phone numbers, and WAIS information source names.

8. HEURISTIC PROGRAMMING PROJECT

    This directory contains, among other things, the HPP FTP files.

9. KSL MAIL ARCHIVES

    This directory contains collections of e-mail messages for various groups within Stanford, CAMIS and the KSL and without (ai-medicine). This archive is currently only available to part of Stanford.

10. NIH, NSF, AND FUNDING

    This directory contains pointers to the NIH Guide, NIH Program Info, a search of NSF Awards, and a link to the National Science Foundation Gopher, among other things.

11. NEWS (STANFORD, USENET, CLARINET)

    This is a pointer to collections of news resources made available to the Stanford University community. Included are Stanford Events, Stanford Press Releases, USENET groups and more.

12. ONLINE LIBRARY CATALOGS

    This directory contains a collection of pointers to library telnet sessions. Instructions for searching on varying different systems are included, as is login information. Launching a telnet session is handled in different ways (or not at all) by different Gopher clients. See client-specific documentation for information about launching telnet sessions.

13. SUMEX-AIM ARCHIVES (INCLUDING INFO-MAC)

    This directory includes the popular INFO-Mac directory of ftp'able files. This directory also contains many of the ftp'able files from the CAMIS community. Different gopher clients handle binhexed files and ftp'ing differently (or not at all). See client-specific documentation for information about ftp and binhex.

14. WORLD FULL OF INFO SOURCES

    This directory is a pointer to the University of Minnesota's collection of pointers to gopher and WAIS servers around the world.

15. MISCELLANEOUS

    This directory contains pointers to selected, interesting information sources cleaned from #13 above. This directory includes weather information, movie reviews, a Webster's Dictionary search, a Roget's Thesaurus search, and more.

URL: `gopher://camis.stanford.edu`

CANCERNET INFORMATION

Description: Gopher Directory

```
PDQ Table of Contents List
PDQ Treatment Information for Physicians
PDQ Treatment Information for Patients
PDQ Cancer Screening Information
PDQ Supportive Care Information
Breast Cancer Prevention Trial (BCPT) Info
PDQ Database Information
Other NCI Information
Design of Clinical Trials
Monthly Updates
Fact Sheets from the NCI
PDQ Drug Information
Search CancerNet Database
```

URL: `gopher://gopher.nih.gov/11/clin/cancernet`

CAOS/CAMM CENTER IN THE NETHERLANDS

Description: The name of the Center derives from Computer Assisted Organic Synthesis and Computer Assisted Molecular Modelling. It is a national expertise center for computer aided chemistry and offers university chemists a package of software tools for remote use on a central computer system.

The emphasis is on easy accessibility, achieved by the application of menu controlled program front-ends and interfaces, and on integration of the various tools and data bases. An example of the latter is the interconversion of molecular structure files between structural data bases, modelling software and computational programs.

An overview of available tools is obtained from the main graphics menu and a hierarchy of alphanumeric menus. Tools are arranged in groups according to their application. Apart from the two subjects mentioned in the name of the Center, other major chemical disciplines covered are biomolecular sequence analysis and computational chemistry. A full description of the menu items is given in the present text. The Center issues a newsletter to keep subscribers informed on changes, additions and Programs are activated either from an alphanumeric menu, or by command, typing the corresponding name. Program input and output is graphical where appropriate.

Through a combination of on-line help facilities, practical courses and the (re)production of manuals the Center supports the use of its tools by chemists without computer experience. A news and conferencing system running on the VAX aims at improving the exchange of information and experience among users, including the Center's staff.

HEALTH SCIENCES

```
Gopher Directory
    About the CAOS/CAMM Center:
    CAMMSA: EMBnet BioInformation Resource the Netherlands
    CAMM Resource
    CAOS Resource
    CompChem Resource
    Genome Data Base Resource
    CAOS/CAMM Network Services
    Miscellaneous Gopher Services
    Chemistry Gophers
    Other Gopher and Information Servers
    The CAOS/CAMM mugshot
```
Access: Gopher
URL: **gopher://camms1.caos.kun.nl**

CASE WESTERN RESERVE UNIVERSITY (CWRU) SCHOOL OF MEDICINE DEPARTMENT OF BIOCHEMISTRY

Description: This Gopher server is being run at the Department of Biochemistry, CWRU School of Medicine. It includes information on the graduate and post-doctoral programs and opportunities available at this department. There are also links to other BioGophers and WAIS servers for searching biological databases such as GenBank, PIR, PDB, TFD etc.

There's also a DBF based approach to searching the Restriction Enzyme Database, maintained by Dr. Richard Roberts of NEB. This approach permits finding compatible over hangs, as well as searching by recognition site, cutting site, or enzyme name.

Contact: Email: **gopher@biochemistry.Bioc.Cwru.Edu**
URL: **gopher://biochemistry.bioc.cwru.edu**

CHEDOKE-MCMASTER HOSPITAL (CANADA) GOPHER

Description: Gopher Directory
```
            About Chedoke-McMaster Hospitals
            About this Gopher server
            About other Internet services
            CMH phone book (experimental)
            CMH Policies and Procedures
            News, Weather, Sports
            Todays events in history
            Internet Assistance
            Federal Government Gophers
            Provincial Government Gophers
            Canadian Gophers
            Other Gopher and Information Servers
            Libraries, reference...
            Healthcare
            Gopher Development
            Faculty of Health Sciences Gopher
```
URL: **gopher://darwin.cmh.mcmaster.ca**

CHEMICAL SUBSTANCE FACT SHEETS

Description: Partial Gopher Directory
```
            1,1,2,2-Tetrachloroethane
```

```
                1,1,2-Trichloro-1,2,2-Trifluoroethane
                1,1,2-Trichloroethane
                1,2,4-Trichlorobenzene
                1,2-Butylene Oxide
                1,2-Dichlorobenzene
                1,2-Dichloroethane
                1,2-Dichloroethylene
                1,2-Dichloropropane
                1,2-Dihydroxybenzene
                1,2-Diphenylhydrazine
                1,2-Oxathiolane-2,2-Dioxide
                1,3-Butadiene
                1,3-Dichlorobenzene
                1,3-Dichloropropene
                1,4-Dichlorobenzene
```
URL: `gopher://ecosys.drdr.Virginia.edu/11/library/factsheets/toxics/`

CO-OPERATIVE HUMAN LINKAGE CENTER (CHLC) GOPHER

Description: Gopher Directory

```
                Welcome: Cooperative Human Linkage Center
                Layout of the Data on this Server
                CHLC Maps
                CHLC Markers
                Integrated Maps
                Genotype Data
                Search CHLC and Marshfield Marker Data
                Search Genotype Data
                Search All Files On This Gopher
                Miscellaneous Genetics Data
                CHLC Newsletters
                Other Bio Gophers
                Other Genetics Gopher Servers
                Other Gopher Servers thru the U. of Minnesota
```
URL: `gopher://gopher.chlc.org`

CODI

Description: CODI: Cornucopia of Disability Information

CODI is a gopher, intended to serve as a community resource for consumers and professionals by providing, via the Internet, disability related information in a wide variety of areas. The information addresses university (SUNY @ Buffalo), local (Buffalo & WNY), state, national and international audiences. Its contents are determined by these communities; their submissions and suggestions are welcome.

Ideally, material should be submitted in computer readable form. However, printed text is also acceptable if the print quality is sufficient for it to be scanned. (Generally, xerox copies scan poorly.) Often, it becomes necessary to rewrite or reformat the material. As a result, errors may appear. Please notify me of these so They may be corrected.

Currently, the material is accessible via 22 main menu items. This article, `About the Cornucopia of Disability Information`, is the first menu item. Due to the continuous addition of new information the organization of the menus is bound to change, along with their contents. Because of

CODI's size and its frequency of change, menu item #2., What's New in Codi, is included for the frequent browser. What's New lists modifications, their dates and locations.

Other options for selection include:

3. Search Menus allows boolean searches of all the CODI menus for keywords using jughead.
4. NY State & Local Services is intended to provide information and directories of services in New York. Comprehensive local servicer information has been gathered by the Independent Living Center of WNY. State wide information has been provided by VESID, Office of Vocational and Educational Services for Individuals with Disabilities, and by the NYS Office of Advocate for the Disabled.
5. College Services and Resources has the membership lists of two area Collegiate Consortium of Disability Advocates. Each of these consortia have approximately 50 instiutional members. These lists are included so that potential students can identify campus contacts who can provide information about accessibility, policy and services. A submenu contains information about SUNY @ Buffalo. Information from other areas and colleges is welcome.
6. National Information Sources on Disabilities is a publication of the NIDRR. It contains 7 national subdirectories: Directory of Organizations, List of Directories Organized by Category, Cross Index of Organizations by Function/Service, Directory of Data Bases, Directory of Hot Lines, Directory of Religious Organizations, and Directory of Sports Organizations.
7. Digest of Data on Persons with Disabilities 1992 is another NIDRR publication. 'This document draws from many sources of published data and narrative explanations issued by federal statistical agencies and other sources on the subject of disability.' Unfortunately, the many tables and graphs lack the quality of the original document.
8. Coming to Terms with Disabilities is a product of the New York State Senate Select Committee on the Disabled: A Compilation of Vocabulary Relating to Visible and Non-Visible Disabilities. It is offered as a primer to further inform those who are interested in learning more about disabilities, and as a catalyst to stimulate awareness in those who may have previously shied away from seeking explanations because of the technical terms involved. The information contained herein is based on a voluminous amount of information which was forwarded to the Committee by people with disabilities, advocates, medical doctors, service agencies, parents, friends, rehabilitation specialists, therapists, educators, counselors and numerous other professionals in the field.
9. WNY TDD Directory is a collection of local, state and national TDD phone numbers. This directory was assembled by Deaf Adult Services of WNY. Additions to the directory are encouraged. For information about other TDD numbers, see under Computing, 'Managing Information Resources for Accessibility' (section 11).
10. Government Documents is intended as a collection of legislation, regulations and legislative summaries. The collection is in the process of being assembled. The Americans with Disabilities Act is actually located on another gopher, infoslug.ucsc.edu. Access is transparent to the CODI reader. Also, see Electronic Resources for access to many other documents located on other gophers and ftp sites.
11. Computing has information relating to adaptive hardware and software. The document, Managing Information Resources for Accessibility, provides a comprehensive overview. Other information includes two articles by Joe Lazzaro which appeared in BYTE magazine plus detailed technology information and directories assembled by the IBM Special Needs Information Referral Center.
12. Legal contains two directories for sources of legal assistance: State Protection and Advocacy Agencies and Legal and Advocacy Organizations. Also, there are a number of publications which were prepared by Mark H. Leeds, Esq. of the Association of the Bar New York City: Its The Law, Rights and Responsibilities, and Rights of People with Disabilities. Its The Law is written for the layman. Rights and Responsibilities is written for agencies and departments of the City of New York. This document can serve as a model for any public institution.
13. Publications currently contains 8 articles of broad interest. Except for Newsletters and Journals, at this time there is no single source of a comprehensive list of publications. However, many focused lists are contained elsewhere in CODI, especially within

14. `Network Resources` has information about FTP sites, bulletin boards and other network resources. In addition, several related gophers are directly accessed: HealthLine, Recordings for the Blind, Deaf Gopher, Medical Resources, and Electronic Rehabilitation Resource Center. Primitive access is available to some FTP sites including Project EASI via other gophers. One subdirectory points to an extensive collection of electronic text found on other gophers and ftp sites.
15. `Other Directories` has the membership list of the President's Committee on Employment of People with Disabilities, two RCEP II directories (CAPs and ILCs) and a national list of support organizations compiled by the IBM Special Needs Information Referral Center.
16. `Independent Living` has the ILRU Directory of Independent Living programs.
17. `Bibliographic Information` has two collections. The History of Disabilities and Social Problems by Gary Woodill represents the results of an extensive library search undertaken in 1987-1988 as part of his research on the history of disabilities and special education. The other is a ftp site with files that contain bibliographies and reference guides prepared by the National Library Service for the Blind and Physically Handicapped (NLS). (The complete data is available via Network Resources, Electronic Rehabilitation Resource Center.)
18. `Heath Resource Center`—Resource Directory The HEATH Resource Directory is a biannual selection of resources in the major areas of interest in the field of postsecondary education and disability.
19. `National Rehabilitation Information Center (NARIC)` contains ABLEDATA Fact Sheets and Top 10 Searches, REHABDATA Top 10 Searches, NARIC Quarterly, a Serials Survey and a number of Resource Guides. This material contains extensive bibliographic and vendor reference material.
20. `Universal Design`
21. `Employment` has some articles on this subject along with access to a national jobs gopher, The Online Career Center.
22. `Announcements` contains contemporary information about meetings, conferences, legislation etc.

Contact: Jay Leavitt `leavitt@ubvmsb`
`leavitt@ubvmsb.cc.buffalo.edu`

URL: `gopher://val-dor.cc.buffalo.edu`

COMPREHENSIVE EPIDEMIOLOGICAL DATA RESOURCE (CEDR) GOPHER

Description: Gopher Directory

```
Introduction—About the CEDR Gopher
The CEDR Catalog: Introduction
The CEDR Catalog: Overview of CEDR Data
The CEDR Catalog: Becoming an Authorized CEDR Data User
The CEDR Catalog: Methods of Accessing CEDR Data
The CEDR Catalog: Individual CEDR Data File Sets
Experimental CEDR Services
```
Non-CEDR Information Services Around the World

URL: `gopher://cedr.lbl.gov`

COMPUTATIONAL BIOLOGY (JOHNS HOPKINS UNIVERSITY)

Description: I. Contents

This gopher hole was first created as a way to provide electronic access to documents pertaining to Computational Biology. However this site has grown dramatically and now contains many other types of services and information, including:

A. Searches of Genbank, Swiss-Prot, PDB, PIR, LiMB, TFD, AAtDB, ACEDB, CompoundKB, PROSITE EC Enzyme Database searches (via Indiana, Houston, Harvard, the Netherlands and NIH);

B. Searches of the following databases:

NRL_3D Protein-Sequence-Structure Database
Eukaryotic Promoter Database (EPD)
Cloning Vector Database
Expressed Sequence Tag Database (ESTDB)
Online Mendelian Inheritance Man (OMIM)
Sequence Analysis Bibliographic Reference Data Bank (Seqanalref),
Database Taxonomy (Genbank, Swiss-Prot), and many more (run here at Welchlab);
C. Direct links to other Gophers which provide information relevant to biology;
D. Links to all other Gophers and Wais servers
E. Links to campus phone books worldwide;
F. Links to Online Library Catalogs all over the world;
H. Links to selected other gophers and services—Physics gophers, Archie (ftp) searches, weather, and Veronica searches of gopher-space;
I. Read and Search Usenet News groups and their FAQs;
J. Links to over 70 ftp sites with data and software for biology;
K. Search and Retrieve Software for all types of machines;
L. Calls for applications from many funding agencies;
M. Searches to help you find other biologists—by name, location and research interests.
N. The first document relevant to Computational Biology to be provided is the book:

URL: `gopher://merlot.welch.jhu.edu`

COMPUTER ASSISTED MOLECULAR MODELING

Description: Gopher Directory

```
Computer Assisted Organic Syntheses
About the CAOS/CAMM Center
CAMMSA: EMBnet BioInformation Resource-The Netherlands
CAMM Resource
CAOS Resource
CompChem Resource
Genome Data Base Resource
CAOS/CAMM Network Services
Miscellaneous Gopher Services
Chemistry Gophers
Other Gopher and Information Servers
The CAOS/CAMM mugshot
```

URL: `gopher://camms1.caos.kun.nl`

COOPERATIVE HUMAN LINKAGE CENTER (CHLC)

Description: The goal of this center is to generate a high resolution map of the human genome and rapidly distribute this information to the genomics community. The project is made up of investigators from the following four institutions: The University of Iowa, Iowa City, Iowa, USA; Harvard Medical School, Boston, Massachusetts, USA; The Marshfield Medical Center, Marshfield, Wisconsin, USA; The Fox Chase Cancer Center, Philadelphia, This Gopher server is maintained as a service of the CHLC informatics core centered at Fox Chase.

The server content consists of the following items:
1. CHLC generated linkage maps and markers,
2. Other information of general interested to human geneticists,
3. Links to other human-oriented genetics gopher servers, and
4. Additional Biological information deemed appropriate to this server.

Additional CHLC generated information will be placed on this gopher as it becomes available. This information is provided free of charge and without any implied commitment by CHLC or its member institutions that the responses will be either correct or useful to you. Any comments addressed to `help@chlc.org` will be read, but there is no commitment to respond in any way. We will try and be as helpful as time and resources permit, but cannot guarantee any level of service.

```
Important: Server Moving, PLEASE READ [20Jan94, 1kb]
Welcome: Cooperative Human Linkage Center
CHLC Maps
CHLC Markers
Integrated Maps
Genotype Data
Search Genotype Data
Search All Files On This Gopher
Search CHLC and Marshfield Marker Data
Miscellaneous Genetics Data
Newsletters
Other Bio Gophers
Other Genetics Gopher Servers
Other Gopher Servers thru the U. of Minnesota.
```

Contact: Primary assistance in gaining access to information or services beyond those described here can be requested via electronic mail (`help@chlc.org`), or via U.S. Mail:

CHLC Informatics Group
c/o Research Computing Services
The Fox Chase Cancer Center
7701 Burholme Avenue
Philadelphia, PA 19111
USA

The Cooperative Human Linkage Center (CHLC) is a federally funded genome center directed by:

Dr. Jeff Murray
Assistant Professor of Pediatrics
The University of Iowa
Iowa City, IA 52242
E-mail: `jeff-murray@umaxc.weeg.uiowa.edu`

URL: `gopher://gopher.chlc.org`

CORNELL MEDICAL COLLEGE

Description: The Cornell University Medical College Gopher is sponsored by the Office of Academic of Computing. Along with information about the College and Faculty, this Gopher also gives access to the NIH Gopher and the Federal Register.

Contact: Email: `steven_erde@qmcumc.Mail.Cornell.Edu`
URL: `gopher://med.cornell.edu`

DANA-FARBER CANCER INSTITUTE

Description: The Dana-Farber Cancer Institute TechInfo Bulletin Board is where the DFCI information is stored. Most of the remaining information is stored on other computers, though that fact is invisible to users of the Gopher service. The menu item Dana-Farber Cancer Institute Positions has been put at the top level to make it easily accessible to outside users.

The NIH Gopher also is accessible at the top level as it contains much that will be of interest to DFCI users. The section on Health and Clinical Information contains the CancerNet information (including the PDQseries), while the AIDS related information contains material of interest to AIDS researchers. Information for Researchers contains material from the Guide to Grants and Contracts and allows searching on keywords. The Molecular Biology Databases can be directly searched.

DFCI users are welcome to make suggestions for improvements to Mohamed Ellozy, either by email or phone (look up his phone number in DFCIonline directory).

URL: `gopher://gopher.dfci.harvard.edu`

DEPARTMENT FOR MEDICAL CYBERNETICS AND ARTIFICIAL INTELLIGENCE

Description: The biology software used here is the GCG program package, and William Pearson's FASTA program suite. The main usage of GCG is currently still VMS bound, therefore, remote submission of jobs from VAX/VMS is possible in a transparent fashion. The Hierarchical Access System for Sequence Libraries in Europe (HASSLE) is developed on this system as far as the UNIX flavor goes.

Contact: Department for Medical Cybernetics and Artificial Intelligence, University of Vienna, and the Austrian Research Institute for Artificial Intelligence, Vienna, Austria

Email: `togopheradmin@ai.Univie.Ac.At`

URL: `gopher://gopher.ai.univie.ac.at`

DNA DATA BANK OF JAPAN (DDBJ)

Description: DDBJ is the sole DNA data bank in Japan. This Gopher is officially certified to collect DNA sequences from researchers and issue accession numbers to data submitters. Data is primarily collected from Japanese researchers. But they also accept data and issue accession numbers to researchers in other countries. Data submission via email is preferable, but submission via floppy diskettes is also accepted. They exchange collected data with the EMBL Data Library and GenBank/NCBI on a daily basis, so that the three data banks share virtually the same data at any moment.

Contact: DDBJ, National Institute of Genetics
Yata, Mishima, 411, Japan
Phone: +81-559-75-0771
Fax: +81-559-75-6040
For inquiries email: `DDBJ@DDBJ.NIG.AC.JP`
For data submission email: `DDBJSUB@DDBJ.NIG.AC.JP`
For citation update email: `DDBJUPDT@DDBJ.NIG.AC.Jp`

URL: `gopher://gopher.nig.ac.jp`

DRUG INFORMATION AND DRUG UTILIZATION CENTER UNIVERSITY OF TENNESSEE, MEMPHIS

Description: Gopher Directory

```
EMBL sequence search in Basel
About_DDBJ
DDBJ_Gopher_WAIS
Other_Gopher
Other_WAIS
Other_ftp
README [ 5Mar93, 3kb]
dna
joho
ls-lR [ 4Feb94, 216kb] [ 4Feb94, 62kb]
protein
pub
```

URL: `gopher://132.192.11.76`

EMBnet (French node)

Description: In the frame of EMBNET this server permits access to daily updated nucleotide sequences.

Contact: Philippe DESSEN Laboratoire de Biochimie
Ecole Polytechnique
91128 PALAISEAU Cedex France
Phone: +33 1 69 33 48 84
Fax: +33 1 69 33 30 13
E-mail: DESSEN@ARTHUR.CITI2.FR
E-mail: DESSEN@COLI.POLYTECHNIQUE.FR

Internet Address:
URL: gopher://coli.polytechnique.fr

EMBnet BIOBOX FINLAND

Description: Partial Directory

```
          *** The BioBox Chronicles ***
              Access to Bionet Newsgroups
              Access to different Libraries
              Bio-Resources on the Network
              Bionaut_software_paradise
              Browse_the_Big_Data_World
              Computing Books from O'Reilly Associates
              European Networking
              FAQ Files
```

URL: gopher://finsun.csc.fi/11/.BioBox

EMBnet Bioinformation Resource EMBL

Description: This BioGopher server is running as part of the EMBnet Bio Information Resources network. The server is maintained by the EMBL Data Library at the European Molecular Biology Laboratory in Heidelberg, Germany. It provides access to a variety of data collections and other information in molecular biology, such as free software for MS-DOS, VAX/VMS, Unix and Macintosh systems, and to other Gophers and BioGophers.

Based on the services of SWITCH, the following services can be offerered. File-Server (anonymous FTP, see README files for non-swiss, non-academics) generic-format sequence databases of biological interest, such as

```
              EMBL DNA sequence database
              SWISS-PROT protein sequence database
              PIR protein sequence database
              GENBANK sequence database
              Weekly updates to EMBL database
              Weekly updates to PIR database
              GCG-/PIR- formatted databases
              EMBL DNA sequence database
              SWISS-PROT Sequence database
              PIR protein sequence database
              GENBANK supplement (EMBL exclusion set)
              Weekly updates to EMBL database
              Weekly recomputed exclusion set of GENBANK databasae
```

Additional databases include:
```
FLYBASE
PROSITE
ENZYME
```

Dates resources are available:

Full databases; at the time of installation either as generic, VAX/VMS or UNIX formatted database. Formats are for PIR (XQS) and GCG software packages.

Weekly updates to EMBL database, either as generic EMBL, or as VAX/VMS or UNIX formatted database.

Genbank exclusion set, weekly updates to EMBL database, either as generic GENBANK, or as VAX/VMS or UNIX formatted database.

Updates to EMBL weekly, either as generic EMBL, or as VAX/VMS or UNIX formatted database.

HASSLE server, details on request. Further databases in development, details on request.

Gopher Directory
```
About Gopher, and this bioftp site
Biology subject tree in Gopher
DIBUG [Discover Insight Biosym User Group] Mailing list
EMBNet BioInformation Resource Switzerland
GCG Software Manual
```

Access: Interactive login:

Those institutions who do not have an own installation will be able to get login permission on the EMBnet system. Access can be achieved via SWITCH on either TCP/IP or DECNET.

Wide Area Information Servers (WAIS):
The GOPHER system is set up and available for browsing via WAIS. WWW capability is also available.

PRICES

EMBnet Switzerland is currently only funded by Basel University, and the Nationalfond (NF). The NF requestedthat the percentage of users who are NF grant holders is outlined explicitly. The service will be free for NF Grant holders. Sites with no NF grant holders will be charged individually. Special arrangements will be made for sites where only part of the users are grant holders of the NF.

Note that this rule also applies for the use of the file server. DATA on this part of the server have been collected as an value-added service; therefore, you are requested to contact the following address if you are NOT swiss-academic:

Dr. Reinhard Doelz
RFC `embnet@comp.bioz.unibas.ch`
Biocomputing FTP and GOPHER server
Biozentrum der Universitaet at `bioftp.unibas.ch`
Klingelbergstrasse 70
FAX x41 61 261-2078 CH 4056 Basel
TEL x41 61 267-2076 or 2247 |

Contact: The EMBL Data Library
Postfach 10.2209
W-6900 Heidelberg
Germany
Phone: +49-6221-387 258
Fax: +49-6221-387 519
E-mail: `DATALIB@EMBL-HEIDELBERG.DE`

URL: `gopher://biox.unibas.ch/1`

EMBNET BIOINFORMATION RESOURCE EMBL AT HEIDELBERG

Description: This is a BioGopher server running as part of the is maintained by the EMBL Data Library at the European Molecular Biology Laboratory in Heidelberg, Germany.

It provides access to a variety of data collections and other information in molecular biology, to free software for MS-DOS, VAX/VMS, Unix and Macintosh systems, and to other gophers and biogophers.

Access: Available via anonymous ftp at `ftp.embl-heidelberg.de` (192.54.41.33).

Additionally, files can be obtained from the EMBL e-mail server. Send mail to `Netserv@EMBL-Heidelberg.DE` and include the word `HELP` on a separate line for more information.

Contact: Contact address:
The EMBL Data Library
Postfach 10.2209
W-6900 Heidelberg Germany
E-mail: `Datalib@EMBL-Heidelberg.DE`
Phone: +49-6221-387 258
Fax: +49-6221-387 519

URL: `gopher://ftp.embl-heidelberg.de/11/`

ENCYCLOPEDIA OF THE MOUSE GENOME

Description: This is a gopher version of the The Encyclopedia of the Mouse Genome. Here you can view the genetic maps of each mouse chromosome, search for specific loci on these maps as well as search for references and notes associated with each locus on the map. In addition you can search the Mouse Locus Catalog which contains detailed information on mouse loci.

Partial Directory

```
About the Encyclopedia of the Mouse Genome
Browse through the Chromosomes
Search Maps for Loci
Notes
References
Mouse Locus Catalog (MLC)
```

URL: `gopher://gopher.gdb.org/11/Database-local/mouse/encyclopedia`

FAM-MED GOPHER

Description: An Internet resource and discussion group on computers in family medicine. FAM-MED contains an electronic conference and file area. Its focus is the use of computer and telecommunication technologies in the teaching and practice of Family Medicine. Besides archives of the FAM-MED & Family-L conferences, this Gopher contains a facinating Medical Reference Section that points to many of the resources listed in this document. The conference and files are accessible to anyone able to send email on Internet, Bitnet, CompuServe, MCIMail, AT&T Mail, SprintMail, America Online, Byte Information Exchange and some FidoNet boards. Everyone is welcome to participate.

FAM-MED GOPHER MENUS

```
Medical References
    1. About Medical References.
    2. Archive: Fam-Med—Computers in Family Medicine
    3. Archive: Family-L—Academic Family Medicine
    4. Archive: Other medically related archives
    5. Gopher: CancerNet from the Nat'l Cancer Institute
    6. Gopher: Healthline—U of Montana Student Health Services
    7. Gopher: National Institute of Allergy & Infectious Disease (NIAID)
    8. Gopher: National Institutes of Health (NIH)
    9. Gopher: National Library of Medicine (NLM)
   10. Gopher: OMIM—Online Mendelian Inheritance in Man
   11. Gopher: Other medically related Gophers
   12. Newsletter: MedNews—Health Info-Com Network Newsletter
```

```
13. Shareware: Macintosh Medical SW, University of Michigan
14. Shareware: Medical SW, Univ of Texas Medical School at Houston
15. Shareware: State University of Campinas, Brazil (unstable)
17. Software Reviews (on Fam-Med)
18. Telnet: Education Technology Network (E.T.Net)
19. Telnet: Food and Drug Administration BBS

Archive: Other medically related archives
    1. AI-Medicine—Artificial Intelligence in Medicine
    2. COCAMED—Computers in Canadian Medical Education
    3. FamlySci— Family Science Network
    4. HealthRe—Health Care Reform

Gopher: Other medically related Gophers
    1. Albert Einstein College of Medicine
    2. American Physiological Society
    3. Anesthesiology Gopher
    4. Austin Hospital, Melbourne, Australia
    5. Baylor College of Medicine
    6. BioInformatics gopher at ANU
    7. Brown Medical School
    8. CAMIS (Center for Advanced Medical Informatics at Stanford)
    9. CWRU Medical School—Department of Biochemistry
   10. Cornucopia of Disability Information
   11. Johns Hopkins University- History of Science and Medicine
   12. NURSING New Gopher Service for Nurses
   13. National Cancer Center, Tokyo JAPAN
   14. Stanford University Medical Center
   15. University of Connecticut Health Center
   16. University of Michigan Medical Center
   17. University of Texas Health Science Center at Houston
   18. University of Texas M. D. Anderson Cancer Center
   19. University of Wisconsin—Madison, Medical School

Shareware: Other medical shareware sites
    1. Handicap directory at Oakland (Michigan) University (PC)
    2. Medical Education Software, Univ of California, Irvine
```

Contact: Paul Kleeberg, M.D.
Email: PAUL@GAC.EDU or PAUL@GACVAX1.BITNET
URL: gopher://gopher.uwo.ca:70/00/.faculties/fammed

GENETHON (HUMAN GENOME RES. CENTER, PARIS, FRANCE)

Description: Genethon est un Centre de Recherche sur le Genome Humain. Le but de ce serveur est de donner acces aux donnees publiques de Genethon.

Genethon is a Human Genome Research Centre. The purpose of this server is to provide access to Genethon's public data.

Ce serveur est encore experimental. J'espere ne pas le casser a chacune de mes modifications.

This server is still experimental. I hope not to break it every time I try something.

Gopher Directory

```
        About Genethon's Gopher
        Biblio
        Bio Catalog
```

```
                    En Francais
                    Genethon Data
                    Links to Wais-sources (Bio)
                    Links to Wais-sources (non bio)
                    Links to other Gophers
                    Search Gopherspace using VERONICA
                    To send mail to gopher admin (only gopher+ clients)
```
URL: **gopher://gopher.genethon.fr/1**

GENOME PROJECT (VIA WELCHLAB/JOHN HOPKINS)
Description: Gopher Directory
```
            TOE Human Genome Program Report
            Human Genome News
            The Genome Data Base (GDB)
            DOE-BioInformatics-Draft, version 2.0
            DOE-BioInformatics-Draft, version 1.0 -Postscript
            Info-Gen: Information in Genetics
```
URL: **gopher://merlot.welch.jhu.edu/11/Genome**

GRANT INFORMATION (University of Texas Gopher)
Description: This section contains information on grants and funding collected from sites all over the U.S. Remember that links to other sites can be down at any time, making some files temporarily unavailable. If you find that a file is consistently unavailable, report it to the address below. If you have or know of information that you would like added here, send electronic mail to: gopher@gopherhost.cc.utexas.edu

The information in this section is maintained by the providers listed below. Providers are responsible for the accuracy and timeliness of their data. Report problems or suggestions to the appropriate provider. Most providers have "About" files that describe their offerings. Read these files for detailed information; brief descriptions are below.

- Deadlines: By Agency

    Deadlines and brief descriptions for funding programs run by over 275 organizations. Maintained by the University of Kentucky.

- Deadlines: By Month

    Deadlines and brief descriptions for funding programs, organized by month of deadline. Maintained by the University of Kentucky.

- FEDIX

    Searchable databases on research and educational programs, contracts, equipment grants, and more from the DOE, FAA, NASA, the Office of aval Research, the Air Force Office of Scientific Research, and other government agencies. Maintained and updated daily by the Federal Information Exchange. Report problems and suggestions to: gopher@fedix.fie.com

- Federal Domestic Assistance Catalog

    A catalog of information on assistance programs of the federal government, published by the U.S. Government Printing Office and updated about every six months. This copy is stored at the University of Tennessee, Knoxville. Report problems and suggestions to the Printing Office at: (202) 783-3238

- NIH

    Contains the NIH Guide to Grants and Contracts, listings of NIH research interests, data on NIH grantees, and other information for researchers. Maintained by the National Institutes of Health. Report problems and suggestions to: `gopher@gopher.nih.gov`

- NSF

    Contains a searchable index to NSF award abstracts and publications, a database of forms for submitting proposals electronically, and much more. Maintained by the National Science Foundation. Report problems and suggestions to: `stis@nsf.gov`

- Other: Funding Programs—Private and Government

    A searchable list and brief descriptions of the funding programs offered by over 300 organizations. Maintained by the University of Wisconsin-Madison. Report problems and suggestions to: `goph_adm@msd.medsch.wisc.edu`

- Other: Funding Programs—Private and Government

    A searchable, menu-driven database of information on state and federal grants, economic data, tax information, and more. Maintained by the Texas Comptroller of Public Accounts. Report problems and suggestions while logged on to the system.

- Other: Funding and Research Database

    A searchable database of over 13,000 funding programs from over 3,000 agencies compiled from various sources. Maintained and updated daily by the University of Tennessee, Knoxville. Off-campus access to some information is prohibited.

- Other: The Foundation Center

    An international network of over 180 libraries that distribute information about organizations giving grants. At UT Austin, the Hogg Foundation for Mental Health (471-5041) is a member of this network. This list is maintained by the University of California, San Francisco. Report problems and suggestions to: `joed@itsa.ucsf.edu`

- U.S. Department of Education

    Announcements (only some of which are related to grants) from the Office of Educational Research and Improvement (OERI) of the U.S. Department of Education. OERI posts this information to `ERL-L@VM.TCS.Tulane.EDU`, a LISTSERV mailing list. These announcements are collected and stored by the University of Wisconsin-Milwaukee. Report problems and suggestions to OERI at: `jbenton@INET.ED.GOV`

- Funding Bulletins from American Psychological Association

    Announcements of funding sources for research and training in psychology, posted to `APASD-L@VTVM2.CC.VT.EDU`, a LISTSERV mailing list. These announcements are collected and stored by the University of Wisconsin-Milwaukee. Report problems and suggestions to the APA at: `APASDDES@GWUVM`

- Templates

    Contains templates from various sources for submitting grant proposals and performing other tasks.

URL: `gopher://bongo.cc.utexas.edu/11/ut-info/department/grants`

GRANTS AND CONTRACTS NIH GUIDE

Description: The information found in this directory is has been taken from the electronic form of the "NIH Guide to Grants and Contracts" available via anonymous ftp from cu.nih.gov.

Each edition of the NIH Guide begins with an index, and may contain one or more of the following:

```
notices
notices of availability (RFPs/RFAs)
ongoing program announcements (PAs)
errata
```

All of the above information has been indexed and is searchable. The logical "and" and "or" operators can be used to do multiple keyword searches.

The six folders listed under this directory are described below:

- About the NIH Guide—this file.
- Search NIH Guide (most recent 6 weeks)—the last six issues of the Guide can be searched here.
- Search NIH Guide (Jan 1992—the present)—searches done here include all Guides back to January 1992.
- NIH Guide—flat text files—each NIH Guide dating back to January 1992 is listed as a directory (by date).
- Request for Applications (RFAs)—Full Text—contains flat text files for each RFA that is available in a full text form (dating back to January 1992). Note—these files can be very long.
- Program Announcements—Full Text—contains flat text files for each Program Announcement that is available in a full text form (dating back to January 1992). These too can be very long.

Questions concerning a specific notice, RFA, RFP or PA should be directed to the contact person listed in that announcement.

General questions concerning the NIH Guide should be directed to the NIH Institutional Affairs Office (301) 496-5366.

Questions regarding gopher should be sent to: gopher@gopher.nih.gov.

Gopher Directory

```
About the NIH Guide
Search NIH Guide (most recent 6 weeks)
Search NIH Guide (Jan 1992-the present)
NIH Guide-Flat Text Files
Request for Applications (RFAs)-Full Text
Program Announcements-Full Text
```

URL: `gopher://gopher.nih.gov/11/res/nih-guide`

GRIN, NATIONAL GENETIC RESOURCES PROGRAM, USDA-ARS

Description: The NGRP gopher server provides germplasm information about plants, animals, microbes and insects within the National Genetic Resources Program of the U.S. Department of Agriculture's Agricultural Research Service (ARS). In addition, connections to other biological gopher servers around the world are provided.

Gopher Directory

```
About the NGRP gopher server
National Plant Germplasm System (NPGS)
National Animal Germplasm (including aquatics)
National Microbial Germplasm
National Insect Genetic Resources
Plant Genome Database gophers
Other biological gophers
Other gopher and information servers
Experimental
```

Contact: The NGRP gopher is still under development and subject to change. Questions or suggestions about the information presented can be sent to Jimmie Mowder at dbmujm@sol.ars-grin.gov.

URL: `gopher://gopher.ars-grin.gov`

HEALTHLINE GOPHER SERVER

Description: University of Montana Student Health Services.

The goal of Healthline is to offer (electronically) many of the same types of information that you'd receive by going to any university health center...and then some. It's NOT designed to replace face-to-face consultation with a doctor or counselor, but to assist in learning and understanding topics of general health/medical interest.

Gopher Directory

```
    About the Student Health Services HEALTHLINE Gopher
    Student Health Service Information
    What's (New) on Healthline
    Calendar/Events/Presentations
    Insurance Information
    General Health Information
    Drug & Alcohol Information
    Sexuality
    Sexual Assault Recovery Service (SARS)
    Internet Health-related Resources
    Search Healthline Files and Menus
```

Access: Gopher

Contact: UM Student Health Service HEALTHLINE Gopher Administrator: `jdc@selway.umt.edu` or `con_jdc@lewis.umt.edu`
  Please mail comments to `health@selway.umt.edu`, or call (406)243-2820.

URL: `gopher://selway.umt.edu:700/1`

HGMP RESOURCE CENTRE COMPUTING FACILITIES GOPHER

Description: The objectives of HGMP-RC computing is to establish and make available databases of genes, genetic markers and map locations, and to develop new computing environments and methods for acquisition and analysis of such data. Computing and networking facilities were developed by the MRC to provide online computing support to the Project. The facilities are connected to a number of other computing systems in centers of genetics and molecular biology research excellence worldwide through national and international wide area networks (WAN's). At present, the HGMP Gopher Service offers access to databases maintained by the Resource Centre. They can be found under the `HGMP Databases` option of the HGMP Gopher Service menu.

To registered users the HGMP-RC computing facilities offer more comprehensive services. Genetics and other databases, application software and miscellaneous services are available on the HGMP servers and other systems around the world through the HGMP-RC Menu system using workstations, personal computers or terminals from variety of manufacturers, equipped with appropriate networking and graphical facilities and connected to a suitable WAN. Several user manuals describing the usage of the HGMP-RC computing facilities have been written and are available to registered users. The user support desk is maintained during working hours, providing practical help with users' problems. A program of courses aimed at giving an understanding of what the facilities can provide are run regularly. A list of forthcoming courses can be found under the "HGMP Training and Seminars" option on the HGMP Gopher Service menu.

For a detailed description of the system and services available see Rysavy, F.R.,Bishop, M.J. et al., The UK Human Genome Mapping Project Online Computing Service. Computer Applications in the Biosciences, Vol.8, no.2. 1992, Pages 149-154. Registration is open to any bonafide academic, whether based in the UK or elsewhere. Registration is not restricted to those directly involved in human genome mapping. To register as a HGMP-RC facilities user retrieve the application from the `HGMP Registration Form` option on the HGMP Gopher Service menu. This defines the terms and conditions of the registration.

Contact: Christine Bates
  The HGMP Resource Centre
  Clinical Research Centre
  Watford Road
  Harrow MIDDX HA1 3UJ

Phone: (081) 869-3446
Fax: (081) 869-3807
URL: `gopher://gopher.hgmp.mrc.ac.uk`

HIVNET (Global Electronic Network for AIDS, Europe

Description: Excellent AIDS information source. Huge collection of documents.
URL: `gopher://gopher.hivnet.org`

IDAHO STATE UNIVERSITY GOPHER SERVER

Description: This server contains information about the schools of Dental Hygiene, Health Care Administration, Nursing, and Speech Pathology and Audiology. In addition the College of Pharmacy allows access to the Pharmacy Mail Exchange (UK), the Brookhaven National Laboratory Protein Data Bank, the Human Genome Mapping Project (UK), the National Institute of Allergy and Infectious Disease (NIAID), the National Institutes of Health (NIH) Gopher, and the National Science Foundation Gopher (STIS).

Contact: Email: `gopher@pharmacy.Isu.Edu`
Phone: (208) 236-2627
URL: `gopher://pharmacy.isu.edu`

IMC: INSTITUTE FOR MEDICAL COMPUTER SCIENCES (AKH WIEN)

Description: These are the services available on the Institute for Medical Computer Sciences Gopher.

```
VM.AKH-Wien.AC.AT Information and Services
Bedienungsanleitung fuer Netzwerkdienste (for Network Services)
Kardiologie AKH-Wien (Cardiology AKH-Vienna)
Other Gopher and Information Servers
University of Minnesota
University of Economics, Vienna
IBM Almaden Research Center
```

URL: `gopher://vm.akh-wien.ac.at`

IST GOPHER SERVER

Description: This is the Gopher Server of the National Institute for Cancer Research (IST) of Genova, Italy. The purpose of Gopher is to make IST data services available to the widest possible body of users and for facilitating access to various Internet services for IST researchers. It includes data from the Interlab Project Databases (biological materials availability in European laboratories) and the Bio-Media Bulletin Board System (biotechnology researchers, projects, fundings and products).

It enables IST researchers to access Gopher servers and WAIS sources, with particular reference to biology and biotechnology.

Contact: Email: `gophman@istge.Ist.Unige.It`.
URL: `gopher://istge.ist.unige.it`

IUBIO ARCHIVE FOR BIOLOGY GOPHER

Description: IUBIO Archive is an archive of biology data and software. The archive includes items to browse, search and fetch molecular data, software, biology news and documents, as well as links to remote information sources in biology and elsewhere. This is a public archive that you will find on the computer with the Internet name of `FTP.BIO.INDIANA.EDU`. (see FTP IUBIO ARCHIVE FOR BIOLOGY) Through Internet Gopher, there are several additional items of general interest to biologists, including GenBank, the data bank of all gene sequences, BIOSCI Network News, Prosite database, the Genome of Drosophila book, and other biology data indexed for keyword searching.

URL: `gopher://ftp.bio.indiana.edu`

MASSACHUSETTS GENERAL HOSPITAL/HARVARD UNIVERSITY GOPHER
Description: Home of the Arabidopsis Research Companion
URL: gopher://weeds.mgh.harvard.edu/1

MEDICAL INFORMATICS GOPHER
Description: Medical Informatics in Goettingen Germany.
Access: Gopher
Contact: Andreas Eichhorn Medical Informatics Goettingen Germany
URL: gopher://serversun.mdv.gwdg.de

NATIONAL CANCER CENTER GOPHER SYSTEM TOKYO JAPAN
Description: This server supports Gopher-mail for people who can only use email (UUCP). This Gopher provides the CancerNet service, Japanese Cancer Research Resources Bank, and National Cancer Center Information. It also allows molecular biological searches.

Access: Send email to GOPHER-MAIL@NCC.GO.JP to retrieve the main menu. Send email to GOPHER-MAIL@NCC.GO.JP with HELP in the Subject: to retrieve the help file.

Contact: H. Mizushima
Email: HMIZUSHI@GAN.NCC.GO.JP
Internet Address: GOPHER-MAIL@NCC.GO.JP

NATIONAL LIBRARY OF MEDICINE GOPHER
Description: The National Library of Medicine's Gopher contains information about the Library and selected references materials. It also provides access to Locator, NLM's online catalog system, and to MEDLARS and TOXNET (for those with access codes). Please note that the NLM Gopher does not provide direct access to the contents of journal articles or books. Articles and books in the NLM collection may be obtained on interlibrary loan through a local or academic library.

The NLM is the world's largest research library in a single scientific and professional field. The Library's computer-based MEDLARS system was established to achieve rapid bibliographic access to NLM's vast store of biomedical information. The Lister Hill National Center for Biomedical Communications and the National Center for Biotechnology Information are research and development divisions within NLM. The Extramural Programs Division of NLM provides a broad variety of grants to support research and development activities leading to the better management, dissemination, and use of biomedical knowledge.

Since September 1992 the NLM has been the site of the National Coordination Office of the multi-agency High Performance Computing and Communications initiative. Dr. Donald Lindberg serves concurrently as Director of the NLM and Director of the National Coordination Office for High Performance Computing and Communications.

Access: Gopher
Contact: admin@gopher.nlm.nih.gov
Additional information may be obtained at the following site:
URL: ftp://nlmpubs.nlm.nih.gov
  gopher://nlm.nih.gov

NIAID—NATIONAL INSTITUTE OF ALLERGY AND INFECTIOUS DISEASE
Description: The NIAID Gopher provides a wide variety of information appealing to both the researcher and the administrator. It has links to the most up-to-date information resources, concentrating on research and reference tools. Of special interest is the AIDS INFORMATION directory, which contains NIAID Press Releases, Center for Disease Control Daily AIDS Summaries, NIAID Protocol Recruitment Sheets, and many more items of an AIDS/HIV nature.

   Directory of National Institute Allergy & Infectious Disease (NIAID)
```
      Welcome to NIAID Gopher
      Read Me! 1/26/93
```

```
              Search for any menu item in NIAID gopher
              Search NIH Phone Book
              Search NIAID Network Userlist
              AIDS Related Information
              Desk Reference Tools
              Research Resources
              NIH Information
              NIH Helix Gopher (DCRT)
              Weather Reports
              Miscellaneous Items
              Other Gophers/WAIS Searches
```

Notice: This gopher is maintained by NIAID. All items in these menus are subject to change. Contributions are welcomed.

Access: Gopher
Contact: Derrick White
    Email: CDW@NIAID.NIH.GOV
    Phone: (301) 402-0980 x424
URL: **gopher://odie.niaid.nih.gov**

NIGHTINGALE

Description: Devoted to nursing.
Access: gopher
URL: **gopher://nightingale.con.utk.edu**

NURSING GOPHER

Description: Devoted to nursing resources.
Access: gopher.csv.warwick.ac.uk 10001
URL: **gopher://crocus.csv.warwick.ac.uk:10001**
    http://crocus.csv.warwick.ac.uk/nursing.html

SCI.MED.TELEMEDICINE GOPHER

Description: A GOPHERMAIL server interface for users without direct INTERNET access or without a GOPHER client nstalled on their machine is under development. An index of this database to it wais searchable is also being developed.

Access: Gopher
    1. gopher solomon.technet.sg 70
    2. select the BioComputing option
    3. select the sci.med.telemedicine option
    4. browse and select the appropriate post of interest.

Contact: WAIS operator waisguy@solomon.technet.sg or Dr Tan Tin Wee
    Department of Biochemistry,
    National University of Singapore.
    Tel 772-3678 Fax 7791453

Internet Address: bchtantw@nuscc.nus.sg
URL: **gopher://solomon.technet.sg**

SERVEUR GOPHER DE GENETHON GENETHON'S GOPHER SERVICE

Description: The purpose of this server is to provide access to Genethon's public data. The language is French.
Access: Gopher
Contact: Email: PATRICIA.RODRIGUEZ-TOME@GENETHON.FR
URL: **gopher://gopher.genethon.fr**

SJU ELECTRONIC REHABILITATION RESOURCE CENTER

Description: Two major software archives available through Gopher. The Handicap News BBS Archive and the U. of Oakland Handicap Archive each contain hundreds of files concerned with all aspects of disabilities and rehabilitation. (Incidentally, that's the University of Oakland in Rochester, Michigan). Both archives can be accessed from the Rehabilitation Resource Center main menu.

Access: Gopher

URL: `gopher://sjuvm.stjohns.edu:70/11/disabled`

THE AUSTRALIAN NATIONAL UNIVERSITY BIOINFORMATICS FACILITY

Description: The Australian National University's BioInformatics Facility is a small group of researchers and programmers located within the Research School of Biological Sciences. It is affiliated with ANU's Centre for Molecular Structure and Function (CMSF), Centre for Information Science Research (CISR), and Supercomputer Facility (ANUSF).

ANU's Bioinformatics Facility provides information on Internet under a number of themes. At present the major themes include:

```
biodiversity
bioinformatics & biocomputing
biomathematics & biostatistics
complex systems
general interest
landscape ecology and the environment
molecular biology
neurosciences
viruses (not computer viruses)
weather & global monitoring
```

Contact: Dr. David Green
BioInformatics Facility
Research School of Biological Sciences
Australian National University
GPO Box 475
Canberra 2601 AUSTRALIA
phone: 61-6-249-2490 or 61-6-249-5031
Fax: 61-6-249-4437
Email: `DAVID.GREEN@ANU.EDU.AU`

URL: `gopher://life.anu.edu.au`

The EMBnet PROJECT (EUROPEAN MOLECULAR BIOLOGY NETWORK)

Description: The European Molecular Biology Network (EMBnet) seeks to provide a communications infrastructure, access to research data and support for bioinformatics research. Further, new topics in this area are to be stimulated by providing a communication and education forum.

Several types of services are provided on national nodes:

1. Daily updates to DNA sequence data are received from EMBL, and properly archived to provide a most up-to date DNA sequence database. Synchronization of the distributed data base is enforced by a quarterly release on tape or CD-ROM. Because of the limited network bandwidth, and the nature of the service, incremental updates are sent as compressed files, which are to be handled individually at the national nodes.
2. Daily DNA sequence updates are forwarded to other national sites who wish to keep their own data set. The mechanisms employed depend on the infrastructure available and range from electronic mailing of abstracts to providing complete binary copies of indexed databases for particular application packages.
3. Login services are provided to researchers who wish to use the national node's infrastructure and facilities for biocomputing. The installations usually offer application software to utilize sequence

data of both public databases and one's own research data. Additionally, electronic mail and Usenet news are available at most of the sites.

Contact: The EMBnet secretary
Email: `LONIGRO@MVX36.CSATA.IT`
Dr. Richard Roberts, Cold Spring Harbor Laboratory
Email: `roberts@cshl.org`

URL: `gopher://bioftp.unibas.ch`

The ICGEB Computer Resource for Molecular Biology (ICGEBnet)

Description: The primary purpose of the ICGEB computer resource (ICGEBnet) is to disseminate the best of currently available computational technology to the molecular biologists of the ICGEB research community. The major objectives are: to provide computational assistance to ICGEB molecular biologists in planning experiments, and analyzing protein and nucleic acid sequences. ICGEBnet provides on-line access to the major sequence data banks among which the EMBL nucleic acid sequence data bank is updated on a daily basis (see below) to promote the rapid sharing of information and collaboration among the ICGEB Member Country scientists through an international computer link, electronic bulletin boards, electronic mail services, and a host of freely available PC software. ICGEBnet is part of EMBnet, the informatics network of the European Molecular Biology Organization.

Access to the ICGEBnet resource is available to all ICGEB Member Country scientists; however, preference will be given to those scientists whose research is directly related to the research goals of ICGEB. The principal mechanism for remote access to the ICGEBnet resource is via the X.25 Public Data Network (PDN). ICGEBnet is connected to the ITAPAC X.25 PDN via a leased data communication line allowing for 16 simultaneous incoming connections.

ICGEBnet is maintained by ICGEB's Computer Services in collaboration with ICGEB's Protein Structure and Function Group. Research is focused on search methods for distant protein sequence homologies. They maintain SBASE, a library of protein domains with over 24,000 entries and are developing methods based on parametric representation and Fourier analysis.

Contact: Gyorgy Simon, Systems Manager ICGEB
Email: `simon@icgeb.trieste.it`
Sandor Pongor Ph.D.
Head, Protein Structure and Function Group and Computer Services
Email: `pongor@icgeb.trieste.it`
Phone: +39-40-3757300

URL: `gopher://genes.icgeb.trieste.it`

RURALNET GOPHER, Marshall University School of Medicine Gopher Server for Rural Health Care Resources & Information

Description: The Marshall University School of Medicine in Huntington, WV, has developed a Gopher Server focused on Rural Health Care. In addition to subject-oriented access to other health care resources, this gopher includes information on the Kellogg Community Partnerships Rural Health Grant in West Virginia, the West Virginia Rural Health Initiative, and rural health programs and research at the Marshall University School of Medicine. Files from the Rural Information Center Health Service and the Food and Nutrition Information Center of FedWorld have been posted as well, including lists of rural health publications, conferences and grant opportunities.

This gopher also archives the session notes from the Kellogg & RHI Multidisciplinary Sessions, rural problem-based-learning sessions for medical, dental, pharmacy, nursing, physical therapy and social work students from all of the health care education institutions within the state.

Contact: Mike McCarthy (`mmccarth@muvms6.wvnet.edu`) or Andy Jarrell (`jarrell@musom01.mu.wvnet.edu`). Your comments and suggestions are welcome.

URL: `gopher://ruralnet.mu.wvnet.edu`

UCLA DISABILITIES AND COMPUTING PROGRAM

Description: UCLA Disabilities and Computing Program (UCLA-DCP) link to the gopher has been added to the SJU Electronic Rehabilitation Resource Center gopher.

The goal for the UCLA-DCP Gopher is to focus on locally developed resources (regional specialties—sounds appetizing!). These are publications, planning documents, annual reports and so forth that come out of our experience here at UCLA. The idea is to share what we've learned. I don't intend to develop a large resource data base of disability resources. Rather we point to CODI and St. Johns and other sites that have large resource gophers that cover this need very well.

Access: Gopher

URL: `gopher://gopher.mic.ucla.edu:4334`

UNIVERSITY OF PENNSYLVANIA POPULATION STUDIES CENTER GOPHER

Description: Gopher Directory

```
1. AMA (American Medical Association)
2. CPS (Current Population Survey)
3. Census Data
4. Heuser Birth Rate Data
5. NHANES (National Health and Nutrition Examination Survey)
6. NLMS (National Longitudinal Mortality Survey)
7. NMIHS (National Maternal and Infant Health Survey)
8. NSFH (National Survey of Families and Households)
9. sipps
```

Access: Gopher

URL: `gopher://lexis.pop.upenn.edu:70`

UNIVERSITY OF TEXAS, HOUSTON, DIAGNOSTIC IMAGING

Description: Welcome to the University of Texas M. D. Anderson Cancer Center Division of Diagnostic Imaging Gopher Server. The Diagnostic Imaging Gopher Server is an electronic information resource dedicated to supporting the activities of the Division of Diagnostic Imaging at the University of Texas M. D. Anderson Cancer Center.

This gopher is currently in an embryonic stage of development. Changes are likely to occur rapidly and without notice.

Gopher Directory

```
About the UTMDACC Division of Diagnostic Imaging Gopher Server
Current Events (news, etc)
Current Time & Weather in Houston, TX, USA
Diagnostic Images Newsletter
Diagnostic Imaging Staff Information Images
Library Information & Resources
Other Gopher and Information Servers
White House Information (Health Care, speeches, etc.)
```

Access: mdaris.mda.uth.tmc.edu

Contact: Questions or comments regarding this server should be directed to Robert Stine at stine@mdaris.mda.uth.tmc.edu

URL: `gopher://utmdacc.uth.tmc.edu`

USDA/CYFER-NET

Description: Gopher Directory

```
1. About the CYFER-NET/ES-USDA Gopher.
2. Extension Service USDA Information/
3. Children Youth Family Education Research Network (CYFER-net)
```

```
                4. Cooperative Extension System: Information Servers /
                5. Information About Gopher/
                6. Libraries/
                7. Other Federal Agencies/
                8. Other Gopher and Information Servers/
                9. public/
```
Access: Gopher
URL: `gopher://cyfer.esusda.gov`

WELCH MEDICAL LIBRARY GOPHER
Description: New medical gopher with a task-based organizational scheme.
```
                Top level menu:
                1. Using this gopher server
                2. Welch Medical Library resources and services
                3. Basic science research resources
                4. Caring for patients
                5. Exploring the Internet
                6. Finding people on the Internet
                7. Funding resources
                8. Health policy resources
                9. Hopkins resources and services
                10. Keeping up with the news
                11. Scientific writing and publishing resources
                12. Teaching, education, and course resources
```
One consequence of this design is that many resources are useful for several tasks and thus there is a lot of redundancy in the resources listed. Gopher points to resources relatively deeply embedded in other gopher servers.

Contact: Karla Hahn
  Internet Services Librarian
  Welch Medical Library
  Johns Hopkins University
  khahn@welchlink.welch.jhu.edu

URL: `gopher://welchlink.welch.jhu.edu`

WHITE HOUSE HEALTH GOPHER
Description: Health reform information from Washington.
Access: Gopher
URL: `gopher://tamu.edu:70/.dir/president.dir`

WORLD HEALTH ORGANIZATION GOPHER
Description: World Health Organization topics.
```
                    About The World Health Organization (WHO)...
                    About This Gopher and WHO's World-Wide-Web Server...
                    WHO's Major Programmes...
                    News; Press Releases & Resolutions of UN agencies, etc.
                    E-mail Directories and Telecomm Catalogues...
                    Other Gopher & Information Servers...
```
Access: Gopher
Contact: WHO Internet Gopher Root Server Administrator
  Information Technology Office (ITO)
  World Health Organization (WHO) Headquarters

CH-1211 Geneva 27
Switzerland
Tel: +41 22 791 2434
Fax: +41 22 791 0746

Internet: `gopher@who.ch`
`akazawa@who.ch`

URL: `gopher://gopher.who.ch`

YALE BIOMEDICAL GOPHER

Description: The Yale biomedical gopher is an effort by the Yale Medical Center to organize biomedical information on the Internet. It is part of YaleInfo, the Yale University gopher. The Yale biomedical gopher has organized Internet biomedical information by specific diseases and biomedical disciplines. We are extremely interested in learning about any biomedical information sources that we can add to augment this gopher.

Contact: gophmed@gopher.cis.yale.edu

URL: `gopher://info.med.yale.edu`

WORLD WIDE WEB SERVERS

HEALTH EDUCATIONAL TECHNOLOGY WEB SERVER

Description: A new Web server on information relevant to educational technology in the health professions is now available. The server is maintained by the Educational Technology Branch (ETB) at the National Library of Medicine. The server features information about Branch research and personnel and provides links to other closely related Web and Gopher servers. ETB runs a Learning Center for Interactive Technology at the NLM in Bethesda, Maryland. Details about the Center and on how to arrange for an appointment to visit us are also provided.

Some of the activities ETB is currently involved in are:

```
Learning Center for Interactive Technology
Interactive Technology Sampler
Educational Technologies
Information Technologies
Monographs
The Learning Center Courseware Database
```

Please contact us if you would like to see something else on this server, including links to other related Web or Gopher servers.

Access: WWW

Contact: Alexa McCray
National Library of Medicine
mccray@nlm.nih.gov

URL: `http://wwwetb.nlm.nih.gov`

LISTER HILL NATIONAL CENTER FOR BIOMEDICAL COMMUNICATIONS (LHNCBC)

Description: The Lister Hill National Center for Biomedical Communications (LHNCBC) was established in 1968 as a research and development arm of the National Library of Medicine, part of the U.S. National Institutes of Health in Bethesda, MD USA.

The LHNCBC is divided into five branches:

Communications Engineering Branch (CEB)

Computer Science Branch (CSB)

Educational Technology Branch (ETB)

Information Technology Branch (ITB)

AudioVisual Program Development Branch (APDB)

One of the activities of the LHNCBC is development of the Unified Medical Language System (UMLS) Project. Other research activity at the LHNCBC includes work on scientific visualization and virtual reality, medical expert systems, natural language processing, computer-aided instruction, machine learning, and biomedical applications of high speed communication techniques.

Contact: Director: Daniel Masys, M.D.

URL: `http://www.nlm.nih.gov/lhc.dir/lhncbc.html`

BOSTON UNIVERSITY SCHOOL OF PUBLIC HEALTH WEB SERVER

Description: Boston University School of Public Health (BUSPH) is pleased to be the first school of public health on the Web. The server offers the School's entire 1994/95 bulletin, current schedule of Public Health Forums, (including a campus map to help get you there), and more. Future additions to the server will include department-specific information, as well as course material (syllabi, notes, etc.) offered by professors to BUSPH students. The server is provided courtesy of the Department of Environmental Health.

Contact: Chris Paulu `cpaulu@bu.edu`
Dept. of Environmental Health/Boston University
School of Public Health

URL: `http://www-busph.bu.edu`

FUNGAL GENETICS STOCK CENTER CATALOGUE ON-LINE

Description: This on-line Hypertext document attempts to emulate the printed catalogue listing strains of Neurospora and Aspergillus preserved and distributed by the Stock Center. It lists mutants, strains collected from nature, plasmids and gene libraries containing sequences isolated from N. crassa and A. nidulans, and general purpose vectors useful in other filamentous fungi.

Access: WWW.

Contact: For any questions about FGSC, contact `fgsc@ukanvm.cc.ukans.edu`

URL: `http://kufacts.cc.ukans.edu/cwis/units/fgsc/main.html`

GNN MEDICAL TABLE OF CONTENTS

Description: WWW links to a variety of internet health resources.

Access: WWW

URL: `http://nearnet.gnn.com/wic/med.toc.html`

JOHNS HOPKINS UNIVERSITY BIOINFORMATICS WEB SERVER

Description: Biological databases (which have links to each other as well as to other databases around the world), electronic publications for biology, a section to help with software needs, and links to other Web servers.

Access: WWW

Contact: Dan Jacobson, `danj@gdb.org`

URL: `http://www.gdb.org/hopkins.html`

NIH MOSIAC WWW

Description: The NIH www server of the Division of Computer Res. and Technology contains biomedical info generated or pertaining to the NIH campus. Most of the accessible items are already being processed by the NIH gopher server. More hypertext specific items will be availble in the near future. The Mosaic home page has a color picture of the NIH campus. Hypertext links exist for the following:

- `Biomedical—health issues and clinical protocols "NIH Grants and Contracts"`
- `Research opportunities at the NIH campus`
- `Molecular biology and modeling topics`

```
    NIH computer and network resources
    NIH calendar
    NIH phone directory
    NIH Bethesda Campus info
    NIH Library
    Other NIH info services
    Access to other info servers
    About this www hypertext server
```

Access: WWW
Contact: Send comments about the www server to gopher@gopher.nih.gov
URL: `http://www.nih.gov/`

ONCOLINK—THE UNIVERSITY OF PENNSYLVANIA MULTIMEDIA ONCOLOGY RESOURCE.

Description: "OncoLink", a WWW-server and gopher server oriented to CANCER. This resource is directed to physicians, health care personnel, social workers, patients and their supporters.

IT CAN BE REACHED AT: `cancer.med.upenn.edu`

This cancer information server is currently under development, with changes made daily. Gopher can reach this resource using Port 80.

The current subject headings are:
```
    medical oncology
    radiation oncology
    pediatric oncology
    surgical oncology
    medical physics
    psychosocial support for oncology patients & families
    links to other oncology centers in the world
```

We shall be exploring interactive BBS and other means of disseminating cancer information throughout the world on the Internet.

Contact: The maintainer of this resource can be contacted at:
Dr. E. Loren Buhle, Jr.
University of Pennsylvania School of Medicine
Rm 440A, 3401 Walnut St.
Philadelphia, PA 19104-6228
Phone: 215-662-3084
FAX: 215-349-5978
buhle@xrt.upenn.edu

URL: `http://cancer.med.upenn.edu`

RNP'S WWW SERVER IN BRAZIL (REDE NACIONAL DE PESQUISA) (NATIONAL RESEARCH NETWORK)

Description: This server offers information about the RNP project and contains links to most ftp, gopher and www servers known in Brazil. It is the central www server for RNP and contains links to all other information servers offered by RNP in the rest of the country.

URL: `http://www.rnp.br/`
`gopher://gopher.rnp.br`

THE WWW VIRTUAL LIBRARY—MEDICINE (BIOSCIENCES)
Description: A comprehensive listing of WWW resources for Biology and Medicine.
URL: `http://golgi.harvard.edu/biopages/medicine.htm`

HEALTH AGENCIES

ARGENTINA
Description: A complete list of Internet nodes for institutions, hospitals, medical schools, sections of the Ministry of Health, etc. is obtainable from Marcela Guissana MD. If you want to reach all these institutes at the same time send a single message to `salud@opsarg.sid.ar`. If you have any questions send a message to `info@pccp.com.ar` In Spanish. 113 nodes.

Access: Electronic Mail

Contact: Here are the server and postmaster's names
Fernando Lopez Guerra `listserv@opsarg.ald.ar` (opsarg= a PAHO office in Buenos Aires).
Dr. Adolfo Galanternik `listserv@dacfyb.sld.ar` (dacfyb= Dpt of Clinical Analysis at Buenos Aires Univ.)
Drs. Marcela Giussani & Alberto Barengols `server@guti.sld.gov.ar` (guti=Hospital de Ninos, Buenos Aires)

AUSTRALIA
Description: AARNet, Australian Academic and Research Network (Frey, Adams, 1989).
Access: +62 493385, `gih900@csc.anu.oz.au`

BRAZIL
Description: Alternex network has an AIDS database.
Contact: Carlos Afonso (Camoes) `labrea.stanford.edu`

CANADA
Description: ONTARIO CANCER INSTITUTE, TORONTO, CANADA
e-mail: `netadmin@utoronto`

COSY at Un. Guelph
`mridley@Mcmaster`

Dept of Communications, Ottawa, Canada
Thomas Erskine, (613) 998-2836, `terskine@doccrc`

CUCHID (Canadian Consortium on Health and International Development)
Sam Lanfranco `lanfran@yorkvm1.bitnet` or `lanfran@vm1.yorku.ca`

Dept. of Health and Welfare
Steve Scantlebury, (613) 954-6449, `steves@hpb.hwc.ca`

EPIX (Emergency Preparedness Information Exchange BBS)
Modem: (604) 291-4921.
Contact: Richard Smith `smith@whistler.sfu.ca`

Ontario Cancer Institute, Toronto, Canada
Norman Housley, (416) 978-4967, `netadmin@utoronto`

Ontario Ministry of Health
Contact: Peter Renzland `peter@ontmoh.uucp` and `renzland@moh.gov.on.ca`, tel: (416) 323-1300.

CROATIA
Description: Nevin Henigsberg MD
Ministry of Health
Republic of Croatia

HEALTH SCIENCES

Office of Cooperation with WHO
8. maja 42
41000 YU-Zagreb.
Tel: +38 41 430 621;
Fax: +38 41 431 067
whocro@uni-zg.ac.mail.yu

CZECHOSLOVAKIA
Description: 3rd Medical School
Charles University
Srobarova 48, 100 42
Praha, Czecho
Milan Jira MD PhD, ulimj@csearn.bitnet

EGYPT
Description: WHO Egypt (Alexandria) system@who.eg
who@egfrcuvx.bitnet
Khaled A. Hadi mondo@egfrcuvx.Bitnet

FRANCE
Description: Institut Pasteur Fondation, Paris, Gerrard Masson, ++33 1 45 6880, gerard@frpstr01
French Communicable Disease Network (INSERM)
Philippe Garnerin, +33 1 43 259226, garnerin@frurbb51

LATIN AMERICA
Description: Request E-mail Lists #23-G and 23-P from Pedro Saizar pedro@ohstpy.bitnet

NAMIBIA
Description: Katatura State Hospital, Windhoek, Namibia
Dr Eberhard Lisse spel@hippo.ru.ac.za

PAN AMERICA
Description: Pan American University (LaQuey, 1990, p22)
BIR: William Morris, (512) 381-2111, wlm3851@panam
INFOREP: Mary Rose
TECHREP: Michael Merold

RUSSIA
Description: Center for Emergency Medicine, Moscow
Ilya V. Zakharov, zakh@home.vega.msk.su
DEMOS networking center networkers@hq.demos.su

UKRAINE
Description: International Information Technology Center
Yuri N. Muraviov myn%myn.computerland.kiev.ua@ussr.eu.net

United States Governmental Agencies
Description: Notes/Code:
BIR= BITNET Institutional Representative;

INFOREP= Local BITNET Support;
TECHREP= for local technical operations.

A. Federal Agencies:

Food and Drug Administration
BIR: Laurence Dusold, (202) 245-1413, `lrd@fdacfsan`
INFOREP: Donna Kovalsky, (202) 472-5382, `dbk@fdacfsan`
TECHREP: Laurence Dusold, (202) 245-1413, `lrd@fdacfsan`

B. Federal Institutions:

CDC Center for Disease Control, Atlanta, GA
Complete list of CDC staff bitnet addresses obtainable from `HSPNET-L@ALBNYDH2` fileserver.
CDC e-mail coordinator—`cdcjuk@emuvm1`
Also call Joan Kennedy at (404) 639-3396 for a directory.

National Institute. of Environmental Health Science
BIR: Art Cullati, (919) 541-3432, `cullati@niehs`
INFOREP: James Dix, (919) 541-3221, `dix@niehs`
TECHREP: Fred Castner, (919) 541-2552, `kastner@niehs`
(Research Triangle Park, NC)

National Institutes of Health
Bethesda, Maryland, USA
Roger Fajman, Postmaster for `CU.NIH.GOV/NIHCU`, `LIST.NIH.GOV/NIHLIST`, `NIH3PLUS`
Telephone: +1 301 402 4265
BITNET: `raf@nihcu`
Internet: `raf@cu.nih.gov`
BIR: Joseph Naughton, (301) 496-5381, `jdn@nihcu`
INFOREP: Roger Fajman, (301) 496-5181, `raf@nihcu`
TECHREP: Roger Fajman, (301) 496-5181, `raf@nihcu`

NIAID
Judy Murphy—Public Information Section
Phone:(301) 496-5717 E-mail: `JM63A@nih.gov`
Deborah Katz—Office of Scientific Information and Reports
Phone:(301) 496-0545 E-mail: `dk30f@nih.gov`
You can also try calling the NLM Medline Help Desk at (301) 496-6095.

National Library of Medicine (NLM)
Robert Mehnert Phone: (301) 496-6308
Office of Public Information
E-Mail: `RM94S@nih.gov`
Carolyn Tilley MEDLARS Management Section
Phone (301) 496-1076
E-mail: `ct32@nih.gov`
Pamela A. Meredith
Head, Reference Section
National Library of Medicine
Internet: `meredith@lhc.nlm.nih.gov`
voice: (301) 496-6097

Naval Health Sciences Med. Data Services (LaQuey, 1990, p78)
   Dennis DePew, (301) 295-0824, `depew@hsetc`

Uniformed Services University of Health Sciences
   (LeQuey, 1990, p136)
   Michael Karas, (202) 295-3304, `karas@usuhs`

US Environmental Protection Agency, (LaQuey, 1990, p27)
   BIR: Bruce P. Almich, `bpa@nccibm1`
   INFOREP: David Best, (919) 541-7862, `dbe@nccibm1`
   TECHREP: David Best, (919) 541-7862, `dbe@nccibm1`

US Public Health Service
   Joycelyn Elders `gateway.Surgeon.Gen@whitehouse.gov`
   Earl Hutchinson, administrator of HCFA's email
   `admin@hcfacom.ssw.dhhs.gov`

National Academy of Sciences (LaQuey, 1990, p20)
   BIR: Tom Wisner, `twisner@nasvm`
   INFOREP: Theresa Lima, (202) 334-3463 `tlima@nasvm`
   TECHREP: Rob FRistom, (202) 334-3592 `rrf@nasvm`

National Science Foundation
   BIR: Fred Wendling, (202) 357-7684, `fwendlin@nsf`
   INFOREP: Theresa Dickson, (202) 357-5933, `tdickson@nsf`
   TECHREP: Lloyd Douglas, `ldouglas@nsf`
   Contact: NSF Network Service Center `NNSC@nnsc.nsf.net`
   (617)873-3400

C. Non-Federal (National Institutions):

   American Medical Informatics Association (AMIA)
      (301) 657-1291,
      `amia@camis.stanford.edu`

   Health Sciences Library Consortium
      Joseph Scorza (215) 222-1532,
      `scorza@shrsys.hslc.org`

   Health Sphere of America, Inc
      Jesse Asher (901) 386-5061
      `jessea@homecare.com`

   Health Sciences Libraries Consortium,
      3600 Market St.
      Suite 550,
      Philadelphia, PA 19104
      (215) 222-1532
      Joseph Scorza
      `scorza@shrsys.hslc.org`

   Health Systems International
      Richard Stevens (602) 297-9416
      `stevens@kohala.Com`

   Salk Institute
      BIR: Anne M. Quinn, (619) 453-4100, `quinn@salk`
      INFOREP: Anne M. Quinn (619) 453-4100, `quinn@salk`
      TECHREP: Anne M. Quinn (619) 453-4100, `quinn@salk`

STATE/PROVINCE -USA
General: Nearly all US State Health Agencies are contracted to the Public Health Foundation Dialcom service
(1220 L Street NW, Ste. 350,
Washington, DC 20005. (202) 898-5600.
Note: Dialcom does not permit connection to Internet.

Arizona:
University of Arizona College of Medicine
Cynthia Tobias, Dir., Office of Medical Computing
`cltobias@arizrvax.bitnet`

Illinois:
State of Illinios School of Medicine
Springfield IL 62794-9230
(217)782-2419
Terri Cameron, Automation Administrator `gh0225@springb`
University of Chicago Medical School (Rockford, Peoria, Champaign/Urbana)
George Yanos, CIO, `u08208@uicvm`

Kansas:
University of Kansas Medical Center
Lee Hancock `Le07144@ukanvm`

New York State:
Albany School of Public Health
Contact person: Barry Krawchuk, (518) 473-1809,
`bdk01@albnydh2`
Albert Einstein College of Medicine
Bronx, NY 10461
(212)430-4211
Robert Lummis, Director of Res.Information Technology,
`bob@aecom.yu.edu`
Columbia University College of Physicians and Surgeons,
Dept of Medicine: Reider Bornholdt,
212) 305-3411,
`reider@cucard`
Health Sciences Campus: Janie Weiss,
(212) 305-7532,
`system@cuhsda`
Cornell Univ. Medical College
Nick Gimbrone, (607) 255-3748, `njg@cornella`
Memorial Sloan Kettering Cancer Center
`Postmast@mskcc`
Mount Sinai School of Medicine
`Postmast@MSRCVX`

New York State Department of Health
   Contact person: Barry Krawchuk, (518) 473-1809,
   `bdk01@albnydh2`
New York University Medical Center, NYC
   Ross Smith `smith@nyumed`
Roswell Park Memorial Institute, Buffalo (microwave link to
   SUNY Albany -no BITNET or Internet node at present. E-mail
   directory in preparation):
   INFOREP: James P. Harlos, Director of Scientific
   Computing, Tower 7,
   RPMI, Buffalo, NY 14263, (716) 845-8647
   `stmjames@ubvmsb.cc.buffalo.edu`
State University of New York (Central),
   BIR: Bruce B. Briggs, (518) 443-5219, `briggs@snycenvm`
State University of NY Health Science Center, Brooklyn
   BIR: Jack Lubowsky (718) 270-3181 `lubowsky@snybksac`
   INFOREP: Jack Lubowsky (718) 270-3181 `lubowsky@snybksac`
   TECHREP: Jack Lubowsky (718) 270-3181 `lubowsky@snybksac`
State University of New York, Syracuse, Health Sciences Center
   Jeannette Stiteler (315) 473-5426 `stiteler@snysyrv1`

North Carolina:
   School of Medicine
      Chapel Hill, NC
      27599-7045
      `request@med.unc.edu`
      Contact: Dr. Kirk Aune, Associate Dean—Information Systems
      `kaune@med.unc.edu`

North Dakota:
   University of N.Dakota School of Medicine
      501 N.Columbia Rd
      Grand Forks, ND 58203.
      Coordinator of Computer Services: Don Larson
      `ud165133@ndsuvm1`
      `ud165133@vm1.nodak.edu`

Ohio:
   Medical College of Ohio, Toledo, OH
      Jerry Levin, Associate Dean for Academic Resources
      `levin%opus@mcoiarc.bitnet`
      INFOREP: Karen E. Torok, Hospital Systems Coordinator,
      (419) 381-5446 `torok%cutter@mcoiarc`
      (also postmaster for MCOIARC)

Pennsylvania:
   Dr.Albert Shar
      Chief Information Officer
      University of Pennsylvnia School of Medicine:

(215) 898-9754.
`shar@mscf.upenn.edu`
Milton Hershey Medical Center
500 University Dr
Hershey, PA 17033
Alton Brantley, CIO `alton@cit.hmc.psu.edu`
University of Pittsburgh Medical Center
Information Services Division,
1400 Penn. Ave
Pittsburgh, PA 15222
(412) 392-6800
Sean McLinden MD, `sean@dsl.pitt.edu`

Texas:
MD Anderson Cancer Center
Houston, TX
(713) 792-6345
Richard Landkamer `mailmnt@uthvm1`
University of Texas Health Science Center at San Antonio
Conni Annabele `annable@thorin.uthscsa.edu`
TRHEX (Texas Rural Hospital Electronic eXchange)
John Oeffinger `cg8061@applelink.apple.com`

Utah:
University of Utah School of Medicine
Salt Lake City, UT 84132
Director, Medical School Computing Center, Clay Epstein
`clay@utahmed.Bitnet`
`clay@msscc.med.utah.edu`

Wisconsin:
State Lab of Hygiene (epidemiology, environment, etc)
(608) 262-0736
Jim Leinweber `jiml@slh.wisc.edu`

WORLD HEALTH AGENCIES
Description: International Red Cross
`Postmaster@verw.switch.ch` Switzerland
Medicins Sans Frontiers, 8 rue Sanin, 75011 PARIS 11eme, France
Tel: 033 1 40 21 29 29, Fax: 033 1 48 06 68 68.
Contact: Dr JF Vibert `vibert@frsim51.bitnet`

WORLD HEALTH ORGANIZATION
Description: WORLD HEALTH ORGANIZATION, GENEVA HEADQUATERS
Mr. Shunichi AKAZAWA, Network Manager `manager@who.ch`
Mr. David BERG, Director, Information Technology Office
`berg@who.ch`

HEALTH SCIENCES 427

Mr. Jim Duppenthaler, Dissemination of Health Statistics
`duppenthaler@who.ch`
Dr. K. Hata, Info Manager, Tropical Diseases Research (TDR)
`hata@who.ch`
Mr. Mark Wallace, Info Technology, Global Programme on AIDS
`wallace@who.ch`

WORLD HEALTH ORGANIZATION, REGIONAL OFFICE FOR THE AMERICAS
PAN-AMERICAN HEALTH ORGANIZATION (PAHO/HEADQUARTERS)

Dr. Carlos Gamboa `gamboaca@pahohq.bitnet`

MISCELLANEOUS

Some reources are difficult to catagorize. So here's a "catch all" section.

ACADLIST KENTVM

Description: A List of ACADEMIC DISCUSSION AND INTEREST GROUPS—Diane Kovacs, editor. Entries are listed under 7 broad subject categories.

> Filename: `ACADLIST.FILE1` to `ACADLIST.FILE7`
> Of interest to the health sciences is: `ACADLIST FILE5`:
> Biological Sciences (entries 1-127)

> These are also available in print as part of the ARL Directory of Electronic Journals.

Access: Email—`KSUVXA.KENT.EDU` with `GET FILENAME` on the first line in the body of the message.
Internet Address: `KSUVXA.KENT.EDU`
URL: `gopher://gopher.cni.org:80/11/cniftp/pub/net-guides/kovacs`

BIOTECHNET ELECTRONIC BUYER'S GUIDE

Description: This guide is divided into 5 individual databases for specific product categories: Molecular Biology, Electrophoresis, Chromatography, Liquid Handling and Instruments & Apparatus. After selecting one of the guides at the prompt, you can search through each database to find either product names and applications, or the name and address of the company that manufactures the product you wish to locate.

Access: telnet
URL: `telnet://biotechnet.com`

Username: `BIOTECH`
Password: `BGUIDE`

CENTER FOR BIOMEDICAL INFORMATICS

Description: The CENTER FOR BIOMEDICAL INFORMATICS maintains a software library with 50 diskettes containing about 150 public-domain medical application programs for IBM PC-compatible microcomputers. Most of these programs are provided in source code (BASIC, Turbo-BASIC, dBASE III and PASCAL). In the last three years, the Center has distributed more than 400 copies to physicians, nurses, dentists, university lecturers and researchers, and other professionals and students in the Health Sciences, in exchange for a small fee per diskette, which is used to expand the public-domain software library. Outside contributions are welcome: if they are accepted, the contributor is entitled to choose any five diskettes from the collection. The majority of the programs are in Portuguese, but some are in English, too. A few of the programs are offered as shareware, meaning there's a small fee to the developer.

Access: To receive the catalog in electronic form, send the following one-line message to the addresses below:

`GET PUBLIC-DOMAIN P` (for version in Portuguese)

> GET PUBLIC-DOMAIN E (for version in English)
>
> Instructions on how to acquire the software are included.

Contact: e-mail

Bitnet Address: `INFOMED@BRUC.BITNET`

Internet Address: `INFOMED@CCVAX.UNICAMP.BR`

CFS/CFIDS/ME RESOURCES

Description: Please note the other Internet resources that focus on CFS/CFIDS/ME Resources on this Listserv and elsewhere. Resources include: a files database; a "Newswire" service for support groups; an electronic newsletter (focusing on medical research); and a general discussion group where advice and information are exchanged among patients each day.

The CFS-FILE list, still in development at this time, will soon host a wide variety of files containing medical journal articles, information on related health issues, advice on coping, social security, related illnesses (candida, Lyme disease, etc.) and others.

To retrieve specific files, note the filenames on the FILELIST and then send the command GET <filename1> <filename2> to the LISTSERV address (each file has a two-part name).

Also, there is a comprehensive list of electronic and other resources contained that all patients should review, contained in the file `CFS-RES.TXT` available at either Listserv.

For electronic journals, see `CFS-WIRE` and `CFS-NEWS` under the `Electronic Publications` category.

For a discussion group, see the CFS-L list.

Other resources include:

> `CFS-D, CFS-D@ALBNYDH2`, Chronic Fatigue Syndrome File Storage
> `CFS-FILE, CFS-FILE@SJUVM`, Chronic Fatigue Syndrome files CFIDS/ME
> `CFS-L, CFS-L@NIHLIST`, Chronic Fatigue Syndrome discussion CFIDS/ME
> `CFS-MED, CFS-MED@NIHLIST`, Chronic Fatigue Syndrome/CFIDS medical list
> `CFS-NEWS, CFS-NEWS@NIHLIST`, Chronic Fatigue Syndrome Newsletter CFIDS/ME
> `CFS-WIRE, CFS-WIRE@SJUVM`, Chronic Fatigue Syndrome NEWSWIRE CFIDS/ME

Access: There is at this time a separate CFS files database at a different Listserv in Albany, New York. For information on that database, send commands just as above to the address `LISTSERV%ALBNYDH2.BITNET@ALBANY.EDU` or to `LISTSERV@ALBANY.BITNET`

Contact: `NIHLIST`

Bitnet Address: `listserv@SJUVM`

Internet Address: `listserv@SJUVM.STJOHNS.EDU`

COLOR AND VISION NETWORK [CVNet]

Description: The CVNet is for scientists working in biological color and/or Vision Korea, Lithuania, Netherlands, New Zealand, Norway, Russia, Scotland, Singapore, Spain, Sweden, Switzerland, the U.S., Wales and Yugoslavia are in the network. They come from, universities, research institutes, national laboratories, military research laboratories and industry.

Access: Scientists working in biological color and/or vision who wish to join should contact:
> `CVNET@VM1.YORKU.CA`

Contact: Peter K. Kaiser, Ph.D.
> CVNet Coordinator
> `CVNET@VM1.YORKU.CA`
> Department of Psychology
> York University
> North York, Ontario M3J 1P3
> Canada

Internet Address: `CVNET@VM1.YORKU.CA`

COLUMBIA PRESBYTERIAN LIBRARY OF MEDICAL LOGIC MODULES (MLM) KNOWLEDGE BASE

Description: The medical knowledge base is composed of units called Medical Logic Modules (MLMs) written in the Arden Syntax. The Arden Syntax for Medical Logic Modules (MLMs) is a language for encoding medical knowledge. Each MLM contains sufficient logic to make a single medical decision. MLMs have been used to generate clinical alerts, interpretations, diagnoses, screening for clinical research, quality assurance functions, and administrative support.

With an appropriate computer program (known as the Event Monitor at CPMC), MLMs run automatically, generating advice where and when it is needed. For example, one MLM warns physicians when a patient develops new or worsening kidney failure.

The Arden Syntax was designed specifically for sharing knowledge. This collection contains MLMs donated by a number of different institutions. Some institutions have supplied only the maintenance and library information from the MLMs for free distribution; the knowledge section is missing. If you want the full versions, contact Johanne La Grange (`lagrang@cpmail-am.cis.columbia.edu`).

Note that these MLMs have a validation level of "testing" and no "domain specialist" has been entered. This means that they are NOT validated for clinical use in their current form. If you use them, you must take responsibility for testing them and making sure they are appropriate for your institution.

Access: FTP and Gopher

Contact: George (George Hripcsak, MD, `hripcsa@cucis.cis.columbia.edu`)

URL: `ftp://cucis.cis.columbia.edu/pub/mlm`
`gopher://cuhsla.cpmc.columbia.edu`
`telnet://cuhsla.cpmc.columbia.edu`

login: `infoseeker`

FINANCIAL ECONOMICS NETWORK

Description: Twenty-five different channels and over 1800 subscribers. The Financial Economics Network provides channels where announcements and messages of interest are posted and ideas exchanged on topics of mutual interest. Additional plans for the Network include: the development of a CSO phonebook for the financial economics profession (broadly defined); usenets to which our discussion lists will be mirrored; a channel or usenet for posting of jobs in financial economics; a channel or usenet for posting resumes; virtual conferences on topics of interest to the financial community; internet finance courses offered by world known faculty; and possible e-journals related to financial economics.

The Network consists of a master subscription, called AFA-FIN, with 21 channels. There are currently 18 channels open to AFA-FIN subscribers, with 3 additional ones coming on line in approximately two weeks. The channels currently operating, which run the gamut of topics in financial economics, are:

The Financial Economics Network is a multi-channel electronic network for scholars and interested individuals in investment banks, banks, companies, government agencies, international agencies and universities. But there are also channels for small investors and people interested in personal finance. Although the Network was formed less than a month ago, there are already nearly 1,800 subscribers, with nearly 100 being added each week. In less than a month, Financial Economics Network has become the largest electronic network in the world linking people with scholarly and practical interests in business and economics. Of interest to the health community are the following:

`AFA-ACCT` (Accounting and Finance)
`AFA-AGE` (Gerontology Finance)
`AFA-HEAL` (Health Finance)
`AFA-INS` (Insurance)
`AFA-INST` (Teaching/Instruction)

Access: Access to the Network is free. But you must request a subscription to be included. Please contact Professor Wayne Marr or Professor John Trimble.

Contact: Founders of the Financial Economics Network Michael Jensen, Harvard University Wayne Marr, First Union Professor of Banking, Clemson University;
marrm@clemson.clemson.edu
(803) 656-0796 (voice)
(803) 653-5516 (fax).

John Trimble, finance faculty at Washington State University;
trimble@vancouver.wsu.edu
telephone: (206) 737-2039

GRANT INFORMATION
Description: A wide variety of public and priviate grant funding information.
Access:Gopher
URL: `gopher://gopher.mountain.net/11/grants`

HEALTH SCIENCE RESOURCES ON BITNET/INTERNET
Description: From the main menu following this path: Departmental Resources/Medical Center Resources
Compiled by Lee Hancock, The University of Kansas Medical Center, this is a comprehensive index of health science resources available on the Internet/Bitnet/Usenet. The list includes Listserv groups, Usenet groups, Freenets, Data Archives, and health science oriented databases. Currently updated 4 or 5 times a year. Also available online at many Gopher sites.

Access: WWW and FTP
Internet Address: `UKANAIX.UKANAIX.CC.UKANS.EDU`
URL: `http://kufacts.cc.ukans.edu/cwis/kufacts_start.html`
`ftp://ftp.sura.net/pub/nic/medical.resources.3-94`

NATIONAL LIBRARY OF MEDICINE EDUCATIONAL TECHNOLOGY NETWORK
Description: A host of forums concerning medical education and the use of multimedia in medical education. These are Compuserve like forums where medical people from all over the world discuss issues concerning the use of computers, laser discs, CD-ROM, etc. in medical education.

Access: telnet
Login: `ETNET`
URL: `telnet://etnet.nlm.nih.gov (or 130.14.1.27)`

NIH EdNnet
Description: An electronic bulletin board at the Bethesda, Maryland campus of NIH. EDNET is set up to allow high school students to ask questions of NIH scientists about current research. There is NO CHARGE to access EDNET. Access is via modem through an tool-free phone number or the Internet. The tool-free number is also for national access which is said to be an international number. If you are interested in receiving an EDNET User's Guide and account, send a personal email message which includes our mailing address to: `VT5@CU.NIH.GOV`

MODEM SETTINGS: 7 data bits, even parity, 1 stop bit (800) 358-2221 (local number is (301) 492-2221)

When you see `connect 2400` on the screen or `connect 1200` depending on your baud rate, type `VT100`

At INITIALS type `NAK`
At ACCOUNT type `ZZYZ`

Continue by following instructions. Select a conference to join and read the messages. All information will be in messages. Leaving a message is somewhat user unfriendly since the user must use Wylbur editing commands. They are described in the User's Guide.

Access: Email—`VT5@CU.NIH.GOV`
Internet Address: `VT5@CU.NIH.GOV`

NIH GRANT LINE (DRGLINE BULLETIN BOARD)

Description: The purpose of NIH GRANT LINE is to make program and policy information for the Public Health Service (PHS) agencies rapidly available to the biomedical research community. Most of the research opportunity information available on this bulletin board is derived from the weekly publication "NIH Guide for Grants and Contracts" consisting of Notices, RFAs, RFPs (announcements of availability), Numbered Program Announcements, and statements of PHS policy. The electronic version known as E-Guide is available for electronic transmission each week, sometimes a day or two in advance of the nominal Friday publication date. The material consists predominantly of statements about the research interests of the PHS Agencies, Institutes, and National Centers that have funds to support research in the extramural community.

Currently under development are 2 new files. One of them will be a monthly listing of new NIH Awards. The other one will be an order form to obtain NIH publications from DRG's Office of Grants Inquiries. The information found on the NIH Grant Line is grouped into three main sections:

1) short News Flashes that appear without any prompting shortly after the user has logs on.
2) Bulletins that are for reading.
3) Files that are intended mainly for downloading.

There are menus and simple English commands, but all the user has to type is the first letter of the commands displayed. Since most of the current as well as archived files are located in the section of the bulletin board called FILES, type F in order to be able to access any of the files which are arranged into directories. To get an overview of the kinds of information available, type D for Directory. Remember that you can mail files (a "download" option) to your Internet address.

Also included is electronic access to NIH guide for grants and contracts. There are two principal methods of accessing the NIH Guide electronically.

1) Via electronic networks to institutional hubs.
2) By accessing NIH GRANT LINE, an electronic bulletin board

The first method is to have someone in your research setting volunteer to receive the NIH Guide, Indices, and Directories automatically via electronic networks each time they are updated then redistribute them locally tobiomedical researchers. These participants are the "institutional hubs." The preferred, and most efficient method of distribution, is for each hub to disseminate the material by existing systems or by methods of their own choosing. To express your interest in serving as the focal point for your organization and to receive a letter of invitation, send an email message in which the responsible person is named to Dr. Claudia Blair whose Bitnet address is Q2C@NIHCU (or Internet Q2C@CU.NIH.GOV).

The other method, which requires active intervention to access the same documents each week, is to get access to the NIH GRANT LINE. Directions for this electronic like bulletin board system are given below. One feature on NIH GRANT LINE is that users have an option of downloading selected documents through a modem, or the rapid transmission of files via Bitnet or Internet to their Bitnet or Internet address. If the connection is to the electronic bulletin board is through a modem, files will download to a PC file. The user can also speed up the process of accessing files in an interactive session by directing mail as indicated below.

To access NIH GRANT LINE:

1) Configure your terminal emulator as: 1200 or 2400 baud, even parity, 7 data bits, 1 stop bit, Half Duplex.
2) Using the procedure specified in the communication software, call (301) 402-2221. When you get a response indicating that you have been connected, then type, GEN1 (the comma is mandatory) and press RETURN; you will be prompted by the NIH system for INITIALS?. Type BB5 and press RETURN. You will then be prompted for ACCOUNT?. Type CCS2 and press RETURN.

Messages and a menu will be displayed that allows the user to read Bulletins, or download Files. It shouldn't take to long to become familiar with the contents of the bulletin board, and the commands to go back and forth from one section to another. On the NIH Grant Line, back issues of the NIH Guide are found in different directories. GUIDE90 has issues going back to July 6, 1990; GUIDE91 has all of the issues in 1991; GUIDE92 has all of the issues in 1992; and GUIDE93 has all issues in 1993.

Remember that although the access is through a modem, transmission of the files selected are much faster through the selection of network transmission. After selecting a file to be "downloaded", chose `2— Transmitted to a NUnet, BITNET, or Internet userid` and then respond with your email address.

Access: telnet

At the `Open` prompt, type `,GEN1` (must include comma)

INITIALS? BB5

ACCOUNT? CCS2

This will get the user into the DRGLINE Bulletin Board (also known as NIH GRANT LINE at NIH).

URL: `telnet://wylbur.cu.nih.gov (128.321.64.82)`

NUS-NCI CANCERNET

Description: As a collaboration between the National University of Singapore and the National Cancer Institute, Bethesda, MA, a new secondary site for the NCI CancerNet files has been set up at biomed.nus.sg in Singapore.

Note that the CancerNet Gopher directory can also be browsed and the CancerNet GOPHER-WAIS be searched via our generic mailgopher service: send email to `bioserve@biomed.nus.sg` or `mailgopher@biomed.nus.sg` with the message GOPHERHELP

The gopher and World Wide Web services are fairly stable and have been online for sometime now.

The following are more recent (please send bug reports):

Mail server: Send the following message to `bioserve@biomed.nus.sg`

CANCERNETHELP

or for `cn-xxxxxx` files, where xxxxxx is the number of the CancerNet file, send the message

cn-xxxxxx

WAIS: This waisindex is accessible from the gopher menu as well as from the web menu. It is of course accessible from a wais client eg. waissearch, xwais, swais, etc.

If you try it, you will find that the titles of the hits are not very meaningful, ie. only the numbers are returned. Work is in progress.

Access: via WAIS, gopher and WWW

Contact: For enquiries about the CancerNet WAIS source, please contact Dr Tan Tin Wee, `bchtantw@leonis.nus.sg`

For enquiries about the CancerNet files, please contact Cheryl Burg, `cheryl@icicb.nci.nih.gov`

Internet Address: `bioserve@biomed.nus.sg`

URL: `gopher://biomed.nus.sg:70`

`http://BIOMED.NUS.SG:80/`

ONTARIO PREVENTION CLEARINGHOUSE

Description: The ONTARIO PREVENTION CLEARINGHOUSE is a provincial agency providing information, support and advice toorganizations and individuals who are working in the areas of prevention and health promotion.

Since it opened its doors in the fall of 1985, the Clearinghouse has been helping to meet the information needs of professionals and other community leaders from the fields of health, human services, and education by providing one easily accessible source for consultation, program data, networking and research.

The Clearinghouse offers a unique and comprehensive combination of services to its users, including:

1. A computerized data bank containing information on such topics as: effective prevention and health promotion programs, program evaluation strategies, funding sources, program resources, support materials, outreach strategies and related research.

2. A collect telephone line and a toll free WATTS line for cost efficient province-wide access to prevention and health promotion information. (Ontario only)
3. Individual consultation on prevention and health promotion programming within Ontario.
4. A bilingual newsletter.
5. Information packages available on Prevention and Health Promotion topics.
6. Regional and topical focus groups.
7. Telecommunications, on-line literature search capability, Internet email access and a fax line.

Access: Email—OPCH@UTORONTO.BITNET or OPC@WEB.APC.ORG

Contact: The Ontario Prevention Clearinghouse is located at:
984 Bay Street #603 Toronto
Ontario M5S 2A5
In Ontario, call toll free (800) 263-2846 or phone
(416) 928-1838 Fax line (416) 928-5975

Bitnet Address: **OPCH@UTORONTO.BITNET**

Internet Address: **OPC@WEB.APC.ORG**

RURAL INFORMATION CENTER (RIC)

Description: Rural Information Center (RIC) within the National Agriculture Library (NAL). RIC operates a sub-specialty service called the Rural Information Center Health Service (RICHS) which provides "customized information products to specific inquiries including assistance in economic revitalization issues; local government planning projects; rural health issues; funding sources; and other related issues for the purpose of monitoring the quality of rural life." Topics include: community development projects; small business; tourism; recycling; water quality; technology transfer; "closures, restructuring and diversification of rural hospitals and clinics; agriculture health and safety; health programs; state initiatives in health delivery. RICHS staff will search various databases for requested information, provide bibliographies, and lists of organizations and experts.

Access: E-mail

Contact: RICHS can be reached at 1-800-633-7701 Mon-Fri, 8 to 4:30 ET.
Mail address is:
Rural Information Center
National Agriculture Library
Room 304
10301 Baltimore Blvd.
Beltsville, MD 20705-2351

Internet Address: **RIC@NALUSDA.GOV**

TEXAS CANCER DATA CENTER

Description: The Texas Cancer Data Center is funded by the Texas Cancer Council as a component of the Texas Cancer Plan to provide computerized information on cancer demographics, resources, services and programs to all who plan, develop, fund, provide, need, and/or use cancer resources in Texas.

```
MAIN MENU
  1. Health Professionals
  2. Health Facilities and Services
  3. Continuing Care Services (Discharge Planning)
  4. Population and Cancer Deaths
  5. Bulletin Board (Read Only) ***NEW FORMAT
  6. Texas Cancer Council Projects
  7. Statistical Topics
  8. Community Resources
  9. TCDC Assistance *** New Fact Sheet Information
```

Access: telnet
Username: TCDC

URL: **telnet://TXCANCER.MDA.UTH.TMC.EDU (129.106.60.97)**

THE SOCIETY OF TEACHERS OF FAMILY MEDICINE
Description: Contact them for more information.
Access: Email
Contact: 0005448812@MCIMAIL.COM or STFM@MCIMAIL.COM.

THE VIRTUAL HOSPITAL (VH)
Description: The Virtual Hospital (VH) is a continuously updated medical multimedia database stored on computers and accessed through high speed networks 24 hours a day. The VH will provide invaluable patient care support and distance learning to practicing physicians. The VH information may be used to answer patient care questions, thus putting the latest medical information at physicians' fingertips. This same information may be used for Continuing Medical Education (CME); delivering CME to physicians' offices and homes at a convenient time and location. The VH is built on pre-existing computer and communication standards and uses the World Wide Web (WWW) software technology to store, organize, and distribute our multimedia textbooks (MMTBs) contained within it. We define a MMTB to be a program that patterns its user interface after a printed textbook. Our MMTBs incorporate functions such as free text searching, the ability to play video and audio clips, and to display an unlimited number of high-resolution images.

Access: The VH can be accessed by any computer connected to the Internet with a Mosaic client.

Contact: For more information, send e-mail to
librarian@indy.radiology.uiowa.edu

URL: `http://indy.radiology.uiowa.edu/VirtualHospital.html`

FREENETS:
Most Freenets have a health or medical section.

FREE-NETS & Community Computing Systems
Description: Big Sky Telegraph
URL: `telnet://192.231.192.1`

login: bbs

Buffalo FREE-NET
URL: `telnet://FREENET.BUFFALO.EDU or 128.205.3.99`

login: freeport

CapAccess: National Capital Area Public Access Network
URL: `telnet://CAP.GWU.EDU or 128.164.140.32`

login: guest
Password: visitor

Cleveland FREE-NET
URL: `telnet://FREENET-IN-B.CWRU.EDU or 129.22.8.32`
URL: `telnet://FREENET-IN-A.CWRU.EDU or 129.22.8.51`
URL: `telnet://HELA.INS.CWRU.EDU or 129.22.8.38`

Login: visitor

Columbia Online Information Network (COIN)
URL: `telnet://BIGCAT.MISSOURI.EDU or 128.206.1.3`

login: guest

Dayton FREE-NET
URL: `telnet://DAYTON.WRIGHT.EDU` or `130.108.128.174`

login: visitor

Denver FREE-NET
URL: `telnet://FREENET.HSC.COLORADO.EDU` or `140.226.1.8`

login: visitor

Heartland FREE-NET
URL: `telnet://HEARTLAND.BRADLEY.EDU` or `136.176.5.114`

Login: bbguest

Huron Valley Free-Net
URL: `telnet://WWW.MPCC.ORG` or `141.211.210.152`

login: visitor

Lorain County FREE-NET
URL: `telnet://FREENET.LORAIN.OBERLIN.EDU` or `132.162.32.99`

login: guest

Milwaukee FREE-NET
URL: `telnet://FREENET.UWM.EDU` or `129.89.70.58`

login: visitor

National Capital Freenet, Ottawa, Canada
URL: `telnet://FREENET.CARLETON.CA` or `134.117.1.12`

login: guest

Rio Grande FREE-NET
URL: `telnet://RGFN.EPCC.EDU` or `192.94.29.9`

login: visitor

SENDIT
URL: `telnet://SENDIT.NODAK.EDU` or `134.129.105.1`

login: bbs
Password: sendit2me
Login: visitor

Tallahassee Free-Net
URL: `telnet://FREENET.FSU.EDU` or `144.174.128.43`

login: visitor

Toledo FREE-NET
URL: `telnet://131.183.4.100`

login: visitor
Password: visitor

Traverse City Free-Net
URL: `telnet://LEO.NMC.EDU` or `192.88.242.239`

login: `visitor`

Tri-State Online (Cincinnati)
URL: `telnet://TSO.UC.EDU`

enter User ID: `visitor`
enter PIN: `9999`
enter Password: (Press return)

Victoria FREE-NET
URL: `telnet://FREENET.VICTORIA.BC.CA` or `134.87.16.100`

login: `guest`

Virginia's Public Education Network
URL: `telnet://VDOE386.VAK12ED.EDU` or `141.104.22.102`

login: `guest`
Password: `guest`

Youngstown FREE-NET
URL: `telnet YFN.YSU.EDU` or `192.55.234.27`

Login: `visitor`

MEDICAL LIBRARIES:

ALBERT EINSTEIN COLLEGE OF MEDICINE
Description: Interface: LIS

Access: telnet—
  To exit: Press the telnet escape key
  At the first screen that says ALT-H PRESENTS A SUMMARY of SPECIAL KEYS Press <return> for logo, and a <return> for the options menu to search the OPAC.

URL: `telnet://LIS.AECOM.YU.EDU`

AUDIE L. MURPHY MEMORIAL VETERANS' ADMINISTRATION HOSPITAL
Description: At the main menu press 3 for Other Library Catalogs. Press 10 for UTHealth Science Center—San Antonio. When it says ENTER LIS type `LIS`

  This brings up the main menu for the University of Texas Health Science Center—San Antonio BLIS.

  Select 1 from the BLIS menu
  Select 0 from the Library Catalogs menu
  Select 3 from the Change Locations menu
  To exit: Press <RETURN> twice, then type `QUIT`

Interface: LIS

Access: telnet
  This connects to the University of Texas-Pan American. At the Username prompt, type `PACKEY`

URL: `telnet://panam2.panam.pdu`

CASE WESTERN RESERVE UNIVERSITY SCHOOL OF MEDICINE
Description: Interface: GEAC

Access: telnet
>   Type library (must be lower case)
>   To exit: x to exit

URL: `telnet://EAGLE.LIT.CWRU.EDU`

COLORADO HEALTH SCIENCES LIBRARIES

Description: Includes the following collections: Association of Operating Room Nurses, C.U. Health Sciences Center, Denver Medical Library, Saint Joseph Hospital, Swedish Medical Center.

Access: telnet
>   To exit: S to stop or switch databases—//EXIT to end session
>   Choose terminal type from list (#5=VT100)
>   Press RETURN twice
>   Choose #1. Library Catalogs Libraries
>   Choose #25. Colorado Health Sciences

URL: `telnet://pac.carl.org`

COLUMBIA UNIVERSITY COLLEGE OF PHYSICIANS AND SURGEONS

Description: Part of the large Columbia University catalog, CLIO.

You can search using MeSH.

Select 3. Clio Plus: Library Catalogs

Select CLIO: Columbia Library

To exit: Q to Quit

Interface: NOTIS

Access: telnet

URL: `telnet://COLUMBIANET.CC.COLUMBIA.EDU`

CORNELL University

Description: To exit: Type STOP

Interface: NOTIS.

Access: telnet—
>   TN3270 emulation is required.
>   At LOGON screen, press return
>   At CP READ screen type Library
>   <RETURN>

URL: `telnet://CORNELLC.CIT.CORNELL.EDU`

DALHOUSIE UNIVERSITY W.K.KELLOGG HEALTH SCIENCES LIBRARY

Description: This library is a member of a consortium currently serving 8 academic institutions. The name of the system is NOVANET. On logging in you are looking at the composite holdings. Items prefaced with the code DALWKK or DALPHARM (acy) are local holdings. Not all member collections contain medical or health material.

> Currently the member institutions are: Dalhousie University Libraries, Technical University of Nova Scotia, St. Mary's University, Mt. St. Vincent University, University College of Cape Breton, University of King's College, Nova Scotia College of Art& Design, Atlantic School of Theology.

To exit: END

Interface: GEAC

Access: telnet
>   If asked "What System?" type NOVANET
>   Option 3—Subject searching: refers to NLM MeSH and to LC subject headings.

URL: `telnet://NOVANET.NSTN.NS.CA`

DANISH NATURAL AND MEDICAL SCIENCE LIBRARY

Description: Welcome to DNLB and COSMOS Online catalog and ordering system.

        CCL> INFO for screens of general information on the system
        CCL> HELP or ? for windows of screen specific help
        CCL> DO or ! for a window of possible commands to type
        CCL> WHY for a window of the last 16 commands entered
        CCL> DIA DAN to change the dialog language to Danish
        CCL> CCL to return to this screen
        CCL> STOP to end the session and logout Interface: Common Command Language.

Access: telnet
    Username: COSMOS
        At the CCL> prompt type DIA ENG for English

URL: **telnet://129.142.160.101**

DANISH VETERINARY AND AGRICULTURAL LIBRARY (AGROLINE)

Description: To exit, type STOP

Access: telnet

login: agroline

Password: agroline

Type DIA ENG for English dialogue

URL: **telnet://AGROLINE.BIB.DK**

DARTMOUTH UNIVERSITY DARTMOUTH MEDICAL SCHOOL

Description: This system also contains two databases of interest; the PILOTS file, an index of literature on Post-traumatic stress, and Project CORK file, which indexes materials on alcohol and substance abuse.

To exit: BYE

Interface: Common Command Language

Access: telnet—
    1. Type your terminal type
    2. Type the command SELECT FILE [name]e.g.,

    e.g., SELECT FILE CATALOG
    SELECT FILE PILOTS
    SELECT FILE CORK

URL: **telnet://lib.dartmouth.edu**

EMORY UNIVERSITY HEALTH SCIENCES CENTER

Description: The Emory University Health Sciences Center library is included in Emory's online catalog, as choice 3 (Health-Sciences Center Library). Please note that this needs tn3270 terminal emulation and that once connected, the logging in and logging out is pretty can be difficult.

To exit: 1. e to end
    2. 4 to logoff
    3. type CSSF and Press <RETURN>
    4. at the point, do whatever necessary to break the connection (usually F-4)

Access: telnet
    Press <RETURN> at the first screen
    When CP READ appears, type DIAL VTAM.
    When VTAM screen appears, type LIB.
    When CICS screen appears, Press ESC and then 1.

URL: **telnet://EMUVM1.CC.EMORY.EDU**

GEORGETOWN UNIVERSITY MEDICAL CENTER

Description: To exit: Press RETURN on the menu. Type Q.

Interface: LIS

Access: telnet
> At the login prompt, Type MEDLIB
> The password is DAHLGREN
> Type NETGUEST
> Press <RETURN> several times
> Select option 1

URL: telnet://GUMEDLIB2.GEORGETOWN.EDU

HAHNEMANN UNIVERSITY

Description: To exit: <ESC>

Interface: LIS

Access: telnet
> Login: HAN

URL: telnet://HAL.HAHNEMANN.EDU

HARVARD UNIVERSITY COUNTWAY LIBRARY OF MEDICINE

Description: The Countway Library of Medicine serves Harvard's schools of medicine, public health and dentistry. The catalog lists books from 1960 to present and journals received from 1981 to 1992 while continuing to addolder holdings. Dissertations are also cataloged on HOLLIS.

Author, Title and Subject searches can be limited to Countway's collection. For author or title, follow your entry with //fa=md. For example: au Harrison p//fa=md will limit the search of author Harrison to Countway's library. Subject searches should be conducted with ME and a medical subject heading; that will automatically limit results to Countway library.

To exit: Exit

Interface: NOTIS

Access: telnet
> At Welcome screen, press <RETURN>
> Type HOLLIS at next screen.
> Select HU for Union Catalog.

Contact: Questions: contact: (617) 495-9388 or LIBRARY@HARVARDA.HARVARD.EDU

URL: telnet://HOLLIS.HARVARD.EDU

HEALTH SCIENCES LIBRARIES CONSORTIUM, INC. (HSLC HEALTHNET)

Description: The Shared Automated Library System, an online catalog of six health sciences institutions, contains the holdings of eight health sciences libraries including:

> College of Physicians of Philadelphia
> Hershey Medical Center/Pennsylvania State University
> George T. Harrell Library, Medical College of Pennsylvania
> Eastern Pennsylvania Psychiatric Institute Library
> Florence A. Moore Library of Medicine
> Philadelphia College of Osteopathic Medicine
> O.L. Snyder Memorial Library
> Philadelphia College of Pharmacy and Science
> Joseph W. England Library
> Temple University Dental/Allied Health/Pharmacy Library
> Health Sciences Center Library.

To exit: Type EX

Interface: SAL

Access: telnet

URL: `telnet://SHRSYS.HSLC.ORG`

INDIANA UNIVERSITY LIBRARIES

Description: IU contains records for more than 2 million items held by the Indiana University Libraries, statewide. IO does not yet contain records for all items owned by the IU Libraries. While many regional campus libraries' entire collections are listed in IO, only 1/3 of the Bloomington Libraries' holdings are listed. It is possible to search by MESH [`sm=(subject-medical)`]

To exit: `STOP`, then `F`, then to exit

Access: telnet
    Type `GUEST` <RETURN> at the user ID prompt
    R3S Information Online

URL: `telnet://IUIS.UCS.INDIANA.EDU`

MCMASTER UNIVERSITY—MORRIS

Description: Once connected: press 9 on your numeric keypad.
    Move the cursor to `MORRIS` and press `S` and then <RETURN>. To exit: `STOP` and then `PF12` (the <CLEAR> key and 2—This varies depending on local systems.)
    Use `sm=` to search for medical subjects. Use `LIBDATA` to check the circulation status of items (type `==n` at the prompt to toggle between `MORRIS` and `LIBDATA`)

Interface: NOTIS

Access: telnet

URL: `telnet://MCMVM1.CIS.MCMASTER.CA`

MEDICAL COLLEGE of WISCONSIN MEDICAL INFORMATION NETWORK

Description: To exit: `Q` to quit from main menu

Interface: INNOPAC

Access: telnet
    Type `LIBRARY`

URL: `telnet://LIB.MCW.EDU`

MUSE

Description: MUSE is the McGill University (Montreal, Quebec) online library catalog. It provides relatively complete access to library holdings of books and serials.

To exit: `STOP`

Interface: NOTIS

Access: telnet
    Press <RETURN> to wake up the system
    Select menu item number 2 <RETURN>
    Press <RETURN> again

URL: `telnet://MVS.MCGILL.CA`

NATIONAL LIBRARY OF MEDICINE LOCATOR

Description: MENU OPTIONS:
```
Keyboard Problems?
Library Hours and Information Books
Audiovisuals
Journal Titles Owned by the National Library of Medicine
Electronic Suggestion Box
Exit
```

The National Library of Medicine has extended its INTERNET reference services to cover inquiries concerning the history of medicine.

Questions only concerning that subject can be sent to: `hmdref@nlm.nih.gov`

This address supplements the main NLM reference address for more general queries: `ref@nlm.nih.gov`

For assistance with Locator, contact the NLM Reference Section. The NLM toll free telephone number is 1-800-272-4787. The Reference Section may also be contacted through Internet at `ref@nlm.nih.gov`.

Keyboard Problems:

The Locator software supports VT100 terminal emulation and uses the F1, F2, and F3 FKEYS (function keys). If your terminal does not have FKEYS or the FKEYS do not function properly, use the following:

> instead of [F1], press [Esc] followed by [1],
> instead of [F2], press [Esc] followed by [2],
> instead of [F3], press [Esc] followed by [3].

If your terminal does not have arrow keys or the arrow keys do not function properly, use the following:

> instead of the up arrow key, press [u]
> instead of the down arrow key, press [d]
> instead of the left arrow key, press [l]
> instead of the right arrow key, press [r]

For more information on terminal emulation press the Help key `[F1]` or `[Esc][1]`.

The National Library of Medicine (NLM) is the world's largest biomedical library, with a collection of over 4.9 million items. NLM is a national resource for all U.S. health sciences libraries and fills over 1/4 million interlibrary loan requests each year for these libraries. The Library is open to the public, but its collection is designed primarily for health professionals.

The Library collects materials comprehensively in all major areas of the health sciences. Housed within the Library is one of the world's finest medical history collections of pre-1914 and rare medical texts, manuscripts, and incunabula. Most materials are in areas which are closed to the public (closed stacks), and may be requested for use in the appropriate Reading Room. Individuals may not borrow materials from the Library.

Access: telnet

Contact: Joyce Backus
  Systems Librarian, Public Services Division
  U.S. National Library of Medicine
  `joyce_backus@occshost.nlm.nih.gov`

URL: `telnet://LOCATOR.NLM.NIH.GOV`

login: `locator`

NATIONAL MEDICAL LIBRARY—HEBREW UNIVERSITY OF JERUSALEM

Description: Available through the Israeli InterUniversity Computerized Catalog System (ALEPH). We are the National Medical Library, Hebrew University of Jerusalem—Hadassah Medical Organization, Jerusalem, Israel.

To exit: `STOP`

Access: telnet
  Username: ALEPH
  From Main ALEPH menu, type LB/MLB (LB is the command to select a library, MLB is the code for the National Medical Library) Select terminal type. 2 = VT100 (Latin only -i.e., no Hebrew fonts) The library is searchable in Hebrew and other soft fonts using VT320 or VT420 terminal emulation. Use terminal type 17,18, or 19.

URL: `telnet://RAM2.HUJI.AC.IL`

NEW YORK UNIVERSITY MEDICAL, DENTAL AND ENVIRONMENTAL MEDICINE LIBRARIES (MEDCAT)

Description: To exit: D to disconnect

Access: telnet LIBRARY

URL: **telnet://MCLIB0.NYU.EDU**

NORTHEASTERN OHIO UNIVERSITIES COLLEGE of MEDICINE

Description: Also contains holdings of 17 affiliated hospitals.

To exit: QUIT [this cannot be abbreviated] and follow the menus.

Access: telnet

    Type neocat (must be lowercase)
    For VT100, just Press return at prompt.

    The sequence of menus for getting into the catalog is obvious and user friendly; the catalog is not. The user is greeted with a ? prompt. Responding with ? <RETURN> will get the first of several help screens. The basic commands needed are r (for retrieve) followed by a word from the catalog (Boolean searching is available) and t (for type) to look at retrieved records in the sets. The command structure is similar to Dialog.

Contact: Monica Unger—MAU@SCOTTY.NEOUCOM.EDU
    Oliver Ocasek Regional Medical Information Center
    Northeastern Ohio Universities College of Medicine
    Rootstown, OH 44272
    (216) 325-2511 ext. 539

URL: **telnet://SCOTTY.NEOUCOM.EDU**

ST. BONIFACE GENERAL HOSIPTAL LIBRARIES

Description: The catalog also includes the collections of the University of Manitoba Libraries and University of Winnipeg Library. The catalog provides access to the collections of three institutions so users should note the online prompt to determine which institution they are searching. If you are using the system for the first time, type: HELP. If you wish to search more than one library at a time in the system, type: HELP SY

To exit: Type $$SofF

Interface: PALS

Access: telnet
    At the UML=> prompt, type BE

URL: **telnet://UMOPAC.UMANITOBA.CA**

STANFORD UNIVERSITY LANE MEDICAL LIBRARY

Description: The catalog includes the holdings of all the Stanford U libraries. After creating a set with the FIND command, type LIMIT LOCATION LANE to limit your results to Lane Medical Library. There is extensive online help.

To exit: END

Interface: Common Command Language.

Access: telnet
    At Account ? type socrates
    At OK to proceed? type YES
    At terminal? type VT100

URL: **telnet://ELF1.STANFORD.EDU**

STATE UNIVERSITY OF NEW YORK AT BUFFALO HEALTH SCIENCES LIBRARY

Description: The Health Sciences Library materials in BISON include all books, journal titles, audiovisuals and the History of Medicine collection. Besides the Health Sciences Library, BISON includes materials from all other University at Buffalo libraries: Science and Engineering Library, Chemistry/Math Library, ArcPress Lecture and Planning Library, Poetry and Rare Books Collection, Lockwood Memorial

Library (social sciences, humanities, business and government documents), the Law Library and the Undergraduate Library.

To exit: Type STOP

Interface: NOTIS

Access: telnet

    At the ATTACHED TO PORT... message, press <RETURN>
    Type terminal type, such as vt100
    At the UB logo, press <RETURN>
    At the Database Selection Menu, type: BAT (BAT is the only choice for remote users.)

URL: `telnet://BISON.CC.BUFFALO.EDU`

THE UNIVERSITY OF WESTERN AUSTRALIA

Description: The UWA Library holds over 1 million volumes, in 11 library locations, including the Medical Library, Biological Sciences Library, Zoology Library, and Dental Library.

To exit: Use <CONTROL>-D or <CONTROL>-Z

Interface: URICA

Access: telnet

    At the Username: prompt, type LIBRARY <RETURN>.
    Answer Y or N to the terminal question.

URL: `telnet://LIBRARY.UWA.OZ.AU`

THOMAS JEFFERSON UNIVERSITY SCOTT MEMORIAL LIBRARY (THOMCAT)

Description: To exit: E to exit at Main Menu

Interface: LIS

Access: telnet

    VT100 emulation required
    At USERNAME prompt type JEFFLINE
    Choose 1. Library Services

URL: `telnet://JEFLIN.TJU.EDU`

UMDNJ UNIVERSITY LIBRARIES HEALTH INFORMATION NETWORK

Description: University of Medicine and Dentistry of New Jersey

To exit: Go to the main menu and type QU at the SELECTION: prompt.

Interface: LIS

Access: telnet

    VT-100 emulation is recommended. At the USERNAME: prompt, type LIBRARY

    You will be prompted to type your last name: After entering your name, set the CAPSLOCK on. At the SELECTION: prompt on the main menu, type OC for the Online Catalog.

    Note that the online catalog defaults to the collection at the George F. Smith Library. It may be changed by choosing CHANGE LOCATIONS from the online catalog menu.

URL: `telnet://LIBRARY.UMDNJ.EDU`

UNIVERSITY OF CALIFORNIA—MELVYL

Description: Includes the collections of all UC libraries. It is possible to limit to just UC San Francisco, all UC medical libraries or all UC medical libraries-excluding UCSF. To restrict your search use the following command: [your search] AT [location] e.g.,

        FIND SU HUMAN GENOME AT UCSF
        FIND SU HUMAN GENOME AT MEDICAL NOT UCSF
        FIND SU HUMAN GENOME AT MEDICAL

Using the SET command will limit your search to a specific library, e.g.,

    `SET LIBRARY MEDICAL`
    `SET LIBRARY UCSF`

Use the `EXPLAIN SET LIBRARY` command for a more detailed explanation. The `EXPLAIN` command will give you access to the very detailed and extensive online help.

The `MAIL` command will send your search results to you via email.

To exit: STOP

Interface: Common Command Language

Access: telnet
    Type your terminal type and press <RETURN>
    At the Welcome screen type: `START TEN` (for the last 10 years) or `START CAT` (for the full catalog) `START PE` (for journal holdings)

URL: **telnet://MELVYL.UCOP.EDU**

UNIVERSITY OF COLORADO HEALTH SCIENCES CENTER

Description: To exit: `S` to stop or switch databases
    `//EXIT` to end session

Access: telnet
    Choose terminal type from list (#5=VT100)
    Press <RETURN> twice
    Choose `#1. Library Catalogs`
    Choose `#9. U of C Health Sciences Center`

URL: **telnet://PAC.CARL.ORG**

UNIVERSITY OF HAWAII MEDICAL LIBRARY

Description: To exit: Type `//EXIT`

Interface: Carl Systems

Access: telnet
    At the `Enter Class` prompt, type `LIB`
    Select your terminal type Select `5. In state Libraries and Databases` Select `1. Hawaii Medical Library Catalog`

URL: **telnet://STARMASTER.UHCC.HAWAII.EDU**

UNIVERSITY OF MARYLAND HEALTH SCIENCES LIBRARY

Description: To exit, hit the Telnet escape key

Access: telnet
    Hit RETURN
    Select `hsl4800`
    Hit RETURN
    Select 1 for online catalog
    At terminal prompt, type `VT100` (upper case)

URL: **telnet://ANNEX.AB.UMD.EDU**

UNIVERSITY OF MIAMI MEDICAL LIBRARY

Description: Catalog of the University of Miami Medical Library. Also provides access to SEFAIN (Southeast Florida Aids Information Network.)

To exit: `D` to disconnect

Interface: INNOPAC

Access: telnet
    login: `library`

Select terminal type RVS for VT100
Type Y to confirm terminal type

URL: `telnet://CALLCAT.MED.MIAMI.EDU`

UNIVERSITY OF MICHIGAN TAUBMAN MEDICAL LIBRARY

Description: Part of the University of Michigan Libraries catalog.
Use sm= to search for medical subjects.

To exit: STOP

Interface: NOTIS

Access: telnet
At which host? Type MIRLYN
Type your terminal type
Press <RETURN> at welcome screen
Type MCAT

URL: `telnet://CTS.MERIT.EDU`

UNIVERSITY OF PENNSYLVANIA—FRANKLIN

Description: The Biomedical Library catalog is part of the larger University of Pennsylvania catalog. It is possible to search by medical subject (MeSH) sm=ou.

To exit: Use the telnet escape key, or Y

Interface: NOTIS

Access: telnet to
Press <RETURN> to wake up the system
Type VT100 <RETURN> whe prompted for a terminal type
Press <RETURN> for list of valid terminal types
Press <RETURN> again.
Select FCAT from the menu.

URL: `telnet://LIBRARY.UPENN.EDU`

UNIVERSITY OF PITTSBURGH—PITTCAT

Description: FALK Library of the Health Sciences WESTERN PSYCHIATRIC INSTITUTE and CLINIC. Part of the larger University of Pittsburgh catalog. Allows searching by medical subject (MeSH) sm=

To exit: Type QUIT from PITTCAT screen X to exit

Interface: NOTIS.

Access: telnet
NOTE: You must have TN3270 Emulation to access PITTCA
Select 1. Libraries
Press <RETURN>
Select PITT

URL: `telnet:// MVS2.CIS.PITT.EDU`

UNIVERSITY OF TENNESSEE, MEMPHIS HEALTH SCIENCE LIBRARY

Description: To exit: Press <RETURN> at the main library menu

Interface: LIS

Access: telnet
VT100 emulation required
At the Username prompt, type HARVEY and press <RETURN>.

URL: `telnet://132.192.1.1`

UNIVERSITY OF TEXAS HEALTH SCIENCE CENTER -SAN ANTONIO

Description: To exit: Press <RETURN> twice, then type QUIT.

Interface: LIS

Access: telnet
>This connets to the University of Texas-Pan American.
>At the `Username` prompt, type `PACKEY`
>At the main menu press 3 for Other Library Catalogs.
>Press 10 for UTHealth Science Center—San Antonio.
>When it says `ENTER LIS` type `LIS`. This brings up the main menu for the University of Texas Health Science Center—San Antonio BLIS.
>Select 1 from the BLIS menu

URL: `telnet://PANAM2.PANAM.EDU`

UNIVERSITY OF TEXAS HEALTH CENTER AT TYLER

Description: To exit: Press <RETURN> twice, then type `QUIT`.

Interface: LIS

Access: telnet
>This connects to University of Texas-Pan American. At the Username prompt, type `PACKEY`.
>At the main menu press 3 for Other Library Catalogs.
>Press 10 for UTHealth Science Center—San Antonio.
>When it says ENTER LIS type `LIS`.
>This brings up the main menu for the University of Texas Health Science Center- San Antonio BLIS.
>Select 1 from the BLIS menu
>Select 0 from the Library Catalogs menu
>Select 2 from the Change Locations menu

URL: `telnet://PANAM2.PANAM.EDU`

UNIVERSITY OF TEXAS MEDICAL BRANCH AT GALVESTON MOODY MEDICAL LIBRARY AUTOMATED CATALOG

Description: To exit: Press the telnet escape key.

Access: telnet
>Type 0 for VT100.
>Type 3 at the enter code prompt.
>Press return as the function code.

URL: `telnet://129.109.1.12`

UNIVERSITY OF TEXAS SOUTHWESTERN MEDICAL CENTER LIBRARY

Description: To exit: Press the ESCAPE key.

Interface: SIRSI.

Access: telnet
>At the login prompt, type `medcat`
>At the password prompt, type `LIBRARY`.
>Press <RETURN> on the next menu.
>If the main menu looks wrong, Press CTRL-0.

Contact: Diane J. Hudson, Systems Librarian
>hudson@library.swmed.edu
>UT Southwestern Medical Center at Dallas
>5323 Harry Hines Blvd.
>(214)648-4723
>Dallas, TX 75235-9049
>(214) 648-3277 (FAX)

URL: `telnet://LIBRARY.SWMED.EDU`

UNIVERSITY OF TORONTO SCIENCE & MEDICINE LIBRARY

Description: Catalog is part of the University of Toronto catalog.

Interface: DRA

To exit: STOP and then #8. Logoff

Access: telnet
>   Username: UTLink
>   Choose DRA System

URL: `telnet://VAX.LIBRARY.UTORONTO.CA`

UNIVERSITY OF UTAH ECCLES HEALTH SCIENCES LIBRARY

Description: To exit: Press the telnet escape key.

Interface: LS/2000

Access: telnet to—
>   At the Username: prompt, type GUEST
>   At the Kermit prompt, Press RETURN
>   At the Select Destination prompt, type CAT96 and press <RETURN>
>   At the TERMINAL: VT100/ prompt, press <RETURN>

Conntact:

URL: `telnet://MED.UTAH.EDU (128.110.78.1)`

UNIVERSITY OF VERMONT LIBRARIES DANA MEDICAL LIBRARY

Description: The Medical Library catalog is part of the larger University of Vermont catalog. It is possible to search by medical subject (MeSH) sm=

To exit: Press the telnet escape key

Interface: NOTIS

Access: telnet
>   Use TAB to move to the COMMAND field
>   Type LUIS <RETURN>
>   When DIALED TO DOSLIBR appears, press <RETURN>

URL: `telnet://UVMVM.UVM.EDU`

UNIVERSITY OF WALES COLLEGE OF MEDICINE

Description: To exit: Select L off the main menu.

Access: telnet
>   At the login prompt, type JANET
>   At the hostname prompt, type UK.AC.UWCM.LIBRARY
>   Type LOGIN OPAC
>   Select 1 for VT100.

URL: `telnet://SUN.NSF.AC.UK (128.86.8.7)`

UNIVERSITY OF WESTERN ONTARIO ALLYN AND BETTY TAYLOR LIBRARY

Description: The Allyn and Betty Taylor Library at the University of Western Ontario serves ALL the sciences, which include all the physical/natural sciences (Chemistry, Geology, Physics, Computer Science, Biology, Zoology, etc.), all the basic health sciences like Anatomy, Biochemistry, Physiology, etc., plus Medicine, Dentistry, Nursing, Occupational Therapy, Physical Therapy and Communicative Disorders.

>   To exit: Ctrl D to exit/disconnect from the system.

Interface: GEAC

Access: telnet—Terminal type VT100
>   Press RETURN (SEND)

URL: `telnet://LIBRARY.UWO.CA (129.100.2.18)`

VIRGINIA HENDERSON LIBRARY INTERNATIONAL NURSING LIBRARY

Description: Sigma Theta Tau International Electronic Library. You need an id and password which costs $20 for a year (individual). E-mail Lorraine Swedberg at the Library (lorrain@stti-sun.iupui.edu)

Access: telnet

Contact: Lorraine Swedberg at the Library (lorrain@stti-sun.iupui.edu)

URL: `telnet://STTI-SUN.IUPUI.EDU`

WASHINGTON UNIVERSITY-ST. LOUIS MEDICAL LIBRARY

Description: The following libraries have their collections listed in the Online Catalog of the Washington University Library and Biomedical Communications Center: Washington University Medical Center Libraries: Washington University Medical Library, Mallinckrodt Institute of Radiology Library, St. Louis Children's Hospital Library, Jewish Hospital Medical Library, Jewish Hospital School of Nursing Library, Barnes College Library, St. Louis area medical center libraries: St. Mary's Health Center Library, St. John's Mercy Medical Center Library, St. Louis College of Pharmacy Library.

To exit: Press the telnet escape key

Access: telnet

At the PLEASE ENTER DESTINATION CODE prompt, type CATALOG

Once at the main catalog menu, you can search individual libraries or ALL.

URL: `telnet://MCFTCP.WUSTL.EDU (128.252.152.1)`

WRIGHT STATE UNIVERSITY FORDHAM HEALTH SCIENCES LIBRARY

Description: Catalog includes WSU's Dunbar Library (general library) as well as several hospital libraries in the Dayton area, including, Children's Medical Center Library; Good Samaritan Hospital Library; Grandview Medical Center Library; Kettering College of Medical Arts; Kettering Medical Center Library; Miami Valley Hospital Library; St. Elizabeth Medical Center Library; Sycamore Medical Center Library and the Veteran's Administration Medical Center Library (Dayton).

To exit: select h (hangup) to log off

Access: telnet

libnet (must be lower case)

URL: `telnet://130.108.120.22`

Guide to Molecular Biology Database

Damian Hayden
School of Library and Information Studies
University of Alberta

TABLE OF CONTENTS

Overview
Sequence Search and Retrieval
Sequence Database CDROMs
Unified Databases
Molecular Biology Servers
Gene Sequence Specialized Databases
Protein Sequence Databases
Human Genome Databases
Animal Genome Databases
Fungal, Prokaryotic and Organellar Databases
Plant Genome Databases
Culture Collections
General Interest Resources

OVERVIEW

This guide provides specific information regarding matters of access to biological sequence information. Many sequence databases are available through the global computer network Internet, so a comprehensive list of molecular biology resources available on the Internet has been included in this guide. The guide has been written for use by biomedical researchers, students and librarians who require an introduction to sequence database resources. Researchers already familiar with database resources will find this guide helpful as well, due to the annotated list of Internet database resources. It is assumed that users of this guide have network access, and be familiar with e-mail and anonymous ftp, as well as URLs (Uniform Resource Locators).

A hypertext (HTML) version and WAIS indexed version of *A Guide To Molecular Biology Databases* may be viewed at the Clearinghouse for Subject-Oriented Internet Resource Guides (University of Michigan) at the URL **http://www.lib.umich.edu/chhome.html**.

An MS Word for Windows 6.0 version of the guide may be obtained by ftp at **ftp.gpu.srv.ualberta.ca/~/rhayden/mbguide/mbguide.doc**. The word processed version may be downloaded for printing, and as it includes discussion of using Internet tools, is meant as a primer for researchers interested in learning about molecular biology database resources and how to access these resources.

The Guide to Molecular Biology Databases was prepared by Damian Hayden while a graduate student at the University of Alberta School of Library & Information Studies. It is anticipated that revisions to this guide will be made on a semi-annual basis, and updates mounted at the University of Michigan Clearinghouse for Internet Guides at the above Internet address. Any suggestions for revision may be sent to Damian Hayden rhayden@gpu.srv.ualberta.ca. Please indicate to the author as well if the guide is used for educational purposes.

August, 1994

Sequence Search and Retrieval

One of the most common activities of molecular biologists is the generation of nucleotide and protein sequences. DNA is now easily and routinely sequenced by most biomedical research laboratories, and isolated proteins sequenced by specially equipped facilities located at most Universities and research centres. One only has to look at the vast amount of sequenced information added daily to union sequence databases such as GenBank to realize the great extent to which sequencing activities occur. Sequence information is usually the result of extended experiments designed to isolate genes or proteins of interest, so interpreting the long strings of letters in nucleotide or amino acid sequences is of paramount importance to typical experiments in molecular biology.

Sequences do not by themselves yield much information, but must be interpreted by comparing them to other well characterized sequences, to learn of their function or degrees of relatedness to other sequences (related functions). For example, a cDNA sequence (an expressed gene) discovered to be relatively abundant in a cancer cell line may be found to be very similar in sequence to a previously characterized protein kinase regulatory factor gene. Research may then proceed to investigate the properties of kinase regulation in the cell line, which may be the direct cause of cells' neoplastic activity. It is interesting to note, however, that while the generation of DNA sequences is routine for many laboratories, the interpretation of such data by comparing them to other sequences is not a practice which is as typically routine or standardized. Following are descriptions of characteristic methods by which gene and protein sequence similarity searches may be performed.

BLAST

The most popular means of performing sequence similarity searches is by way of the BLAST program (Basic Alignment Searching Tool). The BLAST algorithm is a heuristic for finding ungapped, locally optimal sequence alignments, developed by the National Center for Biotechnology Information (NCBI) at the National Library of Medicine (NLM) at the U.S National Institutes of Health (NIH). The BLAST family of programs employs this algorithm to compare an amino acid query sequence against a protein sequence database or a nucleotide query sequence against a nucleotide sequence database, as well as other combinations of protein and nucleic acid. When used as a tool in published research, the designers of the program should be cited (Altschul et al, 1990). C code versions to run on Unix or VMS are available via anonymous ftp from `ftp://nbci.nlm.nih.gov/pub/blast/`.

FASTA

An older related program called FASTA (pronounced fast-ay) is used as well by many researchers, developed by William R. Pearson at the University of Virginia. While FASTA is available for Macintosh and IBM PC formats as well as Unix and VMS, BLAST is many times faster, and provides an important additional feature of statistical significance scores of reported matches (FASTA does have related programs for statistical significance). FASTA programs may be obtained by anonymous ftp from `ftp://uvaarpa.virginia.edu/pub/fasta/`. The GCG (Genetics Computer Group, Madison, WI) set of sequence analysis programs employs FASTA for sequence similarity searching. There are programs for performing multiple sequence alignments as well. While GCG includes a powerful multiple alignment tool, another excellent multiple sequence alignment and editing shareware Windows program, MACAW, is also available by anonymous ftp at `ftp://ncbi.nlm.nih.gov/pub/macaw/`.

Searching and Retrieving Sequences by E-Mail

The following chapters of Internet Resources list various means by which gene and protein sequences may be freely obtained through Internet Gopher, World Wide Web and WAIS connections. However, some users may choose to retrieve sequences simply through e-mail, or through locally mounted databases. Following are descriptions of e-mail servers and available CDROM databases.

NCBI BLAST E-Mail Server

The National Center for Biotechnology Information (NCBI) maintains a BLAST e-mail server which will respond with search results from e-mail messages with specific search queries. The address for this server is `retrieve@ncbi.nlm.nih.gov`. The e-mail server is a computer program which will automatically read and interpret mail messages which contain gene or protein sequence information. The only real limitation to the e-mail server is a 100,000 character limit to mail messages. Information about the BLAST e-mail server, and a manual for formatting e-mail sequence queries is available by sending a message to `blast@ncbi.nlm.nih.gov` with the word `HELP` in the body of the message.

Formatting a BLAST search request consists of a set of search parameters identifying the program to be used (`blastp` for proteins or `blastn` for nucleic acids), the database(s) to be searched, values related to the search parameters, and the query sequence to be used in the search. All of the GenBank and GenBank related databases may be searched. For example, a simple BLAST e-mail query might look like this:

```
PROGRAM blastn
DATALIB nr
BEGIN&gt
MNKSV40 Monkey DNA fragment, Sample 1154
ggttaaaatggtgattttatgctttgtgtatttaccacttttttttttaagg
cagattcctttcaatcatctgagtg
```

The first line specifies the version of BLAST for nucleotide sequences (`blastn`). The second line specifies the non-redundant (`nr`) nucleotide database. Other BLASTable databases include GenBank, EMBLand dbEST. Lines 4-6 are the query sequence in FASTA format. Optional parameters allow the search to be tailored in a number of ways, including specification of the substitution matrix. There are dozens of server directives, search parameters and output options which may be used in the formatting of a message.

If a message is not made to search a specific database with limitations, a searcher may get back hundreds of pages of information. Although often necessary, extensive manual formatting of BLAST messages is difficult. Fortunately, programs are available designed to facilitate the formatting of BLAST e-mail messages.

Macintosh and MS Windows shareware programs ($25 US) are available from NCBI to make formatting of BLAST e-mail messages easier. These may be obtained by anonymous ftp from `ftp://ncbi.nlm.nih.gov/pub`. The advantages of using these programs are that:

1. No prior knowledge is required on how to format a search request. The databases, other options and sequence for comparison are all selected with a mouse. An appropriate search file is automatically written.
2. Examining the output file (returned file) is more convenient than using a text editor. The summary listing, displayed in a separate box, is always visible so that the user can select any alignment with the mouse for quick display.
3. Saving the interesting alignments to a separate file is easy. The alignment alone is saved into a file and no editing is required. Facility to append several alignments to the same file makes it even easier, as the input filename is asked only once.
4. Formatting a request for retrieving database entries is simple and automatic. Entries belonging to the same database may be written to the same file, thereby avoiding repeated file input dialog.
5. A scrolling utility is providing, to allow easy examination of any sequence file.
6. Sequence text files produced by sequence editing programs such as GeneRunner, SeqAid. MacMolly and DNA Strider may be easily uploaded to the programs for formatting of e-mail messages.
7. Automatic sending is provided for users with direct network connections.

NCBI Retrieve E-Mail Server

As with its BLAST sequence similarity searching service, NCBI provides an text-based (vs. sequences) e-mail server which will respond with search results from e-mail messages with specific search queries. The retrieve e-mail server will search for GenBank records in response to queries such as locus name, author, or accession number. Only one database may be searched ata time. The address for this server is `retrieve@ncbi.nlm.nih.gov`. A manual for formatting search queries may be obtained from the server by putting the word HELP in the body of an e-mail message.

A search consists of a mail message with a set of search parameters, each on a separate line, and a query, which can be on one or more lines. The mail message must be in a specific order: a mandatory line (`DATALIB`); any of several optional lines; another mandatory line (`BEGIN`); and the query on a separate line(s). Each search parameter, followed by a space and its value, is entered on a separate line. While troublesome, formatting of e-mail messages for the NCBI retrieve e-mail server is not as complicated as for BLAST. Even so, NCBI has still made available shareware programs for Macintosh and MS Windows ($25 US) to make formatting and sending of messages easier.

These programs, called IRX (Information Retrieval System) may be obtained by anonymous ftp from `ftp://ncbi.nlm.nih.gov/pub`.

As well as facilitating formatting of messages, IRX makes viewing of retrieved results easier as well. It is an information retrieval system that attempts to find a set of documents that best match a user's question. The matching is done probabilistically and therefore the set of retrieved documents is not guaranteed to answer precisely the user's question, but is likely to contain relevant information. The retrieved documents are ordered according to their expected relevance and so a user typically needs to review only a few documents even when the retrieval set is large. IRX may be a preferred means of searching GenBank to using Internet browers such as Mosaic or Gopher.

NCBI provides software for DOS and Macintosh computers designed to facilitate the submission of new sequences to the GenBank set of databases. To retrieve this software via ftp, access `ftp://ncbi.nlm.nih.gov/pub/authorin/`

EMBL E-Mail Servers

There are three e-mail servers for searching data at EMBL, the European Molecular Biology Laboratory: FASTA; BLITZ; QuickSearch. Sequences encoded in mail messages sent to `fasta@EMBL-Heidelberg.de` may be compared to the EMBL set of sequence databases. BLITZ is used for comparing protein sequences with the SWISS-PROT protein database. To execute a search with default settings, a message may be sent to `blitz@embl-heidelberg.de` with the word SEQ on the first line and the sequence on the succeeding lines. EMBL will soon provide a BLITZ e-mail server for nucleotide searches. For more information, send an e-mail message to `blitz@embl-heidelberg` with the word HELP in the body of the message. For Macintosh users, a front-end application (EMBL E-Mail Search) exists for formatting e-mail search queries to the EMBL server at `retrieve@embl-Heidelberg.DE`. EMBL E-Mail Search may be obtained from the EMBL software archives. Another program for use with the GCG set of programs, called Mail-QUICKSEARCH is available as well. Messages formatted with this utility are sent to `quick@EMBL-Heidelberg.DE`. These programs may be obtained from the GCG or EMBL software archives. Detailed information obout these search utilities may be obtained directly by obtaining documents from the following URL links:

Blitz at `gopher://ftp.bio.indiana.edu/00/Gopher%2b/go%2bmolbio/embl/blitz-help`

Quicksearch at `gopher://ftp.bio.indiana.edu:70/00/Gopher%2b/go%2bmolbio/embl/quicksearch-help`

Intelligenetics, which until recently was partly responsible for the organization of GenBank data, also provides a sequence similarity search program called BLAZE. For information about BLAZE, contact `consult@presto.ig.com`.

SEQUENCE DATABASE CDROMS

Sequence database CDROMs are available for researchers without Internet access and for researchers who require comprehensive sequence databases integrated with sequence analysis programs. Also, there have been recent CDROM releases which are very inexpensive, providing convenience of searching at low cost for any user of biological sequence information. CDROMs available for biological sequence databases include CD-SEQ (EMBL), *Entrez* (NCBI GenBank) and IntelliGenetics. Each is discussed below with a summary comparison.

Entrez

Produced by NCBI, *Entrez* is an application program for browsing an interlinked set of several sequence databases. Entrez operates on Macintosh or PC-Windows computers, and uses the BLAST local alignment algorithm for searches of sequence similarity. Entrez is available in three formats: *Entrez* Sequences; NCBI GenBank; and NCBI Sequences. *Entrez* Sequences contains all known gene and protein sequences, with associated bibliographic entries with retrieval software. The DNA and protein sequence data is integrated from a variety of sources, including GenBank, EMBL, DDBJ, PIR and SWISS-PROT. The bibliographic database consists of a sequence related subset of MEDLINE. The DNA sequence, protein sequence and bibliographic data are linked to provide easy transversal among the three databases. The retrieval system allows for traditional keyword searching and uses pre-computed statistical measures of relatedness to allow queries that will find all articles or sequences similar to an article or sequence of interest. A supplementary CDROM is also included which contains a larger subset of molecular sequence-related abstracts from MEDLINE. A users' guide is included. Source code for an X11 version of the software for VMS and Unix platforms is available by anonymous ftp from `ftp://ncbi.nlm.nih.gov/entrez`. Entrez CDROMs are available from the US Government Printing Office (202-783-3238, 202-512-2233 FAX). An annual subscription consisting of six yearly releases is $76 US. Quantity discounts of 25% are available for orders of 100 or more CDROMs at a single address! *Entrez* may be searched through the NLM WWW. To search *Entrez*, or to preview the capabilities of this integrated database, access `http://www.ncbi.nlm.nih.gov`.

NCBI GenBank provides the standard GenBank flat file format. The release contains the standard index files (accession numbers, authors, keywords, gene names and citations). No retrieval software is provided. The annual subscription price is $45 US.

NCBI Sequences provides the integrated sequence dataset used on the Entrez Sequences CDROM in the ISO ASN.1 standard data description format. DNA and protein sequence data is incorporated, non-redundantly, from GenBank, EMBL, DDBJ, SWISS-PROT, PRF and PIR and is linked to journal citations appearing in MEDLINE. The MEDLINE subset currently consists of approximately 50,000 citations. No retrieval software is provided. The annual subscription price is $45 US.

NCBI also provides a Network *Entrez* client program for use with Unix, Macintosh or PC Windows platforms. This is a network service which utilizes a general "service discovery and request" facility called Dispatcher. The Network *Entrez* application provides functionality similar to the Entrez application which is distributed on the Entrez CDROMs. However, no CDROM drive is required to use Network *Entrez*. What is required is a direct Internet connection between NCBI and a local host computer. A local designated administrator acts as support for Network Entrez, registering a central computer and sub network computer IP addresses with NCBI. The Network *Entrez* client applications then operate through a central computer for accessing NCBI databases. For more information on Network *Entrez*, inquire to net-info@ncbi.nlm.nih.gov Users or those interested in Entrez are encouraged to subscribe to NCBI News. Free subscriptions to NCBI News can be obtained by sending one's name and postal mailing address to: info@ncbi.nlm.nih.gov

EMBL

The European Molecular Biology Laboratory (EMBL) distributes a CD-ROM that contains both the complete EMBL DNA sequence database (which should be essentially identical to the GenBank DNA sequence database) and the SWISS-PROT, PROSITE and ENZYME protein sequence databases. The CDROM, called CD-SEQ, is available from EMBL Data Library, Meyerhofstr. 1, D-6900 Heidelberg, Germany. Tel: +49 6221 387258. E-mail: `software@EMBL-Heidelberg.DE`.

The annual costs ($US) of tapes or protein sequence database CD-SEQ is:

	Tape	*CD-ROM*
Academic user (EMBL member state)	75	150
Academic user (non member state)	150	300
Industrial/commercial user	300	600

IntelliGenetics

IntelliGenetics, Inc. offers two related products designed for differing computer platforms. Both CDROMs include NCBI databases, including GenBank and SWISS-PROT. IntelliGenetics Suite is an integrated package of molecular biology software for VAX, MicroVAX, Sun and Solburne computers. The IntelliGenetics Suite is also available on a time-sharing basis through IntelliGenetics and through the GenBank On-Line Service. PC/GENE is the most comprehensive set of integrated programs available for DOS based microcomputers. It performs over sixty different types of protein and nucleic sequence analyses, displaying results with graphic plots. As with IntelliGenetics Suite, these set of programs help molecular biologists plan experiments, analyze protein and nucleic acid sequences, assemble sequencing projects and support multiple alignment searching. The PC/GENE CDROMs include EMBL, PIR and SWISS-PROT databases. Annual subscription to PC/GENE is $2,750 - $3,800 US (Tel 415-962-7300, 415-962-7302 FAX).

GCG

GCG (Genetics Computing Group of Madison, WI) provides a comprehensive set of over 140 gene and protein sequence analysis programs, designed to integrate with EMBL databases on a set of CDROMs. GCG is a powerful and commonly used set of programs, currently used at over 350 institutions. GCG is not sold with any CDROMs, but is commonly used to support EMBL CDROMs, using the FASTA search algorithm.

Unified Databases

Unified databases are the three main government sponsored databases which seek to include all of the world's gene, protein and related sequence information on a daily basis at a single site. These three unified databases include EMBL (European Molecular Biology Laboratory), DDBJ (DNA Data Bank of Japan) and GenBank (National Center for Biotechnology Information - US).

EMBL Data Library

EMNet Directory: `http:/beta.embnet.unibas.ch/embnet/info.html`

Search: `gopher://felix.embl-heidelberg.de/11/EMBnet%20BioInforma tion%20Resource%20EMBL/Databases/Database%20Searches`

Manual: `gopher://biox.embnet.unibas.ch:13021/00/EMBL/Release%20Notes`

Products & Services: `http://beta.embnet.unibas.ch/embnet/embl-datalib.html`

The EMBL Data Library is an enterprise of the European Community, maintained by the European Molecular Biology Laboratory, Heidelberg, Germany and Basel, Switzerland. Since its inception in 1980, the principle role of the EMBL Data Library has been to maintain and distribute a database of nucleotide sequences (EMBL Nucleotide Sequence Database). EMBL also supports and maintains the protein sequence database SWISS-PROT and distrubutes many other molecular biology databases. The Nucleotide Sequence Database is the main activity of the group, done in constant collaboration with GenBank and the DNA Database of Japan (DDBJ). Automated genome projects are now the major source of data, comprising 20% of the entries in the database. The complete database is available every three months on CD-ROM, magnetic tapes, or by ftp. Updates, available by ftp, include entries since the last EMBL CD-ROM.

DDBJ DNA Data Bank of Japan

Directory: `gopher://gopher.nig.ac.jp:1/`

Search: `gopher://gopher.nic.ac.jp/7waissrc%3a/dna/DNA_seq_index_search.src`

DDBJ is maintained by the National Institute of Genetics, Mishima, Japan. DDBJ comprises one of the world's three main genetic databases. DDBJ maintains daily collaboration and exchange of sequences with EMBL and GenBank.

GenBank

Directory: `http://WWW.ncbi.nlm.nih.gov/Genbank/gopher://ncbi.nlm.nih.gov/11/genbank`

Entrez Nucleotide/Protein/Medline Search: `http://ncbi.nlm.nih.gov/Search/Entrez/`

Text Search: `http://www.ncbi.nlm.nih.gov/Search/irx.html`

Listservs: `bionet.molbio.genbank.all`
`bionet.molbio.genbank`
`bionet.molbio.genbank.updates`

On September 30, 1992, the National Center for Biotechnology Information (NCBI) at the National Library of Medicine (NLM) assumed responsibility for the GenBank Sequence Data Bank. At the NLM, sequence entries are created by specialized indexers in the Division of Library Operations. Over 325,000 articles per year from 3400 journals are scanned for sequence data. They are supplemented by journals in plant and veterinary sciences through a collaboration with the National Agricultural Library. As of April 15, 1994, GenBank has 169896 loci, 80,589,455 nucleotides, and 169896 gene sequences entered. These records join the direct submission data stream and submissions from the European Molecular Biology Laboratory (EMBL) Data Library and the DNA Database of Japan (DDBJ) for incorporation within a single union database.

The GenBank sequence database has undergone an expansion in data coverage, annotation content and the development of new services for the scientific community. In addition to nucleotide sequences, data from the major protein sequence and structural databases, and from U.S and European patents is now included in an integrated system. MEDLINE abstracts from published articles describing the sequences provide an important new source of biological annotation for sequence entries. In addition to the continued support of existing services, new CDROM and network-based systems have been implemented for litertaure retrieval and sequence similarity searching. GenBank is an integrated database, including gene sequences fro LANL, EMBL, DDBJ, dbEST, and patents and protein sequences from PIR, SWISS-PROT, PRF and PDB. The integrated database allows NCBI to reduce unnecssary redundancy in the database and thus produce a more useful view of sequence data for researchers. Major releases of GenBank are now more frequent and the data are distributed in several new forms for both end users and software developers.

Molecular Biology Database Servers

Biologists's Control Panel
Directory: `http://gc.bcm.tmc.edu:8088/bio/`

The Biologist's Control Panel is a good starting point for users who need general database access. The Baylor College of Medicine Genome Center WWW site provides searching of CEPH, *Entrez*, ESTdb, GDB, GenBank, PIR, BLAST GenBank, REF52, SWISS-2DPAGE, SWISS-PROT, Tumor Oncogene Database, YAC (Baylor), libraries and literature, and other resources.

DNA and Protein Sequence Databases
Directory: `gopher://genome-gopher.stanford.edu/1/topic/sequence`

This Stanford University molecular biology server is a WAIS searchable gopher of just about all molecular biology databases. Included are dbEST (Arabidopsis cDNA), Blocks, Cloning Vectors, Codon Usage Tables, DDBJ, National Institute of Genetics, Database Taxonomy (Genbank, Swiss-Prot), EMBL, EMBL Updates, EPD, EST, GenBank, Kabat, NRL_3D, NCBI Repository, NDB Rutgers, PIR, REBASE, Ribosomal Database Project, SWISS-PROT, TFD, Tumor Gene Database and wEST.

ExPASy Molecular Biology Server
Directory: `http://expasy.hcuge.ch`

One of the most popular molecular biology servers due to its multimedia capabilities, the ExPASy World Wide Web (WWW) molecular biology server is maintained by the Geneva University Hospital and the University of Geneva. The server is dedicated to the analysis of protein and nucleic acid sequences as well as 2D PAGE. ExPASy allows users to browse through a number of database including SWISS-PROT, SWISS-2DPAGE, PROSITE, REBASE, EMBL, PDB, FLYBASE, OMIM, Crystallized Protein Images and other world wide molecular biology servers. ExPASy currently handles about 1,000 connections per day.

Genome Databases
Directory: `gopher://genome-gopher.stanford.edu/1/topic/genome_db`

This Stanford University molecular biology server provides species-specific directories and databases. Included are AAnDB, ABtDB, ACEDB, Agricultural Genomes, CHLC, Dendrome, Encyclopedia of the Mouse Genome, Flybase, *Drosophila* Genome Database, Genome Data Base, GDB, GrainGenes, Maize, MycDB, OMIM, Organellar Genome Data, Poplar Molecular Network, Portable Dictionary of the Mouse Genome, *Saccharomyces* Information and Soybase.

GenQuest
Directory: `gopher://rdpgopher.life.uiuc.edu/1`

GenQuest is a Johns Hopkins University interface to the sequence comparison server at the Oak Ridge National Laboratory, designed for rapid and sensitive comparison of DNA and protein sequences to existing DNA and protein sequence databases (PDB, SWISS-PROT, Prosite, GSDB) and the rapid retrieval of the full database entries of any sequence found in the course of a search.

GenTools
Directory: `gopher://gopher.gdb.org/77/.INDEX/gentools`

GenTools includes GenBank, GenBank updates, XXEMBL, XEMBL, EMBL, GrainGenes, HDB, Kabat, LimB, TBASE, MycDB, NRL, PDB, PROSITE, REBASE, CCINFO, TFD, Genome of *Drosophila*, Wheat Gene Catalog, wEST.

Johns Hopkins University Bioinformatics Web Server
Directory: `http://WWW.gdb.org/hopkins.html`

This WWW bioinformatics server is a set of databases maintained by the Computational Biology group (Welchlab) at Johns Hopkins University. Databases included are: GenBank, Cloning Vectors, Eukaryotic Promoter Database NRL_3D, OMIM, EST, Kabat, REBASE, EC Enzyme Database, EPD, PDB, GDB, ATCC, ECACC, LISTA, BOING, GenTools and Encyclopedia of the Mouse Genome. Subject specific Molecular Biology bibliographies may also be searched.

ICGEB International Centre for Genetics Engineering and Biotechnology
Directory: `gopher://genes.icgeb.trieste.it/11/dbremote/datafiles`

ICGEB (Trieste, Italy) provides a comprehensive set of databases for biologists of member countries of Europe and the Middle East. The U.S and Canada are not member countries. GCG, Intelligenetics, BLAST and SRS services are provided. Databases include GenBank and GenBank genome subsets, EMBL, PIR, Swis-Prot, VecBase, PROSITE, REBASE, NRL30, TFD

W. M. Keck Center for Genome Informatics
Directory: `http://keck.tamu.edu.cgi/cgi.html`

The Keck Center for Genome Informatics WWW server at the Institute of Biosciences and Technology, Texas A & M University, is dedicated to providing a Mosaic interface to genome databases. It is presently under development. The server currently includes AGsDB, AAnDB, Domestic Animals, Crops and Genome Topographer databases. Database search capabilities are derived from the ACeDB search software.

NIH GenoBase Server
Directory: `http://specter.dcrt.nih.gov:8004/`

The NIH (National Institutes of Health) GenoBase server provides access to GenBank and EMBL entries, organized by genome and then by locus. SWISS-PROT peptides and enzymes, peptide alignments, PROSITE motifs, and enzyme reactions, substrates, products, cofactors and pathways may also be searched.

Other Molecular Biology Servers
ANU Molecular Biology Server (Australian National University)
`http://life.anu.edu.au/molbio.html`

Australian National Genomic Information Service
`http://life.anu.edu.au/molecular/angis.html`

Bioinformatics at The Jackson Laboratory Directory
`http://WWW.informatics.jax.org/tjl.html`

GenBank, Swis-Prot, PIR, PDB (NIH)
`gopher://gopher.nih.gov/7mindex%3a/molbio/all.mindex`

GenBank, PIR, EMBL Updates
`gopher://ftp.bchs.uh.edu:195/77/`

Genome Database Directory
`gopher://gopher.gdb.org/11/Database-local/GDB`

GENE SEQUENCE DATABASES (SPECIALIZED)

AGsDB A Genus Species Database
Directory: `http://keck.tamu.edu/cgi/cgi.html`

AGsDB is a collection of genome databases specific to genera and species, maintained at the Keck Center for Genome Informatics (Texas A & M). Only just recently developed, the database includes information for *Aspergillus nidulans* (AAnDB), *Bos taurus* (Cow), Gossypium *hirsutum* (cotton), *Neurospora crassa, Saccharomyces* and *Homo sapiens*. More will soon be added. AGsDB is based upon ACeDB search software (see Animal Genomes chapter).

dbEST
Directory: `http://WWW/ncbi/nlm`

EST (Expressed Sequence Tag) sequences are 'single pass' partial DNA sequences derived from clones randomly selected from cDNA libraries. EST data are the most repidly expanding source of new genes. dbEST is maintained by NCBI and included in the GenBank database. Because these data differ from tradituional GenBank entries and thus require special processing and annotation, NCBI also makes them available in a separate database, dbEST. As of June, 1993, dbEST included about 20,000 sequences from humans, model organisms for genome research, and other species. dbEST sequences can be searched by the BLAST e-mail server and full reports of EST records can be obtained by querying the e-mail server: `est_report@ncbi.nlm.nih.gov`. The full reports contain information on the availability of physical cDNA clones and mapping data in collaboration with the Genome Data Base at Johns Hopkins University.

dbSTS
Directory: `http://www.ncbi.nlm.nih.gov/dbSTS`

A new NCBI database of short genomic landmark sequences: Sequence Tagged Sites.

Cloning Vectors
Search: `gopher://gopher.gdb.org/77/.INDEX/vector`

Cloning Vectors is a single database of plasmid, cosmid, phage, etc. vector sequences.

Codon Usage Tables
Directory: `gopher://weeds.mgh.harvard.edu/1`
`ftp%3aweeds.mgh.harvard.edu%40/pub/codon_usage_tables`

This Massachusetts General Hospital gopher provides codon usage tables for a comprehensive list of species.

EPD Eukaryotic Promotor Database
Search: `gopher://gopher.gdb.org/77/.INDEX/epd`

EPD is a database of promoter sequences in eukaryotes, defined indirectly by pointers to EMBL sequences.

HGMP Databases - Probes and Primers (UK)
Directory: `gopher://menu.crc.ac.uk/11/HGMP_DBS`

NDBLIB Nucleic Acid Database (Rutgers)
Directory: `gopher://ndb.rutgers.edu:70/11/etc/ndb-link-files`

TFD Transcription Factor Database
Search: `gopher://gopher.nih.gov/77/gopherlib/indices/tfd/index`

The TFD database of transcription factors is maintained by NCBI (National Center for Biotechnology Information).

Tumor Gene Database
Search: `gopher://mbcr.bcm.tmc.edu/77/onc/oncl/indexonc`

The Tumor Gene Database is a database of genes associated with tumorigenesis and cellular transformation. This database includes oncogenes, proto-oncogenes, tumor supressor genes/anti-oncogenes, regulators and substrates of the above, regions believed to contain such genes such as tumor-associated chromosomal break points and viral integration sites, and other genes and chromosomal regions that seem relevant.

The Tumor Gene Database is maintaind by David Steffen, Dept. Cell Biology, Baylor College of Medicine, Houston, TX. The database is not yet fully implemented. A large number of genes and chromosomal regions and some data about all of these genes and regions is included, but the list of genes is not quite complete and there is a significant amount of information about the genes that is still missing. When finished, this database will include a complete list of all tumor-associated genes, an exhaustive list of facts known about these genes (chromosomal location, size of RNA, size of protein, biochemical properties, cooperation with other oncogenes, etc.) with each of these facts associated with appropriate literature references. All current literature references and critical older literature references will be included. In addition, a list of all nucleic acid and protein sequences available for these sequences will be included.

PROTEIN SEQUENCE DATABASES

Blocks
Directory: `gopher://gopher.fhcrc.org:77/shareinfo/biocomp/databases/blocks`

Blocks is operated by the Fred Hutchinson Cancer Research Center. An aid to detection and verification of protein sequence homolgies, Blocks compares a protein or DNA sequence to a database of protein blocks. Blocks are short multiply aligned sequences corresponding to the most highly conserved regions of proteins. The rationale behind searching a database of blocks is that information from multiply aligned sequences is present in a concatonated form, reducing background and increasing sensitivity to distant relationships. Version 7.0 consists of 2605 blocks based on 699 protein groups documented in PROSITE 11.0, keyed to Swiss-Prot 27. The database and PROTOMAT programs used to create it protein blocks as well as the PATMAT searching program are available by anonymous ftp from the NCBI repository: ftp server at `ftp://ncbi.nlm.nih.gov/repository/blocks` An e-mail server is available for searching the Blocks Database. Send the message HELP to blocks@howard.fhcrc.org

EC Enzyme Database
Directory: `http://www.gdb.org/Dan/proteins/ec-enzyme.html`

The EC Enzyme database lists enzyme classes, subclasses and sub-subclasses. It is maintained by Amos Bairoch, Medical Biochemistry Department, University of Geneva, Switzerland. The 1MB database is available by anonymous ftp from `ncbi.nlm.nih.gov/repository.enzyme`. EC Enzyme is also included on the ExPASy molecular biology server, and on NCBI CDROMs.

ENZYME
Search: `gopher://biox.embnet.unibas.ch:163/71/`

ICDB Immunoclone Database
Search: `gopher://arabidopsis.pasteur.fr`

ICDB contains more than 40,000 records of permanent cell lines which produce homogeneous substances of immunological interest (monocloonal antibodies, T-cell receptors, interleukins, macrophage factors, etc.). Updated and validated monthly, each ICDB description includes: reactant(s), non-reactant(s), immunogen, immunocyte donor and immortal partner, type of product, author(s), distributor(s) and literature references. ICDB is maintained by CERDIC, le Centre Europeen de Recherches et de Developpement en Information et Communication Scientifiques, France.

Kabat Database of Proteins of Immunological Interest
Search: `gopher://gopher.gdb.org:70/77/.INDEX/kabat`

The Kabat database of immunological proteins includes amino acid sequences, related nucleotide sequences and aligned sequences. It is maintained by Dr. C. Wu, Technological Institute, Northwestern University. Information for downloading Kabat may be obtained by accessing `gopher://ncbi.nlm.gov/11/repository/kabat`.

NRL_3D Protein Sequence Structure Database
Directory: `http://www.gdb.org/Dan/proteins/nrl3d.html`

NRL_3D is a protein sequence database derived from high resolution x-ray structures of proteins deposited in the Brookhaven National Laboratory's Protein Data Bank (PDB). It is distributed by the Protein Information Resource (PIR), at the National Biomedical Research Foundataion.

OWL
Directory: `http://www.gdb.org/Dan/proteins/owl.html`

OWL is a non-redundant protein sequence database which allows searching of a number of protein databases simultaneously (Swiss-Prot, PIR, GenBank translations, NRL_3D). Hot links to other molecular biology databases are included.

PDB Protein Data Bank
Directory: `gopher://pdb.pdb.bnl/gov/11/`

PDB is a database of crystallographic protein structures, maintained at the Brookhaven National Laboratory, Upton, NY It contains atomic coordinates for the 3-dimensional structure of biomolecules obtained using x-ray, electron or neutron diffraction, nuclear magnetic resonance or molecular modelling. PDB has had a large impact on stimulating theoretical studies toward understanding protein folding and structure. Most journals encourage or require deposition of coordinates data to the Brookhaven Protein Data Bank. PDB is distributed on CDROM together with the MOBY molecular modelling package.

PIR Protein Information Resource
Directory: `http://www.gdb.org/Dan/proteins/pir.html`

PIR is an integrated protein information resource, utilizing information from the DNA Datanase in Japan (DDBJ) and the Martinsried Institute for Protein Sequences (MIPS). It is maintained by the National Biomedical Research Foundation, Washington, DC, and the National Library of Medicine at NIH.

PROSITE
Directory: `gopher://ncbi.nlm.nih.gov/11/repository/prosite`

PROSITE is a dictionary of protein patterns and motifs used for determining function(s) of proteins. It is maintained by Dr. Amos Bairoch, Medical Biochemistry Department, Centre Medical Universitaire, Geneva, Switzerland. PROSITE may be obtained via ftp (information on Gopher).

Quest Protein Database Center
Directory: `http://siva.cshl.org/index.html`

The Quest Protein Database Center is a facility for the construction and analysis of protein databases. The data is generated by two-dimensional (2D) electrophoresis of proteins on polyacrylamide gels. The Quest Protein Database Center is located at the Cold Spring Harbor Laboratory on Long Island, New York. Currently, Quest includes REF52 2D Gel Protein Database (rat). A Mouse Embryo Protein Database and a yeast protein database are being developed.

REBASE Restriction Enzyme Database
Search: `gopher://gopher.gdb.org:70/77.INDEX/rebase`

REBASE restriction enzymes may be searched by enzyme name, prototype, cut site, and recognition sequence. Description of the database is availanle by anonymous ftp from vent.neb.com/pub/rebase/REBASE.DOC. REBASE is supported by the Ribosomal Database Project at University of Illinois-Champaign, IL.

REF52 2D Rat Proteins Database
Directory: `http://siva.cshl.org/REF52.html`

The REF52 2D Gel Protein Database is a rat proteins database whose annotative proteins are graphically available via www. Maintained by the Quest Protein Database Center.

RDP Ribosomal Database Project
Directory: `gopher://rdpgopher.life.uiuc.edu/1`

The Ribosomal Database Project (RDP) at the University of Illinois, Urbana, IL, offers alignments of the various classes of ribosomal RNA sequences, software useful in manipulating the sequence data, and related services to the interested users.

SWISS-2D PAGE
Directory: `http://expasy.hcuge.ch/ch2d/ch2d-top.html`

An ExPASy database of two-dimensional polyacrylamide electrophoresis gels.

SWISS-3D IMAGE
Directory: `http://expasy.hcuge.ch/pub/Graphics`

An ExPASy database of images of crystallized proteins.

SWISS-PROT
Directory: `http://expasy.hcuge.ch/sprot/sprot-top.html`

SWISS-PROT contains all PIR annotated sequence data converted into an EMBL-like format, as well as additional sequences entered by the curators or translated from entries in the EMBL Nucleotide Sequence Database. Cross references to many other databases are included, and nearly all sequence entries are annotated. SWISS-PROT may be searched using the ExPASy World Wide Web server. As of November 1993, there were 33,329 entries in the database. SWISS-PROT is maintained by the EMBL Data Library, Heidelberg. Germany. The SWISS-PROT protein sequence database is available via anonymous FTP from the hosts `ftp://genbank.bio.net` and `ftp://ncbi.nlm.nih.gov`.

HUMAN GENOME DATABASES

CHLC Cooperative Human Linkage Center
Directory: `gopher://gopher.chlc.org:70/1`

The CHLC Gopher includes linkage maps, markers, integrated maps and genotype data.
The Cooperative Human Linkage Center (CHLC) is a federally funded genome center directed by Dr. Jeff Murray, Dept. Pediatrics, University of Iowa. The goal of this center is to generate a high resolution map of the human genome and rapidly distribute this information to the genomics community. This CHLC Gopher server is maintained as a service of the CHLC informatics core, centered at Fox Chase Fox Chase Cancer Center, Philadelphia, PA.

ESTDB Expressed Sequence Tag Database - Human
Search: `gopher://gopher.gdb.org/77/.INDEX/est`

HGP Human Genome Project at Oak Ridge National Labs
Directory: `gopher://gopher.ornl.gov/11/MajorProjects/HGP`

HGP Gopher provides information on the organization and sequencing of the human genome.

OMIM Online Mendelian Inheritance in Man and GDB Genome Database
OMIM, GDB Directory: `gopher://merlot.gdb.org/11/Database-local/GDB`

OMIM Directory: `http://gdbWWW.gdb.org/omimdoc/omimtop.html`

GDB Directory: `http://gdbWWW.gdb.org/`

Human gene loci, polymorphisms, mutations, probes, genetic maps, GenBank, citations and contacts may be searched with the WAIS searchable OMIM and GDB indices. These databases are maintained at the Welch Mecical Library, Johns Hopkins University, Baltimore, MD.

Other Human Genome Information
Baylor College of Medicine Genome Center
`gopher://elegans.cbs.umn.edu:70/1`

Genethon CEPH Human Polymorphism Study Center, France
`gopher://gopher.genethon.fr:70/11`

HGMP (Human Geome Mapping Project - UK)
`gopher://menu.crc.ac.uk:70/11/`

Human Genome Information
`gopher://genome-gopher.stanford.edu/1/topic/human`

Human Genome Newsletter
`gopher://gopher.gdb.org/77/.INDEX/HGN/hgn`

LBL Human Genome Center (Lawrence Berkeley Laboratory)
`http://www-hgc.lbl.gov/GenomeHome.html`

Physical Mapping Data of Cromosome 11 (Salk Institute)
`gopher://gopher.pdb.org:70/7waissrc%3a/Database-Searches/.wais/Salk-Chrom-11.src`

ANIMAL GENOME DATABASES

ACeDB A Caenorhabditis elegans Database & ACeDB WWW Search Program
Search: `gopher://weeds.mgh.harvard.edu/77/.index/Caenorhabditis_elegans_Genome`

ACeDB represents a collection of *Caenorhabditis elegans* gene and protein sequences and references, utilizing integrated search software specially developed for this database, itself called ACeDB.

The Department of Molecular Biology at the Massachusetts General Hospital has developed a powerful interactive, graphical mouse-based search program which can search this and related databases via the X11 network protocol. For appropriate clients, the ACeDB WWW database searching software displays a navy blue menu at the bottom of each page, with five choices in yellow letters (Genbank, Swiss-Prot, PIR, PDB or All). Clicking on an entry goes to the corresponding searchable Gopher interface at the NIH `gopher://gopher.nih.gov`. In the box that appears, enter any search term, and a menu of links to the entrys will be returned. The ACeDB program is meant for Sun Microsystems, NeXT, Silicon Graphic, and Digital Equipment computers, but may now be utilized by standard terminal emulation at the above server, and ones at Stanford University and the Kleck Genome Center. The ACEDB interface supports more powerful query strategies than Gopher or WWW and provides interactive graphical displays of the genetic maps. On the other hand, for many people the Gopher and WWW formats are easier to access, as well as easier to use. ACEDB access requires a Unix machine running the ACEDB software, or a direct network connection (as opposed to a modem connection) to such a machine and an account to use it, and X11 software for your personal computer.

Agricultural Genomes
Directory: `http://probe.nasluda.gov:8000/index.html`

NAGRP represents a national, coordinated effort to map the genomes of the economically important animal species. The Agricultural Genome Gopher Server is a service provided by the USDA, National Agricultural Library in Beltsville, Maryland, USA. Funding is provided through the USDA, National Genetic Resources Program. The information contained on the server consists of genome information for agriculturally important organisms. At this time, mostof the information is provided through the USDA Plant Genome Program. This includes information about genetic maps, loci, probes, references, germplasms, related data, and a subset of the *Agricola* bibliographic database. There is some animal genome information. In time, the server will contain information about insects and microorganisms.

Bos taurus
Search: `gopher://keck.tamu.edu/77/.abtdb.ndx/index`

This database serves as a repository for *Bos taurus* (cow) genome studies. Bos taurus is based upon ACeDB software.

CGC Caenorhabditis Genetics Center
Directory: `gopher://elegans.cbs.umn.edu:70/11`

The CGC acquires, maintains and distributes genetic stocks of *Caenorhabditis elegans* for use by investigators initiating or continuing research on this nematode. The CGC's collection of more than 1900 strains includes one allele of each mapped gene, all available chromosome rearrangements, and selected multiply mutant stocks for genetic mapping.

Encyclopedia of the Mouse Genome
Directory: `gopher://hobbes.informatics.jax.org:70/11/pub/informatics/encyclo`

The Encyclopedia of the Mouse Genome directory contains WAIS searchable indices of loci maps, notes, references and the Mouse Locus Catalog (MLC).

FlyBase (*Drosophila*)
Directory: `gopher://fly.bio.indiana.edu/11/Flybase`

Drosophila melanogaster genome also searchable at:

`gopher://gopher.genethon.fr/7/wasisrc%3a/liens_wais_bio/.IUBio_redbook.src`

`gopher://ftp.bio.indiana.edu/77/.indices/redbook`

FlyBase is a database of genetic and molecular data for *Drosophila*. It contains all the information in the 'Redbook' (D. L. Lindsley and G. G. Zimm, The genome of *Drosophila* melanogaster, Academic Press, 1992) merged with more recently published information, which include gene sequences, clones, P elements, stocks, genetic maps, aberrations, functions, cytological features, species names, researchers, news and a Drosophila bibliography of over 58,000 records. FlyBase data may be accessed via the Internet Gopher or via anonymous ftp from the IUBio server `ftp.bio.indiana.edu/flybase`. A Fylbase user manual is available here in the directory `flybase/docs`. Flybase is maintaind by Biological Laboratories, Harvard University, and researchers at Indiana University and UCLA.

Mouse Genome Informatics Project
Directory: `http://WWW.informatics.jax.org/`

The Mouse Genome Informatics Project is maintained by Jackson Laboratory, in Bar Harbor Maine.

National Insect Genetic Resources
Directory: `gopher://sol.ars-grin.gov/11/nigr`

The National Insect Genetic Resources program will preserve, maintain, distribute the genes, unique genetic combinations, and genetic diversity of beneficial and destructive insect species. Stock centers will preserve the various groups of pests, parasites, and pollinators that are economically important. The information system for the National Insect Genetic Resources program is under development at the present time.

Portable Dictionary of the Mouse Genome
Directory: `http://mickey.utmem.edu/front.html`

The Portable Dictionary of the Mouse Genome is maintained at the University of Tennessee, Memphis, Dept. of Anatomy &amp Neurobiology.

TBASE Transgenic and Targeted Mutation Animal Database
Directory: `gopher://merlot.gdb.org/11/Database-local/mouse/tbase`

TBASE is a database of organisms and gene sequences which have undergone artificially introduced genetic transformations. Data may be searched by accession number, animal, name of line, method used, DNA introduced, genetic background, gene expression, phenotype, integration site, notes, author(s) and citation.

wEST *C. elegans* Expressed Sequence Tag Database
Search: `gopher://gopher.gdb.org/77/.INDEX/west`

wEST is a compilation of Expressed Sequence Tags identified through efforts of sequencing the genome of *Caenorabditis elegans*.

FUNGAL, PROKARYOTIC AND ORGANELLAR DATABASES

AAnDB An Aspergillus nidulans Database
Directory: `http://keck.tamu.edu.cgi/aandb/anid.html`

This WWW server at the Keck Center for Genome Informatics (Texas A&M) contains gene and protein sequence and reference information on the fungus *Aspergillus nidulans*. AAnDB is based upon ACeDB search software capabilities.

Eco *E. coli* Database
FTP Site: `ftp://ncbi.nlm.nih.gov`

Collection of mapped and sequenced *E. coli* genes.

FGSC Fungal Genetics Stock Center
Directory: `gopher://utmmg20.med.uth.tmc.edu/1`

The Fungal Genetics Gopher is a joint project maintained by the faculty and staff of the University of Kansas Fungal Genetics Stock Center and the University of Texas Medical School at Houston Department of Microbiology and Molecular Genetics. The FGSC Gopher facilitates searching of the *Fusarium, Sordaria*, Mitochondrial Mutants, Multiple Mutants, Chromosomal Alterations, Wildtype Strains and Plasmids databases.

MycDB Mycobacterium Database
Directory: `http://kiev.physchem.kth.sc/MycDB.html`

Approximately 10,000 files relating to mycobacteria are included in MycDBm maintained by the Pasteur Institute, France.

LISTA A Compilation of Sequences from Saccharomyces
Search: `gopher://gopher.gdb.org/77/.INDEX/lista`

The LISTA database is a comprehensive compilation of nucleotide sequences encoding proteins from the yeast *Saccharomyces*. It is maintained cooperatively by the Dept. of Microbiology,, Biozentrum, Basel,Switzerland and le Centre de Genetique Moleculaire, Laboratoire propre du CNRS, l'Universite Pierre et Marie Curie, France.

NGDD Normalized Genetic Maps
FTP Site: `ftp://ncbi.nlm.nih.gov`

Normalized genetic maps for *E. coli*, *Salmonella*, *Bacillus subtilus*, *Pseudomonas aeruginosa*, and *Caulobacter crescentus*. Maintained at NCBI by Yvon Abel and Robert Cedergen.

Organellar Genome Data
Directory: `gopher://megasun.bch.umontreal.ca:70//11/Organels`

The Organellar Gopher is a WAIS searchable set of databases which include Images (organisms, genetic maps, etc.), whole genome sequences, Megasequencing Unit data and organelle sequence subsets of GenBank and EMBL. It is maintained by the Megasequencing Center, University of Montreal.

Saccharomyces Genomic Information
Directory: `http: ://genome-gopher.stanford.edu/h0/Saccharomyces/.welcome.html`

The *Saccharomyces* Genome v. 0.0, Olson Physical Map Restriction Fragment Data, GenBank vector sequences, sequenced genes, and LISTA may be searched through the Saccharomyces Genome Information Gopher and HTML servers.

YAC List
Search: `http://gc.bcm.tmc.edu:8088/cgi-bin/lookup-yac.sh`

YAC (Yeast Artificial Chromosomes) may be searched here by YAC name, locus name, chromosome region or primer sequence. YAC List is maintained by the Baylor College of Medicine Genome Center.

PLANT GENOME DATABASES

AAtDB An Arabidopsis Thaliana Database
Directory: `gopher://weeds.mgh.harvard.edu:70/1`

Maintained by the Department of Molecular Biology at the Massachusetts General Hospital, the *Arabidopsis thaliana* database or EAIS (Electronic *Arabidopsis* Information Service) includes gene sequences, alleles and molecular loci, genetic and physical maps, phenotype images, graphic displays of DNA and protein features, autoradiogram imagesand other information. AAtDB utilizes the ACeDB search software. *Arabidopsis* Expressed Sequence Tags (EST's) may be searched by gopher at `gopher://weeds.mgh.harvard.edu:77/.index/Arabidopsis-dbEST`

AIMS
Directory: `gopher://gopher.cps.msu.edu:70/11/cps/aims`

AIMS includes the ABRC Catalog (*Arabidopsis* Biological Resource Center) and images. The service is maintained by Professor Sakti Pramanik of Michigan State University.

Chlamydomonas Genetics Center
Directory: `gopher://atlas.acpub.duke.edu/11/chlamy`

The Chlamydomonas Gopher includes information on *Chlamydomonas* sequences, strains, genetic maps, plasmids, methods, researchers and references. The gopher is maintained by the Duke University Botany Derpartment.

Dendrome A Genome Database for Forest Trees
Directory: `gopher://s27w007.pswfs.gov:70/11/`

Dendrome is a collection of specialized forest tree genome databases which are being developed by the Institute of Forest Genetics. The initial focus of the project is to develop a genome mapping database for loblolly pine (*Pinus taeda L.*) (see TreeGenes). The databases is updtaed and maintained by the Institute of Forest Genetics, USDA Agricultural Research Service.

GrainGenes The Triticae Genome Database
Directory: `http://probe.nalusda.gov:7002/`

GrainGenes, the Triticeae Genome Database, is a compilation of molecular and phenotypic information about wheat, barley, oats, and other small grains. The project is supported by the USDA Plant Genome Research Program. The GrainGenes database is available in three formats: ACEDB, Gopher, and World Wide Web (WWW), and may be searched with WAIS boolean search parameters.

MaizeDB Maize Genome Database
Directory: `gopher://teosinte.agron.missouri.edu/1`

The Maize Genome Database project is part of the National Agricultural Library's Plant Genome Research Program. This gopher server is in an experimental phase, and will undergo frequent changes and enhancements. MaizeDB is searchable under the Maize Genome Database Gopher server, using WAIS search parameters.

PGDIC Plant Genome Data and Information Center
Directory: `http://probe.nalusda.gov:8000/plant`

The Plant Genome Data and Information Center (PGDIC) is a part of the National Agricultural Library (NAL), located in Beltsville, MD. The NAL has established a Gopher server that allows searching a merged database of all the USDA-supported plant genome databases: GrainGenes, AAtDB (Arabidopsis), Maize, Soybase, and TreeGenes. The Center provides access to a variety of information products and services on all aspects of plant and animal genome mapping, including scientific and bibliographic databases.

Poplar Molecular Network
Directory: `gopher://poplar1.cfr.washington.edu:70/1`

Genetic maps, primers, lab protocols and ACeDB database searching is supported for *Voxpop populus* genomic information.

RiceGenes Rice Genome Database
Directory: `gopher://nightshade.cit.cornell.edu:70/1`

RiceGenes is a compilation of molecular and phenotypic information about rice, supported by the USDA Plant Genome Research Program. Maintained at Cornell University, RiceGenes contains gene and protein data, images and maps.

SolGenes
Directory: `gopher://nightshade.cit.cornell.edu:71/1`

Genomic information on *Solonoceae* (tomato, potato, pepper).

SoyBase
Directory: `gopher://probe.nasluda.gov:7005/11/`

The SoyBase provides WAIS searchable indices of soybean gene and allele information, genetic maps, germplasms, pathologies and references. SoyBase is maintained by researchers at Iowa State University.

TreeGenes
Directory: `gopher://s27w007.pswfs.gov/77/.treegenes.ndx/index`

TreeGenes is a sophisticated user interface and genome mapping database for Loblolly pine (*Pinus taeda L.*). TreeGenes displays RFLP and RAPD markers on chromosomal map positions. Many other types of associated information are also included within TreeGenes such as: references, gene sequences, germplasm, segregation data, images, and trait information. TreeGenes uses optional ACEDB software which was originally developed for the *C. elegans* genome project (see ACEDB).

Culture Collections

ATCC American Type Culture Collection
Directory: `gopher://atcc.nih.gov/11/`

The American Type Culture Collection (ATCC) is a unique private, nonprofit resource dedicated to the collection, preservation and distribution of authentic cultures of living microorganisms, viruses, DNA probes, plants, and human and animal cells. The ATCC Gopher has a number of WAIS searchable databases which may be searched in order to find strains, antisera, cell lines, hybridomas, recombinant DNA materials (clones, vectors, libraries, hosts, oligonucleotides) as well as information about the ATCC, ordering information, and an online order form.

ECACC European Collection of Animal Cell Cultures
Directory: `gopher://merlot.gdb.org/11/Database-local/cultures/ecacc`

The European Collection of Animal Cell Cultures (Porton Down, U.K.) is a self financed part of the Centre for Applied Microbiology and Research (U.K.). The above gopher has been made available by the Computational Biology group at Johns Hopkins University. The ECACC gopher includes WAIS searchable databases of cell lines, hybridomas and DNA probes.

WDC World Data Center on Microorganisms (Japan)

CCINFO Strains and Culture Collections (Japan)
WDC Directory: `gopher://fragrans.riken.go.jp/11/databases`

CCINFO Search: `gopher://fragrans.riken.go.jp/7waissrc%3a/databases/CCINFO.src`

WDC (World Data Center on Microorganisms) Strains and Culture Collections (Riken, Japan) is a WAIS searchable directory. WDC includes HDB (Hybridomas Database), a catalogue of hybridoma cell lines and monoclonal antibodies, JTCA (Japan Tissue Culture Association) cell line database, and CCINFO (Culture Collections Database), a comprehensive listing of algal, bacterial and fungal strains. WDC is maintained by the Japan Federation for Culture Collections (JFCC).

General Interest Internet Resources

BioGophers List:
`gopher://gopher.gdb.org/11/biogophers`

Biology Internet Resources Guide:
`gopher://genome-gopher.stanford.edu/11/topic`

Clearinghouse for Subject-Oriented Internet Resource Guides. University of Michigan:
`http://WWW.lib.umich.edu/chhome.html`

FTP Archives for Molecular Biology:
`gopher://genome-gopher.stanford.edu/11/ftp`

Global Biological Information Servers:
`gopher://genome-gopher.stanford.EDU/11/bio`

Gopher+ Molecular Biology Services (Forms based requests):
`gopher://ftp.bio.indiana.edu:70/11/Gopher%2b/go%2bmolbio`

HyperDoc - National Library of Medicine:
http://WWW.nlm.nih.gov

Internet Resources Meta-Index
http://WWW.ncsa.uiuc.edu/SDG/Software/Mosaic/MetaIndex.html

List of Molecular Biology FTP Servers for Databases and Software
gopher://genome-gopher.stanford.edu/0ftp%3aexpasy.hcuge.ch%40/dtabases/info/serv_ftp.txt

Primer on Molecular Genetics
http://WWW.gdb.org/Dan/DOE/intro.html

Search and Retrieve Software
gopher://merlot.gdb.org/11/softsearch

Search BOING (Bio Oriented Internet Gophers)
gopher://gopher.gdb.org:3005/7

Neurosciences Internet Resource Guide

18

Steve Bonario and Sheryl Cormicle
School of Information and Library Studies
University of Michigan

TABLE OF CONTENTS

1.0 About This Guide
2.0 Indexes
3.0 Resources: Description, Evaluation & Internet Location (arranged alphabetically by resource title)

1.0   ABOUT THIS GUIDE

This document, in its many formats, aims to be a guide to free, Internet accessible resources helpful to neuroscientists of all stripes. As biology, chemistry, medicine, engineering, and computer science all increasingly collaborate in the goal to understand the brain, and information technology revolutionizes how everyone communicates and processes information (the Decade of the Brain meets the Information Age), there is a need for mediation and organization. This guide is a tiny step toward meeting that need. We wanted simply to describe what exists. Even that goal is not fully realized. There are gaps and biases—know that now. But we hope you're surprised by what you find here.

As we skimmed the Net, we harvested resources based on their potential value to a neuroscientist—a researcher, educator and/or clinician. Certain disciplines within neuroscience are more involved in the Internet community than others and those variances betray themselves in what we found. If we can be accused of any intentional bias, it would be that we searched harder for underrepresented disciplines in the hope that our work might light some lamps and encourage development.

In particular, we have described some, but not all the resources related to neural networks. There is a wonderful FAQ produced out of the comp.ai.neural-nets usenet group which summarizes many of the best resources in neural networks: `file://rtfm.mit.edu/pub/usenet/news.answers/neural-net-faq`

There is also a hypertext version at: `http://www.eeb.ele.tue.nl/neural/neural_FAQ.html`

Or check out any of several Neural networks home pages mentioned in this guide and you will find much more.

Also, our coverage of medial neuroscience resources is cursory. Lee Hancock's Health Sciences Resources Guide is helpful in this area:

`file://ftp.sura.net/pub/nic/medical.resources.3-94`

We encountered considerable vision and initiative in the neuroscience community concerning Internet use and potential. There is plenty of room to grow. We encourage you to get involved.

2.0   INDEXES

2.1   Alphabetical Listing of Resources

Adaptive Simulated Annealing Resources
ALS (Amyotrophic Lateral Sclerosis) Digest
American Journal of Physiology
Anesthesiology Archive of the New York University Medical Center
Applications of Connectionist Systems in Biomedicine
Australia National University Bioinformatics Facility - Neuroscience Folder
bionet.neuroscience
bionet newsgroup participants
Brain Scan—Dementia

Brain Scan—Epilepsy
Brain Scan—MRI
Brain Scan—Normal
Brain Scan—Normal—Reconstructed in 3D
Brain Scan—Recurrent Tumor
Brain Scan—Recurrent Tumor (Astrocytoma)
Brainbrowser Texts
Brainstack
Cellular Neural Networks
Center for the Neural Basis of Cognition/Neural Processes in Cognition Training Program Home Page
Center for Neural Communication Technology
Center for Theoretical and Applied Neuroscience (CTAN)
Cogneuro
comp.ai.neural-nets
Connectionists
CT Cadaver Head data - A 113-slice MRI data set of a CT study of a cadaver head
Eindhoven University of Technology Electric Circuit Design Home Page - Neural Network Information
Epilepsy List
European Journal of Nuclear Medicine
Experimental Brain Research
Frog-Net
Head Data: A 109-slice MRI data set of a human head
Idealized 3D Anatomical Digital Brain Atlas
Institute for Research in Cognitive Science Home Page
InterPsych
Journal of Neurophysiology
Los Alamos Neural Network Home Page
Manual of Neuroanesthesia
Medical Informatics Home Page at Georgia Tech's Graphics, Visualization and Usability Center
MR Brain data - A 109-slice MRI data set of a head with skull partially removed
Music and Brain Information Database on MuSICA
NASA Ames Biocomputation Center
Neural Computation
Neural Networks at the Austrian Research Institute for Artificial Intelligence (OFAI)
Neural Web
NEURO1-L, the Bitnet Neuroscience Information Exchange Forum
Neuroanatomy Foundations
Neuron-Digest
Neuroprose
Neurotour
NIH Guide to Grants and Contracts
NIH Image
Pacific Northwest Laboratory Neural Network Home Page
Positron Emission Tomography (PET) Home Page
Psyche
Psycholoquy
San Diego 3D Imaging Group
Schiz-L: Clinical And Basic Science Research In Schizophrenia
sci.bio
sci.bio.technology
sci.cognitive
sci.engr.biomed
sci.med
sci.med.pharmacy
sci.med.psychobiology

sci.psychology
Searching for Biologists
Sheep's Brain
Society for Neuroscience Gopher
Stereoscopic Volume Visualization (Lateiner Dataspace)
Stereotaxic Atlases of Pigeon and Electric Fish
University of California at San Diego Neurosciences Gopher
University of California at San Diego NeuroWeb
VOXEL-MAN Atlases

2.2 KEYWORD INDEX FOR SUBJECT, FORMAT, & RESOURCE TYPE

3D
Brain Scan—Normal—Reconstructed in 3D
CT Cadaver Head data - A 113-slice MRI data set of a CT study of a cadaver head
Head data: A 109 slice MRI data set of a human head
Idealized 3D Anatomical Digital Brain Atlas
MR Brain Data - A 109-slice MRI data set of a head with skull partially removed
NASA Ames Biocomputation Center
San Diego 3D Imaging Group
Stereoscopic Volume Visualization (Lateiner Dataspace)
VOXEL-MAN Atlases

ADAPTIVE SIMULATED ANNEALING (ASA)
Adaptive Simulated Annealing Resources

ADDRESSES
Australia National University Bioinformatics Facility - Neuroscience Folder
bionet newsgroup participants
Searching for Biologists
Society for Neuroscience Gopher
University of Californiia at San Diego Neurosciences Gopher

AMPHIBIANS
Frog-Net

AMYOTROPHIC LATERAL SCLEROSIS (ALS)
ALS (Amyotrophic Lateral Sclerosis) Digest

ANESTHESIOLOGY
Anesthesiology Archive of the New York University Medical Center

ATLAS
BrainBrowser Texts
Idealized 3D Anatomical Digital Brain Atlas
Neuroanatomy Foundations
Stereotaxic Atlases of Pigeon and Electric Fish
VOXEL-MAN Atlases

BIBTEX
Neural Computation

BIOMEDICAL ENGINEERING
Applications of Connectionist Systems in Biomedicine
Center for Neural Communication Technology
sci.engr.biomed

BRAIN
Brain Scan—Dementia
Brain Scan—Epilepsy
Brain Scan—MRI
Brain Scan—Normal
Brain Scan—Normal—Reconstructed in 3D
Brain Scan—Recurrent Tumor
Brain Scan—Recurrent Tumor (Astrocytoma)
BrainBrowser Texts
Brainstack
Idealized 3D Anatomical Digital Brain Atlas
MR Brain Data - A 109-slice MRI data set of a head with skull partially removed
Music and Brain Information Database on MuSICA
Neuroanatomy Foundations
Neurotour
Sheep's Brain
VOXEL-MAN Atlases

COGNITION
Cogneuro
Institute for Research in Cognitive Science Home Page
Psyche
sci.cognitive

COMPUTATIONAL NEUROENGINEERING
Center for Neural Communication Technology
Eindhoven University of Technology Electric Circuit Design Home Page - Neural Network Information
NASA Ames Biocomputation Center
Neural Computation
Neural Web
Neuron-Digest
Pacific Northwest Laboratory Neural Network Home Page

DATABASES
Music and Brain Information Database on MuSICA
Neural Networks at the Austrian Research Institute for Artificial Intelligence (OFAI)
Neural Web

DATA SETS
CT Cadaver Head data - A 113-slice MRI data set of a CT study of a cadaver head
Head data: A 109 slice MRI data set of a human head
MR Brain Data - A 109-slice MRI data set of a head with skull partially removed

DIRECTORIES
bionet newsgroup participants
NIH Guide to Grants and Contracts
Searching for Biologists
Society for Neuroscience Gopher
University of California at San Diego Neurosciences Gopher

DISEASES
ALS (Amyotrophic Lateral Sclerosis) Digest
Brain Scan—Dementia
Brain Scan—Epilepsy
Brain Scan—Recurrent Tumor
Brain Scan—Recurrent Tumor (Astrocytoma)
Epilepsy List

EDUCATIONAL SOFTWARE
Brainstack
Neuroanatomy Foundations
Neurotour
Sheep's Brain

ELECTRONIC JOURNALS
Psyche
Psycholoquy

ELECTRONIC NEWSLETTERS
ALS (Amyotrophic Lateral Sclerosis) Digest
Neuron-Digest
Society for Neuroscience Gopher

EPILEPSY
Brain Scan—Epilepsy
Epilepsy List

EVENTS
bionet.neuroscience
Center for the Neural Basis of Cognition/Neural Processes in Cognition Training Program Home Page
comp.ai.neural-nets
Los Alamos Neural Network Home Page
Neural Web
Neuron Digest
sci.bio
University of California at San Diego Neurosciences Gopher

FAQ
bionet.neuroscience
bionet newsgroup participants
comp.ai.neural-nets
Eindhoven University of Technology Electric Circuit Design Home Page - Neural Network Information
Neuroprose
Stereotaxic Atlases of Pigeon and Electric Fish

FTP SITES
Adaptive Simulated Annealing Resources
Anesthesiology Archive of the New York University Medical Center
Center for Neural Communication Technology
Neuroprose

GOPHERS
Australia National University Bioinformatics Facility - Neuroscience Folder
Society for Neuroscience Gopher
University of California at San Diego Neurosciences Gopher

HIGHER EDUCATION
Australia National University Bioinformatics Facility - Neuroscience Folder
Center for the Neural Basis of Cognition/Neural Processes in Cognition Training Program Home Page
Institute for Research in Cognitive Science Home Page
University of California at San Diego Neurosciences Gopher
University of California at San Diego NeuroWeb

HUMAN HEAD
CT Cadaver Head data - A 113-slice MRI data set of a CT study of a cadaver head
Head data: A 109 slice MRI data set of a human head
MR Brain Data - A 109-slice MRI data set of a head with skull partially removed

HYPERCARD
Brainstack
Neuroanatomy Foundations
Neurotour
Sheep's Brain

IMAGES
Brain Scan—Dementia
Brain Scan—Epilepsy
Brain Scan—MRI
Brain Scan—Normal
Brain Scan—Normal—Reconstructed in 3D
Brain Scan—Recurrent Tumor
Brain Scan—Recurrent Tumor (Astrocytoma)
Medical Informatics Home Page at Georgia Tech's Graphics, Visualization and Usability Center
NASA Ames Biocomputation Center
NIH Image
Positron Emission Tomography (PET) Home Page
Stereoscopic Volume Visualization (Lateiner Dataspace)
Stereotaxic Atlases of Pigeon and Electric Fish

IMAGING
Medical Informatics Home Page at Georgia Tech's Graphics, Visualization and Usability Center
NASA Ames Biocomputation Center
NIH Image
Positron Emission Tomography (PET) Home Page
San Diego 3D Imaging Group
Stereoscopic Volume Visualization (Lateiner Dataspace)

JOURNALS
American Journal of Physiology
European Journal of Nuclear Medicine
Experimental Brain Research
Journal of Neurophysiology
Neural Computation
Pacific Northwest Laboratory Neural Network Home Page
Psyche
Psycholoquy

LISTSERVS
ALS (Amyotrophic Lateral Sclerosis) Digest
Cellular Neural Networks
Cogneuro
Connectionists
Epilepsy List
Frog-Net
InterPsych
Neuro1-L, the Bitnet Neuroscience Information Exchange Forum
Neuron-Digest
NIH Image
San Diego 3D Imaging Group
Schiz-L: Clinical And Basic Science Research In Schizophrenia

MAC or MACINTOSH SOFTWARE
Anesthesiology Archive of the New York University Medical Center
Brainstack
Neurotour
NIH Image
Sheep's Brain

MRI
Brain Scan—MRI
CT Cadaver Head data - A 113-slice MRI data set of a CT study of a cadaver head
Head data: A 109 slice MRI data set of a human head
MR Brain Data - A 109-slice MRI data set of a head with skull partially removed

MUSIC
Music and Brain Information Database on MuSICA

NEURAL NETWORKS
Adaptive Simulated Annealing Resources
Applications of Connectionist Systems in Biomedicine
Cellular Neural Networks
comp.ai.neural-nets
Connectionists
Eindhoven University of Technology Electric Circuit Design Home Page - Neural Network Information
Los Alamos Neural Network Home Page
Neural Computation
Neural Networks at the Austrian Research Institute for Artificial Intelligence (OFAI)
Neural Web
Neuron-Digest
Neuroprose
Pacific Northwest Laboratory Neural Network Home Page

NEUROANESTHESIA
Anesthesiology Archive of the New York University Medical Center
Manual of Neuroanesthesia

NEUROANATOMY
bionet.neuroscience
Brain Scan—Dementia
Brain Scan—Epilepsy
Brain Scan—MRI
Brain Scan—Normal
Brain Scan—Normal—Reconstructed in 3D
Brain Scan—Recurrent Tumor
Brain Scan—Recurrent Tumor (Astrocytoma)
BrainBrowser Texts
Brainstack
CT Cadaver Head data - A 113-slice MRI data set of a CT study of a cadaver head
Head Data: A 109-slice MRI data set of a human head
Idealized 3D Anatomical Digital Brain Atlas
MR Brain data - A 109-slice MRI data set of a head with skull partially removed
Neuroanatomy Foundations
Neurotour
Sheep's Brain
Stereoscopic Volume Visualization (Lateiner Dataspace)
Stereotaxic Atlases of Pigeon and Electric Fish
VOXEL-MAN Atlases

NEUROBIOLOGY
Brainstack
Experimental Brain Research
Neurotour
sci.bio
sci.bio.technology
Sheep's Brain

NEUROENGINEERING
Cellular Neural Networks
Center for Neural Communication Technology
Neuron-Digest
sci.engr.biomed

NEUROPHARMACOLOGY
sci.med.pharmacy

NEUROPHYSIOLOGY
American Journal of Physiology
Journal of Neurophysiology

NEUROPSYCHIATRY
InterPsych
Schiz-L: Clinical And Basic Science Research In Schizophrenia
sci.med.psychobiology
sci.psychology

NEUROPSYCHOLOGY
Music and Brain Information Database on MuSICA
Psyche

NEWS/NEWSGROUPS
bionet.neuroscience
comp.ai.neural-nets
Neuro1-L, the Bitnet Neuroscience Information Exchange Forum
sci.bio
sci.bio.technology
sci.engr.biomed
sci.med
sci.med.pharmacy
sci.med.psychobiology
sci.psychology

NUCLEAR MEDICINE
European Journal of Nuclear Medicine

PERCEPTION
Music and Brain Information Database on MuSICA

PET
Positron Emission Tomography (PET) Home Page

PHARMACOKINETICS
Positron Emission Tomography (PET) Home Page

PHOTOGRAPHS
Neuroanatomy Foundations
Sheep's Brain

POSITRON EMISSION TOMOGRAPHY
Positron Emission Tomography (PET) Home Page

PSYCHIATRY
InterPsych
Schiz-L: Clinical And Basic Science Research In Schizophrenia

PSYCHOLOGY
InterPsych
Psyche
Psycholoquy
sci.psychology

PSYCHOPATHOLOGY
InterPsych

RESEARCH PAPERS
Center for the Neural Basis of Cognition/Neural Processes in Cognition Training Program Home Page
Institute for Research in Cognitive Science Home Page
Music and Brain Information Database on MuSICA
Neural Computation
Neural Networks at the Austrian Research Institute for Artificial Intelligence (OFAI)
Neural Web
Pacific Northwest Laboratory Neural Network Home Page
Psyche
Psycholoquy

SAGITTAL
Brain Scan—MRI
BrainBrowser Texts
Stereotaxic Atlases of Pigeon and Electric Fish

SCHIZOPHRENIA
Schiz-L: Clinical And Basic Science Research In Schizophrenia

SKULL
VOXEL-MAN Atlases

SOFTWARE
Anesthesiology Archive of the New York University Medical Center
Brainstack
Neural Web
Neuroanatomy Foundations
Neurotour
NIH Image
Sheep's Brain
Stereoscopic Volume Visualization (Lateiner Dataspace)
VOXEL-MAN Atlases

TABLE OF CONTENTS
American Journal of Physiology
European Journal of Nuclear Medicine
Experimental Brain Research
Journal of Neurophysiology
Pacific Northwest Laboratory Neural Network Home Page

TAPE AVAILABLE
CT Cadaver Head data - A 113-slice MRI data set of a CT study of a cadaver head
Head data: A 109 slice MRI data set of a human head
MR Brain Data - A 109-slice MRI data set of a head with skull partially removed

TEXTUAL DOCUMENTS
Applications of Connectionist Systems in Biomedicine
BrainBrowser Texts
Manual of Neuroanesthesia

THREE DIMENSIONAL
Brain Scan—Normal—Reconstructed in 3D
CT Cadaver Head data - A 113-slice MRI data set of a CT study of a cadaver head
Head data: A 109 slice MRI data set of a human head
Idealized 3D Anatomical Digital Brain Atlas
MR Brain Data - A 109-slice MRI data set of a head with skull partially removed
NASA Ames Biocomputation Center

San Diego 3D Imaging Group
Stereoscopic Volume Visualization (Lateiner Dataspace)
VOXEL-MAN Atlases

UNIX FILE
Idealized 3D Anatomical Digital Brain Atlas
VOXEL-MAN Atlases

USENET GROUPS
bionet.neuroscience
comp.ai.neural-nets
Psycholoquy
sci.bio
sci.bio.technology
sci.cognitive
sci.engr.biomed
sci.med
sci.med.pharmacy
sci.med.psychobiology
sci.psychology

WAIS INDEXED
bionet.neuroscience
Music and Brain Information Database on MuSICA
Neuroprose
Psycholoquy

WORLD WIDE WEB HOME PAGES
Center for the Neural Basis of Cognition/Neural Processes in Cognition Training Program Home Page
Center for Theoretical & Applied Neuroscience (CTAN)
Eindhoven University of Technology Electric Circuit Design Home Page - Neural Network Information
Institute for Research in Cognitive Science Home Page
Los Alamos Neural Network Home Page
Medical Informatics Home Page at Georgia Tech's Graphics, Visualization and Usability Center
NASA Ames Biocomputation Center
Neural Networks at the Austrian Research Institute for Artificial Intelligence (OFAI)
Neural Web
Pacific Northwest Laboratory Neural Network Home Page
Positron Emission Tomography (PET) Home Page
University of California at San Diego NeuroWeb

3.0 RESOURCES
(arranged alphabetically by title)

Adaptive Simulated Annealing Resources
Resource Type: ftp site

URL: `file://ftp.alumni.caltech.edu/pub/ingber`

Description: From the update: The latest Adaptive Simulated Annealing (ASA) code and some related (p)reprints in compressed PostScript format can be retrieved here.

If you do not have ftp access, get information on the FTPmail service by: mail `ftpmail@decwrl.dec.com`, and send only the word `help` in the body of the message.

If any of the above are not possible, and if your mailer can handle large files (please test this first), the code or papers you require can be sent as uuencoded compressed files via electronic mail. If you have gzip, resulting in smaller files, please state this.

Searchable Index: n/a

Manager: Prof. Lester Ingber
Lester Ingber Research
P.O. Box 857
McLean, VA 22101
`ingber@alumni.caltech.edu`
1-800-L-INGBER
Fax: [10ATT]0-700-L-INGBER

To get on or off the ASA e-mail list, just send an email to `asa-request@alumni.caltech.edu` with your request.

Sorry, I cannot assume the task of mailing out hard copies of code or papers. My volunteer time assisting people with their queries on my codes and papers must be limited to electronic mail correspondence.

FAQ: `file://ftp.alumni.caltech.edu/pub/ingber/asa_new`
`file://ftp.alumni.caltech.edu/pub/ingber/00index`

Evaluation: If you need an introduction to ASA and/or the code, this is a good jump off point.

ALS (Amyotrophic Lateral Sclerosis) Digest

Resource Type: listserv

Subscriptions: To subscribe, to unsubscribe, to contribute notes, etc. to ALS Digest, please send e-mail to: `bro@huey.met.fsu.edu` (Bob Broedel)

Postings: All interested people may "broadcast" messages to ALS Digest subscribers by sending to: `als@huey.met.fsu.edu`

Moderator: Bob Broedel
`bro@huey.met.fsu.edu`

Description: From the masthead: This e-mail list has been set up to serve the world-wide ALS community. That is, ALS patients, ALS researchers, ALS support/discussion groups, ALS clinics, etc. Others are welcome (and invited) to join. Currently there are 130+ subscribers.

Archive/Gateway: n/a

Searchable Index: n/a

FAQ: n/a

Evaluation: Lots of news, information resources, and support get passed along here.

American Journal of Physiology

ISSN: 0002-9513

Resource Type: journal

Table of Contents: `gopher://agate.lut.ac.uk:4077/11/American%20Journal%20of%20Physiology%20%20Consolidated%20-%20Including%20Advances%20in%20Physiology%20Education`

Articles (abstracts): n/a

Articles (full-text): n/a

Online Version: not available

Anesthesiology Archive of the New York University Medical Center

Resource Type: FTP archive

URL: `ftp://anes.med.nyu.edu/ps1/pub`

Description: This FTP archive is sponsored by the New York University Medical Center Department of Anesthesiology and offers a collection of goodies for the neuroanesthesiologist, including:

- archives of the Anesthesiology Discussion Group;
- archives of Educational Synopsis in Anesthesia and Critical Care, an electronic journal edited by D. John Doyle;
- ICD-9 codes in German;
- the Pittsburgh Neuroanesthesia Manual;

- the SNACC bibliography in several formats;
- several software programs, including the ECG Interpretation Tutorial (Windows), MS-DOS Medical Statistics Utilities (DOS), ICU Calculation Programs (DOS), ABG and PFT Interpretation Program (DOS), Seldinger Technique HyperCard Stack (MAC), and Steven Shafer's Stanpump Program (DOS).

Searchable Index: Although not searchable, two index texts are worth noting:
```
file://anes.med.nyu.edu/ps1/pub/index.txt
file://anes.med.nyu.edu/ps1/pub/anes/index.txt
```

Manager: For information, finger `info@anes.med.nyu.edu`
    Keith J Ruskin, MD
    Department of Anesthesiology
    NYU Medical Center
    keith@anes.med.nyu.edu
    (212)263-5072

FAQ: n/a

Evaluation: Nice collection and well maintained--all the digests are up to date. Dr. Ruskin has also mounted a hypertext version of the Manual of Neuroanesthesia (see that entry in the guide) and plans a web server.

Applications of Connectionist Systems in Biomedicine

Resource Type: textual document(s)

Date: 9/92

File Format: ASCII

URL: `gopher://info.lanic.utexas.edu/00/la/Brazil/ftp/mirror/Medicine/neuromed.doc`

Author: Renato M.E. Sabbatini, PhD
    Center for Biomedical Informatics
    State University of Campinas
    P.O. Box 6005
    Campinas, Sao Paulo, 13081-970, Brazil
    Tel. +55 192 39-7130
    Fax. +55 192 39-4717
    Tlx. +55 19 1150 uec br

Description: Published in: K.C. Lun, Degoulet, P. & Piemme, T. (Eds.) Proceedings of the 7th International Congress on Medical Informatics. Geneva, Switzerland, September 1992. Amsterdam: North-Holland, 1992, p. 418-425.
    This paper discusses the potential applications and benefits of connectionist systems in Biology and Medicine and reviews the field in its latest developments.

File Size: 35k

Searchable Index: n/a

Evaluation: A nice intro to bridging the gap between neural network modeling and application in the laboratory.

Australia National University Bioinformatics Facility—Neuroscience Folder

Resource Type: gopher

URL: `gopher://life.anu.edu.au/1/neuroscience`

Login Instructions: n/a

Description: This gopher provides extensive information about the neuroscience programs at Australia National University, including descriptions of research projects, e-mail addresses and phone numbers of faculty. There are also some links to archived listservs and newsgroups. Plans for the future include a WWW version, image databases for persons in biological or machine vision, and perhaps an electronic journal.

Searchable Index: n/a

Manager: Dr Ted Maddess
    Visual Sciences Group
    Research School of Biological Sciences

Australian National University
GPO Box 475
nsconv@life.anu.edu.au
phone: 61-6-249-4099

FAQ: `gopher://life.anu.edu.au/00/neuroscience/ArchiveStructure`

Evaluation: Lots of good information about current research. Can't wait for the image database! The other segments of the ANU Bioinformatics Facility are also well worth checking out.

bionet.neuroscience

Resource Type: usenet group

Date: 4/91 to present

Description: From the FAQ: The system is intended to promote communication between professionals in the biological sciences. All postings to the newsgroups should be made in that spirit. While the general public may "listen in" to the discussions, these newsgroups are intended primarily for communications between researchers. There are other forums on USENET such as sci.bio for the asking and answering of biological questions from lay persons.

`Bionet.neuroscience` is one of the many bionet usenet newsgroups. It welcomes input from all disciplines of neuroscience.

Postings can be received via a listserv instead of usenet, but in time this access method will be phased out. See the FAQ if this option is necessary.

Contact: `biosci-help@net.bio.net` for further help.

Archive: The BIOSCI node at `net.bio.net` maintains the entire collection of BIOSCI/bionet messages. They are available via: WAIS (`biosci.src`), Gopher (`net.bio.net port 70`), and anonymous ftp from `net.bio.net` [134.172.2.69].

Searchable Index: `wais://net.bio.net:210/biosci`

FAQ: `gopher://net.bio.net/00/doc/biosci.FAQ`

Evaluation: A very active group—lots of queries and a cooperative atmosphere. One of the best forums for a wide neuroscience audience.

bionet newsgroup participants

Resource Type: directory

Update Frequency: daily

URL: `wais://net.bio.net:210/biologists-addresses`

Contents/Features: From the FAQ: As of May 1993, BIOSCI at `net.bio.net` began running a BIOSCI user address directory which can be accessed through WAIS or waismail. The database serves as a directory that enables biologists, who are currently using (or even just reading) the BIOSCI newsgroups, to look up e-mail addresses and other information about our users. The raw unindexed data is available for FTP from `net.bio.net` and is atomized sufficiently to allow import into your local RDBMS should you so desire. Send the message "`help`" to `waismail@net.bio.net` for instructions on using waismail. Leave the Subject: line in your message blank.

The directory contains information about name, job title, e-mail address, phone number, fax number, address, and research interests.

Searchable?: yes

FAQ: `gopher://net.bio.net/00/doc/biosci.FAQ`

How to Get Listed:
   1) consult the FAQ
   2) a form and instructions are posted periodically to each bionet usenet group
   3) use a gopher to fill out a form:

   `gopher://merlot.gdb.org/11/biol-search/Biosci`

or

   `gopher://gopher.csc.fi/11/tiede/BioBox/faq`

Evaluation: If you know that the person you are looking for participates in the bionet newsgroup, this is a great, quick way to look them up. Also useful for facilitating follow up to usenet articles which do not necessary belong in a public forum or are too complex to deal with electronically.

Searching for research interest keywords could also assemble a quick list of expert contacts. But remember that the info is self-reported and may be out of date.

Brain Scan—Dementia

Resource Type: Image

Image Type: JPEG

URL: `gopher://gopher.austin.unimelb.edu.au/I9/images/petimages/brain_dementia_FDG`

Description: From Austin Hospital Gopher:
    Scan; Brain scan - Dementia
    Location; UCLA
    Scanner; CTI 931
    Radiopharmaceutical; 18F-fluorodeoxyglucose

This scan shows marked hypometabolism in the parietal region with good preservation of the motor strip. There is also slight frontal hypometabolism seen .

File Size: 24K

Hardware/Software Requirements: JPEG file viewing software

Originating Source: UCLA

FAQ: none

Evaluation: Useful for incorporation into compound documents of text and images. Resolution is fairly good, but this resource contains only a JPEG image, which may not be suitable for research purposes.

Brain Scan—Epilepsy

Resource Type: Image

Image Type: JPEG

URL: `gopher://gopher.austin.unimelb.edu.au/I9/images/petimages/brain_epilepsy_FDG`

Description: From Austin Hospital Gopher:
    Scan; Brain scan - Epilepsy
    Location; UCLA
    Scanner; CTI 931
    Radiopharmaceutical; 18F FDG

This is an interictal study (ie. between siezures). The right temporal lobe is hypometabolic. In fact the whole right hemisphere is slightly hypometabolic.

File Size: 52K

Hardware/Software Requirements: JPEG file viewing software

Originating Source: UCLA

FAQ: none

Evaluation: Useful for incorporation into compound documents of text and images. Resolution is fairly good, but this resource contains only a JPEG image, which may not be suitable for research purposes.

Brain Scan—MRI

Resource Type: Image

Image Type: JPEG

URL: `gopher://gopher.austin.unimelb.edu.au/I9/images/petimages/brain_MRI_scan`

Description: From Austin Hospital Gopher: This Brain MRI Scan study shows the sagittal slices of an M.R.I study which can be accessed and displayed by the "ECAT" P.E.T scanner software. Once image files are converted to a compatible format they can be manipulated and processed using the standard "ECAT" software. Overlaying of P.E.T and M.R.I images and reslicing of the M.R.I into different planes are two of the useful options available.

File Size: 183K

Hardware/Software Requirements: JPEG file viewing software

Originating Source: Unknown

FAQ: n/a

Evaluation: Useful for incorporation into compound documents of text and images. The options discussed (reslicing MRI and overlaying MRI and PET images) may prove interesting. Resolution is fairly good, but this resource contains only a JPEG image, which may not be suitable for research purposes.

Brain Scan—Normal

Resource Type: Image

Image Type: JPEG

URL: `gopher://gopher.austin.unimelb.edu.au/I9/images/petimages/brain_normal_FDG`

Description: From Austin Hospital Gopher:
>   Scan; Normal brain -FDG
>   Location; Hammersmith
>   Scanner; Siemens/CTI 953B
>   Radiopharmaceutical; 18F fluorodeoxyglucose
>
>   This is a scan showing the utilization of fluorine-18 labeled glucose by the brain. The intensity at each point reflects the energy being used by that part of the brain while the scan was taken. You can see greater intensity in the outer (or cortical) areas and the deep central structures. This is the grey matter of the brain. The white matter of the brain requires only 1/4 of the energy of the grey matter. The large wedge shaped region in the posterior is called the visual cortex, and is responsible for all of our visual processing. Approximately 25% of the human brain is dedicated to this function. Even though the subject's eyes were closed during the scan the visual areas are still seen to be using a lot of glucose. The deep central structures are responsible for co-ordinating movement, and are involved in cognitive, higher functions. Many structures in the brain are joined through this area as well.

File Size: 89K

Hardware/Software Requirements: JPEG file viewing software

Originating Source: Hammersmith

FAQ: none

Evaluation: Useful for incorporation into compound documents of text and images. Resolution is fairly good, but this resource contains only a JPEG image, which may not be suitable for research purposes.

Brain Scan—Normal—Reconstructed in 3D

Resource Type: Image

Image Type: JPEG

URL: `gopher://gopher.austin.unimelb.edu.au/I9/images/petimages/brain_3D_recon`

Description: From Austin Hospital Gopher:
>   Scan; Normal brainscan reconstructed in 3D.
>   Location; UCLA
>   Scanner; CTI 931
>   Radiopharmaceutical;18F-FDG
>
>   This is a normal FDG brain study which has been reconstructed using volume rendering to create a 3-dimensional display. The individual projections can be linked into a cine display to give the impression of a rotating solid brain.

File Size: 127K

Hardware/Software Requirements: JPEG file viewing software

Originating Source: UCLA

FAQ: none

Evaluation: Useful for incorporation into compound documents of text and images. The options discussed (for creating a rotating solid brain) may prove interesting. Resolution is fairly good, but this resource contains only a JPEG image, which may not be suitable for research purposes.

Brain Scan—Recurrent Tumor

Resource Type: Image

Image Type: JPEG

URL: `gopher://gopher.austin.unimelb.edu.au/I9/images/petimages/brain_tumour2_FDG`

Description: From Austin Hospital Gopher:
> Scan; Brain - Recurrent Tumour
> Location: UCLA
> Scanner; CTI 931
> Radiopharmaceutical; 18F-FDG
>
> There is a hypermetabolic area just lateral to the thalamus on the left side which represents a metabolically active tumour.

File Size: 53K

Hardware/Software Requirements: JPEG file viewing software

Originating Source: UCLA

FAQ: none

Evaluation: Useful for incorporation into compound documents of text and images. Resolution is fairly good, but this resource contains only a JPEG image, which may not be suitable for research purposes.

Brain Scan—Recurrent Tumor (Astrocytoma)

Resource Type: Image

Image Type: JPEG

URL: `gopher://gopher.austin.unimelb.edu.au/I9/images/petimages/brain_tumour1_FDG`

Description: From Austin Hospital Gopher:
> Scan; Brain - Recurrent Tumour (Astrocytoma)
> Location; UCLA
> Scanner; CTI 931
> Radiopharmaceutical; 18F-FDG
>
> There is an obvious cold area in the parieto-occipital region on the right side, where the astrocytoma has been treated. This is probably necrotic tissue. However there is increased metabolic activity on the anterior border of the tumour, probably representing recurrence. Other brain structures on the right side show the effects of radiotherapy ie. decreased metabolism.

File Size: 42K

Hardware/Software Requirements: JPEG file viewing software

Originating Source: UCLA

FAQ: none

Evaluation: Useful for incorporation into compound documents of text and images. Resolution is fairly good, but this resource contains only a JPEG image, which may not be suitable for research purposes.

BrainBrowser Texts

Resource Type: text document(s)

Date: 1989

File Format: ASCII

URL: `file://obex.scripps.edu/pub/shared_data/BrainBrowser`

Author: BrainBrowser was created by Floyd Bloom, Warren Young, and Yuag Kim. This ftp collection of Brain Browser documents is maintained by Warren Young (young@scripps.edu)

Description: BrainBrowser is a commercially available, digitized version of Paxinos and Watson's rat brain atlas. It runs on the Macintosh using Hypercard. The software itself is not available here, but texts produced by the software are. They include a file of over 300 literature references (Reference Reports), "flashcards" from the educational module of BrainBrowser (Learner_Reports), circuitry data (Circuit_Reports), textual descriptions of structures and coordinates in horizontal and saggital slices (Horizontal_Reports and Saggital_Reports), and full descriptions of places in the brain including the entire circuitry chaining (Place_Reports). All of these files are indexed and searchable using the WAIS sources listed below.

File Size: varies

Searchable Index:
> `wais://obex.scripps.edu/BrainBrowserReferences`
> `wais://obex.scripps.edu/BrainBrowserLearner`
> `wais://obex.scripps.edu/BrainBrowserCircuits`
> `wais://obex.scripps.edu/BrainBrowserHorizontal`
> `wais://obex.scripps.edu/BrainBrowserSagittal`
> `wais://obex.scripps.edu/BrainBrowserPlaces`

Evaluation: This is a little known but potentially useful store of information. One drawback is its date. It has not been updated since 1989.

Brainstack

Resource Type: Software

Date/Version: unknown

URL: `file://sunsite.unc.edu/pub/academic/medicine/mac-medical/hypercard/brainstack.cpt.hqx`

Description: Describes different lobes of the brain and specialized regions visually by clicking and highlighting areas. Includes frontal lobe (Broca's area, motor cortex, smell) occipital lobe (primary visual, secondary visual) parietal lobe (primary sensory) temporal lobe (Wernicke's area hearing). Has textual descriptions with hypertext glossary. Several unfinished features promised in the next release.

File Size: 101K in archive

Hardware/Software Requirements:
> Macintosh computer
> Hypercard player
> BinHex compatible decompression software
> Extraction software

Author: For questions concerning the content of this resource, contact:

> John Mack
> 15 Pine Tree Road
> Huntington Station
> New York 11746
> (516) 385-1294
> compuserve: `70411,377`
>
> Robert Slotnick
> NYIT Microcomputer Lab
> 1855 Broadway
> New York, NY 10023
> (212) 399-0790

Evaluation: The content is pretty basic—middle school to bio101 level.

Cellular Neural Networks

Resource Type: Listserv

Subscriptions: `mb@tce.ing.uniroma1.it` (151.100.8.30)

Postings: `cells@tce.ing.uniroma1.it` (151.100.8.30)

Moderator: Marco Balsi
> `mb@tce.ing.uniroma1.it` (151.100.8.30)

Description: From the announcement: We are now announcing the start of a new mailing list dedicated to Cellular Neural Networks. It will give the opportunity of discussing current research, exchanging news, submitting questions. Due to memory shortage, we are currently not able to offer an archive service, and hope that some other group will be able to volunteer for the establishment of this means of fast distribution of recent reports and papers. The list will not be moderated, at least as long as the necessity does not arise.

Cellular Neural Networks (CNN) are continuous-time dynamical systems, consisting of a grid of processing elements (neurons, or cells) connected only to neighbors within a given (typically small) distance. It is therefore a class of recurrent neural networks, whose particular topology is most suited for integrated circuit realization. In fact, while in typical realizations of other neural systems most of silicon area is taken by connections, in this case connection area is neglectible, so that processor density can be much larger.

Archive/Gateway: n/a

Searchable Index: n/a

FAQ: n/a

Evaluation: This list was first announced in late November 1993 and is just getting started. The sponsors will be hosting the next IEEE International Workshop on Cellular Neural Networks and their Applications (CNNA-94), which will be held in Rome, December 18-21, 1994.

Center for the Neural Basis of Cognition/Neural Processes in Cognition Training Program Home Page

Resource Type: web home page

URL: `http://www.cs.cmu.edu:8001/afs/cs/project/cnbc/CNBC.html`

Description: The Center for the Neural Basis of Cognition (CNBC) and the Neural Processes in cognition Training Program (NPC) are joint projects of Carnegie Mellon University and the University of Pittsburgh. Included on their WWW home page are:
- summary information on the CNBC and the NPC training program
- faculty, postdoc, and graduate student lists and research statements
- upcoming talks and colloquia
- local resources such as the connectionists archive and technical reports
- NIPS*94 information, including abstracts when they become available

Manager: David Redish
Dept. of Computer Science
Carnegie Mellon University
5000 Forbes Avenue
Pittsburgh, PA 15213-3891
`David.Redish@cs.cmu.edu`
(412) 268-3074
fax: (412) 681-5739

Evaluation: This site is particularly strong in providing unique resources in addition to pointers to other sites.

Center for Neural Communication Technology

Resource Type: ftp site

URL: `file://hertz.khri.med.umich.edu/pub`

Description: Currently, there is not much here (code for MU, a research proposal, and a schematic in postscript format), but there are plans to develop this site as the communication arm of a proposed Center for Neural Communication Technology at the University of Michigan. Ideas for the future include an electrode catalog; design rules; electronic schematics; data sets, including MU data sets, sampled analog sets, field-potential data, format standards and confocal data sets; various software packages; and a reference database, including citations, conferences, and preprints.

Searchable Index: n/a

Manager: Planning is being headed by:
Ben Clopton
Assoc. Prof Otorhinolaryngology
Univ. of Michigan Medical School

Adj. Assoc. Prof. of Psychology
University of Michigan
`benc@u.washington.edu`

FAQ: n/a

Evaluation: This could be a valuable resource if plans work out.

Center for Theoretical & Applied Neuroscience (CTAN)

Resource Type: web home page

URL: `http://www.yale.edu/HTML/YaleCTAN-Info.html`

Description: From Ted Carnevale: Our specific idea here at CTAN is to post the following kinds of data:

> code for biologically realistic simulations of neurons (using NEURON or GENESIS)
> code that models the biophysics of membrane and cytoplasm (in NMODL for NEURON, tabchannel for GENESIS)
> detailed tables of accurate quantitative morphometric data of the sort generated by B. Claiborne (U Texas San Antonio)
> other code for simulations (e.g., in C, Pascal) for pickup via ftp by anyone who wants to recreate our published simulations or who wishes to create new models for other purposes.

Other types of data might find their way into our ftp repository, as we generate them. Descriptive text will be provided that specifies the empirical basis for these data, points to relevant literature etc.

Author: For more information contact
Ted Carnevale:
`carnevale-ted@CTAN.YALE.EDU`

Evaluation: The CTAN home page provides access to two ftp archives. One archive is a public directory for source code and papers. The other is an archive housing papers and source code for a neuron simulation program. We have not evaluated these resources.

Cogneuro

Resource Type: Listserv

Subscriptions: see below

Postings: see below

Moderator: Kimball Collins

Description: "For more details about the Cognitive Neuroscience Mailing List, including how to subscribe, how to get archives, and posting guidelines, please send email to me at: `cogneuro-request@ptolemy.arc.nasa.gov` with `cogneuro: send info` in the subject line, and I will reply manually with the latest information."

From the announcement: The Cognitive Neuroscience Mailing List is a way to discuss phenomena at the interface of cognitive science (broadly construed) and biology. The discussion is scientific, multi-disciplinary, and academic. Topics include:

- behavioral aspects of neuroanatomy and neurophysiology;
- biological aspects of particular sets of behaviors;
- the neuropsychology of ecology, ethology, genetics, ontogeny, endocrinology, info. science, and pharmacology;
- new imaging, simulation, and measurement techniques;
- books, papers, research directions, and new results;
- curricula, graduate programs, jobs, zeitgeist, and funding.

"Behavior" above is an attempt at a theory-independent, catch-all term for cognition, emotion, volition, and meaningful action in humans and other animals, normal and abnormal, including subjective reports.

Primary emphasis tends to be on science (measurable phenomena) more than philosophy, and on the field itself more than its implications.

Archive/Gateway: `file://ego.psych.mcgill.ca/pub/cogneuro`

Searchable Index: n/a

FAQ: n/a

Evaluation: We have not personally monitored this listserv.

comp.ai.neural-nets

Resource Type: usenet group

Date: unknown

Description: From the FAQ: The newsgroup comp.ai.neural-nets is intended as a forum for people who want to use or explore the capabilities of Artificial Neural Networks or Neural-Network-like structures. Postings may take the form of requests, questions, answers, summaries, announcements, reports, or discussions [more explicit guidelines for these categories are available in the FAQ.] In addition, several regular postings show up here including Paul Bakker's list of conferences and Neuron Digest.

Archive: n/a

Searchable Index: n/a

FAQ: `file://rtfm.mit.edu/pub/usenet/news.answers/neural-net-faq`
`http://www.eeb.ele.tue.nl/neural/neural_FAQ.html`

Evaluation: Great FAQ! A terrific resource for neural network information on the Internet.

Connectionists

Resource Type: Listserv

Subscriptions: `Connectionists-Request@cs.cmu.edu`

Postings: `Connectionists@cs.cmu.edu`

Moderator: Dave Touretzky
David Redish

Description: From a message received when we tried to subscribe:

Connectionists is a restricted mailing list primarily intended for discussion of technical issues relating to neural computation, and dissemination of information directly relevant to researchers in the field. It is NOT a public digest like AIList or the NEURON digest; membership is restricted to students and faculty members who are actively involved in connectionist research. If you would kindly send a list of your papers or other activities in this area, we will be glad to add you to the list. Please include your full name.

Archive/Gateway: `ftp://b.gp.cs.cmu.edu/afs/cs/project/connect/connect-archives`

Searchable Index: n/a

FAQ: n/a

Evaluation: From what we've seen, this list is active and their restrictions on participation keep it focused.

CT Cadaver Head data: A 113-slice MRI data set of a CT study of a cadaver head

Resource Type: data set

Date: n/a

URL: `file://omicron.cs.unc.edu/pub/softlab/CHVRTD/volII`

Description: From announcement at softlab ftp site: A 113-slice MRI data set of a CT study of a cadaver head. Slices are stored consecutively as a 256 x 256 array with dimensions of z-113 y-256 x-256 in z-y-x order. Format is 16-bit integers—two consecutive bytes make up one binary integer. We (Softlabs) do not object to your further distributing these datasets, but we request that full acknowledgement of the source of the data accompany such distribution. If you are going to send a dataset to someone, please also send the accompanying information file. [An installation manual is available in the same folder.] For customers interested in purchasing the datasets on tape, both Volume I and Volume II can be purchased for $50.00 each, or $90.00 as a set. The distribution is available in two different formats. The files on the tape will be written from a DEC VAX computer using the UNIX file copy command `dd` or the UNIX `tar` command. Total block size is 8192 bytes written at 1600 bpi on either a standard

1/2" magnetic tape or a cartridge tape. Please specify your preference when ordering and note that `dd` is not available with the cartridge tape. Installation instructions accompany the distribution.

File Size: 14,811,136 bytes total file size

Hardware/Software Requirements: Software to view these images is not provided with the datasets. When we inquired as to suitable viewing software, we received the following reply from Graham Gash:

> The data we distribute is 3D volume data in raw form. The purpose of our distributing these data sets was to provide a standard suite of data for testing and comparison of various volume visualization methods. Users of these data sets must convert them into whatever format is required by the software they intend to run. Most serious image processing packages provide some capability for making such conversions. The datasets were written on a Digital Equipment Corporation (DEC) VAX computer. Each file contains only pixels, stored in row major order with 2-byte integers per pixel. To use the images on machines that have normal byte order (DECs use reverse byte order), you should swap alternate bytes, for example using the 'dd' command in UNIX. The important thing for those interested in these data sets to realize is that there is a dearth of auxiliary data about them. In particular, practically the only such data available are the dimensions of the images.
>
> In addition, we distribute two packages for image processing, with a somewhat medical slant. The older one, written in C, is called `/usr/image/`. It consists of a small library of file I/O functions, and about 100 application programs built on that library. The other package, called `/usr/Image/`, consists of 6 C++ libraries called DIAL, that perform I/O and a lot more, a few new C++ programs and the original set of programs, which work with the C++ libraries through a "compatibility library". We will eventually convert the C programs to C++. Both of these packages are downloadable via ftp, but they are presently licensed. In the future (probably within 6 months), the C++ libraries (possibly also the programs) will be freely distributable (a la the GNU software).

Originating Source: Data taken on the General Electric CT Scanner and provided courtesy of North Carolina Memorial Hospital. Made available by Softlabs.

> Natalie E. Sipes
> SoftLab Coordinator
> email: `softlab@cs.unc.edu`
> telephone: 919-962-1960
> SoftLab Software Systems Laboratory
> CB# 3175, 361 Sitterson Hall
> University of North Carolina
> Department of Computer Science
> Chapel Hill, North Carolina 27599-3175

> Graham Gash, Ph.D.
> Medical Image Processing Manager
> `gash@cs.unc.edu` or `gash@cv.ruu.nl`
> Department of Computer Science
> Phone: (919) 962-1725
> FAX: (919) 962-1799
> University of North Carolina
> Chapel Hill, N.C. 27599-3175

Evaluation: We have not looked at this dataset personally. E-mail inquiries were handled very expediently, however.

Eindhoven University of Technology Electric Circuit Design Home Page—Neural Network Information

Resource Type: web home page

URL: `http://www.eeb.ele.tue.nl/neural/neural.html`

Description: The sponsors of this resource are interested in the electronic implementation of neural networks using analog hardware. This page provides general information about neural networks as well as more specialized subjects on the electronic implementation. It now contains some general information on neurons, a link to Neuroprose, several reports by members and graduate students of their group on both algorithms and analog electronic implementations, and a hypertext version of the comp.ai.neural-nets FAQ.

Manager: Send any suggestions on information which could also be made public on this page to:
Heini Withagen
`www@eeb.ele.tue.nl`.

Evaluation: It's been fun to watch this resource evolve last two months. The FAQ greatly expands it's scope.

Epilepsy List

Resource Type: listserv

Subscriptions: `listserv@calvin.dgbt.doc.ca`

Postings: `epilepsy-list@calvin.dgbt.doc.ca`

Moderator: Andrew Patrick, Ph.D.
Communications Research Centre,
Ottawa, Canada
`andrew@calvin.dgbt.doc.CA`

Description: This mailing list is intended for discussions about epilepsy and seizure disorders.

Archive/Gateway: n/a

Searchable Index: n/a

FAQ: n/a

Evaluation: We have not personally monitored this list.

European Journal of Nuclear Medicine

ISSN: 0340-6997

Resource Type: journal

Table of Contents: `gopher://trick.ntp.springer.de/11/TOC/259`

Articles (abstracts): not available

Articles (full-text): not available

Subscription Info: not available

Online Version: not available

Other Notes: List of issues presented as a gopher menu organized chronologically by year, month, volume and issue number. Each gopher menu item corresponds to a file containing that issue's table of contents. The table of contents are part of a two-year experiment by publisher Springer-Verlag. Contents are in an ASCII format and tagged to BRS Medline conventions for downloading into personal bibliographic software.

From Springer-Verlag: "The aim of the European Journal of Nuclear Medicine is to provide a forum for the exchange of clinical and scientific information for the nuclear medicine community. The European Journal of Nuclear Medicine will be of primary interest to doctors practising in the field of nuclear medicine, but original works relating to clinical nuclear medicine in physics, dosimetry, radiation biology, computer science, radiopharmacy and radiochemistry are also welcome. The European Journal of Nuclear Medicine also publishes in-depth reviews of topical subjects. Case reports are published only if they are of outstanding interest. All manuscripts should be formulated so that the average reader can at least grasp the general principles of the subject matter."

Experimental Brain Research

ISSN: 0014-4819

Resource Type: journal

Table of Contents: `gopher://morris.lib.udel.edu:70/11/indexes//toc/springer/ebr`

Articles (abstracts): not available

Articles (full-text): not available

Subscription Info: not available

Online Version: not available

Other Notes: List of issues presented as a gopher menu organized chronologically by year, month, volume and issue number. Each gopher menu item corresponds to a file containing that issue's table of contents.

The table of contents are part of a two-year experiment by publisher Springer-Verlag. Contents are in an ASCII format and tagged to BRS Medline conventions for downloading into personal bibliographic software.

From Springer-Verlag: "Experimental Brain Research accepts original contributions on many aspects of experimental research of the central and peripheral nervous system in the fields of morphology, physiology, behaviour, neurochemistry, developmental neurobiology, and experimental pathology relevant to general problems of cerebral function."

Frog-Net

Resource Type: Listserv

Subscriptions: `liaw@rana.usc.edu`

Postings: `frog-net@rana.usc.edu`

Moderator: Jim Liaw
Center for Neural Engineering
Univ. of Southern California
Los Angeles, CA 90089-2520
(213) 740-6991
`liaw@rana.usc.edu`

Description: From the announcement: This mailing list is set up to facilitate the communication and interaction among researchers interested in the behavior and the underlying neural mechanisms in amphibians.

Archive/Gateway: n/a

Searchable Index: n/a

FAQ: n/a

Evaluation: We have not monitored this listserv personally.

Head data: A 109 slice MRI data set of a human head

Resource Type: data set

Date: n/a

URL: `file://omicron.cs.unc.edu/pub/softlab/CHVRTD/volI`

Description: From announcement at softlab ftp site: A 109-slice MRI data set of a human head. Complete slices are stored consecutively as a 256 x 256 array. Pixels consist of 2 consecutive bytes making one binary integer. We (Softlabs) do not object to your further distributing these datasets, but we request that full acknowledgement of the source of the data accompany such distribution. If you are going to send a dataset to someone, please also send the accompanying information file. [An installation manual is available in the same folder.]

For customers interested in purchasing the datasets on tape, both Volume I and Volume II can be purchased for $50.00 each, or $90.00 as a set. The distribution is available in two different formats. The files on the tape will be written from a DEC VAX computer using the UNIX file copy command `dd` or the UNIX `tar` command. Total block size is 8192 bytes written at 1600 bpi on either a standard 1/2" magnetic tape or a cartridge tape. Please specify your preference when ordering and note that `dd` is not available with the cartridge tape. Installation instructions accompany the distribution.

File Size: n/a

Hardware/Software Requirements: Software to view these images is not provided with the datasets. When we inquired as to suitable viewing software, we received the following reply from Graham Gash:

The data we distribute is 3D volume data in raw form. The purpose of our distributing these data sets was to provide a standard suite of data for testing and comparison of various volume visualization methods. Users of these data sets must convert them into whatever format is required by the software they intend to run. Most serious image processing packages provide some capability for making such conversions. The datasets were written on a Digital Equipment Corporation (DEC) VAX computer. Each file contains only pixels, stored in row major order with 2-byte integers per pixel. To use the images on machines that have normal byte order (DECs use reverse byte order), you should swap alternate bytes, for example using the 'dd' command in UNIX. The important thing for those interested in these data sets to realize is that there is a dearth of auxiliary data about them. In particular, practically the only such data available are the dimensions of the images.

In addition, we distribute two packages for image processing, with a somewhat medical slant. The older one, written in C, is called /usr/image/. It consists of a small library of file I/O functions, and about 100 application programs built on that library. The other package, called /usr/Image/, consists of 6 C++ libraries called DIAL, that perform I/O and a lot more, a few new C++ programs and the original set of programs, which work with the C++ libraries through a "compatibility library". We will eventually convert the C programs to C++. Both of these packages are downloadable via ftp, but they are presently licensed. In the future (probably within 6 months), the C++ libraries (possibly also the programs) will be freely distributable (a la the GNU software).

Originating Source: Data taken on the Siemens Magnetom and provided courtesy of Siemens Medical Systems, Inc., Iselin, NJ. Made available by Softlabs.

> Natalie E. Sipes
> SoftLab Coordinator
> email: softlab@cs.unc.edu
> telephone: 919-962-1960
> SoftLab Software Systems Laboratory
> CB# 3175, 361 Sitterson Hall
> University of North Carolina
> Department of Computer Science
> Chapel Hill, North Carolina 27599-3175

> Graham Gash, Ph.D.
> Medical Image Processing Manager
> gash@cs.unc.edu or gash@cv.ruu.nl
> Department of Computer Science
> Phone: (919) 962-1725
> FAX: (919) 962-1799
> University of North Carolina
> Chapel Hill, N.C. 27599-3175

Evaluation: We have not looked at this dataset personally. E-mail inquiries were handled very expediently, however.

Idealized 3D Anatomical Digital Brain Atlas

Resource Type: Software

Date/Version: 1992/1.1 (ongoing)

URL: ftp://etro.vub.ac.be/pub/idDAB

Description: From the Readme file: The accompanied files (sl_m_40 till sl_p_60, grid) contain the data of a digital idealised atlas of the human brain (idDAB). The work is part of an on-going project supported by the European Community, DGFXIII, Framework AIM (Advanced Informatics in Medicine), Contract A2032, Project SAMMIE (Software Applied to MultiModal Images and Education) 92-95.

The file idDAB.doc contains the postscript version of the document delivered to the Commission of the European Communities:

R. Deklerck, F.J Schuier, B. De Cuyper, S. Van Liefferinge, IDEALIZED 3D Anatomical Digital Brain Atlas, Del 05, Project AIM, A2032, 7/92. In this document a detailed description of the contents of the files can be found.

File Size: 557k (tar.Z)

Hardware/Software Requirements: UNIX-based platform

Author: n/a

Evaluation: We have been unable to evaluate this software.

Institute for Research in Cognitive Science Home Page

Resource Type: web home page

URL: http://www.cis.upenn.edu/~ircs/homepage.html

Description: The Institute for Research in Cognitive Science at the University of Pennsylvania is the site of the National Science Foundation Science and Technology Center for Research in Cognitive Science. This WWW page contains information about the center, its faculty, and its activities including the postdoctoral fellow program; short- and long-term visitor program; newsletter series; outreach program; weekly seminar series; technical report series; workshops; and an industrial interaction program.

Manager: `jbkerper@central.cis.upenn.edu`

Evaluation: So far this is primarily a hypertext brochure about the IRCS with the exception of their archive of technical reports.

InterPsych

Resource Type: Listserv

Subscriptions: Each subject area sublist must be subscribed to individually. To join send mail to:
`mailbase@mailbase.ac.uk`

The body of the message should say: join `<listname>` `<firstname>` `<lastname>` (where `<listname>` is the name of the sublist and `<firstname>` `<lastname>` are your first and last names.)

Postings: Postings should be sent to: `<listname>@mailbase.ac.uk` (Where `<listname>` is the name of the sublist.)

Moderator: **`psychiatry-request@mailbase.ac.uk`**
Ian Pitchford
Department of Biomedical Science
University of Sheffield
United Kingdom
`I.Pitchford@Sheffield.ac.uk`

Description: InterPsych is an international electronic forum with the aim of promoting international scholarly collaboration on inter-disciplinary research efforts in the field of psychopathology. A number of electronic mail discussion groups are maintained under the umbrella of InterPsych including:

attachment: This list welcomes discussion on Bowlby-Ainsworth's theory of attachment, from theoretical and philosophical issues, to clinical or applied issues. Particular emphasis is given to socio-affective and defensive processes, and unconscious representations.

transcultural-psychology: Discussion of the delivery of mental health services to diverse cultures. Topics may include cultural differences in views on mental disorders, culture-specific syndromes, collaboration between Western and traditional healers, and cultural variance in symptoms.

psychiatry-resources: This list is intended for those who wish to co-operate in the compilation of a resource guide to enable clinicians and academics in the areas of psychiatry and abnormal psychology to gain maximum benefit from the facilities available over the Internet.

psychiatry: Many research findings and viewpoints in psychiatry are controversial, leaving a gulf between those pursuing radically different approaches to mental illness. This forum will act as a bridge between those taking a biomedical approach and those taking a psychodynamic, existential or behaviourist approach.

depression: This forum exists for scholarly discussion of issues related to mood disorders in clinical and research settings. Integrative biological-psychological contributions are particularly welcome. Topics include causation, correlates, consequences, co-morbidity, treatment/prevention, etc.

helplessness: Learned Helplessness and Explanatory Style was created to discuss the latest research on animals and humans, biological substratum, depression, anxiety, prevention, CAVE, politics, children, personal control, health, battering, bereavement, PTSD, sex differences, pessimism, work, heritability.

traumatic-stress: This list promotes the investigation, assessment, and treatment of the immediate and long-term psychosocial, biophysiological, and existential consequences of highly stressful (traumatic) events. Of special interest are efforts to identify a cure of PTSD (Post-traumatic Stress Disorder).

psychiatry-assessment: This sublist focuses on research and clinical issues related to use of psychological tests (including traditional clinical instruments & normal personality measures) in psychiatry and clinical psychology.

Archive/Gateway: via e-mail: To find out what files are associated with a particular list, send the following command to `mailbase@mailbase.ac.uk:index <listname>`

Files can then be retrieved by sending the command (again to `mailbase@mailbase.ac.uk`): send `<listname><filename>`

via FTP:

`ftp://mailbase.ac.uk/pub/lists/<listname>` where `<listname>` is the name of the list

via gopher:

`gopher://mailbase.ac.uk`

via WWW:

`http://mailbase.ac.uk`

Searchable Index: `gopher://mailbase.ac.uk`
Wais searches are available in the menu for each individual list title.

FAQ: For a FAQ regarding mailbase lists in general, send the following command to `mailbase@mailbase.ac.uk: send user-faq`

Evaluation: We lurked in the shadows of the fledgling stages of this effort. Initial struggles with focus and quantity of messages seems to have been solved with the creation of more narrowly focused subgroups.

Journal of Neurophysiology

ISSN: 0022-3077

Resource Type: journal

Table of Contents: `gopher://oac.hsc.uth.tmc.edu:3300/11/publications/jn`

Articles (abstracts): not available

Articles (full-text): not available

Subscription Info: `gopher://oac.hsc.uth.tmc.edu:3300/00/publications/jn/info`

Online Version: not available

Los Alamos Neural Network Home Page

Resource Type: web home page

URL: `http://laws.lanl.gov/x1_homepage.html`

Description: The Neural Networks project, part of the Simulation and Adaptive Computation Effort in the Applied Theoretical Physics Division at Los Alamos National Laboratories, is serving up two pages of links related to Neural Networks research at Los Alamos and around the world. *Neural Network Theory* provides pointers to background info and resources for the researcher. *Neural Network Announcements* has links to current events information, conferences, journals, etc.

Manager: Roger D Jones
X-1, MS F645
Los Alamos National Laboratory
Los Alamos, NM 87545
`rdj@lanl.gov`
505-667-8979
505-665-3389 (fax)

Evaluation: This is a nice stateside collection of links to other neural network resources. The unique information offered is specific to the work being done at Los Alamos, including a directory of people.

Manual of Neuroanesthesia

Resource Type: text document(s)

Date: 1993-94

File Format: HTML and ASCII

URL (hypertext format): `http://mcan15.med.nyu.edu/neuroman/neuroman.html`

URL (ascii format): `http://mcan15.med.nyu.edu/neuroman/neuroman.txt`

Author: Manual written by Cleveland Waterman for more info contact: Keith J. Ruskin, MD

Department of Anesthesiology
NYU Medical Center
keith@anes.med.nyu.edu

Description: A hypertext or ascii format text describing specific elements of Neuroanesthesia

File Size: 150k (ascii)

Searchable Index: n/a

Evaluation: The subject matter is definitely intended for the specialist. The HTML version is easy to navigate. Since the manual is still considered a work in progress, not all topics are available via hypertext.

Medical Informatics Home Page at Georgia Tech's Graphics, Visualization and Usability Center

Resource Type: web home page

URL: `http://www.gatech.edu/gvu/medical_informatics/medinfo_home_page.html`

Description: The Medical Informatics Group is a part of Georgia Tech's Graphics, Visualization, and Usability Center. The emphasis of their research is on graphics, visualization, animation, computer vision and knowledge based methods to model, simulate, analyze and visualize biomedical processes and structures. This page details their projects, faculty, and students.

Manager: James F. O'Brien
Graphics, Visualization & Usability Center
College of Computing
Georgia Institute of Technology
Atlanta, GA 30332-0280
obrienj@cc.gatech.edu

Evaluation: Although current projects primarily involve the heart, this resource may interest neuroscientists interested in imaging.

MR Brain data: 109-slice MRI data set of a head with skull partially removed to reveal brain

Resource Type: data set

Date: n/a

URL: `file://omicron.cs.unc.edu/pub/softlab/CHVRTD/volII`

Description: From announcement at softlab ftp site: A 109-slice MRI data set of a head with skull partially removed to reveal brain. 256 x 256 array, with dimensions of Z=109 Y=256 X=256 in z-y-x order. Format is 16-bit integers—two consecutive bytes make up one binary integer. We (Softlabs) do not object to your further distributing these datasets, but we request that full acknowledgement of the source of the data accompany such distribution. If you are going to send a dataset to someone, please also send the accompanying information file. [An installation manual is available in the same folder.]

For customers interested in purchasing the datasets on tape, both Volume I and Volume II can be purchased for $50.00 each, or $90.00 as a set. The distribution is available in two different formats. The files on the tape will be written from a DEC VAX computer using the UNIX file copy command `dd` or the UNIX `tar` command. Total block size is 8192 bytes written at 1600 bpi on either a standard 1/2" magnetic tape or a cartridge tape. Please specify your preference when ordering and note that `dd` is not available with the cartridge tape. Installation instructions accompany the distribution.

File Size: 14,286,848 bytes total file size.

Hardware/Software Requirements: Software to view these images is not provided with the datasets. When we inquired as to suitable viewing software, we received the following reply from Graham Gash:

The data we distribute is 3D volume data in raw form. The purpose of our distributing these data sets was to provide a standard suite of data for testing and comparison of various volume visualization methods. Users of these data sets must convert them into whatever format is required by the software they intend to run. Most serious image processing packages provide some capability for making such conversions. The datasets were written on a Digital Equipment Corporation (DEC) VAX computer. Each file contains only pixels, stored in row major order with 2-byte integers per pixel. To use the images on machines that have normal byte order (DECs use reverse byte order), you should swap alternate bytes, for example using the 'dd' command in UNIX. The important thing for those interested in these data sets to realize is that there is a dearth of auxiliary data about them. In particular, practically the only such data available are the dimensions of the images. In addition, we distribute two packages for image processing, with a somewhat medical slant. The older one, written in C, is called `/usr/image/`. It consists of a small library of file I/O functions, and about 100 application programs built on that library. The other package, called `/usr/Image/`, consists of 6 C++ libraries called DIAL, that perform I/O and a lot more, a few new C++ programs and the original set of programs, which work with the C++ libraries through a "compatibility library". We will eventually convert the C programs to C++. Both of these packages are downloadable via ftp, but they are presently licensed. In the future (probably within 6 months), the C++ libraries (possibly also the programs) will be freely distributable (a la the GNU software).

Originating Source: Data taken on the Siemens Magnetom and provided courtesy of Siemens Medical Systems, Inc., Iselin, NJ. Data edited (skull removed) by Dr. Julian Rosenman, North Carolina Memorial Hospital.

>Made available by Softlabs.
>Natalie E. Sipes
>SoftLab Coordinator
>email: `softlab@cs.unc.edu`
>telephone: 919-962-1960
>SoftLab Software Systems Laboratory
>CB# 3175, 361 Sitterson Hall
>University of North Carolina
>Department of Computer Science
>Chapel Hill, North Carolina 27599-3175

>Graham Gash, Ph.D.
>Medical Image Processing Manager
>`gash@cs.unc.edu` or `gash@cv.ruu.nl`
>Department of Computer Science
>Phone: (919) 962-1725
>FAX: (919) 962-1799
>University of North Carolina
>Chapel Hill, N.C. 27599-3175

Evaluation: We have not looked at this dataset personally. E-mail inquiries were handled very expediently, however.

Music and Brain Information Database on MuSICA - the Music and Science Information Computer Archive

Resource Type: database

URL: `telnet://mila.ps.uci.edu`

Login Instructions:
>Telnet: `mila.ps.uci.edu`
>
>login: `mbi`
>
>password: `nammbi`

Modem: 714-856-8960 for 9600 bps modems
>714-856-5661 for 2400 and 1200 bps modems
>>Type `mila.ps.uci.edu`
>
>login: `mbi`
>
>password: `nammbi`

Search Engine: The database software is WAIS (Wide Area Information Servers) with SWAIS interface. New and improved versions of WAIS and SWAIS will be incorporated as they become available. The current version in use is wais-8-b5 which permits Boolean and and not operators. Typing a quote or double-quote around a string of words will elicit a search for documents which contain the exact words located within the quotes. Partial word searches are permitted by using the asterisk symbol(*).

Description: From the announcement: Topics covered are previous and current publications of journal articles and books in the following fields: auditory system, animal and human behavior, cognition, creativity, human brain and neuropsychology of music, effects of music on behavior and physiology, music education, music medicine, musical performance, music therapy, perception and psychophysics. The entire contents of the following journals are being included: Bulletin of the Council for Research in Music Education, Journal of Music Therapy, Journal of Research in Music Education, Music Perception, Psychology of Music, and Psychomusicology. Complete abstracts are included for journal articles, wherever possible. The information base currently has more than 10,000 entries and it is updated continually.

This information is being provided by the Music and the Brain Information Center (MBIC), recently established at the University of California, Irvine and funded by a start-up grant from the National Association of Music Merchants. Its goals are (a) to establish a computer-based bibliographic record of scientific research on music, including its brain substrates, (b) to serve as a clearing house for the newest findings and (c) to foster interdisciplinary knowledge concerning music, behavior, the brain and allied fields.

We invite you to send reprints and preprints for entry into the database and we welcome suggestions concerning all aspects of the database and the MBIC.

Manager: mbic@mila.ps.uci.edu
Norman M. Weinberger
Professor and Scientific Director
Music and the Brain Information Center
Center for the Neurobiology of Learning and Memory
University of California, Irvine
Irvine, California 92717
Phone:(714) 856-5512
Fax: (714) 856-8481

FAQ: n/a

Evaluation: In addition to the literature database, an announcement bulletin board is available with journal tables of contents and conferences. This resource is well thought out and help is graciously offered.

NASA Ames Biocomputation Center

Resource Type: web home page

URL: `http://neuron.arc.nasa.gov`

Description: From the info page: The Biocomputation Center at NASA Ames Research Center is dedicated to computer-based three-dimensional (3-D) visualization of cells, tissues and organs, to mathematically based modeling, and to 3-D simulations of the functioning of living systems from the subcellular and molecular to the organismal level. The emphasis is on teams of broadly based, interdisciplinary investigators and on a union between computational, theoretical and experimental research.

In celebration of the Decade of the Brain, the NASA Biocomputation Center staff is looking forward to interaction with the National Institutes of Health, National Science Foundation, and other government agencies to facilitate computer-based approaches to the study of the nervous system by university investigators.

Author: For more information contact
Dr. Muriel Ross, `muriel_ross@qmgate.arc.nasa.gov`
or
Kevin Montgomery, `kevin@neuron.arc.nasa.gov`

Evaluation: An interesting resource with terrific samples of 3D models available as TIF image files and MPEG movies.

Neural Computation

ISSN: 0899-7667

Resource Type: journal

Table of Contents: `http://www.emsl.pnl.gov:2080/docs/cie/neural/papers/neural_computation.html`

Articles (bibliographic records): `file://mitpress.mit.edu/pub/NeuralComp/NC.bib.Z` (see note below)

Articles (full-text): n/a

Subscription Info: `journals-orders@mit.edu`

Online Version: n/a

Other Notes: Nici Schraudolph has produced a BibTeX database for all articles published in the first five volumes (1989-1993). Abstracts are not included. Copyright permission can be obtained from

> N. Schraudolph
> Computational Neurobiology Lab
> The Salk Institute
> San Diego, CA 92186-5800
> `schraudo@salk.edu`

Neural Networks at the Austrian Research Institute for Artificial Intelligence (OFAI)

Resource Type: web home page

URL: `http://www.ai.univie.ac.at/oefai/nn/nngroup.html`

Description: The Neural Network research group of the Austrian Research Institute for Artificial Intelligence (OFAI) offers information related to their work in four domains:

- practical applications of neural networks
- theoretical research on neural networks
- cognitive modeling with neural networks
- neural network simulation tools

Also available is BIBLIO, a searchable, bibliographic database of neural network books, reports, journal articles, and conferences. It has over 3500 references and is growing. Searching is by author's name or keywords in the title.

Manager: Georg Dorffner
> Austrian Research Institute for Artificial Intelligence
> Schottengasse 3, A-1010 Vienna, Austria
> Tel: +43-1-53532810
> Fax: +43-1-5320652
> `georg@ai.univie.ac.at`

Evaluation: The bibliographic database will make this a popular site. However it requires a browser which supports forms.

Neural Web

Resource Type: web home page

URL: `http://www.erg.abdn.ac.uk/projects/neuralweb`

Description: The Neural Web is an experimental effort to create a comprehensive, one stop shopping resource for the neurocomputing community. It includes pointers to other sites and plans to disseminate unique resources and services, including an updating service. Current offerings include:

- Searching Neural Web database (all papers, reports, profiles and digests) held in the Neural Web
- Online digests - including Neuron Digest.
- Regional information.
- Conferences, workshops and meetings.
- Software archive.
- Document archive.
- Educational material - including hypermedia formats.

Manager: Gary Whittington
> `http://www.erg.abdn.ac.uk/users/gary`

Evaluation: This resource is well planned and organized to grow. Already it has the unique offering of an easily searchable archive of Neuron Digest.

NEURO1-L, the Bitnet Neuroscience Information Exchange Forum

Resource Type: listserv

Date: 11/1/90 to present

Subscriptions:
> **LISTSERV@UICVM.UIC.EDU** (for internet users)
> **LISTSERV@UICVM** (for bitnet users)

Postings:
> NEURO1-L@UICVM.UIC.EDU (for internet users)
> NEURO1-L@UICVM (for bitnet users)

Moderator: E.J. Neafsey, Ph.D.
> NEURO1-L list manager
> #m01ejn@luccpua on Bitnet
> Director, Neuroscience Graduate Program
> Associate Professor
> Department of Cell Biology, Neurobiology & Anatomy
> Loyola University Chicago Medical Center
> 2160 S. First Ave.
> Maywood, IL 60153
> (708) 216-3355

Description: From announcement: "This (unmoderated) forum has several functions. One is to improve everyday communication and interchange between neuroscientists. For example, when a question arises such as "Where can I get an antibody to nerve growth factor" or something like that, simply sending that message to NEURO1-L will, hopefully, address an audience of hundreds or even thousands of neuroscientists, at least a few of whom will be able to send you a reply. I also hope that the forum will promote ongoing discussions of various, more substantial, current issues in Neuroscience: Should some type of National Neural Circuitry Database be established and maintained? What is going on in the field of neuronal transplants? Does the cerebral cortex operate primarily in a hierarchical, sequential manner or in a distributed, parallel fashion? Of course, many other issues also could be discussed. Lastly, I hope that NEURO1-L provides a stimulus for "doing neuroscience" in a more interactive, global way. I am sure my own individual experience of being "overwhelmed" with information is shared by many; perhaps if there is a common forum where open discussion takes place on a regular basis, the "big picture" will become easier to discern, leading to better, more productive neuroscience. Since I hope NEURO1-L becomes a large list, please don't send junk mail because it will clutter up many mailboxes and takes time to read and throw away."

Archive/Gateway: n/a

Searchable Index: n/a

FAQ: n/a

Evaluation: This list is slow. We have received approximately one posting per week for the last month. It seems other avenues of communication are getting more traffic. Content has been solicitations to review articles for Behavioral and Brain Sciences, conference announcements, and an occasional query.

Neuroanatomy Foundations

Resource Type: Software

Date/Version: 1987

URL: **file://orion.oac.uci.edu/med-ed/mac/clinical-science/neuro-foundation-1.stak.sea.hqx**
file://orion.oac.uci.edu/med-ed/mac/clinical-science/neuro-foundation-2.stak.sea.hqx

Description: Neuroanatomy Foundations is a hypercard, introductory atlas to the human brain. By pointing and clicking on pictures and labels, the reader can explore the cerebral hemispheres, the limbic system and subcortical structures, the cerebellum and brainstem, or the major cerebral fiber tracts. There are also text fields connected to labels with more complete information and an index. The images are digitized, black and white photographs from Structure of the Human Brain: A Photographic Atlas by Stephen J. DeArmond, Maeline M. Fusco and Maynard M. Dewey (New York: Oxford University Press, 1976) and The Human Brain: A Photographic Guide by Nedzad Gluhbegovic and Terence H. Williams (Philadelphia: Harper & Row, 1980).

File Size: 900 K (both volumes)

Hardware/Software Requirements: Macintosh computer
>Hypercard player
>BinHex compatible decompression software

Note: Be sure to get both volumes or you will miss out on half the show! After the files are decompressed they are self-extracting.

Author: J. Michael Williams, PhD
>Department of Mental Health Sciences
>Hahnemann University
>Broad & Vine
>Philadelphia, PA 19102

Evaluation: This stack is packed with information! It is relatively easy to navigate with a little common sense and perusal of the intro material. The images don't do justice to the originals, but the tradeoff is a program of reasonable size which is easily transportable and usable on most Macs. Parts of the design are not quite polished, but the volume and quality of the information make up for it. Appropriate for high school and college level.

Neuron-Digest

3/1/89 to present

Resource Type: Listserv

Subscriptions: **neuron-request@psych.upenn.edu**

Postings: neuron-request@psych.upenn.edu

Moderator: Peter Marvit

Description: From the announcement: Neuron-Digest is a list (in moderated, digest form) dealing with all aspects of neural networks (and any type of network or neuromorphic system), especially: natural systems, software simulations, neurobiology, hardware, neuroscience, artificial systems, neural networks, optical, algorithms, cellular automatons. Any contribution in these areas is accepted.

>Any of the following types of items are reasonable: abstracts, reviews, lab descriptions, research overviews, work planned or in progress, half-baked ideas, conference announcements, conference reports, bibliographies, history connectionism, puzzles and unsolved problems, anecdotes, jokes, and poems, queries and requests, address changes.

Archive/Gateway: file://psych.upenn.edu/pub/Neuron-Digest
>That directory contains back issues with the names vol-nn-no-mm (e.g., vol-3-no-02). Neuron-Digest is also posted to the usenet newsgroup comp.ai.neural-networks.
>BITNET and many overseas readers will find the email archive server very useful—to get information and instructions, send a message to archive-server@psych.upenn.edu with the subject line help
>Or try the Web home page for Neuron Digest with search capabilities—details below.

Searchable Index: http://www.erg.abdn.ac.uk/projects/neuralweb/digests

FAQ: n/a

Evaluation: This list is active and well moderated. Lots of conference announcements, calls for papers, book announcements and internet resources. Fair amount of scholarly queries and a collaborative atmosphere. What a wealth of information gets passed along here!

Neuroprose

Resource Type: ftp site

URL: file://archive.cis.ohio-state.edu/pub/neuroprose

Description: From the README: This directory contains technical reports as a public service to the connectionist and neural network scientific community.

>Researchers may place electronic versions of their preprints in this directory, announce availability, and other interested researchers can rapidly retrieve and print the postscripts. This saves copying, postage and handling, by having the interested reader supply the paper. We strongly discourage the

merger into the repository of existing bodies of work or the use of this medium as a vanity press for papers which are not of publication quality.

There are currently well over 300 papers available here. Consult the FAQ for contributor's guidelines.

Searchable Index: `wais://wais.cic.net/neuroprose.src`

This index contains only 137 documents and does not seem to have been updated since 1992. It also indexes only the index page (as opposed to the full text of the articles).

Manager: Jordan Pollack
Assistant Professor
`pollack@cis.ohio-state.edu`
614-292-4890 (then * to fax)
Laboratory for AI Research
2036 Neil Ave.
Columbus, OH 43210

FAQ: `file://archive.cis.ohio-state.edu/pub/neuroprose/README`

Evaluation: Good example of what a research community can do in the name of collaboration. Since the WAIS index is pretty much useless, it's best to occasionally print off the index file and look for new additions or monitor appropriate listservs and usenet groups for announcements of newly available papers.

Neurotour

Resource Type: Software

Date/Version: unknown

URL: `file://sunsite.unc.edu/pub/academic/medicine/mac-medical/hypercard/neurotour.cpt.hqx`

Description: Neurotour begins to cover the basics of neuroanatomy from the macro to the micro level. It starts with a silhouette of a human head, defines 3 sections of brain, zooms in to a diagram of the brain and defines lobes and areas, zooms in to the neuron level and identifies cell parts (some textual description), zooms again to an illustration of the synaptic region, zooms again to transmitter vesicles . . . and stops abruptly. We have not located a finished version to date.

File Size: 361K in archive

Hardware/Software Requirements: Macintosh computer
Hypercard player
BinHex compatible decompression software
Extraction software

Author: The stack was written by Jim Ludtke. We have no other contact information.

Evaluation: Unfinished. What he has is very appealing graphically and his approach is an interesting one, but is simply not very usable in its present form. Middle school to bio101 level.

NIH Guide to Grants and Contracts

Resource Type: directory

Update Frequency: weekly

URL: `gopher://gopher.nih.gov/11/res/nih-guide`

Contents/Features: From the file "`about the NIH Guide`":

The information found in this directory is has been taken from the electronic form of the "NIH Guide to Grants and Contracts" available via anonymous ftp from cu.nih.gov.

Each edition of the NIH Guide begins with an index, and may contain one or more of the following:

- notices
- notices of availability (RFPs/RFAs)
- ongoing program announcements (PAs)
- errata

All of the above information has been indexed and is searchable. The logical and and or operators can be used to do multiple keyword searches.

The folders listed under this directory are described below:

- `Search NIH Guide (most recent 6 weeks)` - the last six issues of the Guide can be searched here.
- `Search NIH Guide (Jan 1992 - the present)` - searches done here include all Guides back to January 1992.
- `NIH Guide - flat text files` - each NIH Guide dating back to January 1992 is listed as a directory (by date).
- `Request for Applications (RFAs) - Full Text` - contains flat text files for each RFA that is available in a full text form (dating back to January 1992). Note - these files can be very long.
- `Program Announcements - Full Text` - contains flat text files for each Program Announcement that is available in a full text form (dating back to January 1992). These too can be very long.

Contacts: Questions concerning a specific notice, RFA, RFP or PA should be directed to the contact person listed in that announcement.

General questions concerning the NIH Guide should be directed to the NIH Institutional Affairs Office:(301) 496-5366.

Questions regarding gopher should be sent to `gopher@gopher.nih.gov`

Searchable?: yes

FAQ: n/a

Evaluation: An excellent resource for keeping up-to-date on NIH research.

NIH Image

Resource Type: Software

Date/Version: V1.55 (V1.56 in beta)

URL: `ftp://zippy.nimh.nih.gov/pub/nih-image`

Description: NIH Image is a public domain image processing and analysis program for the Macintosh. The FTP site above contains the latest version of the program and lots of related resources such as supporting programs, spin-off software, Adobe Photoshop plug-ins, sample images and animations, and supporting documentation.

There is also an e-mail discussion group for users of the software: `nih-image@soils.umn.edu`. Send a subscribe message to `LISTSERV@soils.umn.edu`. It is archived at `ftp://ftp.soils.umn.edu/pub/info/email-lists/nih-image`.

FAQ: `ftp://zippy.nimh.nih.gov/pub/nih-image/documents/faq.txt`

File Size: approx. 412K compressed, 772K uncompressed

Hardware/Software Requirements: Macintosh with a color or grayscale display and at least 1.5MB of free RAM. Sorry, but there is no DOS, Windows or UNIX version.

BinHex and/or MacBinary compatible decompression software.

Author: Wayne Rasband `wayne@zippy.nimh.nih.gov`

Evaluation: This seems to be well supported, public domain imaging software for the Mac platform used by a number of neuroscience labs.

Pacific Northwest Laboratory Neural Network Home Page

Resource Type: web home page

URL: `http://www.emsl.pnl.gov:2080/docs/cie/neural/neural.homepage.html`

Description: Neural network researchers in the Computing and Information Sciences group of the Molecular Sciences Research Center at the Pacific Northwest laboratory sponsor a WWW page with the following resources:

Lists of references to neural network papers in the following areas:

- Chemical Sensor Analysis
- Spectroscopic Analysis
- Chemical Process Control

- Molecular Modeling
- Nuclear Science and Engineering
- Medicine
- Manufacturing
- Optical Neurocomputing
- Description of our work with neural networks
- Links to other neural network and neuroscience resources
- Tables of contents neural network and neuroscience journals

Manager: Sherif Hashem and Paul Keller
Pacific Northwest Laboratory
Richland, Washington, USA
phone: (509) 375-6995 (509) 375-2254
fax: (509) 375-6631
s_hashem@pnl.gov pe_keller@pnl.gov

Evaluation: Wow! The journal tables of contents and gateways to other sites are the most comprehensive we've seen for the neural network community. Check out the map! The unique resources available here are also well presented.

Positron Emission Tomography (PET) Home Page

Resource Type: web home page

URL: http://pss023.psi.ch/index.html

Description: The Paul Scherrer Institute in Switzerland offers a home page with information about their projects and links to other sites with PET resources. Their areas of work include:

- Neuroscience:
- Neuronal Aging
- Movement Disorders Parkinsonism, Huntingtons Chorea
- Temporal Lobe Epilepsy
- Schizophrenia
- Pharmacological studies
- Oncology
- Soft tissue carcinoma follow-up.
- Brain tumor diagnosis

Manager: R Paul Maguire
PET Centre
Paul Scherrer Institute
CH 5232 Villigen PSI
Switzerland
Tel +41 56 99 42 52
Fax +41 56 99 35 15
maguire@cvax.psi.ch

Evaluation: This site has not mounted much unique info (yet), but provides links to other sites with PET info and images. The PET community is poised to take advantage of WWW browsers with graphics capabilities.

Psyche

ISSN: 1039-723X

Resource Type: e-journal

Subscriptions: Subscriptions to the electronic version of PSYCHE may be initiated by sending the one-line message:

SUBSCRIBE PSYCHE-L YourFirstName YourLastName

to LISTSERV@NKI.BITNET or LISTSERV%NKI.BITNET@CUNYVM.CUNY.EDU

Contributions: Read the author's information in the FAQ below. Contributions should be sent to the executive editor.

Editor: Patrick Wilken
>	Department of Psychology
>	Royal Melbourne Institute of Technology
>	BUNDOORA VIC 3083
>	AUSTRALIA
>	`x91007@pitvax.xx.rmit.edu.au`

Description: PSYCHE is a refereed electronic journal dedicated to supporting the interdisciplinary exploration of the nature of consciousness and its relation to the brain. PSYCHE publishes material relevant to that exploration from the perspectives afforded by the disciplines of Cognitive Science, Philosophy, Psychology, Neuroscience, Artificial Intelligence and Anthropology. Interdisciplinary discussions are particularly encouraged. PSYCHE is published four times per year. PSYCHE also publishes a hard-copy version simultaneously with the electronic version. Long articles published in the electronic version may be abbreviated, synopsized or eliminated from the hardcopy version.

Archive/Gateway: `ftp://ftp.cs.monash.edu.au/psyche`
> The archive is also accessible using get commands to `LISTSERV@NKI.BITNET` or `LISTSERV%NKI.BITNET@cunyvm.cuny.edu` More details on this method are in the FAQ.

Searchable Index: n/a

FAQ: `ftp://ftp.cs.monash.edu.au/psyche/PSYFAQ38`

Evaluation: We have not personally monitored this resource.

Psycoloquy

ISSN: 1055-0143

Resource Type: e-journal

Subscriptions: Send email to: `listserv@pucc.bitnet` or `listserv@pucc.princeton.edu`
> containing the following one-line message: `sub psyc Firstname Lastname` (substituting your first and last name, of course).
> PSYCOLOQUY can also be accessed on Usenet as the moderated newsgroup `sci.psychology.digest`

Contributions: Instructions for authors are detailed in the FAQ referenced below. Please submit all material to
> `psyc@pucc.bitnet` or `psyc@pucc.princeton.edu`

Editor: Steven Harnad
>	`harnad@Princeton.edu`

Description: From the announcement: PSYCOLOQUY is a refereed electronic journal sponsoredon an experimental basis by the American Psychological Association and currently estimated to reach a readership of 20,000. PSYCOLOQUY publishes brief reports of new ideas and findings on which the author wishes to solicit rapid peer feedback, international and interdisciplinary ("Scholarly Skywriting"), in all areas of psychology and its related fields (biobehavioral, cognitive, neural, social, etc.) All contributions are refereed by members of PSYCOLOQUY's Editorial Board.
> Target article length should normally not exceed 500 lines [c. 4500 words]. Commentaries and responses should not exceed 200 lines [c. 1800 words].

Archive/Gateway: Anonymous FTP archive is `ftp://princeton.edu/pub/harnad/Psycoloquy`
> The archive is also accessible using get commands to `LISTSERV@PUCC.BITNET`. More details on this method are in the FAQ.

Searchable Index: `gopher://gopher.lib.virginia.edu/77/.indexes/psycoloquy`

FAQ: `ftp://princeton.edu/pub/harnad/Psycoloquy/Instructions`

Evaluation: Psycoloquy is among the first scholarly, refereed e-journals. It has matured gracefully and continues to set the standard. It is available many more places than outlined above.

San Diego 3D Imaging Group

Resource Type: Listserv

Subscriptions: Address message to: `listserver@sdsc.edu`

On first line of message body, left margin, type only: add <user@host> sd3d (do not include < > symbols) where <user@host> is your complete internet address. Do not include anything else in message body with the exception of additional add or delete commands for additional persons. Each add or delete command must occupy its own line. It is not necessary to fill in <subject:> line.

Postings: 3DSD@mailserver.sdsc.edu

Moderator: n/a

Description: From the announcement: The San Diego 3D Imaging Group is a professional forum for keeping up-to-date on all aspects in all disciplines and on all platforms of 3D imaging. In addition to local gatherings in San Diego, an e-mail listserv encourages global discussion. Suggested topics of interest include 3D microscopy, 3D cell and tissue culture, biomedical imaging, holography, reconstruction software, stereoscopic displays, 3D scanning, virtual prototyping, stereo graphics, and virtual reality environments.

Archive/Gateway: n/a

Searchable Index: n/a

FAQ: n/a

Evaluation: We have not personally monitored this listserv.

Schiz-L: Clinical And Basic Science Research In Schizophrenia

Resource Type: Listserv

Subscriptions: **LISTSERV@UMAB.UMD.EDU** or **LISTSERV@UMAB.BITNET**
send the message subscribe schiz-l firstname lastname

Postings: SCHIZ-L@UMAB.UMD.EDU or SCHIZ-L@UMAB.BITNET

Moderator: Steven R. Daviss
Maryland Psychiatric Research Center
PO Box 21247
Baltimore MD 21228 USA
Voice: (410) 455-7624
Fax: (410) 455-7527
sdaviss@cosy.ab.umd.edu

Description: From the announcement: SCHIZ-L is an unmoderated discussion list devoted to schizophrenia research. The objective of the list is to provide a forum for communications among researchers and others interested in this mental illness. It is hoped that this forum will facilitate discussion of both published and unpublished findings and ideas, foster potential collaborations between investigators, and develop into an information resource for those in this field. Topics should relate to basic science and/or clinical science as it applies to schizophrenia, or to items that might be of interest to those in this field. These might include questions, comments, or ideas about:

- epidemiology
- phenomenology/psychopathology
- psychopharmacology
- structural imaging (e.g., CT, MRI, MEG, etc)
- functional imaging (e.g., fMRI, PET, SPECT, CEEG)
- biochemical/neurochemical studies
- neuroanatomy/neuropathology
- postmortem studies
- histological methodologies
- neurodevelopment
- genetics
- neuropsychological assessments
- research ethics
- comments on journal articles
- data analysis

- use of computer resources
- Internet resources
- conferences, meetings

Archive/Gateway: send the message `GET SCHIZ-L LOGyymm` to `LISTSERV@UMAB.UMD.EDU` or `LISTSERV@UMAB.BITNET`, where yy=year and mm=month (e.g., `LOG9401`=Jan 1994)

Searchable Index: n/a

FAQ: n/a

Evaluation: We have not personally monitored this listserv.

sci.bio

Resource Type: usenet group

Date:

Description: This is the general discussion area for biology in the `sci` hierarchy. The volume is high and the topics wide-ranging. There are many queries for information.

Archive: Postings since 12/91:
  `gopher://ftp.bio.indiana.edu/11/Network-News/sci.bio`

Searchable Index: n/a

FAQ: n/a

Evaluation: Neuroscientists who have a biological focus may find monitoring of this group useful for more general concerns. There are more specialized groups which don't have as much "lay" traffic.

sci.bio.technology

Resource Type: usenet group

Date: unknown

Description: This is a subgroup of `sci.bio` which deals with technology issues related to any field in biology.

Archive: `gopher://ftp.bio.indiana.edu/11/Network-News/sci.bio/technology`

Searchable Index: n/a

FAQ: n/a

Evaluation: The volume is small--mostly technical questions and pleas for help. Answers are rarely posted, so it is hard to know if it is effective to field your question to this group.

sci.cognitive

Resource Type: usenet group

Date: 6/92 to present

Description: From the charter: Cognitive science is an inter-disciplinary investigation of cognition, involving cognitive psychology, artificial intelligence, computer science, human-computer interaction, philosophy of mind, philosophy of science, linguistics, neuroscience, cognitive anthropology and other disciplines. The 'mind's new science' has been around since the mid-50's, and has entered an institutional phase with textbooks, journals, centres of research and teaching etc. However, due to its inter-disciplinary and international character, channels of communication devoted specifically to cognitive science are still needed, and the group `sci.cognitive` is intended to serve this end.

The group should serve as an open forum for discussion of all aspects of cognitive science: empirical work, cognitive modeling, theory, methodology, foundational, historical and social issues etc. The group should also facilitate the exchange of information on teaching programmes, conferences, jobs etc. The main language of the group is English, but postings in other languages are also encouraged.

Archive: n/a

Searchable Index: n/a

FAQ: n/a

Evaluation: The volume here is medium (avoiding the perils of non-scientist groups). Content seems to overlap somewhat with `bionet.neuroscience`.

sci.engr.biomed

Resource Type: usenet group

Date: 2/92 to present

Description: The purpose of the group is to facilitate discussions and the exchange of information pertaining to the field of Biomedical Engineering. Biomedical Engineering being (but not limited to): design and manufacture of artificial limbs and organs; scientific research involving medicine/the body and artificial materials; mature discussions on ethical matters; computer programs/hardware related to Biomed Engineering, data collection, and electronic muscle stimulation; modeling/simulation of Biomed systems; and schools/courses involved with Biomedical Engineering.

Archive: n/a

Searchable Index: n/a

FAQ: n/a

Evaluation: We have not monitored this group personally.

sci.med

Resource Type: usenet group

Date: unknown

Description: This is the catch-all group for medical issues in the sci hierarchy. Participation is varied from laypersons to clinicians to researchers.

Archive: n/a

Searchable Index: n/a

FAQ: n/a

Evaluation: This group is high volume—lots of folks seeking diagnoses and advice, but also plenty of clinicians communicating professional and research concerns.

sci.med.pharmacy

Resource Type: usenet group

Date: 8/93 to present

Description: From the charter: The purpose of sci.med.pharmacy is to provide pharmacists with a forum for the discussion of issues related to the teaching and practice of the profession. It is expected that sci.med.pharmacy would attract contributions from all the major disciplines including pharmacology and pharmaceutical chemistry as well as areas with more direct professional implications such as pharmacy practice and legislation. It is proposed that cross posting should occur between the news group and the Pharmacy Mail Exchange List. It is expected that all the postings to the list will be transferred to the news group.

Archive: n/a

Searchable Index: n/a

FAQ: n/a

Evaluation: We have not personally monitored this group.

sci.med.psychobiology

Resource Type: usenet group

Date: 12/93 to present

Description: From Charter: sci.med.psychobiology will be an unmoderated common forum for discussions and announcements among those interested in such scientific aspects of psychiatry as: psychobiology, psychopharmacology, inheritance of psychiatric illness, behavioral genetics, psychoneurobiology, neuropsychiatry, neuropsychology, psychoneuroendocrinology, psychoneuroimmunology, psychosomatics, somatization disorder, psychiatric education and training, research support and funding, research training.

Archive: n/a

Searchable Index: n/a

FAQ: n/a

Evaluation: We have not personally monitored this resource.

`sci.psychology`

Resource Type: usenet group

Date: unknown

Description: This group is the catch-all for psychology in the sci hierarchy. Lots of lay and professional contributions on a wide range of psychological subjects.

Archive: n/a

Searchable Index: n/a

FAQ: n/a

Evaluation: Another high volume group. This one is less research oriented and heavier on theory and "talk". These folks carry a thread longer than most!

Searching for Biologists

Resource Type: directory

Update Frequency: unknown

URL: `gopher://merlot.gdb.org:70/11/biol-search`

Contents/Features: From the file "about-searches":
Looking for someone to collaborate with?
Looking for someone with expertise in a specific field?
Looking for someone's address?

Well here's a good place to start—you can search for people by name, location, and research interests.

What appears here is the pilot project for a database which will help you to find other scientists. At present you can search for:

1. All Researchers funded by the U.S. National Institutes of Health;
2. U.S. Department of Energy - to work on the Genome project;
3. U.S. National Institutes of Health - to work on the Genome project;
4. U.S. National Science Foundation;
5. U.S. Department of Agriculture;
6. Researchers at the National Institutes of Health;
7. Addresses of Chlamydomonas Researchers;
8. E-mail Addresses of Biosci-Bionet Users;
9. E-mail Addresses of Crystallographers;
10. E-mail Addresses of Yeast Reasearchers;
11. Phonebooks of Institutions around the World.

Search 1 supports Booleans (and, or, not), and phrase searches (" "). Searches (2, 3, 6, 7, 8, 9, and 10) support Booleans (and, or, not), phrase searches (" ") and wildcards (*). Search (4) has only simple keyword searching. Search 7) is very experimental and might support Booleans.

The results of the searches in (6) may not have addresses or phone numbers but you may look those up in the NIH phone book and CSO sever that are also provided in (6).

Searchable?: yes

FAQ: none

Evaluation: An easy-to-use resource, but search results vary from database to database. Also, be aware that the databases may not contain up-to-date information.

Sheep's Brain

Resource Type: Software

Date/Version: unknown

URL: `file://ra.nrl.navy.mil/MacSciTech/biology/descriptive/sheepsbrain.cpt.hqx`

Description: Sheep's Brain is a SuperCard stack of labeled B&W photos of sheep brain and various cross sections. It has a self test/quiz feature. A hypertext index of labels will pop you to the appropriate photo, otherwise you are limited to browsing it sequentially. Pictures are used with permission from The Sheep Brain: a Basic Guide by Richard K. Cooley and C. H. Vanderwolf, published by A.J. Kirby Co. Written with Dr. Ross Dingman and Dr. Daniel Moriarity at University of San Diego.

A Thor Production. Portions copyrighted by Silicon Beach Software (a subsidiary of Aldus Corporation).

File Size: 1 M in archive

1.8 M uncompressed

(includes a run-time version of SuperCard)

Hardware/Software Requirements: Macintosh computer

BinHex compatible decompression software

Extraction software

Author: The author, Thor Avidsen, writes in the README file: This is a project I developed which is currently in use at the University of San Diego. Feel free to use it and distribute it any way you like. If you have any questions or bug reports, drop me a line at `Thor@usdcsv.acusd.edu`

Evaluation: This would be a good introduction to a dissection lab. It is complete and well designed. The quiz and the index make it flexible. Some of the photos are not as sharp as they could be.

Society for Neuroscience Gopher

Resource Type: gopher

URL: `gopher://gopher.sfn.org`

Description: This gopher server has been set up by the Society for Neuroscience. As of 6/94 it contains a Neuroscience Newsletter, Membership Directory, and several policy statements, including one on the use of animals in neuroscience research. Future plans include the providing the table of contents for the Journal of Neuroscience.

Searchable Index: n/a

Manager: Questions and comments can be directed to: `gopher-admin@sfn.org`

FAQ: n/a

Evaluation: This gopher is new and still under construction. Nevertheless, it should be valuable to those looking for information and contacts beyond a local gopher or home page.

Stereoscopic Volume Visualization (Lateiner Dataspace)

Resource Type: web home page

URL: `http://www.dataspace.com/WWW/documents/stereoscopic.html`

Description: The Stereoscopic Volume Visualization home page describes the Lateiner Dataspace project known as The Vox-L Stereoscopic Workstation: Stereoscopic Interactive Volume Visualization for Medical Data. The project was presented in January 1994 at the Medicine Meets Virtual Reality II conference in San Diego.

From the home page: An interactive visualization system for medical data is proposed as a clinical diagnostic and research tool. The combination of an intuitive, graphical interface, interactive stereoscopic rendering, and powerful volume manipulation algorithms provides an environment for efficient interpretation of data generated by modern medical imaging hardware (confocal microscopes, MRI, PET, and CAT-scanners). This increased interpretive power has the potential to streamline diagnosis and patient care, creating significant opportunities for enhanced data utilization and reduced cost.

Manager: Joshua S. Lateiner

Lateiner Dataspace

500 West Cummings Park

Technology Development, Suite 1700

Woburn, MA 01801

Tel 617-937-8330

Fax 617-937-8331
Net `lateiner@dataspace.com`

Evaluation: This homepage is actually a detailed ad for and exhibition of the Vox-L Workstation. As an exhibition, it includes excellent inline graphic images and informative text. The text describes the advantages of 3-dimensional modeling in clinical and research applications, discussing advances in technology which enhance a doctor's access to data. Working models of the software are available for ftp from ftp.dataspace.com.

This Internet resource is aimed chiefly at clinical neuroscientists, but should be of interest to anyone exploring image-analysis equipment.

Stereotaxic Atlases of Pigeon and Electric Fish

Resource Type: image

Date: n/a

URL: `file://obex.scripps.edu/pub/shared_data/Karten`

Description: These Canvas files are Harvey Karten's attempts to convert traditional paper based stereotaxic atlases into digital format. There are 3 sets of plates from Karten and Hodos Stereotaxic Atlas of the Pigeon and 1 set of plates from the Maler atlas of Apteronotus, a weakly electric fish. (There is also a tempting folder entitled "Squirrel" which won't open.) The sets are meant to be viewed as layers in Canvas, a graphics program.

File Size: Pigeon Anterior: 58 files, each 46-89K
Pigeon Posterior: 19 files, each 56-88K
Pigeon Saggital: 11 files, each 52-119K
Electric Fish: 3 files, each 307-327K

Hardware/Software Requirements: Canvas 3.0 or higher

Originating Source: Harvey J. Karten
`kartenh@sdsc.edu`
619-534-4938
Dept. of Neurosciences
UCSD
La Jolla, CA 92093-0608

FAQ: `file://obex.scripps.edu/pub/shared_data/Karten/Read_Me_first.txt`
`file://obex.scripps.edu/README`

Evaluation: We don't have access to Canvas, so we were unable to take a look.

University of California at San Diego Neurosciences Gopher

Resource Type: gopher

URL: `gopher://salk.edu`

Description: This gopher server has been set up by the UCSD Neurosciences graduate programme using computing facilities of the Computational Neurobiology Laboratory at the Salk Institute. It contains information about the graduate and undergraduate offerings in neuroscience at UCSD, lists of faculty with research interests and publications, and postings concerning lectures on neuroscience topics in the San Diego area.

Searchable Index: n/a

Manager: Questions, comments, and gripes about the information available here can be sent to:
`neuro-students-request@ucsd.edu`

FAQ: n/a

Evaluation: Although the lectures are primarily of local interest, the faculty and institutional information can be of general interest.

University of California at San Diego NeuroWeb

Resource Type: web home page

URL: `http://salk.edu/NeuroWeb/`

Description: From the info page: The goals of this server are:
> 1. to provide relevant and valuable internet information to UCSD students and faculty,
> 2. to provide similar information to all interested in neuroscience,
> 3. to provide non-UCSD people with information on the neuroscience program here at UCSD.

Author: For more information contact Preston Holmes, pholmes@sdcc3.ucsd.edu

Evaluation: The UCSD NeuroWeb page is still under construction, but it already points to a number of resources available through the world-wide-web. It also provides access to the UCSD Neurosciences Gopher.

VOXEL-MAN Atlases

Resource Type: Software

Date/Version: 1993 (ongoing)

URL: **n/a**

Description: From a posting to MEDINF: As some of you may know we (K.H. Hohne et al.) are working on a true 3D interactive atlas of the human body(VOXEL-MAN). The present versions of VOXEL-MAN/brain and VOXEL-MAN/skull may now be usefully applied. People interested in getting the programs or information about them may contact me.

References:

K. H. Hohne, M.Bomans, M.Riemer, R.Schubert, U.Tiede, and W.Lierse, "A 3D anatomical atlas based on a volume model," IEEE Comput. Graphics Appl., vol.12, no.4, pp.72--78, 1992.

K.H. Hohne, A.Pommert, M.Riemer, T.Schiemann, R.Schubert, U.Tiede, and W.Lierse, "Eine modellbasierte Multimediatechnik zur Erzeugung von dreidimensionalen medizinischen Atlanten," it-Informationstechnik, vol.35, no.3, pp.26--30, 1993.

R.Schubert, K.H. Hohne, A.Pommert, M.Riemer, T.Schiemann, and U.Tiede, "Spatial knowledge representation for visualization of human anatomy and function," in Information Processing in Medical Imaging, Proc. IPMI '93 (H.H. Barrett, A.F. Gmitro, eds.), pp.168--181, Berlin: Springer-Verlag, 1993.

U.Tiede, M.Bomans, K.H. Hohne, A.Pommert, M.Riemer, T.Schiemann, R.Schubert, and W.Lierse, "A computerized three-dimensional atlas of the human skull and brain," Am. J. Neuroradiology, vol.14, pp.551--559, 1993.

D. A. Charletta "A computerized three-dimensional atlas of the human skull and brain(Commentary)" Am. J. Neuroradiology, vol.14, pp.560--561,1993.

File Size: 400 MB

Hardware/Software Requirements: VOXEL-MAN/Atlases run under a MOTIF user-interface presently on the following UNIX-Workstations:

- DECstation 5000/xxx (preferably /240)
- DEC 3000 AXP("alpha")
- SUN Sparcstation
- Silicon Graphics Iris

The following minimum configuration is required:

- color display(8 bit frame buffer is sufficient, 24 bit is better)
- >=96 Mbytes of main memory
- >=400 Mbytes of disk storage
- installation medium e.g., DEC TLZ04 tape, etc.
- X11 window system

Compatibility with other workstations like Hewlett-Packard 7xx (portation progress) and IBM RS/6000 is planned for the future.

Author: Karl Heinz Hoehne
Inst. of Math. and Computer Science in Medicine
University Hospital
Eppendorf
Martinistrasse 52
20246 Hamburg

Phone(business):(040)4717-3698
Fax:(040)4717-4882
Tel.(home):(04101)25464

Evaluation: We have not looked at this resource personally (we don't have 400 MB just laying around) See the list of references in the description for reviews. This is obviously a big ticket item to put on your department wish list.

Index

Recommended Resources

These are some of our favorite Internet resources; we hope you'll find them as useful as we do.

Academe (Chronicle of Higher Education) 158
Agricola (US National Agricultural Database) 205

Biology, World Wide Web Virtual Library 176

CancerNet 176, 207
CIA World Fact Book 240
CIESIN (Consortium for International Earth Science Information Network) 164, 258
Clearinghouse for Subject-Oriented Internet Resource Guides 148, 220
COSMIC (Computer Software Management and Information Center) 62

DIALOG Information Servcies 210

EcoGopher 196, 262, 266
EiNet (Engineering International Internet Services) 210, 223
EnviroGopher 196, 239
ERIN (Environmental Resources Information Network) 151, 165, 223, 259, 261

Federal Register 275
FEDIX 137, 166
FedWorld 137, 264

Geographic Name Server 239
Geography, World Wide Web Virtual Library 222
Gopher Jewels 97, 16

HPCC (National Coordination Office for High Performance Computing and Communications) 56, 62

Library of Congress 63, 138, 153, 168

Medicine, World Wide Web Virtual Library 176

NASA (National Aeronautics and Space Administration) 68, 217, 224, 253
NIH (National Institutes of Health) 140, 154, 217
NLM (National Library of Medicine) 139, 154, 217
NSF (National Science Foundation) 170, 197, 217

PENpages 140, 155, 171, 263

STIS (Science and Technology Information Service) 141, 154, 224
SunSITE Archives 156

UNCOVER (CARL) 134, 200, 216
US Census Bureau 236
USDA Extension Service 128, 166, 173

Index

Subject

(Bold-faced numbers pertain to subjects areas which have their own chapter.)

3-D analysis 242
3-D imaging 504
4-H Clubs 137

abnormal psychology 338
abortion 354
acid precipitation 264
acid rain 259
activism 143, 145
acute respiratory infections 375
ADA (Americans with Disabilities Act) 288
adaptation 101, 319
adaptive simulated annealing 478
addiction 288
adolescent rights 352
adopted children 295
aeronautics 63, 64, 67
aerospace engineering **53-70**
aerospace notices 60
aerospace vehicles 62
Africa, ecology 276
aging 131, 144, 288, 319
aging, research 331
agricultural engineering 73, 135, 175
agricultural genomes 461
agricultural management 73
agricultural production 73
agriculture 141, 158, 171, 179, 200, 205
agriculture, education 135
agriculture, market prices 127
agriculture, Netherlands 127
agriculture, sustainable 121, 143, 272

agroforestry 144
AIDS 74, 139, 145, 287, 289, 321, 351, 354, 361, 389, 410
AIDS and health care workers 358
AIDS, communications 320
AIDS, Florida 379
AIDS, statistics 289
air flow 62
air pollution 259, 264
air sampling 215
aircraft 64
alcoholism 290, 375
alcoholism, database 368
algae 131, 144, 200, 202
allergies 169, 320, 411
ALS (Amyorophic Lateral Sclerosis) 290, 358, 478
alternative energy 260
amalgam, dental 290
American Astronomical Society 63
American Chemical Society 205, 212
American Institute of Physics 63, 205
American Medical Informatics Association 290-291
American Physiological Society 159, 387, 389
American Psychological Association 75
American Sign Language 291
American type culture 159
Ames Research Center 57, 60
amino acid sequences 459
amphibians 97, 145
amphibians, urodele 134
analytical chemistry 205
anesthesiology 75, 291, 380, 390, 479
animal alternatives 74

animal behavior 72, 94, 144, 163
animal care 112
animal consciousness 145
animal ethology 76
animal genetics 73
animal genome databases 461
animal rights 73, 77. 145, 146
animal science 75
animal-related resources, bulletin board systems 180-192
animals **71-193**
anonymous FTP 13
anthropology, biological 100, 319
anthropology, historical 89
anti-vivisection 73
APA (American Psychology Association) 291
applications, networked 60
aquaculture 76, 104, 106, 196, 202
aquariums 76, 104, 143-146, 162, 202
aquatic biology **195-204**
aquatic conservation 129
aquatic larvae 76
aquatic science, libraries 101
Arabidopsis 387, 390, 411
Arabidopsis Genome Project 131, 144
Arabidopsis Thaliana genomes 464
ARC/Info 234, 235
archaeology 89, 230
Archie **31-34**
archives 378, 381
archosaurs 90
arctic wildlife 203
arthritis 352
arthritis, rheumatoid 334
arthropods 200
artificial intelligence 74, 145, 401, 498
artificial intelligence and medicine 288
artificial intelligence, software 62
Aspergillus genomes 463
astrocytoma 484
astronautics 64
astronomy 63, 252
astronomy, classification 214
astrophysics 58, 61, 63, 252
astrophysics, preprints 62
astrophysics, ultraviolet 63
atmospheric research 224
atmospheric science 198
audiology 410
auditory perception 292
Australia, science 78
Australia, wildlife 274

autism 292, 354
aviation 62-67
aviation, military 66
aviation, students 67
axolotls 134

back pain 292
badgers 143
bats 79
beef specialists 79
bees 79, 145
behavioral biology 366
behavioral disorders, children 292
behavioral ecology 94, 144
behavioral psychology 338
benthology 200
biodiversity 388
biodiversity 80, 146, 159, 160, 196, 198, 202
biodiversity, fish 197
bioinformatics 130, 146, 153, 158, 160, 175, 196, 238, 392, 413, 418, 456
biological anthropology 100, 319
biological chemistry 206
biological conservation 299
biological race 319
biological societies 102
biological systematics 121
biological timing 170
biology 117, 158, 161, 176, 196-199, 206, 222
biology and computing 160, 362, 368, 380, 383, 398, 497
biology and ethics 81, 129, 159, 368-371
biology and information theory 144
biology and mathematics 160
biology and technology 354
biology and women 132, 144
biology archives 168
biology journals 353
biology, aquatic **195-204**
biology, behavioral 366
biology, Canada 133
biology, computer applications 204
biology, conservation 87-88, 202, 227, 274
biology, crustacean 202
biology, databases 144, 353, 385, 410
biology, deep sea 89
biology, education 80, 82, 206, 292
biology, employment 144
biology, evolutionary 89
biology, experimental 166
biology, funding 204

SUBJECT INDEX

biology, gravitational 59
biology, journals 131, 144, 204, 362-363
biology, literature 371
biology, marine 196, 197
biology, mathematical 120, 153, 155
biology, molecular 92, 103, 131, 146, 206, 212, 306, 310, 414, **449-467**
biology, morphometrics 107, 328
biology, oxygen free radical 335
biology, plant 132, 144
biology, population 132, 204, 337
biology, primate 319
biology, sea turtles 202
biology, skeletal 319
biology, software 131, 305, 380, 383
biology, theoretical 88
biology, tropical 132, 144, 204
biology, wildlife 126
biomaterials 81
biomechanics 81, 293
biomedical communications 293, 417
biomedical engineering 145, 507
biomedical ethics 293
biomedical informatics 147, 325
biomedical libraries 359
biomedicine 59, 106, 480
biomedicine, education 319
biometrics 206
Biophysical Society 144
biophysics 131, 216
biosciences 363
biosciences, Philippines 113
biosciences, policy 160
biosphere 82, 144, 202
biotechnology 59, 82, 129, 147, 456
biotechnology, marine 106
biothermokinetics 131
birds 82-84, 118, 145, 159, 161
birds, Europe 94
birds, hole-nesting 122
birds, mid-Atlantic 105
birds, migratory 139
birds, neotropical 78
birds, Oregon 110
birds, Washington state 122
birth parents 295
bisexuality 293-294
BLAST (Basic Alignment Searching Tool) 450
blindness 294, 302, 367
Bos taurus genomes 462
Braille 294
brain 294

brain and music 496
brain atlas 492
brain injury 346-347
brain research 490
brain scans 482-485
brain tumors 294
brain, sheep 508
brine shrimp 84
Brookhaven National Laboratory 392
Buckyballs 207

Caenorhabditis elegans genomes 461-462
CAI (computer aided instruction) 227
California, ecology 276
California, health initiative 355
camels 84
Canada, biology 133
Canada, ecology 276
cancer 295, 297, 371, 394, 411, 419
cancer research 131
cancer resources 139, 147, 162, 164, 171, 207
cancer, treatment 134
Candida 320
capillary electrophoretic methods 209
carpal tunnel syndrome 344, 367
cartographic data 246-251
cartography 229
cartography, dynamic 231
CASS (Center for Advanced Space Studies) 252
cats 95, 145
CDC (Centers for Disease Control) 135, 361, 372
cell biology 131
cellular aging 353
cellular automatons 109
cellular bioprocesses 144
cellular neural networks 485
census data 235, 379
cerebro vascular accidents 345
cetaceans 92, 202
chemical engineering 207, 208, 212
chemical management 209
chemical management and tracking systems 297
chemical physics 206, 212
chemical substances 395
chemical tracking 209
chemical visualization 209
chemistry **205-218**
chemistry and computers 205
chemistry and materials 208
chemistry textbooks 208
chemistry, analytical 205

chemistry, biological 206
chemistry, computational 207-209
chemistry, directory 212
chemistry, education 207-209, 212
chemistry, medicinal 206
chemistry, organic 213
chemistry, quantum 213, 214
chemometrics 211
child abuse 287, 340
child support 310
children's rights 352
children, behavioral and emotional disorders 292
children/youth and marine science 203
chinchillas 143
Chlamydomonas 131
Chlamydomonas genomes 464
Chromosome 22 353
chromosomes 131, 144
chromosomes, artificial 134
Chronic Fatigue Syndrome 296, 320, 359-360
cigarette addiction 343
ciliates 132, 144
circadian rhythms 85
city locations 238
classification, biological 85
clay 209
clean air 259
Clearinghouse for Subject-Oriented Internet Resource Guides **49-50**
clients 7
climate 57, 198, 201, 226, 259, 264
climatic datasets 255
clinical alerts 139
clinical laboratories 325
clinical trials 366
coal technologies 264
coastal management 85, 101, 135, 226
cognition, neural processes 486
cognition, spatial 231
cognitive neuroscience 86, 148, 487
cognitive rehabilitation 342
cognitive science 298, 506
cold fusion 63
communication disorders 296
comparative medicine 86, 148, 298
Compendex 210
complexity 362
computational biology 164, 398
computational chemistry 207-209
computational engineering 59
computational fluid dynamics, software 62
computer-mediated communication 222

computing and biology 160, 368, 380, 383
computing, parallel 59
condensed matter theory 210
confocal microscopy 299
conformal theory 210
Congress 173, 174
connectionist systems 480
consciousness 338, 366
conservation biology 87-88, 202, 227, 274, 299
conservation, aquatic 129, 201
consumerism 325
coordinate conversion 235
corrosion 209
cosmology 89
COSTAR (COmputer STored Ambulatory Records) 299
county data 235
cows 143
Cray 59
crayfish 200
creationism 119, 343
Crohn's Disease 320
crustaceans 88, 202
cryonics 300
crypto-zoology 119, 343
crystallographic data 207
crystallographic protein structures 459
crystallography 132, 144, 209, 216, 240
culture collections 466
custody 310
cyanobacteria 202
cyanobacterial toxins 301
cybernetics 401
cystic fibrosis 301
cystic fibrosis (French) 329
cytoskeleton 131

dairy cattle 89, 149
dairy science 75
deafness 302, 354, 360
deep sea biology 89
deep sea vents 196, 202
Delauney Triangle algorithm 234
dementia 482
demographic modeling 244
dendromes 464
dental hygiene 410
dentistry, databases 302
dentistry, education 348
dentistry, research 302
dentistry, testing 302

Department of Health 316
developing countries, health 296
diabetes 303
diagnostic imaging 415
diarrhoea 303
diatoms 201, 202
diet 90, 303
digital elevation models 236-238
digital imaging processing 228
dinosaurs 90
disabilities 288, 302, 354, 367, 382
disabilities and computing 415
disabilities, access 328
disabilities, education 323, 352
disabilities, history and analysis 363
disabilities, public policy 324
disabilities, research 304
disabilities, technology 361, 363
disability information 396-398
disabled students 304
disabled, access to libraries 305
disaster research 360
diseases 135
diseases, tropical 121, 346
diving medicine 319
divorce 310
DNA 129, 401, 455
DNA, polymorphic 132, 144
dogs 84, 97, 110, 145, 149, 150, 165
dogs, guard 115
dogs, guide 152
dolphin slaughter 119
dolphins 143, 202
domain names 3
drift nets 119
Drosophila
Drosophila 90, 131, 144, 151, 362, 383
Drosophila genomes 462
drug abuse 290, 304
drug development 75
drug information 401
drugs and politics 355
Dryden Flight Research Facility 67
dynamic cartography 231

e-mail addresses 4
E. coli genomes 463
earth images 252, 263
earth science 199, **219-256**, 258
earth science, bulletin board systems 233
earth science, data sets 224

earth science, employment 233
earth science, software 223
earthquakes 229, 240, 241
earthquakes, Oklahoma 240
echinoderms 120, 202
Ecological Society of America 91, 144, 261
ecology 196
ecology (Spanish language) 91
ecology, behavioral 94, 144
ecology, conservation 201
ecology, education 98, 266-267
ecology, fish 96, 167
ecology, freshwater 202
ecology, landscape 122, 160, 238
ecology, research 145
ecology, software reviews 267
ecology, trends 92
ecology, tropical 204
ecology, US midwest 275
ecosystem modeling 92, 202
ecosystem theory 202
ecosystems 201
education, biology 206
EGRET 305
EINet Galaxy 20
electric circuits 489
electromagnetics 63, 133, 306
Electron Spin Resonance 292
electronic records 378, 381
element percentages 218
elevation data 221
EMBNet (European Molecular Biology Network)
    306, 353, 362, 388, 392, 402-404, 413, 452-454
emergency medicine 296, 306-307
emergency medicine, rural 321
emergency services 306, 354
emotional disorders, children 292
employment, earth science 233
employment, US federal government 233
endangered species 150, 261
endometriosis 351
energy 227, 259
energy, alternative 260
engineering 210
engineering and women 127
engineering, aerospace **53-70**
engineering, agricultural 135, 175
engineering, biomedical 145, 507
engineering, chemical 207, 208, 212
engineering, computational 59
entomology 93, 151, 165, 177, 196, 198, 200-203
Entrez 452

environment 196-199, 223, **257-285**
environment and human behavior 307
environment and politics 91
environment and women 264
environment, education 93
environment, employment 261
environment, library catalogs 276-281
environment, US northwest 276
environmental alerts 259
environmental education 262, 266-267
environmental health 305
environmental history 78, 266
environmental journalism 266
environmental medicine 111
environmental planning 238
environmental regulation 274
environmental safety 116, 136, 275
environmental stress 319
enzyme databases 458
enzymes 379
EPA (Environmental Protection Agency) 136, 151, 165, 216, 258
epidemiological data 398
epidemiology 321
epidemiology, nutritional 333
epidemiology, software 305
epilepsy 482, 490
equestrians 93
ethics 120, 300
ethology 103, 203, 204
eukaryote chromosomes 131, 144
eukaryotes 457
European Synchotron Radiation Facility 210
evolution, human 98, 101, 319
evolutionary biology 89
evolutionary medicine 101
exercise 345
expert systems and vision 350
Explorer 55
expressed sequence tag 457
eye movement 307, 350

facilities 307
falconry 143
family medicine 308, 404
family science 308
family therapy 308
FAO (Food and Agriculture Organization) 308
farming 143, 145
FASTA 450
fathers' rights 310

FDA 374
feminism 309
ferrets 95
fetal physiology 309
fibromyalgia 95, 309
fibrositis 95, 309
field theory 210
finger 22
finite element structural analysis, software 62
finite elements, geologic 241
fire, effects of 265
fish 145, 177, 201
Fish and Wildlife Service 199, 256
fish, bettas 79
fish, ecology 96, 167
fisheries 96, 200, 203
fisheries, computing and statistics 126
fishing 77, 143
fitness 309-310
fleas 151
flight, space 56, 58
Florida, environment and ecology 119, 275
fluid dynamics, geophysical 226
fluid flow analysis, software 62
flyfishing 145
food 167
Food and Drug Administration 136, 166
forensic anthropology 319
forensic medicine 310
forestry 131, 135, 164, 196, 239, 267-268
forestry, Canada 268, 274
FORTRAN 59
foxes 143
Free-Nets, medical 434-436
frogs 97, 491
FTP (File Transfer Protocol) **12-15**
Fuller, Buckminster 206, 207
Fullerenes 207, 210
funding 97, 116, 132, 144, 154, 158, 167, 406
fungal databases 463
fungal genetics 418
fungi, filamentous 132, 144
fungus 201, 203
fusion, cold 63

galactic data 253
galaxy formation 62
GAO (General Accounting Office) 374, 382
gays 297
GenBank 454
GenBank nucleic acid 353

gender 309, 311
gene sequence databases 457-458
genetic algorithms 210
genetic databases, Johns Hopkins 377
genetic linkage 131, 144, 353, 396, 399
genetic research (French) 412
genetic sequences 144
genetic stock 98
genetics 76, 138, 206, 319
genetics engineering 456
genetics resources 167, 408-409
genetics, clinical 311
genetics, fungal 418
genetics, software 310
Genome Data Bank 144
genome databases 131, 210
genome informatics 456
genome research 405-406
genomes, agricultural 461
genomes, Arabidopsis Thaliana 464
genomes, Aspergillus 463
genomes, Bos taurus 462
genomes, Caenorhabditis elegans 461-462
genomes, Chlamydomonas 464
genomes, Drosophila 462
genomes, E. coli 463
genomes, Maize 465
genomes, mouse 106, 137, 138, 151, 153, 168, 462-463
genomes, mycobacteria 463
genomes, Pinus taeda L. 465
genomes, plant 464
genomes, Saccharomyces 463-464
genomes, Somonoceae 465
genomes, soy 465
genomes, Triticae 464
genomes, Voxpop populus 465
geochemistry 243
geochronology 230
geodesy 246
geographic data 220
geographic names 239
geography 222, 227, 229
geography, education 239
geography, historical 89
geography, Japan 239
geologic faults 241
geologic finite-elements 241
geologic software 242
geologic survey, Oklahoma 225
geologic surveys 242
Geological Survey 222

geology 63, 201, 221-230, 252
geology, historical 89
geology, mathematical 234
geomagnetism 240
geomorphology 230
geophysical fluid dynamics 226
geophysics 63, 223, 252
geoscience 223, 230
geoscience and computers 233
geoscience librarians 227
GeoSim 244
geriatric health care 312
GIS (Geographic Information Systems) 122, 221-231, 244-246, 255
GIS and user interface 231
GIS, bulletin board systems 233
glaciers 243
global change 199, 223
Goddard Space Flight Center 56, 58, 67
Gopher 9, **16-18**
GPO (Government Printing Office) 142
GPS (Global Positioning System) 225, 226, 228
grants 97, 98
grants, federal government 145, 197
grants, NIH 140
GRASS 228, 244, 245
grasses 133
Grateful Med 312
gravitational biology 59
grazing, impacts 121
Great Lakes 167, 196, 197, 200, 276
groundwater discharge 226
groundwater recharge 202
groundwater research 244
growth 319
growth inhibitory molecules 321
guides to the Internet **49-50**

handicap see disabilities
Hawaii, ecology 276
hazardous substances 139, 155, 172, 263, 270
health 90
health agencies 420-427
health agencies, e-mail addresses 378
health and minorities 327
health care administration 10, 314, 317, 327
health care and communication 299
health care reform 315, 324
health care, finance 309
health care, geriatric 312
health care, residential 341

health care, rural 414
health care, telecommunications 315
health expectancy 341
health fraud 343
health informatics, Brazil 367
health promotion 313
health research, women 351
health science 99, 145, 152, **287-448**
health science, education 335, 417
health science, history 295
health science, librarians 325
health science, libraries 312, 324, 351
health service, students 342
health statistics, Cuba 376
health, communication 321
health, education 314
health, native peoples 329
HEASARC (High Energy Astrophysics Science Archival Research Center) 58
herpetology 99
high performance computing 56, 62
high temperature materials 216
higher education 120
higher education, employment 158
historical anthropology 89
historical geography 89
historical geology 89
historical linguistics 89
HIV 131, 144, 145, 353-354
HL-7 317, 382
holistics 318
homosexuality and medical profession 312
hormonal manipulation 76
horse racing 90, 152
horses 100, 112, 145, 151
horses, model 107
hospitals 318
HPCC (High Performance Computing and Communications Program) 56, 62
HTML (HyperText Markup Language) 18
Hubble Space Telescope 62, 63
human DNA 129
human gene mapping 316
Human Genome Program 312, 353
human genomes 362, 460-461
human resource development 348
human resources 375
hunting 77, 101, 145
hydrogen 260
hydrologic units 236
hydrology 226, 228, 246
hydrothermal vents 196, 202

hyperbaric medicine 319
Hypoglycemia 320

ice coverage 243
IDRISI 228, 245
image processing 145
immune-system breakdowns 320
immunization, tracking 320, 383
immunoclone database 458
immunology 90, 131, 144, 353
immunology, veterinary 124
incest 340
India, digital data 236
industrial psychology 322
infectious diseases 169, 411
inflammatory bowel diseases 320
ingestive disorders 321
insect genetics 462
insects, social 120
interfacial phenomena 211
interleukins 458
Internet addresses 4
Internet guides **49-50**
Internet searching **43-47**
investment, space 64
IP (Internet Protocol) 3
IP addresses 4
irreproducible results 106
isotope patterns 218
Israel, ecology and environment 238

Japan, geography 239
Japan, primates 102
Jet Propulsion Laboratory 55, 253
Joel's Hierarchical Subject Index 20
Johnson Space Center 67
JumpStation 20

Kennedy Space Center 67
killifish 102
kinetics 131, 144

laboratories, diagnostics 287
laboratories, veterinary 302, 323
laboratory animals 298
laboratory primates 103, 324
laboratory safety 212, 215

lactic acid 102, 322
Lake Superior 275
lampreys 143
land coverage maps 236
land information 223
land use maps 236
landscape ecology 122, 160, 238
Langley Research Center 56, 59, 67
LAS (Land Analysis System) 235
lasers and medicine 323
leishmaniasis 103
lemmings 143
lesbians 297
Lewis Research Center 59
life sciences 59, 265
limnology 106, 203
Linear Time algorithm 234
linguistics, historical 89
Lister Hill National Center for Biomedical
    Communications 417
LISTSERVs 24
livestock reports 127
Lou GehrigÕs Disease 290, 358
lunar studies 63
Lupus 320
LYCOS 20
Lyme Disease 103, 153, 364
Lynx 18

macromolecules 144
macrophage factors 458
Magellan mission 56, 251
magnetic fields 243
mailing lists **24-27**, 168
Maize genome 465
malnutrition 376
mammalogy 104
    marine facilities 104
mammals 203
mammals, marine 105
map datasets 237
MapInfo 229, 247
mapping software 246-251
mapping standards 253-255
mapping tools 246-251
maps, Canada 251
maps, history 229
maps, land coverage 236
maps, land use 236
maps, Mid-East 250
maps, US 250

marine biology 196, 197
marine biology, Adriatic Sea 106
marine biotechnology 106
marine organisms 200
marine science 153
marine science, libraries 101
marine studies 104
marine technology 104
marriage therapy 308
material database 213
materials safety 168, 213
math education 117
math, computer applications 204
mathematical biology 120, 153, 155, 160
mathematical psychology 329
mathematics, education 211
medical applications, NeXT 331
medical decision-making 343
medical education, Ontario 313
medical informatics 134, 162, 288, 290-291, 320,
    393, 495
medical informatics, eastern Europe 327
medical informatics, education 327
medical libraries 436-448
medical logic 429
medical pharmacy 113
medical products 318
medical research 154
medical research, gophers 387-389
medical schools 387
medical science (Spanish) 303
medical students, Canada 297
medical students, Europe 307
medical telecommunications 105
medicinal chemistry 206
medicinal plants 316
medicine 145
medicine and computers 87, 295, 298, 410
medicine and physics 326
medicine, comparative 86, 298
medicine, Croatia 300
medicine, education and computers 298
medicine, environmental 111, 333
medicine, evolutionary 101
medicine, family 404
medicine, journals 139, 322, 363
medicine, lasers 323
medicine, nuclear 332, 490
medicine, occupational 111, 333
medicine, questions 322
medicine, software 383-386
medicine, students 325, 326

medicine, telecommunications 326
medicine, veterinary 350
MEDLARS 213, 377
MEDLINE 139, 377
Mendelian Inheritance 461
menopause 327
mental health 171
mentoring 305
metabolism 204
metals 216
meteorology 222, 226, 255, 269
microbiology, oral 90
microbiology, veterinary 125, 350
microbiota, oral 301
microgravity 59
microorganisms 389
microscopy 145
microscopy, confocal 299
Middle East, water resources 106
midwifery 365
migration patterns 244
mineralogy 240
mining, impacts 121
minorities, education 58
missing children 377
modeling, demographic 244
modeling, ecosystem 92, 202
modeling, pollution 266
molecular biology 92, 103, 131, 144, 146, 206, 212, 306, 310, 353-354, 414, **449-467**
molecular biology (French) 340
molecular biology, databases 383, 454-465
molecular biology, laboratory 374
molecular diagnoses 329
molecular evolution 131, 144
molecular modeling 394, 399
molecular science 212
mollusks 107
monoclonal antibodies 458
morbidity 168, 361
morphology, quantitative 116, 340
morphometrics, biological 107, 328
mortality 168, 361
Mosaic 18
motor skills 328
mouse DNA 129
mouse genomes 106, 137, 138, 151, 153, 168, 404, 462-463
movement science 293
MRI (Magnetic Resonance Imaging) 482, 491, 495
multiple sclerosis 329
music and the brain 496

music therapy 496
music, education 496
music, perception 497
mustelidae 143
mycobacteria genomes 463
mycobacterium 388
mycology 132
mycoplasma, veterinary 125

NAL (National Agriculture Library) 140, 168
NASA (National Space and Space Administration) 55-70, 208, 217, 224, 253, 378, 381
National Institute of Allergy and Infectious Disease 169
National Institute of Environmental Health Sciences 169, 217
National Institute of Mental Health 169
National Oceanographic Data Center 170, 178, 197
National Space Science Data Center 57
native peoples, health 329
native peoples, Latin America 375
natural resources, libraries 108
Naval Observatory 224
NCAR (National Center for Atmospheric Research) 224
NCBI (National Center for Biotechnology Information) 450, 457
neotropical birds 78
Netfind 22
neural communications 486
neural computation 488, 497
neural networks 109, 145, 154, 488, 494, 498, 502
neural networks, cellular 485
neural processes and cognition 486
neuroanatomy 499
neuroanesthesia 494
neurobiology 109
neurophysiology 159, 494
neuroscience 108, 117, 132, 144, 172, 330, 338, 357, 366, **469-512**
neuroscience, applied 487
neuroscience, Chile 108, 330
neuroscience, cognitive 487
neuroscience, theoretical 487
New York, Bureau of Health Resource Development 292
New York, Department of Health 288, 291, 304, 323, 328, 330, 340
New York, ecology 276
newts 134
NIAID (National Institute of Allergy and Infectious Disease) 411

NIH (National Institutes of Health) 109, 110, 131, 144, 169, 217, 296, 331-332, 385
NIH funding 331, 407, 431, 501
NIH, research 364
NISS (National Information Services & Systems, UK) 208
NIST (National Institute for Standards and Technology) 63, 169, 217
nitrogen fixation 132, 144
NLM (National Library of Medicine) 169, 217, 365, 385, 454
NOAA (National Oceanographic and Atmospheric Administration) 169, 271
nondestructive testing 216
Nova-Links 20
NSF, grants 313
NTIS 374
nuclear magnetic resonance 133
nuclear medicine 332, 490
nucleic acids 138, 213
nucleotide sequences 375, 450-453
nudibranchs 200
nurses, Canada 297
nursing 332-333, 366, 410, 412
nursing informatics 332
nursing, practicing 313
nursing, students 310, 344
nutrient cycling 330
nutrition 90, 366, 375
nutritional epidemiology 333

Oak Ridge National Laboratories 460
occupational injuries 354
occupational medicine 111
oceanography 140, 149, 155, 164, 171, 196-200
oceanography, mapping 248
online catalogs 222
oral microbiology 90, 301
oral radiology 334
Oregon, environment 276
organ transplants 348
organellar databases 463
organic chemistry 213
organic chemistry, theoretical 218
organic synthesis 394
organizational psychology 322
ornithology 108
OSHA (Occupational Safety and Health Administration) 270, 275
outdoors 111
overpopulation 77

oxygen free radical biology 335
ozone depletion 269

paleoanthropology 319
paleodemography 319
paleoenvironment 230
paleomagnetic data 243
paleontology 89, 145, 197, 230, 251
paleontology, invertebrate 199
paleopathology 319
palynology 230
Pan American Health Organization 351
parallel computing 59
paranormal 343
parapsychology 119
parasitology 132, 144, 155
parenting 375
paridae 122
park rangers 112
Parkinson's Disease 335
Patent and Trademark Office 217, 218
patents 211, 214, 217
patents, international 210
pathology 112, 179, 329
patient records 300
pediatrics 336
perinatal data 337
perinatal physiology 309
periodic table 214, 216, 218
periodontal disease 302
periphytons 200
pest management 135
PET (Positron Emission Tomography) 503
pharmaceutical research 291
pharmacology 206
pharmacy 336, 507
pharmacy, education 342
pharmacy, medical 113
pharmacy, veterinary 121
Philippines, biosciences 113
philosophy of science 99
photogrammetry 251
photosynthesis 132, 144, 204
phycology 202
phylogeny 85, 89
physician's data 139
physics 63, 205
physics and medicine 326
physics, chemical 206, 212
physics, classification 214
physics, polymer 214

physiology 159, 336
physiology, fetal and perinatal 309
physiology, thermal 347
physiotherapy 336
pigs 113
Pinus taeda L. genomes 465
planetary studies 63
planets 251
plant biology 132, 144
plant genomes 464
plants, New World 196
plasma membranes 131, 144
play 336
Point in Polygon 234
pollutants, reactive 215
pollution 202
pollution modeling 266
pollution, acid 260
pollution, air 264
pollution, water 226
polygons 234
polymer physics 214
polymorphic DNA 132, 144
polymorphism, human 388
population 366
population biology 132, 204, 337
population ecology 114
population genetics 114
population growth 375
population studies 415
pork 143
postdoctoral positions 214
poultry 75, 113
primate behavior 319
primate biology 319
primates 114, 141, 155, 172, 179
primates, Japan 102
primates, laboratory 103, 324
prokaryotic databases 463
promoter sequences 457
PROSITE 459
protein data bank 392
protein science 362
protein sequence database 458
protein sequences 138, 375, 450-453
proteins 132
protists 132, 144
psychiatry 115, 145, 338
psychobiology 145, 507
psychology 115, 338, 354, 366-367
psychology and the arts 338
psychology and the law 339

psychology, abnormal 338
psychology, behavioral 338
psychology, collaboration 319
psychology, education 347
psychology, industrial 322
psychology, mathematical 329
psychology, measure development 349
psychology, organizational 322
psychology, sports 345
psychology, students 338, 367
psychology, testing 349
psychology, validation 349
psychomusicology 496
Psycoloquy 115, 145, 366
public health 179, 345-346, 418
pychology, research 291

qualitative research 340
quantitative morphology 340
quantum chemistry 213, 214
Quarternary period 230

rabbits 112, 143, 145
radiation 57, 210
radiochemistry 215
radiology 145, 340
radiology, oral 334
railroads 230
rape prevention 345
recovery programs 352
recycling 136, 271
rehabilitation 413
reincarnation 119
remote sensing 122, 251
repetitive strain injury 367
repetitive stress injuries 294
reptiles 145
research administration 340
research funding 341
research methodology 145
residential health care 341
respiratory health 329
restriction enzyme database 379
rheumatoid arthritis 334
ribozymes 134
risk management 341
RNA 134
roots 203
rural health care 414

Saccharomyces genomes 463-464
safety 172, 270
safety, campus 341
safety, environmental 116
salamanders 134
satellite altimetry 226
satellite images 251
satellite launches 226
schizophrenia 342, 505
Schmidt nets 242
science and philosophy 145
science and women 127
science awareness 341
science education 78, 117, 140, 145, 211
science, philosophy of 99, 100
scientific fraud 117
scientific visualization 223
scientific visualization, software 62
Scotland, ecology 276
Scripps Institution of Oceanography 111, 149, 164, 197, 198
scuba diving 118, 144, 145, 195, 197
sea turtles 89, 202, 274
seal hunting 119
searching the Internet 43-47
seismology 230, 240
self-help 343
Senate 156
senior citizens 305-306, 342
sequence databases 452-453
servers 7
sexual abuse 340
sexuality 311, 345-346
Share Medical Systems 344
shipboard education 104
shrimp, brine 84, 202
Siberia, ecology 276
Sierra Club 119
sign language 291
skeletal biology 319
skepticism 119, 343
skunks 143
sleep disorders 343
Smithsonian Institution 88, 156, 172, 197, 199
snow cover satellite images 252
social deviants 303
social sciences and computers 301
social work 344
software 156
software reviews, ecology 267
software simulations 109
soil science 230, 243

solar collectors 269
solar energy 267
Somonoceae genomes 465
soy genomes 465
space 60
space development 61
space exploration 61
space flight 56, 58
space geodesy 226
space physics 253
space science, software 223
space shuttle 59, 252
spatial cognition 231
spatial data 229, 254
spatio-temporal reasoning 231
specimen collections 201
spectroscopy 210, 215, 226
spectroscopy, NMR 133
speech pathology 410
sports psychology 345
statistics education 203
stemmatics 89
stereonets 242
stereoscopic volume visualization 509
stereotaxic atlases 510
string theory 210
strokes 345
stuttering 345
substance abuse, education 342
sunrise and sunset calculations 243
Supreme Court 156, 173
surface temperature 249
survey, geological 222, 242
sustainable agriculture 121, 143, 272
systematics 89

T-cell receptors 458
TCP (Transmission Control Protocol) 3
technology and social behavior 305
technology transfer 60
tectonics 232
telemedicine 347
telescope, space 62, 63
Telnet **11-12**
tendonitis 344
Texas, environment 276
textual transmission 89
The Scientist 142, 156, 173, 199, 202, 265, 362, 386
theoretical biology 88
thermal flow analysis, software 62
thermal physiology 347

thermodynamics 131, 204
Thiessen polygons 234
ticks 151
tidal heights 249
tides 202
timber harvesting, impacts 121
time zone data 236
tissue interactions 81
tobacco deaths 375
topographic analysis 235
topography 232
topography, time dependent 243
tourism, impacts 121
toxic substances 270
toxicology 139
toxicology, veterinary 126
toxics 259, 264
toxins, cynobacterial 301
training 348
transcription factors 457
transplantation, behavioral research 295
transplants 348
transportation 255
transportation planning 231
trapping 77
traumatic brain injury 346-347
Triticae genomes 464
tropical biology 132, 144, 204
tropical databases 359
tropical diseases 121, 346
tropical ecology 204
tropical studies 111
tumor gene 458
tumor, brain 482
twins 348

UFOs (Unidentified Flying Objects) 119
Ulcerative Colitis 320
UN (United Nations) 173
UN Environmental Summit 268
unemployment 322
urban life 348
urban planning 231
URL (Uniform Resource Locator) 4
US (see agency name)
USDA (US Department of Agriculture) 142, 157, 161
Usenet 26
user interface, GIS 231

vector sequences 457
veganism 91
vegetarianism 77, 95, 122, 123, 142, 157, 313, 349
vehicles, aerospace 62
vents, deep-sea 196, 202
vents, hydrothermal 196
Veronica **35-37**
vertebrates 174
Veterans Administration 362
veterinary health information 78
veterinary hospitals 123, 349
veterinary immunology 124
veterinary informatics 72, 124
veterinary laboratories 72, 302, 323
veterinary medicine 125, 134, 154, 164, 350
veterinary medicine, education 123
veterinary medicine, librarians 125
veterinary microbiology 125, 350
veterinary mycoplasma 125
veterinary pharmacy 121
veterinary resources 170
veterinary science 94
veterinary science and computers 78
veterinary students 126
veterinary toxicology 126
Vietnam, science 78
Viewshed algorithms 234
Viking mission 56
virology 132, 144, 157, 158, 174
virtual reality 145, 231
viruses 307
vision 324
vision and expert systems 350
volcanoes 231
Voronoi polygons 234
Voronoi tessellation 234
Voxel-man 3D 386, 511
Voxpop populus genomes 465
Voyager mission 251
VT100 emulation 8

WAIS **39-41**, 180, 218
water 197
water pollution 226
water quality 199, 244, 272-275
water resources, Middle East 106
Web Crawler 20
weight loss 303

wetlands 106, 256, 273
whaling 119
White House 142, 174
White House, health plan 315, 324, 355-358
White House, press releases 275
WHO (World Health Organization) 158, 175, 262, 362, 415
Whole Internet Catalog 20
wildlife 256, 274
wildlife biology 126
wildlife refuges 256
Wildlife Society 121, 122
wildlife, Australian 274
witchcraft 343
wolves 144
Woods Hole Oceanographic Institution 175, 197, 199, 271
World Bank 263, 366
Wulff nets 242
WWW (World Wide Web) 9, **18-20**
WWW Virtual Library 20
WWW Worm 20

yeast 132, 134, 144
yeast artificial chromosomes 464
young scientists 127

zoology, comparative 201
zoology, invertebrate 201
zoos 162

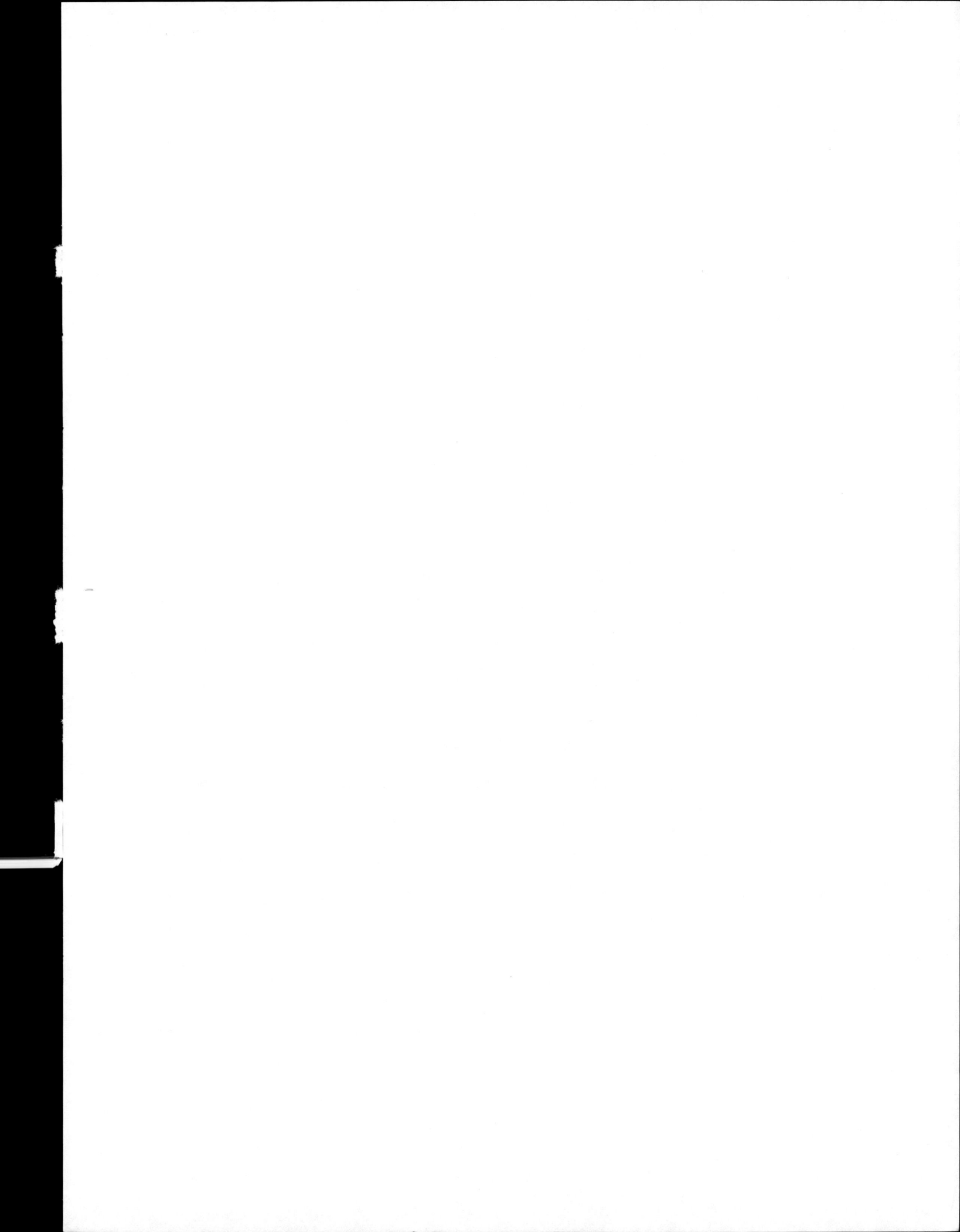